Handbook for

Brunner & Suddarth's
Textbook of Medical-Surgical Nursing

ELEVENTH EDITION

Joyce Young Johnson, RN, PhD
Dean and Professor
College of Sciences and Health Professions
Albany State University
Albany, Georgia

D1495562

Wolters Kluwer | Lippincott Williams & Wilkins
Health

Philadelphia · Baltimore · New York · London
Buenos Aires · Hong Kong · Sydney · Tokyo

Acquisitions Editor: Hilarie Surrena
Managing Editor: Melanie Cann
Senior Project Editor: Tom Gibbons
Director of Nursing Production: Helen Ewan
Senior Managing Editor/Production: Erika Kors
Design Coordinator: Joan Wendt
Senior Manufacturing Manager: William Alberti
Indexer: Ken Hassman
Compositor: Techbooks
Printer: R. R. Donnelley-Crawfordsville

11th Edition

9   8   7

Library of Congress Cataloging-in-Publication data available upon request.

ISBN-13: 978-0-7817-6749-1
ISBN-10: 0-7817-6749-0

Care has been taken to confirm the accuracy of the information presented and to
describe generally accepted practices. However, the authors, editors, and
publisher are not responsible for errors or omissions or for any consequences
from application of the information in this book and make no warranty, express
or implied, with respect to the content of the publication.

The authors, editors, and publisher have exerted every effort to ensure that
drug selection and dosage set forth in this text are in accordance with the current
recommendations and practice at the time of publication. However, in view of
ongoing research, changes in government regulations, and the constant flow of
information relating to drug therapy and drug reactions, the reader is urged to
check the package insert for each drug for any change in indications and dosage
and for added warnings and precautions. This is particularly important when the
recommended agent is a new or infrequently employed drug.

Some drugs and medical devices presented in this publication have Food and
Drug Administration (FDA) clearance for limited use in restricted research
settings. It is the responsibility of the health care provider to ascertain the FDA
status of each drug or device planned for use in his or her clinical practice.

*All praises, honor, glory and thanks to God
and our Lord Jesus Christ!*

*To my husband, Larry, and my children,
Virginia and Larry Jr.,
who are my joy and inspiration.
To my family and friends,
who are my support and strength.*

*To my students, past and future,
who are my hope for Nursing's future.*

Preface

This *Handbook for Brunner & Suddarth's Textbook of Medial Surgical Nursing,* 11th edition, is a comprehensive yet concise clinical reference designed for use by students and nurses. Perfect for both the hospital and community setting, the *Handbook* presents need-to-know information on nearly 200 commonly encountered diseases and disorders in an easy-to-use, colorful, alphabetized outline format. Each entry is formatted consistently for quick access to vital information on

- Disease (Pathophysiology)
- Clinical Manifestations
- Assessment and Diagnostic Methods
- Medical, Surgical, and Pharmacological management
- Nursing Management according to the Nursing Process

For readers requiring more in-depth information, the *Handbook* is completely cross-referenced to chapters in *Brunner & Suddarth's Textbook of Medical Surgical Nursing,* 11th edition, by Suzanne C. Smeltzer and Brenda G. Bare.

Special Features

The *Handbook* places special emphasis on Home and Community Based nursing practice, Patient Education, and Expected Outcomes of care as more and more patients in the 21st century receive health care outside of hospitals and clinics. Additional features include:

  Gerontologic Considerations—Thumbnail descriptions and interventions related to the care of the older adult population, whose health care needs continue to expand at a rapid rate.

! Nursing Alerts—Instant notes focused on priority care issues and hazardous or potentially life-threatening situations.

Selected **tables and boxes**—At-a-glance presentations of additional diseases, disorders, measurements, and the like.

Up-to-date **appendices** for use in clinicals, on the unit, and at home or in the community. These include

- Acronyms and abbreviations
- Important lab values
- Current nursing diagnoses

This pocket-sized, flexible handbook has been compiled and written to provide content that nurses need to know. I hope it will be a valuable guide that will help you in your education and nursing practice.

—*Joyce Young Johnson, RN, PhD*

Contents

A

Acquired Immunodeficiency Syndrome
(HIV Infection) 1

Acute Respiratory Distress Syndrome 18

Addison's Disease (Primary Adrenocortical
Insufficiency) 21

Alzheimer's Disease 26

Amyotrophic Lateral Sclerosis 31

Anaphylaxis 33

Anemia 35

Anemia, Aplastic 40

Anemia, Iron-Deficiency 42

Anemia, Megaloblastic (Vitamin B12 and Folic
Acid Deficiency) 45

Anemia, Sickle Cell 48

Aneurysm, Aortic 54

Aneurysm, Intracranial 58

Angina Pectoris 63

Aortic Insufficiency (Regurgitation) 68

Aortic Stenosis 69

Appendicitis 71

Arterial Embolism and Arterial Thrombosis 73

Arteriosclerosis and Atherosclerosis 75

Arthritis, Rheumatoid 77

Asthma 84

Asthma: Status Asthmaticus 87

B

Back Pain, Low 90

Bell's Palsy 94

Benign Prostatic Hyperplasia and Prostatectomy 96

Bone Tumors 98

Bowel Obstruction, Large 104

Bowel Obstruction, Small 106

Brain Abscess 108

Brain Tumors 109

Bronchiectasis 114

Bronchitis, Chronic 115

Buerger's Disease (Thromboangiitis Obliterans) . . . 117

Burn Injury 119

C

Cancer 136

Cancer of the Bladder 156

Cancer of the Breast 159

Cancer of the Cervix 168

Cancer of the Colon and Rectum
    (Colorectal Cancer) 172

Cancer of the Endometrium 179

Cancer of the Esophagus 180

Cancer of the Kidneys (Renal Tumors) 185

Cancer of the Larynx 188

Cancer of the Liver 195

Cancer of the Lung (Bronchogenic Carcinoma) 200

Cancer of the Oral Cavity 203

Cancer of the Ovary 208

Cancer of the Pancreas 210

Cancer of the Prostate 213

Cancer of the Skin (Malignant Melanoma) 220

Cancer of the Stomach (Gastric Cancer) 226

Cancer of the Testis 231

Cancer of the Thyroid 233

Cancer of the Vagina 234

Cancer of the Vulva 235

Cardiac Arrest 239

Cardiomyopathies 240

Cataract 245

Cerebral Vascular Accident (Ischemic Stroke) 248

Cholelithiasis (and Cholecystitis) 260

Chronic Obstructive Pulmonary Disease (COPD) . . 267

Cirrhosis, Hepatic 274

Constipation 279

Contact Dermatitis 281

Coronary Atherosclerosis and Coronary
   Artery Disease 283

Cushing's Syndrome 286

Cystitis (Lower Urinary Tract Infection) 292

D

Diabetes Insipidus 297

Diabetes Mellitus 299

Diabetic Ketoacidosis 312

Diarrhea 316

Disseminated Intravascular Coagulopathy 321

Diverticular Disorders 325

E

Emphysema, Pulmonary 331

Empyema 333

Endocarditis, Infective 334

Endocarditis, Rheumatic 337

Endometriosis 339

Epididymitis 342

Epilepsies 343

Epistaxis (Nosebleed) 350

Esophageal Varices, Bleeding 351

Exfoliative Dermatitis 355

F

Fractures 358

G

Gastritis 377

Glaucoma 382

Glomerulonephritis, Acute 386

Glomerulonephritis, Chronic 388

Gout 391

Guillain-Barré Syndrome (Polyradiculoneuritis) 394

H

Headache 401

Head Injury (Brain Injury) 407

Heart Failure (Cor Pulmonale) 420

Hemophilia 429

Hepatic Encephalopathy and Hepatic Coma 434

Hepatic Failure, Fulminant 436

Hepatitis, Viral: Types A, B, C, D, E, and G 437

Hiatal Hernia 443

Hodgkin's Disease 447

Huntington's Disease 450

Hyperglycemic Hyperosmolar Nonketotic
    Syndrome (HHNKS) 453

Hypertension (and Hypertensive Crisis) 455

Hyperthyroidism (Graves' Disease) 461

Hypoglycemia (Insulin Reaction) 468

Hypoparathyroidism 472

Hypopituitarism 474

Hypothyroidism and Myxedema 475

I

Idiopathic Thrombocytopenia Purpura 482

Impetigo 484

Increased Intracranial Pressure 486

Influenza 492

K

Kaposi's Sarcoma 494

L

Leukemia 497

Leukemia, Lymphocytic, Acute 504

Leukemia, Lymphocytic, Chronic 506

Leukemia, Myeloid, Acute 507

Leukemia, Myelogenous, Chronic 509

Lung Abscess 511

Lymphedema and Elephantiasis 513

M

Mastoiditis and Mastoid Surgery 516

Ménière's Disease 520

Meningitis 525

Mitral Regurgitation (Insufficiency) 529

Mitral Stenosis 530

Mitral Valve Prolapse 531

Multiple Myeloma 533

Multiple Sclerosis 534

Muscular Dystrophies 542

Musculoskeletal Trauma (Contusions, Strains,
     Sprains, and Joint Dislocations) 544

Myasthenia Gravis 548

Myocardial Infarction 554

Myocarditis 560

N

Nephrotic Syndrome 562

O

Obesity, Morbid 564

Osteoarthritis (Degenerative Joint Disease) 567

Osteomalacia 569

Osteomyelitis 572

Osteoporosis 576

Otitis Media, Acute 581

Otitis Media, Chronic 583

P

Pancreatitis, Acute 585

Pancreatitis, Chronic 592

Parkinson's Disease 594

Pelvic Infection (Pelvic Inflammatory Disease) 600

Pemphigus 603

Peptic Ulcer 607

Pericarditis (Cardiac Tamponade) 615

Perioperative Nursing Management 619

Peripheral Arterial Occlusive Disease 647

Peritonitis 651

Pharyngitis, Acute 653

Pharyngitis, Chronic 655

Pheochromocytoma 656

Pituitary Tumors 659

Pleural Effusion 661

Pleurisy 663

Pneumonia 665

Pneumothorax and Hemothorax 670

Polycythemia 674

Prostatitis 676

Pruritus 678

Psoriasis 680

Pulmonary Edema, Acute 687

Pulmonary Embolism 689

Pulmonary Heart Disease (Cor Pulmonale) 695

Pulmonary Hypertension 698

Pyelonephritis, Acute 701

Pyelonephritis, Chronic 702

R

Raynaud's Disease 704

Regional Enteritis (Crohn's Disease) 705

Renal Failure, Acute 707

Renal Failure, Chronic (End-Stage Renal Disease) .. 713

S

Seborrheic Dermatoses 719

Shock, Cardiogenic 720

Shock, Hypovolemic 723

Shock, Septic 725

Spinal Cord Injury 727

Syndrome of Inappropriate Antidiuretic
    Hormone Secretion 738

Systemic Lupus Erythematosus 739

T

Thrombocytopenia 743

Thyroiditis, Acute 744

Thyroiditis, Chronic (Hashimoto's Thyroiditis) 746

Thyroid Storm (Thyrotoxic Crisis) 747

Toxic Epidermal Necrolysis and Stevens-Johnson
    Syndrome 748

Transient Ischemic Attack 753

Trigeminal Neuralgia (Tic Douloureux) 756

Tuberculosis, Pulmonary 759

U

Ulcerative Colitis 765

Unconscious Patient 773

Urolithiasis 780

V

Vein Disorders 787

Appendix A: Selected Lab Values 793

Appendix B: NANDA-Approved Nursing Diagnoses
    2005–2006 797

Appendix C: Key Health Care Abbreviations
    and Acronyms 802

Index 827

Acquired Immunodeficiency Syndrome (HIV Infection)

Acquired immunodeficiency syndrome (AIDS) is defined as the most severe form of a continuum of illnesses associated with human immunodeficiency virus (HIV) infection. HIV belongs to a group of viruses known as retroviruses. These viruses carry their genetic material in the form of ribonucleic acid (RNA) rather than deoxyribonucleic acid (DNA). Infection with HIV occurs when it enters the host CD4 (T) cell and causes this cell to replicate viral RNA and viral proteins, which in turn invade other CD4 cells.

The stage of HIV disease is based on clinical history, physical examination, laboratory evidence of immune dysfunction, signs and symptoms, and infections and malignancies. The stage of primary infection is acute and spans the time from infection to antibody development. Four categories of infected states have been denoted:

- Primary infection (part of CDC Category A: dramatic drop in CD4 T-cell counts from normal level between 500 and 1500 cells/mm^3)
- HIV asymptomatic (CDC Category A: more than 500 CD4+ T lymphocytes/mm^3)
- HIV symptomatic (CDC Category B: 200–499 CD4+ T lymphocytes/mm^3)
- AIDS (CDC Category C: fewer than 200 CD4+ T lymphocytes/mm^3)

Risk Factors

HIV is transmitted through bodily fluids by high-risk behaviors such as heterosexual intercourse with an HIV-infected partner, injection drug use, and male homosexual relations. Also at risk are people who received transfusions of blood or blood products contaminated with HIV, children born to mothers with HIV infection, breast-fed infants of HIV-infected mothers, and health care workers exposed to needle-stick injury associated with an infected patient.

Clinical Manifestations

Symptoms are widespread and may affect any organ system. Manifestations range from mild abnormalities in immune response without overt signs and symptoms to profound immunosuppression, life-threatening infection, malignancy, and the direct effect of HIV on body tissues.

Respiratory

- Shortness of breath, dyspnea, cough, chest pain, and fever are associated with opportunistic infections, including *Pneumocystis jiroveci* pneumonia (PCP), the most common infection, and the immune reconstitution syndromes, such as *Mycobacterium avium complex* (MAC)/*Mycobacterium avium intracellulare* (MAI), which is a leading bacterial infection in AIDS patients. Legionella and CMV are other opportunistic organisms.
- HIV-associated tuberculosis occurs early in the course of HIV infection, often preceding a diagnosis of AIDS.

Gastrointestinal

- Loss of appetite
- Nausea and vomiting
- Oral and esophageal candidiasis (white patches, painful swallowing, retrosternal pain, and possibly oral lesions)
- Chronic diarrhea, possibly with devastating effects (eg, weight loss, fluid and electrolyte imbalances, perianal skin excoriation, weakness, and inability to perform activities of daily living)

Wasting Syndrome (Cachexia)

- Multifactorial protein-energy malnutrition
- Profound involuntary weight loss exceeding 10% of baseline body weight
- Chronic diarrhea, chronic weakness, and documented intermittent or constant fever with no concurrent illness
- Anorexia, diarrhea, gastrointestinal malabsorption, lack of nutrition, and for some patients a hypermetabolic state

Neurologic

Neurologic complications involve central, peripheral, and autonomic functions.

- HIV encephalopathy (AIDS dementia complex [ADC]) occurs in two thirds of patients with AIDS. Symptoms include memory deficits, headache, lack of concentration, progressive confusion, psychomotor slowing, apathy and ataxia, and in later stages global cognitive impairments, delayed verbal responses, spastic paraparesis, hyperreflexia, psychosis, seizures, incontinence, mutism, and death.
- HIV-related peripheral neuropathy is thought to be a demyelinating disorder; it is associated with pain and numbness in the extremities, weakness, diminished deep tendon reflexes, orthostatic hypotension, and impotence.
- *Cryptococcus neoformans*, a fungal infection (fever, stiff neck, nausea and vomiting, seizures).
- Central and peripheral neuropathies, including vascular myelopathy (spastic paraparesis, ataxia, and incontinence)
- Progressive multifocal leukoencephalopathy (PML), a central nervous system demyelinating disorder, can occur.
- Other neurologic disorders include *Toxoplasma gondii*, CMV, and *Mycobacterium tuberculosis* infection, with symptoms ranging from confusion to blindness, aphasia, paresis, and death.

Integumentary

- Kaposi's sarcoma (KS), herpes simplex and herpes zoster viruses, and various forms of dermatitis associated with painful vesicles
- Folliculitis, associated with dry flaking skin or atopic dermatitis (eczema or psoriasis)

Reproductive (Female)

- Persistent recurrent vaginal candidiasis may be the first sign of HIV infection.
- Ulcerative sexually transmitted diseases, such as chancroid, syphilis, and herpes, are more severe in women with HIV.
- Venereal warts and cervical cancer/cervical intraepithelial neoplasia (CIN) may be noted.
- Women with HIV have a higher incidence of pelvic inflammatory disease (PID) and menstrual abnormalities (amenorrhea or bleeding between periods).

Hematologic/Lymphatic

B–cell lymphomas, such as non-Hodgkin's lymphoma, are the second most common AIDS-related cancer (the first is KS). These lymphomas usually differ from those in the general population because they develop outside the lymph nodes (mostly in the brain, bone marrow, and GI tract), grow aggressively, affect multiple organs, and exhibit resistance to treatment, which may be complicated by severe hemotologic toxicity.

Other: Chronic Illness and Cancers

Early diagnosis and treatment of opportunistic diseases and antiviral therapy have brought HIV infection into the chronic illness category. Additional clinical manifestations follow:

- Fatigue, headache, profuse night sweats, unexplained weight loss, dry cough, shortness of breath, extreme weakness, diarrhea, decreased endurance, edema, blindness, swallowing difficulties, and possible neurologic

involvement resulting in dementia, hemiplegia, spastic paraparesis, painful neuropathies, proximal and distal muscle weakness, and persistent lymphadenopathy
- Higher than usual incidence of cancer, including KS, B-cell lymphomas, and carcinomas of cervix, skin, stomach, pancreas, rectum, and bladder
- Depressive symptoms from multiple causes, including preexisting mental illness, neuropsychiatric disturbances, and psychosocial factors
- Irrational guilt, shame, loss of self-esteem, helplessness, worthlessness, and suicidal ideation

Assessment and Diagnostic Methods

Confirmation of HIV antibodies is done using enzyme immunoassay (EIA; formerly enzyme-linked immunosorbent assay [ELISA]), Western blot assay, and viral load tests such as target amplification methods.

Medical Management

Currently there is no cure for HIV or AIDS, although researchers continue to work on developing a vaccine. Treatment decisions for an individual patient are based on three factors: HIV RNA (viral load), CD4 T-cell counts, and the clinical condition of the patient (severity of symptoms and patient's commitment to participate in lifelong therapy). The goals of treatment are maximal and durable suppression of viral load, restoration and/or preservation of immunologic function, improvement of quality of life, and reduction of HIV-related morbidity and mortality. To determine and evaluate the treatment plan, viral load testing is recommended at diagnosis and then every 3 to 4 months thereafter in the untreated person. CD4+ T-cell counts should be measured at diagnosis and generally every 3 to 6 months thereafter.

Combination therapy is defined as a regimen containing at least two antiretroviral agents; highly active antiretroviral therapy (HAART) includes at least one nucleoside reverse transcriptase inhibitor plus various other drug combinations. As new medications are developed, the number of combinations continues to increase. High cost of medications, difficulties with adherence to the regimen, drug resistance, and drug toxicities present problems in drug therapy. Intermittent therapy is under investigation as an alternative regimen.

Pharmacologic Therapy

Antiretroviral Therapy (ART)

(For combination regimens with at least three medications)

- Nucleoside/nucleotide reverse transcriptase inhibitors (NRTI)
- Non-nucleoside reverse transcriptase inhibitors (NNRTI)
- Protease inhibitors (PI)
- Fusion inhibitors (FI)

Drug Resistance Testing

Helps determine which antiretroviral agents to eliminate from the antiretroviral regimen (rather than which agents should be used)

Treatment Interruption and Reinstitution

Depending on the patient and CD4 cell count, ART may be temporarily discontinued when immune competence recurs and stabilizes (eg, sustained CD4 count between 500 and 800 cells/mm^3). Then, when CD4 counts fall between 350 and 400 cells/mm^3, ART should restart.

Medications for HIV-Related Infections

- PCP: trimethoprim-sulfamethoxazole (TMP-SMZ) and antibacterial agents, such as dapsone; alternatively, pentamidine, an antiprotozoal agent
- MAC: treatment for MAC infections involves use of either clarithromycin (Biaxin) or azithromycin (Zithromax). The combination of azithromycin with rifabutin (Mycobutin) is more effective but costly, with more adverse effects and interactions.

- Cryptococcal meningitis: intravenous amphotericin B with or without antifungal agents, such as fluconazole (Diflucan) or flucytosine (Ancobon).
- CMV retinitis: ganciclovir, foscarnet, or cidofovir
- Encephalitis: pyrimethamine (Daraprim) and sulfadiazine or clindamycin (Cleocin)
- Candidiasis: clotrimazole (Mycelex), ketoconazole, or fluconazole

Anticancer Agents

- KS: alpha-interferon, surgical excision of lesions, liquid nitrogen to lesions, vinblastine injected into intraoral lesions, interferon; chemotherapy with doxorubicin (Adriamycin), bleomycin, and vincristine (ABV); radiation
- Lymphomas: limited successful treatment; chemotherapy and radiation therapy may be used

Immunomodulators

- Alpha-interferon
- Other substances under evaluation (interleukin-2, interleukin-12, and other cytokines and lymphokines)

Antidepressants

Psychotherapy is integrated with pharmacology (imipramine [Tofranil], desipramine [Norpramin], fluoxetine [Prozac], methylphenidate [Ritalin]; electroconvulsive therapy if depression is severe).

Antidiarrheal Agents and Appetite Stimulants

Octreotide acetate (Sandostatin) is given to treat diarrhea and megestrol acetate (Megace) or dronabinol (Marinol) to stimulate appetite.

Supportive Care and Alternative Therapies

- Spiritual: laughter, hypnosis, faith healing, guided imagery, positive affirmations

- Nutritional: Goal is to attain or maintain ideal weight and decrease risk for infections. Appetite stimulants (megestrol [Megace]) have been successful; dronabinol (Marinol), which contains synthetic tetrahydrocannabinol (THC), the active ingredient in marijuana, has been effective when used to relieve nausea and vomiting. Alternative nutritional measures include oral supplements, such as Advera, and parenteral nutrition as well as vegetarian and macrobiotic diets, vitamin C or beta-carotene supplements, turmeric (curcumin), and Chinese herbs.
- Administration of intravenous fluid and electrolyte replacement may treat imbalances.
- Drug and biologic: medicines not approved by the FDA; oxygen, ozone, and urine therapy
- Physical forces and devices: acupuncture, acupressure, massage therapy, yoga, therapeutic touch, reflexology, crystals

NURSING PROCESS: The Patient with HIV/AIDS

Assessment

Identify potential risk factors, including sexual practices and IV/injection drug use history. Assess physical and psychological status. Thoroughly explore factors affecting immune system functioning.

Nutritional Status

- Obtain dietary history.
- Identify factors that may interfere with oral intake, such as anorexia, nausea, vomiting, oral pain, or difficulty swallowing.
- Assess patient's ability to purchase and prepare food.
- Measure nutritional status by weight, anthropometric measurements (triceps skin-fold measurement), and blood urea nitrogen, serum protein, albumin, and transferrin levels.

Skin and Mucous Membranes

- Inspect daily for breakdown, ulceration, and infection.
- Monitor oral cavity for redness, ulcerations, and creamy-white patches (candidiasis).
- Assess perianal area for excoriation and infection.
- Obtain wound cultures to identify infectious organisms.

Respiratory Status

- Monitor for cough, sputum production, shortness of breath, orthopnea, tachypnea, and chest pain; assess breath sounds.
- Assess other parameters of pulmonary function (chest x-rays, arterial blood gases, pulmonary function tests).

Neurologic Status

- Assess mental status as early as possible to provide a baseline. Note level of consciousness and orientation to person, place, and time and the occurrence of memory lapses.
- Observe for sensory deficits, such as visual changes, headache, and numbness and tingling in the extremities.
- Observe for motor impairments, such as altered gait and paresis.
- Observe for seizure activity.

Fluid and Electrolyte Status

- Examine skin and mucous membranes for turgor and dryness.
- Assess for dehydration by observing for increased thirst, decreased urine output, low blood pressure, weak rapid pulse, or urine specific gravity.
- Monitor electrolyte imbalances (laboratory studies show low serum sodium, potassium, calcium, magnesium, and chloride).
- Assess for signs and symptoms of electrolyte depletion, including decreased mental status, muscle twitching, muscle cramps, irregular pulse, nausea and vomiting, and shallow respirations.

Level of Knowledge

- Evaluate patient's knowledge of disease and transmission.
- Assess level of knowledge of family and friends.
- Explore patient's reaction to the diagnosis of HIV infection or AIDS.
- Explore how patient has dealt with illness and major life stressors in the past.
- Identify patient's resources for support.

Use of Alternative Therapies

- Question patient about use of alternative therapies.
- Encourage patient to report any use of alternative therapies to primary health care provider.
- Become familiar with potential side effects of alternative therapies; if side effect is suspected to result from alternative therapies, discuss with patient and primary and alternative health care providers.
- View alternative therapies with an open mind, and try to understand the importance of the treatment to patient.

Diagnosis

Nursing Diagnoses

- Impaired skin integrity related to cutaneous manifestations of HIV infection, excoriation, and diarrhea
- Risk for infection related to immunodeficiency
- Activity intolerance related to weakness, fatigue, malnutrition, impaired fluid and electrolyte balance, and hypoxia associated with pulmonary infections
- Disturbed thought processes related to shortened attention span, impaired memory, confusion, and disorientation (HIV encephalopathy)
- Ineffective airway clearance related to PCP, increased bronchial secretions, and decreased ability to cough related to weakness and fatigue
- Imbalanced nutrition: Less than body requirements related to decreased oral intake
- Diarrhea related to enteric pathogens or HIV infection

- Pain related to impaired perianal skin integrity secondary to diarrhea, KS, and peripheral neuropathy
- Social isolation related to stigma of the disease, withdrawal of support systems, isolation procedures, and fear of infecting others
- Anticipatory grieving related to changes in lifestyle and roles and unfavorable prognosis
- Deficient knowledge related to self-care and preventing HIV transmission

Collaborative Problems/Potential Complications

- Opportunistic infections
- Impaired breathing or respiratory failure
- Wasting syndrome and fluid and electrolyte imbalance
- Adverse reaction to medications

Planning and Goals

Goals include improved airway clearance, achievement and maintenance of skin integrity, resumption of usual bowel patterns, absence of infection, relief of pain and discomfort, improved nutritional status, activity tolerance, improved thought processes, increased socialization, expression of grief, absence of complications, and increased knowledge of disease prevention and self-care.

Nursing Interventions

Improving Airway Clearance

- At least daily, assess respiratory status, mental status, and skin color.
- Note and document presence of cough and quantity and characteristics of sputum; send specimen for analysis as ordered.
- Encourage adequate rest to minimize energy expenditure and prevent fatigue.
- Provide pulmonary therapy, such as coughing, deep breathing, postural drainage, percussion, and vibration,

every 2 hours to prevent stasis of secretions and promote airway clearance.

- Assist patient into a position (high- or semi-Fowler's) that facilitates breathing and airway clearance.
- Evaluate fluid volume status; encourage intake of 3 liters daily.
- Provide humidified oxygen, suctioning, intubation, and mechanical ventilation as necessary.

Promoting Skin Integrity

- Assess skin and oral mucosa for changes in appearance, location and size of lesions, and evidence of infection and breakdown; encourage regular oral care.
- Encourage patient to balance rest and mobility whenever possible; assist immobile patients to change position every 2 hours.
- Use devices such as alternating-pressure mattresses and low-air-loss beds.
- Encourage patient to avoid scratching, to use nonabrasive and nondrying soaps, and to use nonperfumed skin moisturizers on dry skin; administer antipruritic agents, antibiotic medication, analgesic agents, medicated lotions, ointments, and dressings as prescribed; avoid excessive use of tape.
- Keep bed linen free of wrinkles, and avoid tight or restrictive clothing to reduce friction to skin.
- Advise patient with foot lesions to wear white cotton socks and shoes that do not cause feet to perspire.

Maintaining Perianal Skin Integrity

- Assess perianal region for impaired skin integrity and infection.
- Instruct patient to keep the area as clean as possible, to cleanse after each bowel movement, to use sitz bath or irrigation, and to dry the area thoroughly after cleaning.
- Assist debilitated patient in maintaining hygiene practices.
- Promote healing with prescribed topical ointments and lotions.
- Culture wounds if infection is suspected.

Promoting Usual Bowel Habits

- Assess bowel patterns for diarrhea (frequency and consistency of stool, pain or cramping with bowel movements).
- Assess factors that increase frequency of diarrhea.
- Assess self-care strategies patient uses to control diarrhea.
- Measure and document volume of liquid stool as fluid volume loss; obtain stool cultures.
- Counsel patient about ways to decrease diarrhea (rest bowel, avoid foods that act as bowel irritants, including raw fruits and vegetables); encourage small, frequent meals.
- Administer prescribed medications, such as anticholinergic antispasmodic medications or opiates, antibiotic medications, and antifungal agents.

Preventing Infection

- Instruct patient and caregivers to monitor for signs and symptoms of infection. Recommend strategies to avoid infection (upper respiratory infections).
- Monitor laboratory values that indicate the presence of infection, such as white blood cell count and differential; assist in obtaining culture specimens as ordered.
- Strongly urge patients and sexual partners to avoid exposure to body fluids and to use condoms for any sexual activities.
- Strongly discourage IV/injection drug use because of risk to patient of other infections and transmission of HIV infection.
- Maintain strict aseptic technique for invasive procedures.

> **!** **NURSING ALERT** Observe universal precautions in all patient care. Teach colleagues and other health care workers to apply precautions to blood and all body fluids, secretions, and excretions except sweat (eg, cerebrospinal fluid; synovial, pleural, peritoneal, pericardial, amniotic, and vaginal fluids; semen). Consider all body fluids to be potentially hazardous in emergency circumstances when differentiating between fluid types is difficult.

Relieving Pain and Discomfort

- Assess patient for quality and severity of pain associated with impaired perianal skin integrity, KS lesions, and peripheral neuropathy.
- Explore effects of pain on elimination, nutrition, sleep, affect, and communication, along with exacerbating and relieving factors.
- Encourage patient to use soft cushions or foam pads while sitting and topical anesthetics or ointments as prescribed.
- Instruct patient to avoid irritating foods and to use antispasmodic agents and antidiarrheal preparations if necessary.
- Administer nonsteroidal anti-inflammatory agents and opiates, and use nonpharmacologic approaches, such as relaxation techniques.
- Administer tricyclic antidepressants and recommend elastic stockings as prescribed to help alleviate neuropathic pain.

Improving Nutritional Status

- Assess weight, dietary intake, anthropometric measurements, serum albumin, blood urea nitrogen, protein, and transferrin levels.
- Instruct patient about ways to supplement nutritional value of meals (eg, add eggs, butter, milk).
- Based on assessment of factors interfering with oral intake, implement specific measures to facilitate oral intake; consult dietitian to determine nutritional requirements.
- Control nausea and vomiting; encourage patient to eat easy-to-swallow foods; encourage oral hygiene before and after meals.
- Encourage rest before meals; do not schedule meals after painful or unpleasant procedures.
- Provide enteral or parenteral feedings to maintain nutritional status, as indicated.

Improving Activity Tolerance

- Monitor ability to ambulate and perform daily activities.
- Assist in planning daily routines to maintain balance between activity and rest.

- Instruct patient in energy conservation techniques (eg, sitting while washing or preparing a meal).
- Decrease anxiety that contributes to weakness and fatigue by using measures such as relaxation and guided imagery.
- Strategize with other health care team members to uncover and address factors associated with fatigue (eg, epoetin alfa [Epogen] for fatigue related to anemia).

Maintaining Thought Processes

- Assess for alterations in mental status.
- Reorient to person, place, and time as necessary; maintain and post a regular daily schedule.
- Give instructions, and instruct family to speak to patient, in a slow, simple, and clear manner.
- Provide night lights for bedroom and bathroom. Plan safe leisure activities that patient previously enjoyed.

 NURSING ALERT Provide around-the-clock supervision as necessary for patients with HIV encephalopathy.

Decreasing Sense of Social Isolation

- Provide an atmosphere of acceptance and understanding of AIDS patients, their families, and partners.
- Assess patient's usual level of social interaction early to provide a baseline for monitoring changes in behavior.
- Encourage patient to express feelings of isolation and aloneness; assure patient that these feelings are not unique or abnormal.
- Assure patients, family, and friends that AIDS is not spread through casual contact.

Coping With Grief

- Help patients explore and identify resources for support and mechanisms for coping.
- Encourage patient to maintain contact with family, friends, and coworkers and to continue usual activities whenever possible.
- Encourage patient to use local or national AIDS support groups and hotlines and to identify losses and deal with them when possible.

Monitoring and Managing Complications

- Respiratory failure and impaired breathing: monitor arterial blood gas values, oxygen saturation, respiratory rate and pattern, and breath sounds; provide suctioning and oxygen therapy; assist patient on mechanical ventilation to cope with associated stress.
- Inform patient that signs and symptoms of opportunistic infections include fever, malaise, difficulty breathing, nausea or vomiting, diarrhea, difficulty swallowing, and any occurrences of swelling or discharge. These symptoms should be reported to the health care provider immediately.
- Wasting syndrome and fluid and electrolyte disturbances: monitor weight gain or loss, skin turgor and dryness, ferritin levels, hemoglobin and hematocrit, and electrolytes. Assist in selecting foods that replenish electrolytes. Initiate measures to control diarrhea. Provide intravenous fluids and electrolytes as prescribed.
- Side effects of medications: provide information about purpose, administration, side effects (those reportable to physician), and strategies to manage or prevent side effects of medications. Monitor laboratory test values.

Promoting Home and Community-Based Care

Teaching Patients Self-Care

- Thoroughly discuss the disease and all fears and misconceptions; instruct patient, family, and friends about the transmission of AIDS.
- Discuss precautions to prevent transmission of HIV: use of condoms during vaginal or anal intercourse; using dental dam or avoiding oral contact with the penis, vagina, or rectum; avoiding sexual practices that might cut or tear the lining of the rectum, vagina, or penis; and avoiding sexual contact with multiple partners, those known to be HIV positive, those who use illicit injectable drugs, and those who are sexual partners of people who inject drugs.
- Teach patient and family how to prevent disease transmission, including hand hygiene and methods of safely handling items soiled with bodily fluids.

- Instruct patient not to donate blood.
- Emphasize importance of taking medication as prescribed. Assist patient and caregivers in fitting the medication regimen into their lives.
- Teach medication administration, including intravenous preparations.
- Teach guidelines about infection, follow-up care, diet, rest, and activities.
- Instruct patient and family how to administer enteral or parenteral feedings, if applicable.
- Offer support and guidance in coping with this disease.

Continuing Care

- Refer patient and family for home care nursing or hospice for physical and emotional support.
- Assist family and caregivers in providing supportive care.
- Assist in administration of parenteral antibiotics, chemotherapy, nutrition, complicated wound care, and respiratory care.
- Provide emotional support to patient and family.
- Refer patient to community programs, housekeeping assistance, meals, transportation, shopping, individual and group therapy, support for caregivers, telephone networks for the homebound, and legal and financial assistance.
- Encourage patient and family to discuss end-of-life decisions.

Evaluation

Expected Patient Outcomes

- Maintains skin integrity
- Resumes usual bowel habits
- Experiences no infections
- Maintains adequate level of activity tolerance
- Maintains usual level of thought processes
- Maintains effective airway clearance
- Experiences increased sense of comfort, less pain
- Maintains adequate nutritional status
- Experiences decreased sense of social isolation

- Progresses through grieving process
- Reports increased understanding of AIDS and participates in self-care activities as possible
- Remains free of complications

For more information, see Chapter 52 in Smeltzer and Bare: *Brunner and Suddarth's Textbook of Medical-Surgical Nursing*, 11th edition. Philadelphia: Lippincott Williams & Wilkins, 2008.

Acute Respiratory Distress Syndrome

Acute respiratory distress syndrome (ARDS; noncardiogenic pulmonary edema) is a clinical syndrome characterized by sudden and progressive edema, increasing bilateral infiltrates, reduced lung compliance, and hypoxemia refractory to oxygen supplementation. ARDS results from an inflammatory trigger that causes injury to the alveolar capillary membrane. People at risk for ARDS are those experiencing direct injury to the lungs (eg, aspiration, smoke inhalation) or indirect insult to the lungs (eg, shock). Death results mainly from multi-system organ failure with sepsis. The mortality rate of ARDS may be as high as 50% to 60%.

Clinical Manifestations

- Rapid onset of severe dyspnea, usually 12 to 48 hours after an initiating event
- Intercostal retractions and crackles
- Arterial hypoxemia not responsive to oxygen supplementation
- Labored breathing and tachypnea

Assessment and Diagnostic Findings

- Based on clinical criteria: history of risk factors, acute onset of respiratory distress, bilateral pulmonary infiltrates,

absence of left heart failure, and severe refractory
hypoxemia (PaO_2/FiO_2 < 200 mm Hg)
- Chest x-ray shows bilateral infiltrates and pulmonary edema.

Medical Management

- Identify and treat the underlying condition; ensure early
  detection; use aggressive supportive treatment; prevent
  infection (intubation and mechanical ventilation).
- As disease progresses, use positive end-expiratory pressure
  (PEEP).
- Neuromuscular blocking agents such as pancuronium
  (Pavulon) and vecuronium (Norcuron) may be used to
  paralyze patient for easier ventilation.
- Monitor arterial blood gas values, pulse oximetry, and
  pulmonary function testing.
- Provide circulatory support; treat hypovolemia carefully;
  avoid overload.
- Provide adequate fluid management; administer
  intravenous solutions.
- Provide nutritional support (35 to 45 kcal/kg daily).
- Pharmacologic therapy may include human recombinant
  interleukin-1 receptor antagonist, neutrophil inhibitors,
  pulmonary-specific vasodilators, surfactant replacement
  therapy, antisepsis agents, antioxidant therapy, and
  corticosteroids (late in the course of ARDS).

NURSING PROCESS: The Patient with ARDS

Assessment

- Monitor patient closely because ARDS can quickly progress
  to a life-threatening situation.
- Note agitation and anxiety, and minimize.

Nursing Diagnoses

- Impaired gas exchange related to congestion
- Anxiety related to fear of death

Planning and Goals

The goals of patient care may include achieving adequate spontaneous, nonlabored ventilation; maintaining arterial blood gas values within normal limits for patient without ventilator assistance; and ensuring that patient experiences minimal anxiety.

Nursing Interventions

Promoting Adequate Ventilation

- Facilitate respiratory management: position patient to maximize respiration, oxygen, endotracheal intubation, tracheostomy, suctioning, and mechanical ventilation with sedation and paralytics as needed.
- Chest physiotherapy (monitor closely for deterioration in oxygenation with changes in position)
- Provide safety interventions related to ventilator care.
- Encourage rest to limit oxygen consumption.
- Encourage oral fluid intake if patient is not ventilated.

Minimizing Anxiety

- Provide emotional support and reduce patient anxiety.
- Explain all procedures and deliver care in calm, reassuring manner.

Evaluation

Expected Outcomes

- Nonlabored spontaneous respirations
- Arterial blood gases, pulse oximetry, and pulmonary function tests within normal limits

---

For more information, see Chapter 23 in Smeltzer and Bare: *Brunner and Suddarth's Textbook of Medical-Surgical Nursing*, 11th edition. Philadelphia: Lippincott Williams & Wilkins, 2008.

Addison's Disease (Primary Adrenocortical Insufficiency)

Addison's disease is caused by a deficiency of cortical hormones. It results when the adrenal cortex function is inadequate to meet the patient's need for cortical hormones. Autoimmune or idiopathic atrophy of the adrenal glands is responsible for 80% to 90% of cases. Other causes include surgical removal of both adrenal glands or infection (tuberculosis or histoplasmosis) of the adrenal glands. Inadequate secretion of adrenocorticotropic hormone (ACTH) from the primary pituitary gland results in adrenal insufficiency. Symptoms may also result from sudden cessation of exogenous adrenocortical hormonal therapy, which interferes with normal feedback mechanisms.

Clinical Manifestations

Chief clinical manifestations include muscle weakness, anorexia, gastrointestinal symptoms, fatigue, emaciation, dark pigmentation of the skin and mucous membranes, hypotension, low blood glucose, low serum sodium, and high serum potassium. The onset usually occurs with nonspecific symptoms. Mental changes (depression, emotional lability, apathy, and confusion) are present in 60% to 80% of patients. In severe cases, disturbance of sodium and potassium metabolism may be marked by depletion of sodium and water and severe, chronic dehydration.

Addisonian Crisis

This medical emergency develops as the disease progresses. Signs and symptoms include:

- Cyanosis, fever, and classic signs of circulatory shock: pallor, apprehension, rapid and weak pulse, rapid respirations, and low blood pressure

- Headache, nausea, abdominal pain, diarrhea, confusion, and restlessness
- Slight overexertion, exposure to cold, and acute infections decrease salt intake and may lead to circulatory collapse, shock, and death.
- Stress of surgery or dehydration from preparation for diagnostic tests or surgery may precipitate addisonian or hypotensive crisis.
- Decreased blood glucose and sodium levels, increased serum potassium (hyperkalemia), and leukocytosis

Assessment and Diagnostic Findings

Primary adrenocortical insufficiency; greatly increased plasma ACTH (>22.0 pmol/L); serum cortisol low normal or lower than normal (<165 nmol/L); decreased blood glucose (hypoglycemia) and sodium (hyponatremia) levels, increased serum potassium (hyperkalemia) level, and increased white blood cell count (leukocytosis).

Medical Management

Immediate treatment is directed toward combating shock.

- Restore blood circulation, administer fluids, monitor vital signs, and place patient in a recumbent position with legs elevated.
- Administer intravenous hydrocortisone, followed by 5% dextrose in normal saline.
- Vasopressor amines may be required if hypotension persists.
- Antibiotics may be prescribed for infection.
- Oral intake may be initiated as soon as tolerated.
- If adrenal gland does not regain function, lifelong replacement of corticosteroids and mineralocorticoids is required.
- Dietary intake should be supplemented with salt during times of gastrointestinal losses of fluids through vomiting and diarrhea.

NURSING PROCESS: The Patient with Addison's Disease

Assessment

Assessment focuses on fluid imbalance and stress.

- Check blood pressure from a lying to standing position; check pulse rate.
- Assess skin color and turgor.
- Assess history of weight changes, muscle weakness, and fatigue.
- Ask patient and family about onset of illness or increased stress that may have precipitated crisis.

Diagnosis

Nursing Diagnoses

- Deficient fluid volume related to inadequate fluid intake and fluid loss secondary to inadequate adrenal hormone secretion
- Deficient knowledge about need for hormone replacement and dietary modification

Collaborative Problems/Potential Complications

Addisonian crisis

Planning and Goals

Goals may include improving fluid balance, improving response to activity, decreasing stress, increasing knowledge about need for hormone replacement and dietary modifications, and ensuring absence of complications.

Nursing Interventions

Restoring Fluid Balance

- Record weight changes daily.
- Assess skin turgor and mucous membranes.

- Instruct patient to report increased thirst.
- Monitor lying, sitting, and standing blood pressures frequently.
- Assist patient in selecting, and encourage patient to consume, food and fluids that assist in restoring and maintaining fluid and electrolyte balance (eg, foods high in sodium during gastrointestinal disturbances and very hot weather). Include a dietitian for added guidance.
- Assist patient and family in learning to administer hormone replacement and to modify dosage during illness and stress.
- Provide written and verbal instructions about mineralocorticoid and glucocorticoid therapy.

Improving Activity Tolerance

- Avoid unnecessary activities and stress that might precipitate a hypotensive episode.
- Detect signs of infection or presence of stressors that may have triggered the crisis.
- Provide a quiet, nonstressful environment during acute crises; carry out all activities for patient.
- Explain all procedures to reduce fear and anxiety.
- Explain rationale for minimizing stress during acute crisis.

Monitoring and Managing Complications (Addisonian Crisis)

- Assess for signs and symptoms of crisis: circulatory collapse and shock.
- Avoid physical and psychological stress, including exposure to cold, overexertion, infection, and emotional distress.
- Initiate immediate treatment with intravenous fluid, glucose, and electrolytes, especially sodium; corticosteroid supplements; and vasopressors.
- Avoid patient exertion; anticipate and take measures to meet patient's needs.
- Monitor symptoms, vital signs, weight, and fluid and electrolyte balance to evaluate return to precrisis state.
- Identify factors that led to crisis.

Promoting Home and Community-Based Care

Teaching Patients Self-Care

- Give patient and family explicit verbal and written instructions about the rationale for replacement therapy and proper dosage.
- Teach patient and family how to modify drug dosage and increase salt in times of illness, very hot weather, and stressful situations.
- Instruct patient to modify diet and fluid intake to maintain fluid and electrolyte balance.
- Provide patient and family with a syringe and vial of injectable steroid (Solu-Cortef) for emergency use and instruct when and how to use.
- Advise patient to inform health care providers (eg, dentists) of steroid use. Urge patient to wear a medical alert bracelet.
- Teach patient and family signs of excessive or insufficient hormone replacement.
- Instruct patient regarding modification of diet (sodium) during illness and hot weather to maintain fluid and electrolyte balance.

Continuing Care

- Encourage patients to weigh themselves daily to detect significant changes in weight that indicate fluid loss (due to too little hormone) or retention (due to too much hormone).
- If patient cannot return to work and family responsibilities after hospital discharge, refer to home health care nurse.
- Assess recovery, monitor hormone replacement, and assess stress in the home.
- Assess patient's plans for follow-up visits to clinic or physician's office.

For more information, see Chapter 42 in Smeltzer and Bare: *Brunner and Suddarth's Textbook of Medical-Surgical Nursing*, 11th edition. Philadelphia: Lippincott Williams & Wilkins, 2008.

Alzheimer's Disease

Alzheimer's disease (AD) is one of the most common, irreversible, degenerative neurologic dementias. Dementia is an acquired syndrome of progressive deterioration in global intellectual abilities. The deterioration interferes with the person's customary occupational and social performance. In AD, specific neuropathologic and biochemical changes are thought to result in decreased brain size and decreased acetylcholine production. The disease begins insidiously and is characterized by gradual loss of cognitive and functional abilities and disturbances in behavior and affect.

Combined factors are thought to cause AD, including genes, neurotransmitter changes, vascular abnormalities, stress hormones, circadian changes, head trauma, and seizures.

The role of inflammation and oxidative stress and the contribution of brain infarctions are being explored as contributory factors to AD. Death occurs as a result of a complicating condition such as pneumonia, malnutrition, or dehydration.

Clinical Manifestations

Symptoms are highly variable; some include:

- In early disease there is forgetfulness and subtle memory loss, although social skills and behavior patterns remain intact. Forgetfulness is manifested in many daily actions with progression of the disease (eg, the patient gets lost in a familiar environment or repeats the same stories).
- Ability to formulate concepts and think abstractly disappears.
- Patient may exhibit inappropriate impulsive behavior.
- Personality changes are evident; patient may become depressed, suspicious, paranoid, hostile, and combative.
- Speaking skills deteriorate to nonsense syllables; agitation and physical activity increase.
- Voracious appetite may develop from high activity level; dysphagia is noted with disease progression.

- Eventually patient requires help with all aspects of daily living, including toileting because incontinence occurs.
- Terminal stage may last for months.

Assessment and Diagnostic Findings

The diagnosis, which is one of exclusion, is confirmed at autopsy.

- Clinical symptoms are found through health history, including physical findings and results from functional abilities assessments (eg, Mini-Mental Status Examination)
- Electroencephalography (EEG)
- Computed tomography (CT) scan
- Magnetic resonance imaging (MRI)
- Laboratory tests, primarily blood and cerebrospinal fluid (CSF)

Medical Management

Without a cure or a way to slow progression of AD, treatment relies on managing cognitive symptoms with cholinesterase inhibitors, such as donepezil (Aricept), rivastigmine (Exelon), and galantamine (Reminyl). These drugs enhance acetylcholine uptake in the brain to maintain memory for a while. Memantine (Namenda) was recently approved for use to reduce clinical deterioration in moderate to severe AD.

NURSING PROCESS: The Patient with Alzheimer's Disease

Assessment

Obtain health history with mental status exam and physical examination, noting symptoms indicating dementia. Report findings to physician. As indicated, assist with diagnostic evaluation, promoting calm environment to maximize patient safety and cooperation.

Nursing Diagnoses

- Impaired thought processes related to decline in cognitive function
- Risk for injury related to decline in cognitive function
- Anxiety related to confused thought processes
- Imbalanced nutrition: less than body requirements related to cognitive decline
- Activity intolerance related to imbalance in activity/rest pattern
- Deficient self-care, bathing/hygiene, feeding, toileting related to cognitive decline
- Impaired social interaction related to cognitive decline
- Deficient knowledge of family/caregiver related to care for patient as cognitive function declines
- Ineffective family processes related to decline in patient's cognitive function

Planning and Goals

Goals for the patient may include supporting cognitive function, physical safety, reduced anxiety, adequate nutrition, improved, activity tolerance, self-care, and socialization, support, and education of caregivers.

Nursing Interventions

Supporting Cognitive Function

Provide a calm, predictable environment to minimize confusion and disorientation. Help patient feel a sense of security with a quiet, pleasant manner, clear, simple explanations, and use of memory aids and cues.

Promoting Physical Safety

- Provide a safe environment to allow patient to move about as freely as possible and relieve family's worry about safety.
- Prevent falls and other accidents by removing obvious hazards and providing adequate lighting.
- Monitor intake of medications and food.

- Allow smoking only with supervision.
- Reduce wandering behavior with gentle persuasion and distraction. Supervise all activities outside the home to protect patient. As needed, secure doors leading from the house. Ensure that patient wears an identification bracelet or neck chain.
- Avoid restraints, because they may increase agitation.

Reducing Anxiety and Agitation

- Give emotional support to support a positive self-image.
- When skill losses occur, adjust goals to fit patient's declining ability and structure activities to help prevent agitation.
- Keep the environment simple, familiar, and noise-free; limit changes.
- Remain calm and unhurried, particularly if the patient is experiencing a combative, agitated state known as catastrophic reaction (overreaction to excessive stimulation).
- Use easy-to-understand sentences to convey messages.

Promoting Adequate Nutrition

- Keep mealtimes simple and calm; avoid confrontations.
- Cut food into small pieces to prevent choking, and convert liquids to gelatin to ease swallowing. Offer one dish at a time.
- Prevent burns by serving typically hot food and beverages warm.

Balancing Activity and Rest

- Help patient to relax to sleep with music, warm milk, or a back rub.
- To enhance nighttime sleep, provide sufficient opportunities for daytime exercise. Discourage long periods of daytime sleeping.
- Assess and address any unmet underlying physical or psychological needs that may prompt wandering or other inappropriate behavior.

Promoting Independence in Self-Care Activities

- Simplify daily activities into short achievable steps so that patient feels a sense of accomplishment.
- Maintain patient's personal dignity and autonomy.
- Encourage patient to make choices when appropriate and to participate in self-care activities as much as possible.

Meeting Socialization Needs

- Encourage visits, letters, and phone calls (visits should be brief and nonstressful, with one or two visitors at a time).
- Advise that the nonjudgmental friendliness of a pet can provide satisfying activity and an outlet for energy.
- Encourage spouse to talk about any sexual concerns, and suggest sexual counseling if necessary.

Promoting Home and Community-Based Care

Be sensitive to the highly emotional issues that the family is confronting. Encourage early visits to explore long-term care facilities to minimize "crisis relocation" if and when it becomes necessary. Refer family to the Alzheimer's Association for assistance with family support groups, respite care, and adult day care services.

Evaluation

Expected Patient Outcomes

- Patient maintains cognitive, functional, and social interaction abilities for as long as possible.
- Patient remains free of injury.
- Patient demonstrates minimal anxiety and agitation.
- Patient receives adequate nutrition, activity and rest.
- Patient's socialization needs are met.
- Patient and family caregivers are knowledgeable about condition and treatment and care regimens.

For more information, see Chapter 12 in Smeltzer and Bare: *Brunner and Suddarth's Textbook of Medical-Surgical Nursing*, 11th edition. Philadelphia: Lippincott Williams & Wilkins, 2008.

Amyotrophic Lateral Sclerosis

Amyotrophic lateral sclerosis (ALS) is a disease of unknown cause in which there is a loss of motor neurons (nerve cells controlling muscles) in the anterior horns of the spinal cord and the motor nuclei of the lower brain stem. As these cells die, the muscle fibers that they supply undergo atrophic changes. The degeneration of the neurons may occur in both the upper and lower motor neuron systems. ALS affects more men than women, with onset occurring usually in the fifth or sixth decade of life. In the United States, it is often referred to as Lou Gehrig's disease. Death occurs from infection, respiratory failure, or aspiration. The average time from onset to death is about 3 years.

Clinical Manifestations

Clinical features of ALS depend on the location of the affected motor neurons. In most patients, the chief symptoms are progressive muscle weakness, cramps, incoordination, atrophy, and fasciculations (twitching).

Loss of Motor Neurons in Anterior Horns of Spinal Cord

- Progressive weakness and atrophy of the arms, trunk, or leg muscles
- Spasticity; deep tendon stretch reflexes are brisk and overactive.
- Anal and bladder sphincters not affected

Weakness in Muscles Supplied by Cranial Nerves (25% of Patients in Early Stage)

- Difficulty talking, swallowing, and ultimately breathing
- Soft palate and upper esophageal weakness, causing liquids to be regurgitated through nose
- Impaired ability to laugh, cough, or blow the nose

Bulbar Muscle Impairment

- Progressive difficulty in speaking and swallowing, and aspiration
- Nasal voice and unintelligible speech
- Emotional lability, but intellectual function unimpaired
- Eventually, compromised respiratory function

Assessment and Diagnostic Methods

Diagnosis is based on signs and symptoms because no clinical or laboratory tests are specific for this disease. Electromyographic (EMG) studies and magnetic resonance imaging may be helpful.

Medical Management

No specific treatment for ALS is available. See below for symptomatic treatment.

Supportive and Rehabilitative Measures

- Baclofen, dantrolene sodium, or diazepam for spasticity
- Quinine for muscle cramps
- Riluzole (a glutamate antagonist)
- Enteral feedings (percutaneous endoscopic gastrostomy [PEG]) for patients with aspiration or swallowing difficulties

Mechanical Ventilation

- Decision is based on patient and family's understanding of the disease, prognosis, and implications of initiating such therapy.
- Encourage patient to complete an advance directive or "living will" to preserve autonomy.

Nursing Management

The nursing care of the patient with ALS is generally the same as the basic care plan for patients with degenerative neurologic disorders (see Myasthenia Gravis). Encourage patient and family to contact the ALS Association for information and support.

For more information, see Chapter 65 in Smeltzer and Bare: *Brunner and Suddarth's Textbook of Medical-Surgical Nursing*, 11th edition. Philadelphia: Lippincott Williams & Wilkins, 2008.

Anaphylaxis

Anaphylaxis is a severe, life-threatening allergic response to an immunologic reaction (type I hypersensitivity) between a specific antigen and an immunoglobulin E (IgE) antibody. Type I hypersensitivity requires previous exposure to the specific antigen through inhalation, injection, ingestion, or skin contact. An anaphylactoid (anaphylaxis-like) reaction is clinically similar to anaphylaxis. Anaphylaxis may occur with medications, food, latex, insect stings, and cytotoxic antibody transfusions. Reactions may be local or systemic. Local anaphylactic reactions usually involve urticaria (hives) and angioedema (swelling) at the exposure site. The reaction can be severe but is rarely fatal. Systemic reactions occur in major organ systems within minutes of exposure.

Clinical Manifestations

Clinical symptoms are determined by the amount of the allergen, the amount of mediator released, the sensitivity of the target organ, and the route of allergen entry. Type I hypersensitivity reactions may include both local and systemic anaphylaxis.

Mild

Symptoms include peripheral tingling; a warm sensation; fullness in the mouth and throat; nasal congestion; periorbital swelling, pruritus, sneezing, and tearing eyes. Symptoms begin within 2 hours of exposure.

Moderate

May include any of the mild symptoms plus anxiety, bronchospasm, and edema of the airways or larynx with dyspnea, cough, and wheezing. Symptom onset is the same as that of a mild reaction.

Severe

An abrupt onset with the same signs and symptoms described above, progressing rapidly to bronchospasm, laryngeal edema, severe dyspnea, cyanosis, and hypotension. Dysphagia, abdominal cramping, vomiting, diarrhea, and seizures are additional symptoms, with cardiac arrest and coma occurring rarely.

Assessment and Diagnostic Methods

Diagnostic evaluation of the patient with allergic disorders commonly includes blood tests (CBC with differential, high total serum IgE levels), smears of body secretions, skin tests, and the radioallergosorbent test (RAST).

Prevention

Prevention by avoidance of allergens is of utmost importance. Health care providers should always obtain a careful history of any sensitivities before administering medications. Venom immunotherapy may be given to people who are allergic to insect venom. Insulin-allergic diabetic patients or penicillin-sensitive patients may require desensitization as well.

Medical Management

Respiratory and cardiovascular functions are evaluated and cardiopulmonary resuscitation (CPR) is initiated in cases of cardiac arrest. Oxygen is administered in high concentrations during

CPR or when the patient is cyanotic, dyspneic, or wheezing. Patients with mild reactions need to be educated about the risk for recurrences. Patients with severe reactions need to be observed for 12 to 14 hours.

Pharmacologic Therapy

- Epinephrine, antihistamines, and corticosteroids may be given to prevent recurrences of the reaction and to relieve urticaria and angioedema.
- Aminophylline may be administered if indicated.
- Volume expanders and vasopressor agents may be used to maintain blood pressure and normal hemodynamic status; glucagon also may be used.

Nursing Management

- Teach people who are sensitive to insect bites and stings, certain medications, or foods, and people who have idiopathic or exercise-induced anaphylactic reactions to avoid exposure to allergens.
- Instruct patient always to carry an emergency kit that contains injectable epinephrine.
- Provide verbal and written instruction about the emergency kit.
- Ensure that patient can perform correct self-injection.
- Encourage patient always to wear or carry medical identification.

For more information, see Chapter 53 in Smeltzer and Bare: *Brunner and Suddarth's Textbook of Medical-Surgical Nursing*, 11th edition. Philadelphia: Lippincott Williams & Wilkins, 2008.

Anemia

Anemia is a condition of lower-than-normal red blood cell (RBC) count and hemoglobin (Hgb) level. It is often not a specific disease state but a sign of an underlying disorder. Anemia results in a diminished amount of oxygen delivery to body tissues. There are many different kinds of anemia, but all can be classified as being due to a decrease in the production of RBCs (hypoproliferative), excessive destruction of RBCs (hemolytic), or a loss of RBCs (eg, gastrointestinal bleeding). Other etiologic factors include deficits in iron and nutrients, hereditary factors, and chronic diseases. Complications of severe anemia include heart failure, paresthesias, confusion, and other problems specific to the type of anemia.

Clinical Manifestations

Several factors influence symptom development from anemia, including its severity, speed of development (the faster the onset, the more severe the symptoms), and duration (eg, its chronicity; long-term anemia may produce few or no symptoms); the patient's metabolic requirements and concurrent disorders or disabilities (eg, cardiopulmonary disease); and special complications or features of the condition that produced the anemia. Pronounced symptoms of anemia include the following:

- Dyspnea, chest pain, muscle pain or cramping, tachycardia
- Weakness, fatigue, general malaise
- Pallor of the skin and mucous membranes (sclera, oral mucosa)
- Jaundice (megaloblastic or hemolytic anemia)
- Smooth, red tongue (iron-deficiency anemia)
- Beefy-red, sore tongue (megaloblastic anemia)
- Angular cheilosis (ulceration of the corner of the mouth)
- Brittle, ridged, concave nails and pica (unusual craving for starch, dirt, ice) in patients with iron-deficiency anemia

Assessment and Diagnostic Methods

- Complete hematologic studies (eg, Hgb, hematocrit, reticulocyte count, and RBC indices, particularly mean corpuscular volume)

- Iron studies (serum iron level, total iron-binding capacity, percentage saturation, and ferritin)
- Serum vitamin B12 and folate levels; haptoglobin and erythropoietin levels
- Bone marrow aspiration and biopsy
- Other studies as indicated to determine underlying illness

Gerontologic Considerations

Anemia is the most common hematologic condition affecting elderly people. In this population, bone marrow typically has a decreased ability to respond to the body's need for blood cells. The inability to increase blood cell production adequately in cases of increased need seriously affects cardiopulmonary function. Because elderly people with a concurrent cardiac or pulmonary problem may be unable to tolerate anemia, a prompt, thorough evaluation of the anemia is warranted.

Medical Management

The goal is to correct or control the cause of the anemia and replace lost or destroyed RBCs by transfusing packed RBCs. In elderly patients it is important to identify and treat the cause of anemia rather than considering it a consequence of aging.

NURSING PROCESS: The Patient with Anemia

Assessment

- Obtain a health history, perform a physical examination, and obtain laboratory values.
- Ask patient about extent and type of symptoms experienced and impact of symptoms on lifestyle; medication history; alcohol intake; athletic endeavors (extreme exercise).
- Ask patient about any loss of blood (eg, excessive menses or vaginal bleeding), use of iron supplements during pregnancy.

- Ask about family history of inherited anemias.
- Perform nutritional assessment: ask about dietary habits resulting in nutritional deficiencies, such as iron, vitamin B12, and folic acid.
- Monitor relevant laboratory test results; note changes.
- Assess cardiac status (for symptoms of increased workload or heart failure): tachycardia, palpitations, dyspnea; dizziness, orthopnea, exertional dyspnea; cardiomegaly, hepatomegaly, peripheral edema.
- Assess for neurologic deficits (important with pernicious anemia): presence and extent of peripheral numbness and paresthesias; ataxia and poor coordination; confusion.
- Assess for gastrointestinal function: nausea, vomiting; diarrhea, melena or dark stools, occult blood; anorexia, glossitis.

Diagnosis

Nursing Diagnoses

- Fatigue related to the blood's decreased hemoglobin and diminished oxygen-carrying capacity
- Imbalanced nutrition: Less than body requirements related to inadequate intake of essential nutrients
- Ineffective tissue perfusion related to inadequate blood volume or hematocrit
- Noncompliance with prescribed therapy

Collaborative Problems/Potential Complications

- Heart failure
- Angina
- Paresthesias
- Confusion

Planning and Goals

The major goals may include decreased fatigue, attainment or maintenance of adequate nutrition, maintenance of adequate tissue perfusion, adherence to prescribed therapy, and absence of complications.

Nursing Interventions

Managing Fatigue

- Assist patient to prioritize activities and establish a balance between activity and rest.
- Encourage patient with chronic anemia to maintain physical activity and exercise to prevent deconditioning.
- Use safety precautions to prevent falls from poor coordination, paresthesias, and weakness.

Maintaining Adequate Nutrition

- Encourage a well-balanced diet high in protein, calories, fruits, and vegetables.
- Teach patient to avoid or limit intake of alcohol and spicy (irritating) and gas-producing foods.
- Plan dietary teaching sessions for patient and family; consider cultural aspects of nutrition.
- Discuss dietary supplements (eg, vitamins, iron, folate) as prescribed.

Maintaining Adequate Perfusion

- Monitor vital signs closely, and adjust or withhold medications (antihypertensives) as indicated.
- Administer supplemental oxygen, transfusions, and intravenous fluids as ordered.

Monitoring and Managing Complications

- Assess patient with anemia for heart failure.
- Decrease activities and stimuli that cause an increase in heart rate and cardiac output.
- Encourage patient to identify situations that precipitate palpitations and dyspnea.
- Administer oxygen; elevate head of bed for dyspnea.
- Monitor vital signs and observe for indications of fluid retention.
- Administer diuretic agents as ordered.
- Monitor for signs of paresthesia, poor coordination, ataxia, and confusion.
- Implement safety measures to prevent injury.

Promoting Home and Community-Based Care

- Teach patient and family purpose of prescribed medication, how and how long to take it, and how to manage side effects of therapy.
- Assist patient in developing ways to incorporate therapeutic plan into lifestyle.
- Inform patient that abruptly stopping some medications may have serious consequences.

Evaluation

Expected Patient Outcomes

- Reports less fatigue and tolerates activity at level that is safe and acceptable
- Attains and maintains adequate nutrition
- Maintains adequate perfusion
- Experiences no or minimal complications

For more information, see Chapter 33 in Smeltzer and Bare: *Brunner and Suddarth's Textbook of Medical-Surgical Nursing*, 11th edition. Philadelphia: Lippincott Williams & Wilkins, 2008.

Anemia, Aplastic

Aplastic anemia (hypoproliferative) is a rare disease caused by a decrease in or damage to marrow stem cells in the bone marrow and replacement of the marrow with fat, resulting in markedly reduced hematopoiesis. Significant neutropenia and thrombocytopenia (a deficiency of platelets) are also seen. Aplastic anemia can be congenital or acquired. It may be idiopathic, it may result from certain infections or from pregnancy, or it may be caused by medications, chemicals, or radiation damage. The most common offenders are antimicrobials (chloramphenicol), benzene and benzene derivatives (airplane glue), pesticides, inorganic arsenic, anticonvulsants, phenylbutazone, sulfonamides, and gold compounds. A prompt and complete recovery may be anticipated if exposure is terminated early. Death is usually caused by hemorrhage or infection.

Clinical Manifestations

- Gradual onset marked by complications: infection, fatigue, and pallor; dyspnea on exertion
- Purpura (bleeding); retinal hemorrhages are common
- Repeated throat infections with possible lymphadenopathy and splenomegaly

Assessment and Diagnostic Methods

- Complete blood count and analysis
- Diagnosis is made by bone marrow aspirate and biopsy (marrow replaced with fat).

Medical Management
Prevention

Potentially toxic medications are used only when alternative therapies are not available. In patients receiving potentially bone marrow–toxic drugs, such as chloramphenicol, blood cell counts are monitored. Some patients benefit from bone marrow transplantation or peripheral blood stem cell transplantation and administration of immunosuppressive therapy with antithymocyte globulin (ATG) and cyclosporine.

Supportive Therapy

Offending drugs are discontinued. Symptoms may be prevented with transfusions of red blood cells and platelets. Patients with pronounced leukopenia are protected from contact with people who have infections.

Nursing Management

See Nursing Management under Anemia for additional information.

- Preserve patient's energy by planning care, depending on the degree of weakness and fatigue.
- Assess for signs of infection and bleeding; provide meticulous care of intravenous sites or wounds, and avoid trauma.
- Guard against any wound, abrasion, or ulcer of mucous membrane or skin as a potential site of infection.
- Encourage and assist with meticulous body and oral hygiene (with soft toothbrush, no floss).
- Avoid trauma when possible (avoid subcutaneous and intramuscular injections, pad side rails, avoid suctioning) when thrombocytopenia is present.

Promoting Home and Community-Based Care

- Teach patient importance of regular atraumatic bowel movements. Urge use of stool softeners and oral laxatives because hemorrhoids can develop and become infected or bleed.
- Protect patients with pronounced leukopenia from contact with people who have infections.
- Teach patients taking toxic drugs on a long-term basis the need for periodic blood studies and symptoms that should be reported.

For more information, see Chapter 33 in Smeltzer and Bare: *Brunner and Suddarth's Textbook of Medical-Surgical Nursing*, 11th edition. Philadelphia: Lippincott Williams & Wilkins, 2008.

Anemia, Iron-Deficiency

Iron-deficiency anemia is a condition in which the total-body iron content is decreased below a normal level and iron stores are depleted. It is the most common type of anemia in the world. It typically results when the intake of dietary iron is inadequate to maintain the level necessary for hemoglobin synthesis. For most adults, blood loss is the cause of this anemia. Risk factors include a history of ulcers, gastritis, intestinal hookworm, gastrointestinal tumors, malabsorption, or diet very high in fiber (prevents iron absorption). The most frequent cause in men and postmenopausal women is bleeding; in premenopausal women the most common cause is menorrhagia. Chronic alcoholism often causes inadequate iron intake and loss of iron through blood from the gastrointestinal tract.

Clinical Manifestations

- Symptoms of anemia: fatigue, irritability, numbness, and tingling of extremities
- Symptoms in more severe cases: smooth, sore tongue; brittle and ridged nails; angular cheilosis (mouth ulceration)
- Pica (unusual cravings, such as for clay, ice, or laundry starch), history of multiple pregnancies, or gastrointestinal bleeding
- Hemoglobin proportionately lower than hematocrit and red blood cell count
- Serum iron concentration low
- Total iron-binding capacity high; serum ferritin low

Assessment and Diagnostic Methods

- Bone marrow aspiratation
- Laboratory values, including serum ferritin levels (indicates iron stores), blood count (hemoglobin, hematocrit, red blood cell count, mean corpuscular volume), serum iron level, and total iron-binding capacity
- Colonoscopy and/or endoscopy or other radiographic examination of the gastrointestinal tract to detect ulcerations, gastritis, polyps, or cancer (particularly for people 50 years or older)

Medical Management

- Search for the cause, which may be a curable gastrointestinal cancer or uterine fibroids.

- Test stool specimens for occult blood.
- Administer prescribed iron preparations (oral, intramuscular, or intravenous).
- Avoid tablets with enteric coating; may be poorly absorbed.
- Continue iron for 6 to 12 months.

Nursing Management

See Nursing Management under Anemia for additional information.

- Administer intramuscular or intravenous iron in some cases when oral iron is not absorbed, is poorly tolerated, or is needed in large amounts.
- Administer a small test dose before intramuscular injection to avoid risk of anaphylaxis (greater with intramuscular than with intravenous injections).
- Advise patient to take iron supplements an hour before meals. If gastric distress occurs, suggest taking the supplement with meals and, after symptoms subside, resuming between-meal schedule for maximum absorption.
- Inform patient that iron salts change stool to dark green or black.
- Advise patient to brush and floss teeth frequently because ferrous sulfate is likely to be deposited on the teeth and gums; take liquid iron through a straw and rinse mouth with water.
- Teach preventive education, because iron-deficiency anemia is common in menstruating and pregnant women.
- Educate patient regarding foods high in iron (eg, organ and other meats, beans, leafy green vegetables, raisins, molasses).
- Advise patient to take iron-rich foods with vitamin C to enhance absorption.
- Instruct patient to avoid taking antacids or dairy products with iron (diminishes iron absorption).
- Provide nutritional counseling for those whose normal diet is inadequate.

- Encourage patient to continue iron therapy for total therapy time (6 to 12 months), even when fatigue is no longer present.

For more information, see Chapter 33 in Smeltzer and Bare: *Brunner and Suddarth's Textbook of Medical-Surgical Nursing*, 11th edition. Philadelphia: Lippincott Williams & Wilkins, 2008.

Anemia, Megaloblastic (Vitamin B12 and Folic Acid Deficiency)

The anemias caused by deficiencies of the vitamins B12 and folic acid show identical bone marrow and peripheral blood changes. Both vitamins are essential for DNA synthesis.

Pathophysiology

The two vitamin deficiencies may coexist. In each case, hyperplasia of the bone marrow occurs, and the precursor erythroid and myeloid cells are large and bizarre in appearance. The RBCs produced are abnormally large (megaloblastic). A pancytopenia (a decrease in all myeloid-derived cells) develops.

Vitamin B12 deficiency can occur from inadequate intake in strict vegetarians; faulty absorption from the gastrointestinal tract; absence of intrinsic factor (pernicious anemia); disease involving the ileum or pancreas, which impairs B12 absorption; and gastrectomy. People with pernicious anemia have a higher incidence of gastric cancer than the general public.

Folic acid deficiency occurs when intake of folate is deficient or the requirement is increased. People at risk include those who rarely eat uncooked vegetables or fruits, primarily elderly people living alone or people with alcoholism. Alcohol use, hemolytic anemia, and pregnancy increase folic acid requirements. Patients with malabsorptive or small bowel disease may not absorb folic acid normally.

Clinical Manifestations

Symptoms are progressive and may be marked by spontaneous partial remissions and exacerbations.

- Gradual development of signs of anemia (weakness, listlessness, and pallor)
- Possible development of a smooth, sore, red tongue and mild diarrhea (pernicious anemia)
- Possible development of confusion; more often, paresthesias in the extremities and difficulty keeping balance; loss of position sense
- Lack of neurologic manifestations with folic acid deficiency alone
- Vitiligo (patchy loss of skin pigmentation) and prematurely graying hair (often seen in pernicious anemia)
- Without treatment, patients die, usually as a result of congestive heart failure from anemia.

Assessment and Diagnostic Findings

- Schilling test (primary diagnostic tool)
- Complete blood count (Hgb value as low as 4 to 5 g/dL, WBC count 2,000 to 3,000/mm^3, platelet count less than 50,000/mm^3; MCV is very high, usually exceeding 110)
- Serum levels of folate and vitamin B12 (folic acid deficiency and deficient vitamin B12)

Medical Management: Vitamin B12 Deficiency

- Oral supplementation with vitamins or fortified soy milk (strict vegetarians)
- Intramuscular injections of vitamin B12 for defective absorption or absence of intrinsic factor
- Prevention of recurrence with lifetime vitamin B12 therapy for patient who has had pernicious anemia or noncorrectable malabsorption

Medical Management:
Folic Acid Deficiency

- Intake of nutritious diet and 1 mg folic acid daily
- Intramuscular folic acid for malabsorption syndromes
- Folic acid taken orally as a separate tablet (except prenatal vitamins)
- Folic acid replacement stopped when hemoglobin level returns to normal, with the exception of alcoholics, who continue replacement as long as alcohol intake continues

Nursing Management

See Nursing Management under Anemia for additional information.

- Assess patients at risk for megaloblastic anemia for clinical manifestations (eg, inspect the skin, sclera, and mucous membranes for jaundice, note vitiligo or premature graying or smooth, red, sore tongue).
- Perform careful neurologic assessment (eg, note gait and stability; test position and vibration sense).
- Assess need for assistive devices (eg, canes, walkers) and need for support and guidance in managing activities of daily living and home environment.
- Ensure safety when position sense, coordination, and gait are affected.
- Refer for physical or occupational therapy as needed.
- When sensation is altered, instruct patient to avoid excessive heat and cold.
- Advise patient to prepare bland, soft foods and to eat small amounts frequently.
- Explain that other nutritional deficiencies, such as alcohol-induced anemia, can induce neurologic problems.
- Instruct patient in complete urine collections for the Schilling test. Also explain the importance of the test and of complying with the collection.

- Teach patient about chronicity of disorder and need for monthly vitamin B12 injections even when patient has no symptoms. Instruct patient how to self-administer injections, when appropriate.
- Stress importance of ongoing medical follow-up and screening, because gastric atrophy associated with pernicious anemia increases the risk of gastric carcinoma.

For more information, see Chapter 33 in Smeltzer and Bare: *Brunner and Suddarth's Textbook of Medical-Surgical Nursing*, 11th edition. Philadelphia: Lippincott Williams & Wilkins, 2008.

Anemia, Sickle Cell

Sickle cell anemia is a severe hemolytic anemia resulting from the inheritance of the sickle hemoglobin gene (HbS), which causes a defective hemoglobin molecule.

Pathophysiology

The defective hemoglobin molecule assumes a sickle shape when exposed to low oxygen tension. These long, rigid red blood cells become lodged in small vessels and can obstruct blood flow to body tissue, causing ischemia and possibly necrosis ("sickling crisis"). The HbS gene is inherited, with some people having the sickle cell trait (a carrier, inheriting one abnormal gene) and some having sickle cell disease (inheriting two abnormal genes). Sickled RBCs have a shortened life span, resulting in anemia. Sickle cell disease is found predominantly in people of African descent and less often in people descended from the Mediterranean countries, the Middle East, or aboriginal tribes of India.

Clinical Manifestations

Symptoms and complications result from chronic hemolysis or thrombosis.

- Anemia, with hemoglobin values in the 7 to 10 g/dL range
- Jaundice is characteristic, usually obvious in the sclera.
- Bone marrow expands in childhood, sometimes causing enlargement of bones of the face and skull.
- Tachycardia, cardiac murmurs, and often cardiomegaly are associated with chronic anemia.
- Dysrhythmias and heart failure may occur in adults.
- There is severe pain in various parts of the body. All tissues and organs are vulnerable and susceptible to hypoxic damage or true ischemic necrosis at any time.
- Sickle cell crisis: sickle crisis, aplastic crisis, or sequestration crisis
- Acute chest syndrome: rapidly falling hemoglobin level, tachycardia, fever, and bilateral infiltrates seen on chest x-ray films

Assessment and Diagnostic Findings

- Hemoglobin and hematocrit levels, blood smear (usually normal)
- Diagnosis is confirmed with hemoglobin electrophoresis.
- Isoelectric focusing, high-performance liquid chromatography techniques
- Sickling occurs whether patient has sickle trait or sickle cell anemia; only electrophoresis shows a distinction.

Medical Management

- Many antisickling drugs are undergoing trial; hydroxyurea has been effective (increases fetal hemoglobin production). Arginine is also used.
- Bone marrow transplantation is a potential cure but is limited because of lack of donors or organ damage.
- Chronic transfusions with red blood cells are administered to relieve anemia, prevent complications, or improve response to infection.
- Pulmonary function is monitored and pulmonary hypertension is treated early if found. Infections and acute chest syndrome, which predispose to crisis, are treated

promptly. Incentive spirometry is performed to prevent pulmonary complications; bronchoscopy is done to identify source of pulmonary disease.

- Fluid restriction may be beneficial. Corticosteroids may be useful.
- Folic acid is administered daily for increased marrow requirement.
- Supportive care involves pain management (aspirin or NSAIDs, morphine, and patient-controlled analgesia [PCA]), oral or intravenous hydration, chelation therapy, supplemental oxygen, physical and occupational therapy, physiotherapy, cognitive and behavioral intervention, and support groups. If possible, the patient is supported with corticosteroids (prednisone), intravenous immunoglobulin (IVIG; Gammagard, Sandoglobulin, Venoglobulin), and erythropoietin (Epogen, Procrit).

NURSING PROCESS: The Patient with Sickle Cell Crisis

See Nursing Management under Anemia for additional information.

Assessment

- Question patients in crisis about factors that could have precipitated the crisis and measures used to prevent crisis.
- Assess all body systems, with particular emphasis on pain (0-to-10 scale, quality, and frequency), swelling, fever (all joint areas and abdomen).
- Elicit symptoms of cerebral hypoxia by careful neurologic examination.
- Carefully assess respiratory system, including breath sounds and oxygen saturation levels.
- Assess for signs of cardiac failure (edema, increased point of maximal impulse, and cardiomegaly) by radiography.
- Assess for signs of dehydration and history of fluid intake; examine mucous membranes, skin turgor, urine output, serum creatinine, and BUN values.

- Assess current and past history of medical management, particularly chronic transfusion therapy, hydroxyurea use, and prior treatment for infection.
- Assess for signs of any infectious process (examine chest and long bones and femoral head, because pneumonia and osteomyelitis are common).
- Monitor hemoglobin, hematocrit, and reticulocyte count and compare with baseline levels.
- Discuss history of alcohol intake.

Diagnosis

Nursing Diagnoses

- Acute pain related to tissue hypoxia due to agglutination of sickled cells within blood vessels
- Risk for infection
- Risk for powerlessness related to illness-induced helplessness
- Deficient knowledge regarding prevention of crisis

Collaborative Problems/Potential Complications

- Hypoxia, ischemia, infection, and poor wound healing leading to skin breakdown and ulcers
- Dehydration
- Cerebrovascular accident (stroke)
- Renal dysfunction
- Heart failure, pulmonary hypertension, and acute chest syndrome
- Impotence

Planning and Goals

The major goals include relief of pain, decreased incidence of crisis, enhanced sense of self-esteem and power, and absence of complications.

Nursing Interventions

Managing Pain

- Use patient's subjective description of pain and pain rating on a pain scale to guide the use of analgesic agents.

- Support and elevate any joint that is acutely swollen until swelling diminishes.
- Teach patient relaxation techniques, breathing exercises, and distraction to ease pain.
- When acute painful episode has diminished, implement aggressive measures to preserve function (eg, physical therapy, whirlpool baths, and transcutaneous nerve stimulation).

Preventing and Managing Infection

- Monitor patient for signs and symptoms of infection.
- Initiate prescribed antibiotics promptly.
- Assess patient for signs of dehydration.
- Teach patient to take prescribed oral antibiotics at home, if indicated, emphasizing the need to complete the entire course of antibiotic therapy. Assist patient to identify a feasible administration schedule.

Promoting Coping Skills

- Enhance pain management to promote a therapeutic relationship based on mutual trust.
- Focus on patient's strengths rather than deficits to enhance effective coping skills.
- Provide opportunities for patient to make decisions about daily care to increase feelings of control.

Increasing Knowledge

- Teach patient about situations that can precipitate a sickle cell crisis and steps to take to prevent or diminish such crises (eg, keep warm, maintain adequate hydration, avoid stressful situations).
- Arrange for group education, when possible, carried out by members of the community who are from the same ethnic group as patient.

Promoting Self-Care

Management measures for many of the potential complications are delineated in the previous sections; additional measures should be taken to address the following issues.

Leg Ulcers

- Protect the leg from trauma and contamination.
- Use scrupulous aseptic technique to prevent nosocomial infections.

Priapism Leading to Impotence

- Teach patient to empty the bladder at the onset of the attack, to exercise, and then to take a warm bath.
- Inform patient to seek medical attention if an episode persists more than 3 hours.

Chronic Pain

- Emphasize the importance of complying with prescribed treatment plan.
- Use a nonjudgmental attitude, and actively seek involvement from patient in establishing a treatment plan and developing useful strategies.
- Promote trust with patient through adequate management of acute pain during episodes of crisis.
- Suggest to patient that receiving care from a single provider over time is much more beneficial than receiving care from rotating physicians and staff in an emergency department.
- When a crisis arises, emergency department staff should contact patient's primary health care provider for optimal management.
- Promote continuity of care and establish written contracts with patient.

Promotion Home and Community-Based Care

Teaching Patients Self-Care

- Involve the patient *and family* in teaching about the disease, treatment, assessment, and monitoring needed to detect complications. Also teach about care of PCA access device and chelation therapy.
- Advise health care providers, patients, and families to communicate regularly.
- Provide guidelines regarding when to seek urgent care.

Evaluation

Expected Patient Outcomes

- Reports control of pain
- Is free of infection
- Expresses improved sense of control
- Increases knowledge about disease process
- Experiences absence of complications

For more information, see Chapter 33 in Smeltzer and Bare: *Brunner and Suddarth's Textbook of Medical-Surgical Nursing*, 11th edition. Philadelphia: Lippincott Williams & Wilkins, 2008.

Aneurysm, Aortic

An aneurysm is a localized sac or dilation of an artery formed at a weak point in the vessel wall. The most common cause is atherosclerosis. Saccular and fusiform are the most common forms of aneurysm. Saccular aneurysms project from one side of the vessel only; fusiform aneurysms involve dilation of an entire arterial segment. Mycotic aneurysms are small aneurysms due to local infections. Aortic aneurysms are usually classified as thoracic, abdominal, or dissecting. Other causes include trauma to the wall of the artery, infection (pyogenic or syphilitic), and congenital defects of the artery wall. Men are affected more often than women. Rupture can lead to hemorrhage and death.

Thoracic aortic aneurysms occur most frequently in men between the ages of 40 and 70 years. The thoracic area is the most common site for the development of a dissecting aneurysm. About one third of patients die from rupture.

🌿 Gerontologic Considerations

Abdominal aortic aneurysms are more common among patients between the ages of 60 and 90 years. Risk factors include genetic predisposition, smoking, and hypertension. If surgical complications are expected to be life-threatening, repair may be delayed until the aneurysm is about 5.5 cm (2″) wide.

A dissecting aneurysm of the aorta is caused by rupture in the intimal layer, resulting in blood dissecting the vessel layers. It is often associated with poorly controlled hypertension and is three times more common in men between ages 50 and 70. Early diagnosis is difficult because of a variable clinical picture.

Clinical Manifestations

Symptoms are variable and depend on how rapidly the aneurysm dilates and affects surrounding intrathoracic structures.

Thoracic Aortic Aneurysm

Some do not produce symptoms.

- Constant, boring pain, which may occur only when supine (prominent symptom)
- Dyspnea, cough (paroxysmal and brassy), or stridor
- Hoarseness, weak voice or aphonia (complete loss of voice)
- Dysphagia
- Dilated superficial veins on chest, neck, or arms
- Edematous areas on chest wall
- Cyanosis
- Unequal pupils

Abdominal Aortic Aneurysm

- Patient complains of "heart beating" in abdomen when lying down or a feeling of an abdominal mass or abdominal throbbing.
- Possibly, "blue-toe syndrome" (occlusion of a digital vessel) if aneurysm is associated with thrombus.
- Severe back pain or abdominal pain is a sign of impending rupture.

Dissecting Aneurysm

- Sudden onset with severe and persistent pain described as "tearing" or "ripping" in anterior chest or back, extending to

shoulders, epigastric area, or abdomen (may be mistaken for acute myocardial infarction)
- Pallor, sweating, and tachycardia
- Blood pressure elevated or markedly different from one arm to the other
- Death usually caused by external rupture of the hematoma

Assessment and Diagnostic Findings

- Chest radiograph, angiogram, transesophageal echocardiography, and magnetic resonance imaging (MRI)
- Duplex ultrasonography or computed tomography (CT) scan to determine size, length, and location of aneurysm
- In abdominal aortic aneurysms, a pulsatile mass in middle and upper abdomen; a systolic bruit may be auscultated over the mass.

Medical Management

Medical or surgical treatment depends on the type of aneurysm. For a ruptured aneurysm, prognosis is poor and surgery is performed immediately. When surgery can be delayed, medical measures include:

- Strict control of blood pressure and reduction in pulsatile flow
- Systolic pressure maintained at 100 to 120 mm Hg with antihypertensive drugs, such as nitroprusside
- Pulsatile flow reduced by medications that reduce cardiac contractility, such as propranolol

Surgical Management

Removal of the aneurysm and restoration of vascular continuity with a graft (resection and bypass graft or endovascular grafting) is the goal of surgery and the treatment of choice for abdominal aortic aneurysms larger than 5.5 cm (2 inches) in diameter or those that are enlarging. Intensive monitoring in the critical care unit is required.

Nursing Management

See Preoperative and Postoperative Nursing Management for additional information.

Preoperative Assessment

- Assessment is guided by the fact that the aneurysm may rupture (signs include persistent or intermittent back or abdominal pain that may be localized in the middle or lower abdomen or lower back).
- Establish functional capacity of all organ systems, recognizing possible cerebral, cardiovascular, pulmonary, and renal impairment due to atherosclerosis.
- Implement medical therapies to stabilize patient.

Postoperative Assessment

- Intensely monitor the pulmonary, cardiovascular, renal, and neurologic systems.
- Monitor for complications: arterial occlusion, hemorrhage, infection, ischemic bowel, renal failure, and impotence.
- Prescribe an exercise schedule after the acute recovery phase.
- Discourage prolonged sitting.

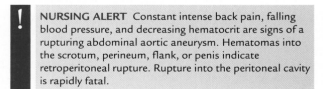

> **!** **NURSING ALERT** Constant intense back pain, falling blood pressure, and decreasing hematocrit are signs of a rupturing abdominal aortic aneurysm. Hematomas into the scrotum, perineum, flank, or penis indicate retroperitoneal rupture. Rupture into the peritoneal cavity is rapidly fatal.

For more information, see Chapter 31 in Smeltzer and Bare: *Brunner and Suddarth's Textbook of Medical-Surgical Nursing,* 11th edition. Philadelphia: Lippincott Williams & Wilkins, 2008.

Aneurysm, Intracranial

An intracranial (cerebral) aneurysm is a dilation of the walls of a cerebral artery that develops as a result of weakness in the arterial wall. Its cause is unknown, but it may be due to atherosclerosis, a congenital defect of the vessel walls, hypertensive vascular disease, head trauma, or advancing age. Most commonly affected are the internal carotid, anterior or posterior cerebral, anterior or posterior communicating, and middle cerebral arteries. Symptoms are produced when the aneurysm enlarges and presses on nearby cranial nerves or brain tissue, or ruptures, causing subarachnoid hemorrhage. Prognosis depends on the age and neurologic condition of the patient, associated diseases, and the extent and location of the aneurysm.

Clinical Manifestations

- Rupture of the aneurysm causes sudden, unusually severe headache; often, loss of consciousness for a variable period; pain and rigidity of the back of the neck and spine; and visual disturbances (visual loss, diplopia, ptosis). Tinnitus, dizziness, and hemiparesis may also occur.
- If the aneurysm leaks blood and forms a clot, patient may show little neurologic deficit, or severe bleeding, resulting in cerebral damage followed rapidly by coma and death.

Assessment and Diagnostic Methods

- Computed tomography (CT) scan, cerebral angiography, and lumbar puncture are diagnostic procedures used to confirm an aneurysm.
- The Hunt-Hess Classification System of Clinical Grades is a guide for diagnosing the severity of subarachnoid hemorrhage after an aneurysm bleeds.

Medical Management

- Allow the brain to recover from the initial insult (bleeding).
- Prevent or minimize the risk of rebleeding.

- Prevent or treat other complications: rebleeding, cerebral vasospasm, acute hydrocephalus, and seizures.
- Provide bed rest with sedation to prevent agitation and stress.
- Maintain cerebral blood flow and oxygenation; maintain hemoglobin and hematocrit levels and adequate hydration. Avoid blood pressure extremes (hypertension or hypotension).
- Manage vasospasm with calcium-channel blockers, such as nimodipine (Nimotop), verapamil (Isoptin), and nifedipine (Procardia). Endovascular techniques may also be used.
- Institute surgical treatment (arterial bypass) or medical treatment to prevent rebleeding.
- Manage increased intracranial pressure (ICP) by draining cerebrospinal fluid (CSF) via lumbar puncture or ventricular catheter drainage.
- Administer mannitol to reduce ICP, and monitor for signs of dehydration and rebound elevation of ICP.
- Administer antifibrinolytic agents to delay or prevent dissolution of the clot if surgery is delayed or contraindicated.
- Manage systemic hypertension with antihypertensive therapy, blood pressure monitoring by intravascular arterial line; prophylactic anticonvulsant therapy; stool softeners to prevent straining and elevation of blood pressure; analgesic therapy for head and neck pain; and prevention of deep vein thrombosis with graded-pressure elastic stockings.

NURSING PROCESS: The Patient with an Intracranial Aneurysm

Assessment

- Perform a complete neurologic assessment: level of consciousness, pupillary reaction (sluggishness), motor and sensory function, cranial nerve deficits (extraocular eye movements, facial droop, ptosis), speech difficulties, visual disturbance or headache, and nuchal rigidity or other neurologic deficits.

- Document and report neurologic assessment findings, and reassess and report any changes in patient's condition.
- Detect subtle changes, especially altered levels of consciousness (earliest signs of deterioration include mild drowsiness and slight slurring of speech).

Diagnosis

Nursing Diagnoses

- Ineffective tissue perfusion (cerebral) related to bleeding or vasospasm
- Disturbed sensory perception due to the restrictions of aneurysm precautions
- Anxiety due to illness or restrictions of aneurysm precautions

Collaborative Problems/Potential Complications

- Seizures
- Vasospasm
- Hydrocephalus
- Aneurysm rebleeding
- Hyponatremia

Planning and Goals

Patient goals include improved cerebral tissue perfusion, relief of sensory and perceptual deprivation, relief of anxiety, and absence of complications.

Nursing Interventions

Improving Cerebral Tissue Perfusion

- Monitor closely for neurologic deterioration, and maintain a neurologic flow record.
- Check blood pressure, pulse, level of consciousness, pupillary responses, and motor function hourly; monitor respiratory status and report changes immediately.

- Implement aneurysm precautions (immediate and absolute bed rest in a quiet, nonstressful setting; restrict visitors, except for family).
- Elevate head of bed 15 to 30 degrees or as ordered.
- Avoid any activity that suddenly increases blood pressure or obstructs venous return (eg, Valsalva maneuver; instruct patient to exhale during voiding or defecation to decrease strain), eliminate caffeine, administer all personal care, and minimize external stimuli.
- Apply elastic compression stockings or sequential compression boots. Observe legs for signs and symptoms of deep vein thrombosis (tenderness, swelling, warmth, and positive Homans' sign).

Relieving Sensory Deprivation

- Keep sensory stimulation to a minimum.
- Explain restrictions to help reduce patient's sense of isolation.

Relieving Anxiety

- Inform patient of plan of care.
- Provide support and appropriate reassurance to patient and family.
- Provide reality orientation.

Monitoring and Managing Potential Complications

- Maintain seizure precautions. Also maintain airway and prevent injury if a seizure occurs. Administer antiseizure medications and fluids as prescribed (phenytoin [Dilantin] is medication of choice).
- Assess for and immediately report signs of possible vasospasm, which may occur several days after surgery or on the initiation of treatment (intensified headaches, decreased level of responsiveness, or evidence of aphasia or partial paralysis). Also administer calcium-channel blockers or fluid-volume expanders as prescribed.
- Monitor for onset of symptoms of hydrocephalus, which may be acute (first 24 hours after hemorrhage), subacute (days later), or delayed (several weeks later). Report

symptoms immediately: acute hydrocephalus is characterized by sudden stupor or coma; subacute or delayed is characterized by gradual onset of drowsiness, behavioral changes, and ataxic gait.

- Monitor for and report symptoms of aneurysm rebleeding. Rebleeding occurs most often in the first 2 weeks. Symptoms include sudden severe headache, nausea, vomiting, decreased level of consciousness, and neurologic deficit. Administer medications to maintain blood pressure and antifibrinolytics as ordered to delay lysis of the clot.

- Hyponatremia: monitor laboratory data often because hyponatremia (serum sodium level under 135 mEq/L) affects 10% to 40% of patients. Report low levels persisting for 24 hours, as syndrome of inappropriate antidiuretic hormone (SIADH) or cerebral salt wasting phenomenon (kidneys connot conserve sodium) may develop.

Teaching Patients Self-Care

Provide patient and family with information to promote cooperation with the care and required activity restrictions and prepare them for patient's return home. Identify the causes of intracranial hemorrhage, its possible consequences, and the medical or surgical treatments that are implemented. Discuss the importance of interventions taken to prevent and detect complications (eg, aneurysm precautions, close monitoring of patient). As indicated, facilitate transfer to a rehabilitation unit or center.

Continuing Care

Urge patient and family to follow recommendations to prevent further complications and to schedule and keep follow-up appointments. Refer for home care if warranted, and encourage health promotion and screening practices.

Evaluation

Expected Patient Outcomes

- Demonstrates intact neurologic status and normal vital signs and respiratory patterns
- Demonstrates normal sensory perceptions

- Exhibits reduced anxiety level
- Is free of hyponatremia and other complications

For more information, see Chapter 62 in Smeltzer and Bare: *Brunner and Suddarth's Textbook of Medical-Surgical Nursing*, 11th edition. Philadelphia: Lippincott Williams & Wilkins, 2008.

Angina Pectoris

Angina pectoris is a clinical syndrome characterized by paroxysms of pain or a feeling of pressure in the anterior chest. The cause is insufficient coronary blood flow, resulting in an inadequate supply of oxygen to meet the myocardial demand. Angina is usually a result of atherosclerotic heart disease and is associated with a significant obstruction of a major coronary artery. Factors affecting anginal pain are physical exertion, exposure to cold, eating a heavy meal, stress, or any emotion-provoking situation that increases myocardial workload. Atypical angina is not associated with the above and may occur at rest. Diabetic neuropathy can interfere with neuroreceptors, thus dulling the patient's perception of pain.

Clinical Manifestations

- Pain varies from a feeling of indigestion to a choking or heavy sensation in the upper chest to agonizing pain. The patient with diabetes mellitus may not experience severe pain with angina.
- Angina is accompanied by severe apprehension and a feeling of impending death.
- The pain is usually retrosternal, deep in the chest behind the upper or middle third of the sternum.
- Discomfort is poorly localized and may radiate to the neck, jaw, shoulders, and inner aspect of the upper arms (usually the left arm).

- Patient feels a tightness, heavy choking, or strangling sensation with a viselike, insistent quality. Shortness of breath, pallor, diaphoresis, dizziness, light-headedness, nausea, and vomiting may be noted (called angina-like signs if noted alone; may represent myocardial infarction).
- Angina is accompanied by a feeling of weakness or numbness in the arms, wrists, and hands.
- An important characteristic of anginal pain is that it subsides when the precipitating cause is removed or with nitroglycerin.

Assessment and Diagnostic Methods

- Evaluation of clinical manifestations of pain and patient history
- Electrocardiogram changes (12-lead ECG), stress testing, blood tests
- Echocardiogram, nuclear scan, or invasive procedures such as cardiac catheterization and coronary artery angiography

🌿 Gerontologic Considerations

The elderly person who experiences angina may not exhibit the typical pain profile because of age-related changes in neuroceptors. In older patients, pain may be sensed in the jaw or fainting may occur. Advise patient to recognize feelings of weakness as an indication for rest or taking prescribed medications. During exposure to cold temperature, elderly patients may experience anginal symptoms more quickly than younger people. Encourage these patients to wear warm clothing as appropriate.

Medical Management

The goals of medical management are to decrease the oxygen demands of the myocardium and to increase the oxygen supply through pharmacologic therapy and risk factor control (see Modifiable Risk Factors under Coronary Artery Disease for additional information).

Surgical Management

Frequently, therapy includes a combination of medicine and surgery. Surgically, the goals of management include revascularization of the blood supply to the myocardium.

- Coronary artery bypass surgery or minimally invasive direct coronary artery bypass (MIDCAB)
- Percutaneous transluminal coronary angioplasty (PTCA) or percutaneous transluminal myocardial revascularization (PTMR)
- Application of intracoronary stents and atherectomy to enhance blood flow
- Lasers to vaporize plaques
- Percutaneous coronary endarterectomy to extract obstruction

Pharmacologic Therapy

- Nitrates, the mainstay of therapy (nitroglycerin)
- Beta-adrenergic blockers (metoprolol [Toprol])
- Calcium ion antagonists and calcium-channel blockers (amlodipine [Norvase] and diltiazem [Cardizem])
- Antiplatelet and anticoagulant medications (aspirin, clopidogrel [Plavix], ticlopidine [Ticlid], or heparin)
- Oxygen therapy

NURSING PROCESS: The Patient with Angina

Assessment

Observe and record facts about pain (location, description, and intensity) and patient activities that precede and precipitate attacks of anginal pain (from patient history).

Diagnosis

Nursing Diagnoses

- Ineffective cardiac tissue perfusion secondary to coronary artery disease as evidenced by chest pain (or equivalent symptoms)
- Death anxiety
- Deficient knowledge about underlying disease and methods for avoiding complications
- Noncompliance, Ineffective therapeutic regimen management or Noncompliance related to nonacceptance of necessary lifestyle changes

Collaborative Problems/Potential Complications

Potential complications of angina include myocardial infarction and its complications: acute pulmonary edema, heart failure, cardiogenic shock, dysrhythmias and cardiac arrest, myocardial rupture, pericardial effusion, and cardiac tamponade.

Planning and Goals

Goals may include pain relief and absence of return of pain, reduction of anxiety, awareness of the underlying nature of the disorder, understanding of the prescribed care, adherence to the self-care program, and absence of complications.

Nursing Interventions

An overall goal of ongoing intervention is to design a logical program of prevention using data collected during the nursing assessment.

Preventing Pain

- Teach patient to understand the symptom complex and avoid activities known to cause anginal pain (Box A-1).
- Direct patient to stop all activities and sit or rest in bed in a semi-Fowler's position if chest pain is sensed.
- If patient has frequent pain or pain with minimal activity, discuss ways to alternate rest and activity periods.

BOX A–1 Factors that Trigger Angina Episodes

- Sudden or excessive exertion
- Exposure to cold
- Tobacco use
- Heavy meals
- Excessive weight
- Some over-the-counter drugs, such as diet pills, nasal decongestants, or drugs that increase heart rate and blood pressure

---

- Assess pain and vital signs, noting respiratory distress, and ST segment on ECG.
- Administer nitroglycerin (up to 3 doses) and oxygen.

Reducing Anxiety

- Explore implications that the diagnosis has for patient.
- Provide essential information about the illness and methods of preventing progression. Explain importance of following prescribed directives for the ambulatory patient at home.
- Explore various stress reduction methods with patient (eg, music therapy).

Teaching Patients Self-Care

- Educate patient about basic nature of the illness.
- Furnish facts needed to reorganize living habits in order to reduce the frequency and severity of anginal attacks, to delay underlying disease, and to protect against other complications.
- Collaborate on a self-care program with patient, family, or friends.
- Plan activities to minimize angina episodes.
- Teach patient that any pain unrelieved within 30 minutes by the usual methods should be treated at the closest emergency center. Patient should call 911 for assistance.

Evaluation

Expected Patient Outcomes

- Reports that pain is relieved promptly
- Reports and demonstrates less anxiety
- Understands ways to avoid complications and demonstrates freedom from complications
- Complies with self-care program

For more information, see Chapter 28 in Smeltzer and Bare: *Brunner and Suddarth's Textbook of Medical-Surgical Nursing*, 11th edition. Philadelphia: Lippincott Williams & Wilkins, 2008.

Aortic Insufficiency (Regurgitation)

Aortic insufficiency is the flow of blood back into the left ventricle from the aorta during diastole. The result is left ventricular dilation and hypertrophy. It may be caused by inflammatory lesions that deform the leaflets of the aortic valve. The lesions prevent complete sealing of the aortic orifice during diastole. This disorder may result from endocarditis, congenital abnormalities, or conditions such as blunt chest trauma, syphilis, and dissecting aneurysm that cause dilation or tearing of the ascending aorta.

Clinical Manifestations

- Develops insidiously (without symptoms in most patients)
- Earliest manifestation: increased force of heartbeat—that is, visible or palpable pulsations over the temporal arteries (head) and at the neck (carotid)
- Exertional dyspnea and easy fatigability
- Signs and symptoms of left ventricular failure (orthopnea, paroxysmal nocturnal dyspnea)
- Widened pulse pressure
- Water-hammer pulse (pulse strikes the palpating finger with quick, sharp strokes and then suddenly collapses)

Assessment and Diagnostic Methods

ECG, radionuclide imaging, MRI, echocardiogram, and cardiac catheterization are used in the diagnosis.

Medical Management

- Antibiotic prophylaxis is used before invasive and dental procedures.
- Heart failure and dysrhythmias are treated.
- Treatment of choice is aortic valve replacement; surgery is recommended in the presence of left ventricular hypertrophy.
- Valve repair (valvuloplasty commissurotomy) may be performed instead of replacement. Repaired valves function longer than replaced valves, and continuous anticoagulation is not required.

Nursing Management

See Preoperative and Postoperative Nursing Management for additional information.

- Teach patient about wound care, diet, activity, medication, and self-care.
- Instruct patient on importance of antibiotic prophylaxis to prevent endocarditis.
- Reinforce all new information and self-care instructions for 4 to 8 weeks after the procedure.

For more information, see Chapter 29 in Smeltzer and Bare: *Brunner and Suddarth's Textbook of Medical-Surgical Nursing*, 11th edition. Philadelphia: Lippincott Williams & Wilkins, 2008.

Aortic Stenosis

Aortic valve stenosis is the narrowing of the orifice between the left ventricle and the aorta. In adults, the stenosis may be congenital, or it may be a result of rheumatic endocarditis or cusp calcification of unknown cause. There is progressive narrowing of the valve orifice over a period of several years to several decades. The heart muscle increases in size (hypertrophy) in response to all degrees of obstruction; clinical signs of heart failure occur when compensatory mechanisms of the heart fail.

Clinical Manifestations

- Exertional dyspnea
- Dizziness and syncope (fainting)
- Angina pectoris
- Blood pressure possibly low but usually normal
- Low pulse pressure (30 mm Hg or less)
- Physical examination: loud, rough, systolic murmur heard over the aortic area; vibration over the base of the heart

Assessment and Diagnostic Methods

- 12-lead ECG and echocardiogram
- Left heart catheterization

Medical Management

Antibiotic prophylaxis is provided to prevent endocarditis. Medications for left ventricular failure or dysrhythmia are administered as needed. Surgical replacement of the aortic valve is the favored definitive treatment. Uncorrected condition can lead to irreversible heart failure. Patients who are symptomatic and are not surgical candidates may benefit from one- or two-balloon percutaneous valvuloplasty procedures.

Nursing Management

See Preoperative and Postoperative Nursing Management for additional information.

For more information, see Chapter 29 in Smeltzer and Bare: *Brunner and Suddarth's Textbook of Medical-Surgical Nursing*, 11th edition. Philadelphia: Lippincott Williams & Wilkins, 2008.

Appendicitis

The appendix is a small, finger-like appendage attached to the cecum just below the ileocecal valve. Because it empties into the colon inefficiently and its lumen is small, it is prone to becoming obstructed and is vulnerable to infection (appendicitis). The obstructed appendix becomes inflamed and edematous and eventually fills with pus. It is the most common cause of acute inflammation in the right lower quadrant of the abdominal cavity and the most common cause of emergency abdominal surgery. Males are affected more than females, teenagers more frequently than adults; the highest incidence is in those between the ages of 10 and 30 years.

Clinical Manifestations

- Lower right quadrant pain usually accompanied by low-grade fever, nausea, and sometimes vomiting
- At McBurney's point (located halfway between the umbilicus and the anterior spine of the ilium), local tenderness with pressure and some rigidity of the lower portion of the right rectus muscle
- Rebound tenderness may be present; location of appendix dictates amount of tenderness, muscle spasm, and occurrence of constipation or diarrhea.
- Rovsing's sign (elicited by palpating left lower quadrant, which paradoxically causes pain in right lower quadrant)
- If appendix ruptures, pain becomes more diffuse; abdominal distention develops from paralytic ileus, and condition worsens.

Assessment and Diagnostic Findings

- Diagnosis is based on a complete physical examination and laboratory and radiologic tests.
- Leukocyte count greater than 10,000/mm^3; neutrophil count greater than 75%; abdominal radiographs, ultrasound

studies, and CT scans may reveal right lower quadrant density or localized distention of the bowel.

Gerontologic Considerations

In the elderly, signs and symptoms of appendicitis may vary greatly. Signs may be very vague and suggestive of bowel obstruction or another process; some patients may experience no symptoms until the appendix ruptures. The incidence of perforated appendix is higher in the elderly because many of these people do not seek health care as quickly as younger people.

Medical Management

- Surgery (conventional or laparoscopic) is indicated if appendicitis is diagnosed and should be performed as soon as possible to decrease risk of perforation.
- Administer antibiotics and intravenous fluids until surgery is performed.
- Analgesic agents can be given after diagnosis is made.

Complications of Appendectomy

- The major complication is perforation of the appendix, which can lead to peritonitis or an abscess.
- Perforation generally occurs 24 hours after onset of pain; symptoms include fever (37.7°C [100°F] or greater), toxic appearance, and continued pain or tenderness.

Nursing Management

- Nursing goals include relieving pain, preventing fluid volume deficit, reducing anxiety, eliminating infection due to the potential or actual disruption of the gastrointestinal tract, maintaining skin integrity, and attaining optimal nutrition.
- Preoperatively, prepare patient for surgery, start intravenous line, administer antibiotic, and insert nasogastric tube (if evidence of paralytic ileus). Do not administer an enema or laxative (could cause perforation).

- Postoperatively, place patient in high Fowler's position, give narcotic analgesic as ordered, administer oral fluids when tolerated, give food as desired on day of surgery (if tolerated). If dehydrated before surgery, administer intravenous fluids.
- If a drain is left in place at the area of the incision, monitor carefully for signs of intestinal obstruction, secondary hemorrhage, or secondary abscesses (eg, fever, tachycardia, and increased leukocyte count).

Promoting Home and Community-Based Care

Teaching Patients Self-Care

- Teach patient and family to care for the wound and perform dressing changes and irrigations as prescribed.
- Reinforce need for follow-up appointment with surgeon.
- Discuss incision care and activity guidelines.
- Refer for home care nursing as indicated to assist with care and continued monitoring of complications and wound healing.

For more information, see Chapter 38 in Smeltzer and Bare: *Brunner and Suddarth's Textbook of Medical-Surgical Nursing,* 11th edition. Philadelphia: Lippincott Williams & Wilkins, 2008.

Arterial Embolism and Arterial Thrombosis

An arterial embolus is a vascular occlusion. It arises most commonly from thrombi that develop in the chambers of the heart as a result of atrial fibrillation, myocardial infarction, infective endocarditis, or chronic heart failure.

Arterial thrombosis is a slowly developing clot in a degenerated vessel that can itself occlude an artery. Thrombi also become detached and are carried from the left side of the heart into the arterial system, where they cause obstruction. The immediate effect is cessation of distal blood flow. Secondary vasospasm can contribute to ischemia. Emboli tend to lodge at arterial bifurcations and areas of atherosclerotic narrowing (cerebral, mesenteric, renal, and coronary arteries). Acute thrombosis frequently occurs in patients with preexisting ischemic symptoms.

Clinical Manifestations

The symptoms of arterial emboli depend primarily on the size of the embolus, the organ involved, and the state of the collateral vessels.

- Symptoms can generally be described as the six "P"s: pain, pallor, pulselessness, paresthesia, poikilothermia (coldness), and paralysis.
- The part of the limb below the occlusion is markedly colder and paler than above as a result of ischemia.

Assessment and Diagnostic Methods

- Sudden or acute onset of symptoms and apparent source for the embolus is diagnostic.
- Two-dimensional echocardiography, transesophageal echocardiography, chest x-ray, ECG, noninvasive duplex and Doppler ultrasonography, and arteriography might be used.

Medical Management

- In cases of acute embolic occlusion, heparin therapy is initiated immediately, followed by emergency embolectomy as the surgical procedure of choice only if the involved extremity is viable. Percutaneous thrombectomy devices, which require inserting a catheter into the obstructed artery, may also be used.
- When collateral circulation is affected, the anticoagulant heparin is administered intravenously. Intra-arterial thrombolytic therapy may be administered with agents such

as streptokinase, reteplase, staphylokinase, or urokinase and others. Contraindications to thrombolytic therapy are internal bleeding, stroke, recent major surgery, uncontrolled hypertension, and pregnancy.

Nursing Management

- Encourage movement of the leg to stimulate circulation and prevent stasis.
- Continue anticoagulants to prevent thrombosis of the affected artery and to diminish development of subsequent thrombi.
- Assess surgical incision frequently for potential hemorrhage.

For more information, see Chapter 31 in Smeltzer and Bare: *Brunner and Suddarth's Textbook of Medical-Surgical Nursing*, 11th edition. Philadelphia: Lippincott Williams & Wilkins, 2008.

Arteriosclerosis and Atherosclerosis

Arteriosclerosis, or "hardening of the arteries," is the most common disease of the arteries. It is a diffuse process whereby the muscle fibers and the endothelial lining of the walls of small arteries and arterioles become thickened.

Atherosclerosis primarily affects the intima of the large and medium-sized arteries, causing changes that include the accumulation of lipids (atheromas), calcium, blood components, carbohydrates, and fibrous tissue on the intimal layer of the artery. Although the pathologic processes of arteriosclerosis and atherosclerosis differ, rarely does one occur without the other. The terms are used interchangeably. The most common direct results of atherosclerosis in the arteries include narrowing (stenosis) of the lumen and obstruction by thrombosis, aneurysm, ulceration, and rupture; ischemia and necrosis occur if the supply of blood, nutrients, and oxygen is severely and permanently disrupted.

Atherosclerosis can develop anywhere in the body but is most common in bifurcation or branch areas of blood vessels. The fibrous plaques are predominantly found in the abdominal aorta and coronary, popliteal, and internal carotid arteries.

Risk Factors

Many risk factors are associated with atherosclerosis; the greater the number of risk factors, the greater the likelihood of developing the disease.

- Smoking (strongest risk factor)
- High fat intake (suspected risk factor, along with high serum cholesterol and blood lipid levels)
- Hypertension
- Diabetes
- Obesity, stress, and lack of exercise

Clinical Manifestations

Clinical features depend on the tissue or organ affected: heart (angina and myocardial infarction due to coronary atherosclerosis), brain (transient ischemic attacks and stroke due to cerebrovascular disease), peripheral vessels (includes hypertension and symptoms of aneurysm of the aorta, renovascular disease, atherosclerotic lesions of the extremities). See specific condition for greater detail.

Gerontologic Considerations

Atherosclerotic cardiovascular disease is found in 80% of the population older than 65 years of age and is the most common condition of the arterial system in elderly people.

Management

Traditional management of atherosclerosis includes risk factor modification, medication administration, a controlled exercise program, interventional or surgical graft procedures (inflow or outflow procedures), and nursing measures related to the resulting diseases.

Several radiologic techniques are important adjunctive therapies to surgical procedures. They include arteriography, percutaneous transluminal angioplasty, stents and stent grafts, and rotational atherectomy.

For more information, see Chapter 31 in Smeltzer and Bare: *Brunner and Suddarth's Textbook of Medical-Surgical Nursing*, 11th edition. Philadelphia: Lippincott Williams & Wilkins, 2008.

Arthritis, Rheumatoid

Rheumatoid arthritis (RA) is an inflammatory disorder that primarily involves the synovial membrane of the joints. RA occurs between the ages of 30 and 50 years, with peak incidence between 40 and 60 years of age. Women are affected two to three times more frequently than men. RA is believed to be an autoimmune response to unknown antigens. The stimulus may be viral or bacterial. There may be a predisposition to the disease.

Clinical Manifestations

Clinical features are determined by the stage and severity of the disease.

- Joint pain, swelling, warmth, erythema, and lack of function are classic clinical features.
- Palpation of joints reveals spongy or boggy tissue.
- Fluid can usually be aspirated from the inflamed joint.

Characteristic Pattern of Joint Involvement

- Begins with small joints in hands, wrists, and feet
- Progressively involves knees, shoulders, hips, elbows, ankles, cervical spine, and temporomandibular joints

- Symptoms are usually acute in onset, bilateral, and symmetric.
- Joints may be hot, swollen, and painful; morning stiffness lasts for more than 30 minutes.
- Deformities of the hands and feet can result from misalignment and immobilization

Extra-Articular Features

- Fever, weight loss, fatigue, anemia, sensory changes, and lymph node enlargement
- Raynaud's phenomenon (cold- and stress-induced vasospasm)
- Rheumatoid nodules, nontender and movable; found in subcutaneous tissue over bony prominences
- Arteritis, neuropathy, scleritis, pericarditis, splenomegaly, and Sjögren's syndrome (dry eyes and mucous membranes)

Assessment and Diagnostic Methods

- Several factors contribute to an RA diagnosis: rheumatoid nodules, joint inflammation, laboratory findings, extra-articular changes.
- Rheumatoid factor (RF) is present in more than 80% of patients.
- Red blood count and C4 complement component are decreased; erythrocyte sedimentation rate is elevated.
- C-reactive protein (CRP) and antinuclear antibody (ANA) may be positive.
- Arthrocentesis and radiographs may be performed.

Medical Management

Treatment begins with education, a balance of rest and exercise, and referral to community agencies for support.

- Early RA: medication management involves therapeutic doses of salicylates or nonsteroidal anti-inflammatory drugs (NSAIDs); includes new COX-2 inhibitors, antimalarials, gold, penicillamine, or sulfasalazine; methotrexate; biologic response modifiers and antitumor necrosis factor receptors (TNFR) are helpful; analgesic agents for periods of extreme pain.

- Moderate, erosive RA: formal program of occupational and physical therapy; an immunomodulator such as cyclosporine may be added.
- Persistent, erosive RA: reconstructive surgery and corticosteroids
- Advanced unremitting RA: immunosuppressive agents such as methotrexate, cyclophosphamide, and azathioprine (highly toxic, can cause bone marrow suppression). Also promising for refractory RA is an FDA-approved apheresis device: a protein A immunoadsorption column (Prosorba) that binds circulating immune system complex (IgG).
- RA patients frequently experience anorexia, weight loss, and anemia, requiring careful dietary history to identify usual eating habits and food preferences. Corticosteroids may stimulate appetite and cause weight gain.
- Low-dose antidepressant medications (amitriptyline) are used to reestablish adequate sleep pattern and manage pain.

NURSING PROCESS: The Patient with Rheumatoid Arthritis

Assessment

- Assess patient's self-image related to musculoskeletal changes. Determine whether patient is experiencing unusual fatigue, weakness, pain, morning stiffness, fever, or anorexia.
- Assess skin, hair, ears, mouth, chest, abdomen, genitalia, and cardiovascular, pulmonary, neurologic, renal, and musculoskeletal systems.
- Assess joints by inspecting, palpating, and inquiring about tenderness, swelling, and redness in the affected joints.
- Assess joint mobility, range of motion, and muscle strength.
- Focus on identifying patient problems and factors, abilities, past experiences, preconceptions, and fears.

Diagnosis

Nursing Diagnoses

- Pain related to inflammation, increased disease activity, tissue damage, fatigue, and lowered tolerance
- Fatigue related to increased disease activity, pain, inadequate rest, deconditioning, inadequate nutrition, emotional stress, depression
- Impaired physical mobility related to muscle weakness, pain on movement, lack of or improper use of ambulatory devices
- Deficient self-care (feeding, bathing, dressing, toileting) related to contractures, fatigue, or loss of motion
- Disturbed sleep pattern related to pain and fatigue
- Disturbed body image related to physical and psychological changes and dependency imposed by chronic illness
- Ineffective coping related to actual or perceived lifestyle or role changes

Collaborative Problems/Potential Complications

Side effects of medications

Planning and Goals

Patient goals may include relief of pain and discomfort, relief of fatigue, optimal functional mobility, maintenance of self-care, improved body image, optimal level of independence in activities of daily living, improved sleep, increased knowledge regarding self-management, a positive self-concept, and absence of complications.

Nursing Interventions

Relieving Pain and Discomfort

- Question carefully to distinguish pain from stiffness.
- After administering medication, reassess pain levels at intervals. With persistent pain, compare assessment findings with baseline pain measurements and evaluations.

- Teach and use pain management techniques for immediate short-term management (ie, heat and cold, joint protection and support with splints and braces, rest, and analgesic agents).
- Educate patient regarding long-term pain management (ie, anti-inflammatory medications, exercise regimen for maintaining joint mobility, and relaxation techniques).
- Provide comfort measures while giving care.
- Set realistic expectations so that patient and significant others realize pain can be controlled depending on disease activity.

Reducing Fatigue

- Educate patient on biologic, psychological, social, and personal factors related to RA that cause or contribute to fatigue.
- Teach the patient how to use level of fatigue to monitor the disease and balance physical activities accordingly.
- Encourage patient to use naps, nighttime sleep, and splints for joints to provide rest to system and joints.
- A sleep-inducing routine, medications, and comfort measures may help improve the quality of sleep.

Increasing Mobility

- Teach patient to support all joints in a position of optimal function: lie on a firm mattress with feet against a footboard, only one pillow under head.
- Instruct patient to lie prone (on the abdomen) several times daily to prevent hip flexion contracture.
- Encourage active range-of-motion exercises to prevent joint stiffness.
- Understand that deformity does not equate with disability and patient's ability to perform self-care.
- Relieve persistent pain and morning stiffness to increase patient's mobility and self-care.
- Provide assistive devices and assist the patient in learning to use them properly (cane held in hand opposite affected side, forearm-trough style crutches if disease involves hands and wrists).

Facilitating Self-Care

- Be sensitive to patient's feelings, demonstrating acceptance and positive attitudes about using assistive devices.
- Help preserve patient's independence in inpatient and home settings by making available adaptive equipment for eating, toileting, bathing, and dressing.

Improving Sleep

- Identify the cause of a sleep problem.
- Adjust anti-inflammatory and analgesic administration times.
- Encourage and provide a sleep-inducing routine, medications, and comfort measures to help improve quality of sleep.

Improving Body Image and Coping Skills

- Try to understand patient's emotional reactions to the disease.
- Encourage communication, so that patient and family verbalize feelings, perceptions, and fears related to the disease.
- Help patient and family identify areas in which they have some control over disease symptoms and treatment.
- Encourage patient and family to commit to the management program for more positive outcomes.

Monitoring and Managing Potential Complications

- Work with physician and pharmacist to help patient recognize and deal with side effects from medications.
- Monitor for medication side effects, including gastrointestinal bleeding or irritation, bone marrow suppression, kidney or liver toxicity, increased incidence of infection, mouth sores, rashes, and changes in vision. Other signs and symptoms include bruising, breathing problems, dizziness, jaundice, dark urine, black or bloody stools, diarrhea, nausea and vomiting, and headaches.
- Monitor closely for systemic and local infections, which often can be masked by high doses of corticosteroids.

Increasing Knowledge of Disease Management

- Tailor education to patient's knowledge base, interest level, degree of comfort, and social or cultural influences.
- Instruct patient on basic disease management, medications, and necessary adaptations in lifestyle.
- Encourage patient to practice new self-management skills.

Promoting Home and Community-Based Care

Teaching Patients Self-Care

- Focus patient teaching on the disease, possible changes related to it, the prescribed therapeutic regimen, side effects of medications, strategies to maintain independence and function, and safety in the home.
- Encourage patient and family to verbalize their concerns and ask questions.
- Address pain, fatigue, and depression before initiating a teaching program, because they can interfere with patient's ability to learn.
- Instruct patient about basic disease management and necessary adaptations in lifestyle.

Continuing Care

- Refer for home care as warranted (eg, frail patient with significantly limited function).
- Note that problems caused by RA may interfere with treatment of a primary condition, and treatment of a primary condition may cause or increase problems related to RA.
- Identify any barriers to compliance, and make appropriate referrals.
- Assess patient's need for assistance in the home, and supervise home health aides.
- Make referrals to physical and occupational therapists as problems are identified and limitations increase.
- Alert patient and family to support services such as Meals on Wheels and local Arthritis Foundation chapters.
- Emphasize the importance of follow-up appointments to the patient and family.

Evaluation

Expected Patient Outcomes

- Experiences relief of pain or improved comfort level
- Experiences reduction in fatigue
- Increases or maintains mobility
- Maintains self-care activities
- Experiences improved body image and coping
- Experiences absence of complications

For more information, see Chapter 54 in Smeltzer and Bare: *Brunner and Suddarth's Textbook of Medical-Surgical Nursing*, 11th edition. Philadelphia: Lippincott Williams & Wilkins, 2008.

Asthma

Asthma is a chronic inflammatory disease of the airways characterized by hyperresponsiveness, mucosal edema, and mucus production. Inflammation leads to obstruction from mucosal edema, reducing airway diameter, and contraction of bronchial smooth muscle. Acute exacerbations last from minutes to hours to days, and are interspersed with symptom-free periods.

Asthma can begin at any age. It is the most common chronic disease of childhood. Risk factors for asthma include family history, allergy (strongest factor), and chronic exposure to airway irritants or allergens (eg, grass, weed pollens, mold, dust, or animals). Common triggers for asthma symptoms and exacerbations include airway irritants (eg, pollutants, cold, heat, strong odors, smoke, perfumes), exertion, stress, sinusitis, and esophageal reflux.

Clinical Manifestations

- Most common symptoms of asthma are cough (with or without mucus production), dyspnea, and wheezing (first on expiration, then possibly during inspiration as well).

- Asthma attacks frequently occur at night or in the early morning.
- An asthma exacerbation is frequently preceded by increasing symptoms over days, but it may begin abruptly.
- Chest tightness and dyspnea occur.
- Expiration requires effort and becomes prolonged.
- As exacerbation progresses, central cyanosis secondary to severe hypoxia may occur.
- Additional symptoms, such as diaphoresis, tachycardia, and a widened pulse pressure, may occur.
- A severe, continuous reaction, status asthmaticus, may occur. It is life-threatening.
- Eczema, urticaria, and temporary edema are allergic reactions that may be noted with asthma.

Assessment and Diagnostic Methods

- Family, environment, and occupational history is essential.
- During acute episodes, sputum and blood test, pulse oximetry, arterial blood gases (ABGs), and hypocapnia and respiratory alkalosis and pulmonary function (FEV & FVC decreased) tests are performed.

Medical Management

Pharmacologic Therapy

There are two classes of medications—long-acting control and quick-relief medications—as well as combination products.

- Leukotriene modifiers inhibitors/antileukotrienes block receptors to prevent bronchoconstriction.
- Beta-adrenergic agonists
- Methylxanthines
- Anticholinergics
- Corticosteroids: metered-dose inhaler (MDI)
- Mast cell inhibitors

NURSING PROCESS: The Patient with Asthma

Assessment

- Evaluate and identify substances that precipitate attacks (obtain history of exacerbations, family, environment, health history).
- Monitor respiratory status for progression or resolution of asthma attack (eg, breath sounds, pulse oximetry, vital signs, peak flow)—daily monitoring.
- Obtain medical history and history of medication allergy.

Nursing Diagnoses

- Ineffective airway clearance related to airway constriction and excess mucus production
- Anxiety related to fear of death
- Risk for ineffective management of treatment regimen

Planning and Goals

Goals may include unlabored breathing, clear breath sounds, pulmonary studies within normal limits, and knowledge of self-care regimen for prevention and treatment of asthma exacerbations.

Nursing Interventions

Promoting Airway Clearance

- Administer prescribed therapy, and monitor patient responses.
- Administer fluids and antibiotics (if infection present).
- Assist with intubation and respiratory support as needed.

Minimizing Anxiety

- Provide nursing care, using a calm approach.
- Keep patient and family informed about procedures.

Promoting Home and Community-Based Care

Teaching Patients Self-Care

- Teach patient and family about asthma (chronic inflammatory), purpose and action of medications, triggers to avoid (eg, exposure to offending pollens—stay in air-conditioned rooms during pollen season or, if feasible, change climate zone).
- Instruct patient and family about peak-flow monitoring.
- Teach patient how to implement an action plan and how and when to seek assistance.
- Emphasize adherence to prescribed therapy, preventive measures, and need for follow-up appointments.

Continuing Care

- Refer for home health nurse as indicated.
- Home visit to assess for allergens may be indicated (with recurrent exacerbations).
- Encourage patient to maintain good physical and mental health because attacks may be induced by suggestion alone.
- Refer patient to community support groups.

For more information, see Chapter 24 in Smeltzer and Bare: *Brunner and Suddarth's Textbook of Medical-Surgical Nursing*, 11th edition. Philadelphia: Lippincott Williams & Wilkins, 2008.

Asthma: Status Asthmaticus

Status asthmaticus is severe persistent asthma that is unresponsive to conventional therapy; it can last longer than 24 hours. Infection, anxiety, nebulizer abuse, dehydration, increased adrenergic block, and nonspecific irritants may contribute to these episodes. An acute episode may be precipitated by hypersensitivity to aspirin. Two predominant pathologic problems occur: a decrease in bronchial diameter and a ventilation-perfusion abnormality.

Clinical Manifestations

- Same as those in severe asthma
- No correlation between severity of attack and number of wheezes; with greater obstruction, wheezing may disappear, possibly signaling impending respiratory failure

Assessment and Diagnostic Findings

- Primarily pulmonary function studies and ABG analysis
- Respiratory alkalosis most common finding

 NURSING ALERT Rising PCO_2 to normal or higher is a danger sign, signaling respiratory failure.

Medical Management

- Initial treatment: Beta-adrenergic agonists, corticosteroids, supplemental oxygen and IV fluids to hydrate patient. Sedatives are contraindicated.
- Start with low-flow humidified oxygen by mask or nasal catheter; flow rate determined by ABG values (PaO_2 65 to 85 mmHg).
- Hospitalization if blood gas levels deteriorate or pulmonary function scores are low
- Mechanical ventilation if patient is tiring or in respiratory failure or if condition does not respond to treatment

NURSING PROCESS: The Patient with Status Asthmaticus

Assessment

Assess for signs of dehydration by checking skin turgor. Also monitor respiratory status constantly for the first 12 to 24 hours, or until status asthmaticus stops.

Nursing Diagnoses

- Ineffective airway clearance related to airway constriction and thick secretions
- Deficient fluid volume related to decreased hydration from insensible losses

Planning and Goals

Major goals include unlabored breathing, clear breath sounds, and pulmonary function within normal limits.

Nursing Interventions

Promoting Airway Clearance

Keep patient's room quiet and free of respiratory irritants (flowers, smoke, perfumes); use nonallergenic pillows and bedding.

Promoting Adequate Hydration

- Combat dehydration with adequate fluid intake to loosen secretions and facilitate expectoration.
- Administer prescribed IV fluids (3,000 to 4000 mL/day unless contraindicated).

Promoting Home and Community-Based Care

Teach patient self-care measures to minimize recurrences. See Nursing Process under Asthma for additional information.

Evaluation

Expected Patient Outcomes

- Breathes freely and clearly
- Experiences no respiratory failure or other complications.
- Carries out self-care measures effectively

For more information, see Chapter 24 in Smeltzer and Bare: *Brunner and Suddarth's Textbook of Medical-Surgical Nursing*, 11th edition. Philadelphia: Lippincott Williams & Wilkins, 2008.

B

Back Pain, Low

Most cases of low back pain are caused by disk degeneration and overstretching of spinal supports secondary to musculoskeletal problems (eg, acute lumbosacral strain, unstable lumbosacral ligaments and weak muscles, osteoarthritis of the spine, spinal stenosis, intervertebral disk problems, unequal leg length). Older patients may have back pain associated with osteoporotic vertebral fractures or bone metastasis. Many other medical and psychosomatic conditions are causes of back pain. Obesity, stress, and occasionally depression may contribute to low back pain. Patients with chronic low back pain may develop a dependence on alcohol or analgesic agents.

Clinical Manifestations

- Acute or chronic back pain (lasting more than 3 months without improvement) and fatigue
- Pain radiates along a nerve root (radiculopathy; sciatica) and is accentuated by movement.
- Pain is associated with straight-leg raising (spinal root irritation).
- Paravertebral muscle spasm (greatly increased muscle tone of back postural muscles) occurs, with loss of normal lumbar curve and possible spinal deformity.
- Back pain is aggravated by activity (usually from musculoskeletal rather than other conditions).

Assessment and Diagnostic Methods

- Health history and physical examination (back exam, neurologic testing)

- Spinal x-ray
- Computed tomography (CT) scan
- Magnetic resonance imaging (MRI)
- Bone scan and blood studies
- Electromyography and nerve conduction studies

Medical Management

Supportive treatment focuses on relief of pain and discomfort, activity modification, and patient education. Bed rest is a treatment of choice if pain is severe. Patient is positioned in bed to increase lumbar flexion. The head of the bed is elevated 30 degrees, and knees are slightly flexed to avoid the prone position. Analgesic agents, stress reduction, and relaxation supplement bed rest. Discomfort is usually self-limiting and resolves within 4 weeks. Physical therapy, intermittent pelvic traction, heat or cold therapy, and manipulation may be helpful in the absence of radiculopathy symptoms; other treatment methods include whirlpool, exercise program, and low back supports and braces.

Pharmacologic Therapy

- Analgesic agents (mild or opioids)
- Muscle relaxants
- Tranquilizers
- Anti-inflammatory agents and nonsteroidal anti-inflammatory drugs (NSAIDs)

NURSING PROCESS: The Patient with Back Pain

Assessment

- Encourage patient to describe the discomfort (onset, severity, duration, characteristics, radiation, weakness in the legs, location).
- Obtain history of pain origin, previous pain control, and how back problem is affecting lifestyle.

B

- Observe patient's posture, position changes, and gait.
- Assess spinal curves, pelvic crest, leg length discrepancy, and shoulder symmetry.
- Palpate paraspinal muscles and note spasm and tenderness.
- Note discomfort and limitations in movement when bending forward and laterally.
- Evaluate nerve involvement by assessing for abnormal sensations, muscle weakness or paralysis, and back and leg pain with straight-leg raises, and deep tendon reflexes.
- Assess for obesity and perform nutritional assessment.

Nursing Diagnoses

- Pain related to musculoskeletal problems
- Impaired physical mobility related to pain, muscle spasm, and decreased flexibility
- Imbalanced nutrition: More than body requirements related to excess food intake for activity level
- Impaired social interaction related to impaired mobility, chronic pain, and altered role performance
- Deficient knowledge related to body mechanics

Planning and Goals

Goals for the patient include relief of pain, improved mobility, healthful nutrition and weight reduction, improved role performance, and proper use of body mechanics.

Nursing Interventions

Relieving Pain

- Encourage patient to reduce stress on the back and to change position frequently.
- Decrease pain through therapies such as diaphragmatic breathing, relaxation, guided imagery, and diversions (eg, reading, watching television).
- Advise patient that intermittent heat or cold may reduce pain.
- Assess response to each medication prescribed.

Improving Mobility

- Encourage patient to alternate lying, sitting, and walking activities. Advise patient to avoid sitting, standing, and walking for long periods. Encourage patient to resume self-care activities and exercise as pain subsides.
- Advise patient to rest on a firm, nonsagging mattress. With severe pain, limit activity for 1 to 2 days.
- Encourage patient to adhere to prescribed exercise program, to avoid twisting and jarring motions, and to maintain proper posture with chest up and abdomen tucked in.

Modifying Nutrition for Weight Reduction

- Provide a sound nutritional plan that includes a change in eating habits to maintain desirable weight.
- Monitor weight loss, and note achievements.
- Provide encouragement and positive reinforcement, and facilitate adherence.

Preventing Social Isolation

- Assist patient and support people to recognize continued dependency to help patient cope.
- Monitor for "low back neurosis." Help patient to cope with specific stressors and control stressful situations.
- Refer for counseling or psychotherapy if needed.

Promoting Proper Body Mechanics

Teach patient how to stand, sit, lie, and lift properly:

- Shift weight frequently when standing and rest one foot on a low stool; wear low heels.
- Sit with knees and hips flexed and knees level with hips or higher. Keep feet flat on the floor. Use chair with arm rests and place soft support to small of back.
- Sleep on side with knees and hips flexed or supine with knees flexed and supported; avoid sleeping prone.
- Lift objects using thigh muscles, not back. Stand with wide base of support, and lift objects close to the body. Wear a back brace or support belt when lifting, and avoid lifting more than one third of own weight.

B

- Practice protective and defensive postures, positions, and body mechanics to strengthen the back and to diminish chance of recurrence of back pain.

Evaluation

Expected Patient Outcomes

- Experiences pain relief
- Demonstrates resumption of mobility
- Achieves desired nutritional status and weight
- Resumes role-related responsibilities
- Demonstrates back-conserving body mechanics

For more information, see Chapter 68 in Smeltzer and Bare: *Brunner and Suddarth's Textbook of Medical-Surgical Nursing*, 11th edition. Philadelphia: Lippincott Williams & Wilkins, 2008.

Bell's Palsy

Bell's palsy (facial paralysis) is due to peripheral involvement of the seventh cranial nerve on one side, which results in weakness or paralysis of the facial muscles. The cause is unknown, but possible causes may include vascular ischemia, viral disease (herpes simplex, herpes zoster), autoimmune disease, or a combination. Bell's palsy may represent a type of pressure paralysis in which ischemic necrosis of the facial nerve causes a distortion of the face, increased lacrimation (tearing), and painful sensations in the face, behind the ear, and in the eye. The patient may experience speech difficulties and may be unable to eat on the affected side owing to weakness.

Medical Management

The objectives of management are to maintain facial muscle tone and to prevent or minimize denervation. Steroidal therapy may be initiated to reduce inflammation and edema, which reduces vascular compression and permits restoration of blood circulation to the nerve. Early administration of corticosteroids appears to diminish severity, relieve pain, and minimize denervation. Facial pain is controlled with analgesic agents or heat applied to the involved side of the face. Additional modalities may include electrical stimulation applied to the face to prevent muscle atrophy, or surgical exploration of the facial nerve. Surgery may be performed if a tumor is suspected, for surgical decompression of the facial nerve, and for surgical rehabilitation of a paralyzed face.

Nursing Management

Patients need reassurance that a stroke has not occurred and that spontaneous recovery occurs within 3 to 5 weeks in most patients. Teaching patients with Bell's palsy to care for themselves at home is an important nursing priority.

Teaching Eye Care

Because the blink reflex is diminished, the involved eye may not close completely and needs to be protected to prevent corneal irritation and ulceration. Inform the patient of potential complications, including corneal irritation and ulceration, overflow of tears, and absence of blink reflex. Key teaching points include:

- Cover the eye with a protective shield at night.
- Apply eye ointment to keep eyelids closed during sleep.
- Close the paralyzed eyelid manually before going to sleep.
- Wear wrap-around sunglasses or goggles to decrease normal evaporation from the eye.

Teaching About Maintaining Muscle Tone

- Show patient how to perform facial massage with gentle upward motion several times daily when the patient can tolerate the massage.
- Demonstrate facial exercises, such as wrinkling the forehead, blowing out the cheeks, and whistling, in an effort to prevent muscle atrophy.

B

- Instruct patient to avoid exposing the face to cold and drafts.
- Remind patient and family of the importance of participating in health promotion activities and recommended health screening practices.

For more information, see Chapter 64 in Smeltzer and Bare: *Brunner and Suddarth's Textbook of Medical-Surgical Nursing*, 11th edition. Philadelphia: Lippincott Williams & Wilkins, 2008.

Benign Prostatic Hyperplasia and Prostatectomy

Benign prostatic hyperplasia (BPH) is enlargement, or hypertrophy, of the prostate. The prostate gland enlarges, extending upward into the bladder and obstructing the outflow of urine. Incomplete emptying of the bladder and urinary retention leading to urinary stasis may result in hydronephrosis, hydroureter, and urinary tract infections. The cause is uncertain, but evidence suggests hormonal involvement. BPH is common in men older than 50 years of age.

Clinical Manifestations

The prostate is large, rubbery, and nontender. Prostatism (obstructive and irritative symptom complex) is noted. Symptoms include:

- Hesitancy in starting urination, increased frequency of urination, nocturia, urgency, abdominal straining
- Incomplete bladder emptying with urinary tract infections possibly resulting from urinary stasis
- Decrease in volume and force of urinary stream, interruption of urinary stream, dribbling
- Sensation of incomplete emptying of the bladder, acute urinary retention (more than 60 mL), and recurrent urinary tract infections

Fatigue, anorexia, nausea and vomiting, and epigastric discomfort are also reported, and ultimately azotemia and renal failure result with chronic urinary retention and large residual volumes.

Assessment and Diagnostic Methods

- Physical examination, including digital rectal examination (DRE)
- Urinalysis and urodynamic studies to determine obstructed flow
- Renal function tests, including serum creatinine levels
- Complete blood studies, including clotting studies

Medical Management

The treatment plan depends on the cause, severity of obstruction, and condition of the patient. Treatment measures include:

- Immediate catheterization if patient cannot void (a urologist may be consulted if an ordinary catheter cannot be inserted). A suprapubic cystostomy is sometimes necessary.
- "Watchful waiting" to monitor disease progression
- Balloon dilation or alpha-1 adrenergic receptor blockers (terazosin) to relax smooth muscle of the bladder neck and prostate
- Hormonal manipulation with antiandrogen (finasteride [Proscar]) decreases the size of the prostate and improves urinary flow.
- Saw palmetto is a botanical remedy for mild to moderate BPH.

Surgical Management

- Transurethral laser resection with ultrasound guidance
- Transurethral needle ablation (spares urethra, nerves, muscles, and membranes)
- Microwave thermotherapy (using transurethral probe) applied to hypertrophied tissue, which then becomes necrotic and sloughs off

B

Surgical procedures such as prostatectomy can be used to remove the hypertrophied portion of the prostate gland. Other kinds of surgery include:

- Transurethral resection of the prostate (TUR or TURP); urethral endoscopic procedure is most common approach
- Suprapubic prostatectomy (via abdominal incision)
- Perineal prostatectomy (perineal incision); incontinence, impotence, or rectal injury may be complications
- Retropubic prostatectomy (low abdominal incision)

Nursing Management

See Nursing Process: The Patient Undergoing Prostatectomy under Cancer of the Prostate for additional information.

For more information, see Chapter 49 in Smeltzer and Bare: *Brunner and Suddarth's Textbook of Medical-Surgical Nursing*, 11th edition. Philadelphia: Lippincott Williams & Wilkins, 2008.

Bone Tumors

Neoplasms of the musculoskeletal system are of a variety of types. They include osteogenic, chondrogenic, fibrogenic, muscle, and marrow cell tumors as well as nerve, vascular, and fatty cell tumors. They may be primary tumors or metastatic tumors from primary cancers elsewhere in the body (eg, breast, lung, prostate, kidney). Metastatic bone tumors are more common than primary bone tumors. Tumors cause bone destruction and weaken the bone structure, resulting in fracture.

Benign Bone Tumors

Benign bone tumors are slow-growing and well circumscribed. They produce few symptoms and do not cause death. Benign primary neoplasms of the musculoskeletal system include osteochondroma, enchondroma, osteoid osteoma, bone cyst, rhabdomyoma, and fibromas. Benign tumors of the bone and soft tissue are more common than malignant tumors.

Bone cysts are expanding lesions within the bone (eg, aneurysmal and unicameral). Osteochondroma, the most common benign bone tumor, may become malignant. Enchondroma is a common tumor of the hyaline cartilage of hand, ribs, leg, humerus, or pelvis. Osteoid osteoma is a painful tumor that occurs in children and young adults. Osteoclastomas (giant cell tumors) are benign for long periods but may invade local tissue and cause destruction. These tumors may undergo malignant transformation and metastasize.

Malignant Bone Tumors

Primary malignant musculoskeletal tumors are rare and arise from connective and supportive tissue cells (sarcomas) or bone marrow elements (myelomas). Soft tissue sarcomas include liposarcoma, fibrosarcoma, and rhabdomyosarcoma. Metastasis to the lungs is common. Osteogenic sarcoma (osteosarcoma) is the most common and is often fatal owing to metastasis to the lungs. It is seen most frequently in rapidly growing bones (boys aged 10 to 25 years), older people with Paget's disease, and patients exposed to radiation. Common sites are distal femur, proximal tibia, and proximal humerus.

Chondrosarcoma, the second most common primary malignant bone tumor, is a large, bulky, slow-growing tumor that affects adults (men more frequently). Tumor sites may include pelvis, ribs, femur, humerus, spine, scapula, and tibia. Tumors may recur after treatment.

Metastatic bone tumors (secondary bone tumors) are more common than any primary malignant bone tumor. Tumors that metastasize to bone most frequently include carcinomas of the kidney, prostate, lung, breast, ovary, and thyroid. Metastatic tumors frequently attack the skull, spine, pelvis, femur, and humerus.

Clinical Manifestations

Bone tumors present with a wide range of associated problems:

- Asymptomatic or pain (mild, occasional to constant, severe)
- Varying degrees of disability; at times, obvious bone growth

B

- Weight loss, malaise, and fever may be present.
- Pain, swelling, and limitation of motion; the bony mass may be palpable, tender, and fixed; common sites are distal femur, proximal tibia, and proximal humerus
- Spinal metastasis results in cord compression and neurologic deficits.

Assessment and Diagnostic Findings

- May be diagnosed incidentally after pathologic fracture
- Computed tomography (CT), bone scans, myelography, magnetic resonance imaging (MRI), arteriography, x-ray studies
- Biochemical assays of the blood and urine (alkaline phosphatase levels are frequently elevated with osteogenic sarcoma; serum acid phosphatase levels are elevated with metastatic carcinoma of the prostate; hypercalcemia is present with breast, lung, and kidney cancer bone metastases)
- Surgical biopsy for histologic identification; staging based on tumor size, grade, location, and metastasis

Medical Management

The goal of treatment is to destroy or remove the tumor. This may be accomplished by surgical excision (ranging from local incision to amputation and disarticulation), radiation, or chemotherapy.

- Soft tissue sarcomas are treated with radiation, limb-sparing excision with grafting as needed, and adjuvant chemotherapy.
- Metastatic bone cancer treatment is palliative; therapeutic goal is to relieve pain and discomfort as much as possible.
- Internal fixation of pathologic fractures, arthroplasty, or methylmethacrylate (bone cement) minimizes associated disability and pain in metastatic disease.

NURSING PROCESS: The Patient with a Bone Tumor

Assessment

- Ask patient about onset and course of symptoms. Note patient's and family's understanding of disease, coping skills, and pain management.
- Palpate mass gently. Note size and associated soft tissue swelling, pain, and tenderness.
- Assess neurovascular status and range of motion of extremity.
- Evaluate mobility and ability to perform activities of daily living.

Diagnosis

Nursing Diagnoses

- Deficient knowledge related to disease process and therapeutic regimen
- Pain related to pathologic process and surgery
- Risk for injury: pathologic fracture related to tumor
- Ineffective coping related to fear of the unknown, perception of disease process, and inadequate support system
- Risk for low situational self-esteem related to loss of body part or changing role

Collaborative Problems/Potential Complications

- Delayed wound healing
- Nutritional deficiency
- Infection
- Hypercalcemia

Planning and Goals

The major goals include knowledge of disease process and treatment regimen, control of pain, absence of pathologic fractures,

B

effective patterns of coping, improved self-esteem, and absence of complications.

Nursing Interventions

Promoting Understanding

- Explain diagnostic tests, treatments, and expected results.
- Reinforce and clarify information provided by the physician.
- Encourage independence and function as long as possible.
- Postoperatively, monitor vital signs; assess blood loss and development of complications (eg, deep vein thrombosis, pulmonary emboli, infection, contracture, and disuse atrophy).
- Elevate affected part to control swelling; assess neurovascular status of extremity; immobilize the area with splints, casts, or elastic bandages until the affected area heals.

Controlling Pain

- Use nonpharmacologic and pharmacologic pain management techniques, including external radiation with systemic radioisotopes.
- Work with patient to design the most effective pain management regimen.
- Prepare patient and give support during painful procedures.

Preventing Pathologic Fracture

- Support affected bones and handle gently during nursing care.
- Use external supports (eg, splints) for additional protection.
- Follow prescribed weight-bearing restrictions.
- Show patient how to use ambulatory assistance devices safely and how to strengthen unaffected extremities.

Enhancing Effective Coping

- Encourage patient and family to verbalize fears, concerns, and feelings honestly.
- Support and accept patient and family as they deal with the impact of the malignant bone tumor.

- Expect feelings of shock, despair, and grief.
- Refer to health professionals and clergy for specific psychological help.

Promoting Self-Esteem

- Support family in working through adjustments that must be made, specifically changes in body image due to surgery and possible amputation.
- Provide realistic reassurance about the future and resumption of role-related activities; encourage self-care and socialization.
- Involve patient and family throughout treatment to encourage confidence and restoration of self-concept, and promote a sense of control.

Monitoring and Managing Potential Problems

- Minimize pressure on wound site to promote circulation.
- Promote healing with an aseptic, nontraumatic wound dressing.
- Monitor and report laboratory findings.
- Reposition patient frequently to prevent skin breakdown; use therapeutic bed when indicated.

Monitoring for and Managing Hypercalcemia

Recognize symptoms: muscle weakness, incoordination, anorexia, nausea and vomiting, constipation, ECG changes, and altered mental status.

Achieving Adequate Nutritional Status

- Give antiemetics and provide relaxation techniques to reduce gastrointestinal reaction.
- Control stomatitis (resulting from cancer therapies) with anesthetic or antifungal mouthwash.
- Provide adequate hydration, nutritional supplements, or total parenteral nutrition.

Managing Osteomyelitis and Wound Infections

- Use prophylactic antibiotics and strict aseptic dressing techniques.

- Prevent other infections (eg, upper respiratory), so that hematogenous spread does not result in osteomyelitis.
- Monitor white blood cell count, and instruct patient to avoid contact with people who have colds or infections.

Promoting Home and Community-Based Care

- Prepare and coordinate continuing health care and direct patient education toward medications, dressings, treatment regimens, weight-bearing limitations, and physical and occupational therapy programs.
- Teach signs and symptoms of complications to patient and family.
- Arrange for home care, and advise patient to keep telephone numbers of contact people readily available.
- Emphasize the need for long-term health supervision to ensure cure or to detect tumor recurrence or metastasis.
- Explore end-of-life issues if patient has metastatic disease.

For more information, see Chapter 68 in Smeltzer and Bare: *Brunner and Suddarth's Textbook of Medical-Surgical Nursing*, 11th edition. Philadelphia: Lippincott Williams & Wilkins, 2008.

Bowel Obstruction, Large

Intestinal obstruction (mechanical or functional) occurs when blockage prevents the flow of contents through the intestinal tract. Large bowel obstruction results in an accumulation of intestinal contents, fluid, and gas proximal to the obstruction. Obstruction in the colon can lead to severe distention and perforation unless gas and fluid can flow back through the ileal valve. Dehydration occurs more slowly than in small bowel obstruction. If the blood supply is cut off, intestinal strangulation and necrosis occur; this condition is life-threatening.

Clinical Manifestations

Symptoms develop and progress relatively slowly.

- Constipation may be the only symptom for days (obstruction in sigmoid colon or rectum).
- Abdomen eventually becomes markedly distended, loops of large bowel become visibly outlined through the abdominal wall, and patient has crampy lower abdominal pain.
- Fecal vomiting develops; symptoms of shock may occur.

Assessment and Diagnostic Methods

Symptoms plus radiologic studies (flat and upright abdominal radiographs; barium studies are contraindicated)

Medical Management

- Colonoscopy to untwist and decompress the bowel, if obstruction is high in the colon
- Cecostomy may be performed for patients who are poor surgical risks and urgently need relief from the obstruction.
- Rectal tube to decompress an area that is lower in the bowel
- Usual treatment is surgical resection to remove the obstructing lesion; a temporary or permanent colostomy may be necessary; an ileoanal anastomosis may be performed if entire large colon must be removed.

Nursing Management

- Monitor symptoms indicating worsening intestinal obstruction.
- Provide emotional support and comfort.
- Administer intravenous fluids and electrolyte replacement.
- Prepare patient for surgery if no response to medical treatment.
- Provide preoperative teaching as patient's condition indicates.

- Give general abdominal wound care postoperatively.
- Provide routine postoperative nursing care.

For additional information, see Preoperative and Postoperative Nursing Management. Also see Chapter 38 in Smeltzer and Bare: *Brunner and Suddarth's Textbook of Medical-Surgical Nursing*, 11th edition. Philadelphia: Lippincott Williams & Wilkins, 2008.

Bowel Obstruction, Small

Most bowel obstructions (85%) occur in the small intestine. Intestinal contents, fluid, and gas accumulate above the intestinal obstruction. Distention and retention reduce the absorption of fluids and stimulate gastric secretion. Reflux vomiting may also occur. Fluids and electrolytes are lost. Dehydration and acidosis develop because of water and sodium loss. With acute fluid losses, hypovolemic shock may occur. Increasing distention and pressure within the intestinal lumen cause a decrease in venous and arteriolar capillary pressure, resulting in edema, congestion, necrosis, and eventual rupture or perforation of the intestinal wall, with resultant peritonitis. Adhesions are the most common (60%) cause of obstruction. Other causes include hernias, neoplasms, intussusception, volvulus, and paralytic ileus.

Clinical Manifestations

- Initial symptom is usually crampy pain that is wavelike and colicky. Patient may pass blood and mucus but no fecal matter or flatus. Vomiting occurs.
- Peristaltic waves become extremely vigorous and assume a reverse direction, propelling intestinal contents toward the mouth, if the obstruction is complete.
- If the obstruction is in the ileum, fecal vomiting takes place.
- Dehydration results in intense thirst, drowsiness, generalized malaise, and aching.
- Tongue and mucous membranes become parched; abdomen becomes distended (the lower the obstruction in the gastrointestinal tract, the more marked the distention).

B

- If uncorrected, shock occurs due to dehydration and loss of plasma volume.

Assessment and Diagnostic Findings

Symptoms plus radiologic studies (abnormal quantities of gas and/or fluid in bowel) and laboratory studies (electrolytes and complete blood count show dehydration and possibly infection)

Medical Management

Decompression of the bowel may be achieved through a nasogastric or small bowel tube. However, when the bowel is completely obstructed, the possibility of strangulation warrants surgical intervention. Surgical treatment depends on the cause of obstruction (eg, hernia repair). Before surgery, intravenous therapy is instituted to replace water, sodium, chloride, and potassium.

Nursing Management

- Maintain the function of the nasogastric tube. Assess and measure nasogastric output. Assess for fluid and electrolyte imbalance.
- Monitor nutritional status. Assess for improvement in bowel function (ie, return of normal bowel sounds, decreased abdominal distention, improvement in abdominal pain and tenderness, passage of flatus or stool).
- Report discrepancies in intake and output, worsening of pain or abdominal distention, and increased nasogastric output.
- If patient's condition does not improve, prepare him or her for surgery.
- Provide postoperative nursing care similar to that for other abdominal surgeries (see Preoperative and Postoperative Nursing Management for additional information).

For more information, see Chapter 38 in Smeltzer and Bare: *Brunner and Suddarth's Textbook of Medical-Surgical Nursing*, 11th edition. Philadelphia: Lippincott Williams & Wilkins, 2008.

Brain Abscess

A brain abscess is a collection of infectious material within the tissue of the brain. It may occur by direct invasion of the brain from intracranial trauma or surgery, by spread of infection from nearby sites (eg, sinuses, ears, teeth, tongue), or by spread of infection from other organs (lung abscess, infective endocarditis). It can be a complication associated with some forms of meningitis. It can also be a complication in patients whose immune systems have been suppressed through therapy or disease.

Prevention

To prevent brain abscesses, treat otitis media, mastoiditis, sinusitis, dental and oral infections, and systemic infections promptly.

Clinical Manifestations

- Generally, symptoms result from edema, brain shift, infection, or the location of the abscess.
- Headache, usually worse in morning, is the most continuing symptom.
- Vomiting and focal neurologic signs (weakness of an extremity, decreasing vision, seizures) may occur, depending on the site of the abscess.
- Change in mental status may occur (eg, lethargic, confused, irritable, or disoriented behavior).
- Fever may or may not be present.

Assessment and Diagnostic Methods

- Computed tomography (CT) scan to locate the site of the abscess and to determine the best time for surgical intervention
- Magnetic resonance imaging (MRI) to obtain images of the brain stem and posterior fossa
- Laboratory studies (blood) and chest x-ray to rule out infections

Complications

Neurologic deficits following treatment may include hemiparesis, seizures, visual defects, and cranial nerve palsies. Relapse is common, with a high mortality rate.

Medical Management

The goal is to eliminate the abscess. Treatment modalities include antimicrobial therapy, surgical incision, or aspiration (CT-guided stereotactic needle). Medications used include corticosteroids to reduce the inflammatory cerebral edema and anticonvulsant medications for prophylaxis against seizures (phenytoin, phenobarbital). Abscess resolution is monitored with CT scans.

Nursing Management

Nursing interventions support the medical treatment, as do patient teaching activities that address neurosurgical procedures. Patients and families need to be advised of neurologic deficits that may remain after treatment (hemiparesis, seizures, visual deficits and cranial nerve palsies). The nurse assesses the family's ability to express their distress at the patient's condition, cope with the patient's illness and deficits, and obtain support. See Nursing Management under associated neurologic conditions (eg, Epilepsies, Meningitis, or Increased Intracranial Pressure).

For more information, see Chapter 64 in Smeltzer and Bare: *Brunner and Suddarth's Textbook of Medical-Surgical Nursing*, 11th edition. Philadelphia: Lippincott Williams & Wilkins, 2008.

Brain Tumors

A brain tumor is a localized intracranial lesion that occupies space within the skull. Primary brain tumors originate from cells and structures within the brain. Secondary, or metastatic,

B

brain tumors develop from structures outside the brain (lung, breast, lower gastrointestinal tract, pancreas, kidney, and skin [melanomas]) and occur in 10% to 20% of all cancer patients. The highest incidence of brain tumors in adults occurs between the fifth and seventh decades, with a slightly higher incidence in men. Brain tumors rarely metastasize outside the central nervous system but cause death by impairing vital functions (respiration) or by increasing intracranial pressure (ICP). Brain tumors are classified as follows: (1) dural meningiomas, those arising from the covering of the brain; (2) acoustic neuromas, those developing in or on the cranial nerves; (3) various gliomas, those originating in the brain tissue; and (4) metastatic lesions originating elsewhere in the body. Tumors of the pineal gland, pituitary, and cerebral blood vessels are also included in the types of brain tumors. Tumors may be benign or malignant. A benign tumor may occur in a vital area and have effects as serious as a malignant tumor.

Types of Tumors

- Meningiomas are common benign encapsulated tumors of arachnoid cells on the meninges. They are slow-growing and occur most often in middle-aged women.
- An acoustic neuroma is a tumor of the eighth cranial nerve (hearing and balance). It may grow slowly and attain considerable size before it is correctly diagnosed.
- Gliomas, the most common brain neoplasms, cannot be totally removed without causing damage, because they spread by infiltrating into the surrounding neural tissue.
- Pituitary adenomas may cause symptoms as a result of mass effects (pressure) on adjacent structures (eg, optic nerve or third ventricle) or hormonal changes (eg, galactorrhea or Cushing's disease).
- Angiomas are masses composed largely of abnormal blood vessels and are found in or on the surface of the brain; they may never cause symptoms, or they may give rise to symptoms of brain tumor. The walls of the blood vessels in angiomas are thin, increasing the risk for cerebral vascular accident (stroke).

Clinical Manifestations

Generalized (Increasing ICP) Symptoms

- Headache, although not always present, is most common in the early morning and is made worse by coughing, straining, or sudden movement. Headaches are usually described as deep, expanding, or dull but unrelenting. Frontal tumors produce a bilateral frontal headache; pituitary gland tumors produce bitemporal pain; in cerebellar tumors, the headache may be located in the suboccipital region at the back of the head.
- Vomiting, seldom related to food intake, is usually due to irritation of the vagal centers in the medulla.
- Papilledema (edema of the optic nerve) is associated with visual disturbances.
- Mental changes (eg, dullness and giddiness) are often general but can be localized.
- Pituitary adenomas may cause symptoms of hormone imbalance and Cushing's disease (eg, fat redistribution, hypertension, elevated serum glucose) in addition to general symptoms.

Localized Symptoms

The progression of the signs and symptoms is important because it indicates tumor growth and expansion. The most common focal or localized symptoms are hemiparesis, seizures, and mental status changes.

- Tumor of the motor cortex: convulsive movements localized to one side of the body (jacksonian seizures)
- Occipital lobe tumors: visual manifestations, such as contralateral homonymous hemianopsia (visual loss in half of the visual field on the opposite side of tumor) and visual hallucinations
- Tumors of the cerebellum/cerebellopontine angle: tinnitus and vertigo followed by progressive deafness, numbness and tingling of the face followed by motor function disturbance (dizziness, ataxic or staggering gait, with

B

    tendency to fall toward side of lesion; marked muscle incoordination; and nystagmus)
- Tumors of the frontal lobe: personality disorders, changes in emotional state and behavior, and an uninterested mental attitude
- Tumors of the acoustic nerve may result in loss of hearing, tinnitus, vertigo, staggering gait, painful sensations of the face (numbness, tingling) and tongue, progressing to weakness and paralysis of the face.

Assessment and Diagnostic Methods

- History of the illness and manner in which symptoms evolved
- Neurologic examination indicating areas involved
- CT, MRI, computer-assisted stereotactic (three-dimensional) biopsy, positron-emission tomography (PET), cerebral angiography, electroencephalogram (EEG), and cytologic studies of the cerebrospinal fluid

Medical Management

A variety of medical treatments, including chemotherapy and external-beam radiation therapy, are used by themselves or in combination with surgical resection.

Surgical Management

The objective of surgical management is to remove or destroy all of the tumor or as much as possible without increasing the neurologic deficit (paralysis, blindness) or to achieve relief of symptoms by partial tumor removal (decompression), radiation therapy, chemotherapy, or a combination of these. Evaluation and treatment should be done as soon as possible before irreversible neurologic damage occurs. Most patients undergo a neurosurgical procedure, followed by radiation and possibly chemotherapy.

Other Therapies

- Corticosteroids to prevent postoperative swelling
- Intravenous autologous bone marrow transplantation for marrow toxicity associated with high doses of drugs and radiation
- Radioisotopes (131-I) implanted directly into the brain tumor (brachytherapy)
- Gene-transfer therapy (currently being tested)
- Photodynamic therapy (investigational) to destroy tumor but conserve healthy tissue

Nursing Management

- Evaluate gag reflex and ability to swallow preoperatively.
- Teach patient to direct food and fluids toward the unaffected side. Assist patient to an upright position to eat, offer a semisoft diet, and have suction readily available if gag response is diminished.
- Reassess function postoperatively.
- Perform neurologic checks. Monitor vital signs. Maintain a neurologic flow record. Space nursing interventions to prevent rapid increase in ICP.
- Reorient patient when necessary to person, time, and place. Use orienting devices (personal possessions, photographs, lists, clock). Supervise and assist with self-care. Monitor and intervene to prevent injury.
- Monitor patients with seizures.
- Check motor function at intervals; assess sensory disturbances.
- Evaluate speech.
- Assess eye movement, pupil size, and reaction.

For more information, see Chapter 65 in Smeltzer and Bare: *Brunner and Suddarth's Textbook of Medical-Surgical Nursing*, 11th edition. Philadelphia: Lippincott Williams & Wilkins, 2008.

B

Bronchiectasis

Bronchiectasis is a chronic, irreversible dilation and impaired mucociliary clearance of the bronchi and bronchioles. The result is retention of secretions, obstruction, and eventual alveolar collapse. Bronchiectasis may be caused by a variety of conditions, including pulmonary infections and obstruction of the bronchus; diffuse airway injury; genetic disorder (eg, cystic fibrosis); and abnormal host defense (eg, humoral immunodeficiency). Bronchiectasis is usually localized in a lobe or segment of a lung (frequently the lower lobes). A person may be predisposed to bronchiectasis (history of recurrent respiratory infections, measles, influenza, tuberculosis, and immunodeficiency disorders). Patients with bronchiectasis almost always have bronchitis.

Clinical Manifestations

- Chronic cough and production of copious purulent sputum, which has a quality of "layering out" into three layers on standing: a frothy top layer, a middle clear layer, and a dense particulate bottom layer
- Hemoptysis, clubbing of the fingers, and repeated episodes of pulmonary infection

Assessment and Diagnostic Findings

- Definite diagnostic clue is prolonged history of productive cough, with sputum consistently negative for tubercle bacilli.
- Diagnosis is established on the basis of computed tomography (CT) scan.

Medical Management

- Objectives of treatment are to prevent and control infection and to promote bronchial drainage.
- Chest physiotherapy with percussion; postural drainage, expectorants, or bronchoscopy to remove bronchial secretions

- Antimicrobial therapy guided by sputum sensitivity studies
- Year-round regimen of antibiotics, alternating types of drugs at intervals
- Vaccination against influenza and pneumococcal pneumonia
- Bronchodilators; sympathomimetics (beta-adrenergic agonists)
- Increased oral fluid intake
- Smoking cessation
- Surgical intervention (segmental resection of lobe or lung removal), used infrequently
- In preparation for surgery: vigorous postural drainage, suction through bronchoscope, and antibacterial therapy

Nursing Management

See Nursing Management and Patient Education under Chronic Obstructive Pulmonary Disease and Preoperative and Postoperative Nursing Management for additional information.

For more information, see Chapter 24 in Smeltzer and Bare: *Brunner and Suddarth's Textbook of Medical-Surgical Nursing*, 11th edition. Philadelphia: Lippincott Williams & Wilkins, 2008.

Bronchitis, Chronic

Chronic bronchitis is defined as a productive cough that lasts 3 months a year for 2 consecutive years, with other causes excluded. Chronic exposure to smoke or another pollutant irritates the airways, resulting in hypersecretion of mucus and inflammation, thickened bronchial walls, and narrow bronchial lumen. Risk factors include cigarette smoking (major risk factor) or exposure to pollution or hazardous airborne substances. Patients have increased susceptibility to recurring infections of the lower respiratory tract.

B

Clinical Manifestations

- Chronic, productive cough in winter months, earliest sign; cough is exacerbated by cold weather, dampness, and pulmonary irritants
- History of cigarette smoking, frequent respiratory infections

Assessment and Diagnostic Methods

- History, including family; exposure to irritants, including smoking
- Pulse oximetry, arterial blood gases, chest radiograph, pulmonary function studies, blood counts

Medical Management

Prevention

- Smoking cessation
- Minimize exposure to environmental irritants.
- Prophylactic vaccination against influenza and pneumonia
- Antimicrobial therapy at first sign of purulent sputum

Treatment

Main objectives of treatment are to keep the bronchial tubes open and functioning, facilitate removal of secretions, and prevent disability.

- Note changes in sputum (nature, color, amount, thickness) and in the cough pattern.
- Treat recurrent bacterial infections with antibiotic therapy.
- Facilitate removal of secretions (bronchodilators).
- Provide for postural drainage and chest percussion.
- Give fluids orally or parenterally to liquefy secretions.
- Use steroid therapy when conservative measures fail. Patient must stop smoking (causes bronchoconstriction).
- Counsel patient to avoid respiratory irritants (eg, tobacco smoke).

- Immunize against common viral agents (influenza, pneumonia).
- Treat acute upper respiratory infections (antimicrobial therapy and sensitivity studies).

Nursing Management

See Preoperative and Postoperative Nursing Management and Patient Education under Chronic Obstructive Pulmonary Disease for additional information.

For more information, see Chapter 24 in Smeltzer and Bare: *Brunner and Suddarth's Textbook of Medical-Surgical Nursing*, 11th edition. Philadelphia: Lippincott Williams & Wilkins, 2008.

Buerger's Disease (Thromboangiitis Obliterans)

Buerger's disease is a recurring inflammation of the intermediate and small arteries and veins of the lower or rarely the upper extremities. It results in thrombus formation and occlusion of the vessels. It is believed to be an autoimmune vasculitis. It occurs most often in men between the ages of 20 and 35 years and has been reported in all races in many areas of the world. There is considerable evidence that heavy smoking or chewing tobacco is either a causative or aggravating factor. Involvement is generally bilateral and symmetric with focal lesions. Superficial thrombophlebitis may be present.

Clinical Manifestations

- Pain is the outstanding symptom. Patients complain of cramps in the feet, particularly the arches, after exercise (instep claudication). Pain is relieved by rest. Involvement is usually bilateral and symmetric.

B

- Burning pain aggravated by emotional disturbances, nicotine, or chilling; digital rest pain (fingers or toes); and a feeling of coldness or sensitivity to cold may be early symptoms.
- Various types of paresthesia may develop; radial and ulnar artery pulses are absent or diminished.
- Color changes (rubor) of the feet progress to cyanosis (in only one extremity or certain digits) that appears when the extremity is in a dependent position.
- Eventually ulceration and gangrene occur.

Assessment and Diagnostic Methods

Segmental limb blood pressure, duplex ultrasonography, and contrast angiography are used to identify occlusions.

🌿 Gerontologic Considerations

In older patients, Buerger's disease may be followed by athero-sclerosis of the larger vessels after involvement of the smaller vessels.

Medical Management

Main objectives are to improve circulation to the extremities, prevent progression of the disease, and protect extremities from trauma and infection. (See Medical Management under Peripheral Arterial Occlusive Disease for additional information.) Treatment measures include:

- Completely stopping use of tobacco
- Regional sympathetic block or ganglionectomy produces vasodilation and increases blood flow.
- Conservative débridement of necrotic tissue is used in treatment of ulceration and gangrene.
- If gangrene of a toe develops, usually a below-knee amputation, or occasionally an above-knee amputation, is necessary. Indications for amputation are worsening

gangrene (especially if moist), severe rest pain, or sepsis secondary to gangrene.

- Vasodilators are rarely prescribed (cause dilation of healthy vessels only).

Nursing Management

See Nursing Management under Peripheral Arterial Occlusive Disease for additional information.

For more information, see Chapter 31 in Smeltzer and Bare: *Brunner and Suddarth's Textbook of Medical-Surgical Nursing*, 11th edition. Philadelphia: Lippincott Williams & Wilkins, 2008.

Burn Injury

Burns are caused by a transfer of energy from a heat source to the body. The depth of the injury depends on the temperature of the burning agent and the duration of contact with it. Burns are categorized as thermal (including electrical burns), radiation, or chemical burns. They disrupt the skin, which leads to increased fluid loss, infection, hypothermia, scarring, compromised immunity, and changes in function, appearance, and body image. Young children and elderly people are at higher risk for burn injury, and those younger than 5 years and older than 40 years are at higher risk for death after burn trauma. Inhalation injuries in addition to cutaneous burns worsen the prognosis.

Burn Depth and Breadth
Depth

The depth of a burn injury depends on the type of injury, causative agent, temperature of the burn agent, duration of contact with the agent, and the skin thickness. Burns are classified according to the depth of tissue destruction:

B

- Superficial partial-thickness burns (similar to first-degree), such as sunburn: the epidermis and possibly a portion of the dermis are destroyed.
- Deep partial-thickness burns (similar to second-degree), such as a scald: the epidermis and upper to deeper portions of the dermis are injured.
- Full-thickness burns (third-degree), such as a burn from a flame or electric current: the epidermis, entire dermis, and sometimes the underlying tissue are destroyed.

Extent of Surface Area Burned

How much surface area is burned is determined by one of the following methods:

- Rule of Nines: an estimation of the total body surface area (BSA) burned by assigning percentages in multiples of nine to major body surfaces.
- Lund and Browder method: a more precise method of estimating the extent of the burn; takes into account that the percentage of the surface area represented by various anatomic parts (head and legs) changes with growth.
- Palm method: used to estimate percentage of scattered burns, using the size of the patient's palm (about 1% of body surface area) to assess the extent of burn injury.

🌿 Gerontologic Considerations

Elderly people are at higher risk for burn injury because of reduced mobility, changes in vision, and decreased sensation in feet and hands. The morbidity and mortality associated with burns are often much greater than with younger patients. Thinning and loss of elasticity of the skin in elderly people predispose them to a deep injury from a thermal insult that might cause a less severe burn in a younger person.

Chronic illness decreases the older person's ability to withstand the multisystem stressors of burn injury, so older patients with even small burns require close observation during the emergent and acute phases. Acute oliguric renal failure is more common in elderly people than in those younger than 40 years of age. Suppressed immunologic response, a high incidence of malnutrition, and inability to withstand metabolic stressors (cold environment) further compromise the patient's ability to heal. Eschar separation in full-thickness burns is delayed.

> **NURSING ALERT** For elderly burn patients, the nursing focus should include particular attention to pulmonary function, response to fluid resuscitation, and signs of mental confusion or disorientation. A careful history of preburn medications and preexisting illnesses is essential.

Medical Management

Four major goals relating to burn management are prevention, institution of life-saving measures for the severely burned person, prevention of disability and disfigurement, and rehabilitation.

NURSING PROCESS: Emergent and Resuscitative phase

Assessment

- Review the initial assessment data obtained by prehospital providers. If needed, further assess the time of injury, mechanism of burn, whether the burn occurred in a closed space, the possibility of inhalation of noxious chemicals, and any related trauma.
- Focus on the major priorities of any trauma patient: Airway, Breathing, Circulation (also cervical spine immobilization and cardiac monitoring), Disability, Exposure, and Fluid resuscitation. The burn wound is a secondary consideration, although aseptic management of burn wounds is continued.
- Assess respiratory status as first priority (airway patency and breathing adequacy).

B

- Note any increased hoarseness, stridor, abnormal respiratory rate and depth, or mental changes from hypoxia.
- Evaluate circulation (apical, carotid, and femoral pulses). Start cardiac monitoring if indicated (eg, electrical injury, history of cardiac or respiratory problems or dysrhythmia).
- Check vital signs frequently, using an ultrasound device if necessary.
- Check peripheral pulses on burned extremities hourly; use Doppler as needed.
- Monitor fluid intake (intravenous fluids) and output (urinary catheter) and measure hourly. Assess urine specific gravity, pH, protein, and hemoglobin. Note amount of urine obtained when catheter is inserted (indicates preburn renal function and fluid status).
- Arrange for patients with facial burns to be assessed for corneal injury.
- Assess body temperature, body weight, history of preburn weight, allergies, tetanus immunization, past medical-surgical problems, current illnesses, and use of medications.
- Assess depth of wound, and identify areas of full- and partial-thickness injury.
- Assess neurologic status: consciousness, psychological status, pain and anxiety levels, and behavior.
- Assess patient's and family's understanding of injury and treatment. Assess patient's support system and coping skills.

Diagnosis

Nursing Diagnoses

- Impaired gas exchange related to carbon monoxide poisoning, smoke inhalation, and upper airway obstruction
- Ineffective airway clearance related to edema and effects of smoke inhalation
- Fluid volume deficit related to increased capillary permeability and evaporative fluid loss from burn wound
- Hypothermia related to loss of skin microcirculation and open wounds

- Pain related to tissue and nerve injury and emotional impact of injury
- Anxiety related to fear and emotional impact of injury

Collaborative Problems/Potential Complications

- Acute respiratory failure
- Distributive shock
- Acute renal failure
- Compartment syndrome
- Paralytic ileus
- Curling's ulcer

Planning and Goals

The major goals for the emergent and resuscitative phase include a patent airway and tissue oxygenation, optimal fluid and electrolyte balance and perfusion of vital organs, adequate body temperature, minimal pain and anxiety, and absence of complications.

Nursing Interventions

Promoting Gas Exchange and Airway Clearance

- Provide humidified oxygen, and monitor arterial blood gases (ABGs), pulse oximetry, and carboxyhemoglobin levels.
- Assess breath sounds, respiratory rate, rhythm, depth, and symmetry; monitor for hypoxia.
- Observe for signs of inhalation injury: blistering of lips or buccal mucosa, singed nostrils, burns of face, neck, or chest, increasing hoarseness, or soot in sputum or respiratory secretions.
- Report labored respirations, decreased depth of respirations, or signs of hypoxia to physician immediately; prepare to assist with intubation and escharotomies.
- Monitor mechanically ventilated patient closely.
- Institute aggressive pulmonary care measures: turning, coughing, deep breathing, periodic forceful inspiration using spirometry, and tracheal suctioning.

- Maintain proper positioning to promote removal of secretions and patent airway and to promote optimal chest expansion; use artificial airway as needed.
- Maintain asepsis to prevent contamination of the respiratory tract and infection, which increases metabolic requirements.

Restoring Fluid and Electrolyte Balance

- Insert large-bore intravenous catheters and an indwelling urinary catheter.
- Monitor vital signs and urinary output (hourly), central venous pressure, pulmonary artery pressure, and cardiac output. Note and report signs of hypovolemia or fluid overload.
- Provide intravenous fluids as prescribed, and titrate with urinary output. Document intake and output and daily weight.
- Elevate head of bed and burned extremities.
- Monitor serum electrolyte levels (eg, sodium, potassium, calcium, phosphorus, bicarbonate); recognize developing electrolyte imbalances.

Maintaining Normal Body Temperature

- Provide warm environment: use heat shield, space blanket, heat lights, or blankets.
- Assess core body temperature frequently.
- Work quickly when wounds must be exposed to minimize heat loss from the wound.

Minimizing Pain and Anxiety

- Use a pain scale to assess pain level (ie, 1 to 10).
- Perform a respiratory assessment before giving analgesic agents to nonventilated patients.
- Administer intravenous analgesics as prescribed, and assess response to medication.
- Assess patient and family understanding of burn injury, coping strategies, family dynamics, and anxiety levels. Provide individualized responses to support patient and family coping.

- Provide emotional support, reassurance, and simple explanations about procedures.
- Provide pain relief, and give antianxiety medications if patient remains highly anxious and agitated after psychological interventions.

Monitoring and Managing Potential Complications

- Acute respiratory failure: Assess for increasing dyspnea, stridor, changes in respiratory patterns; monitor pulse oximetry and ABG values to detect problematic oxygen saturation and increasing CO_2; monitor chest x-rays; assess for cerebral hypoxia (eg, restlessness, confusion); report deteriorating respiratory status immediately to physician; and assist as needed with intubation or escharotomy.
- Distributive shock: Monitor for early signs of shock (decreased urine output, cardiac output, pulmonary artery pressure, pulmonary capillary wedge pressure, blood pressure, or increasing pulse) or progressive edema. Administer fluid resuscitation as ordered in response to physical findings; continue monitoring fluid status.
- Acute renal failure: Monitor and report abnormal urine output and quality, blood urea nitrogen (BUN) and creatinine levels; assess for urine hemoglobin or myoglobin; administer fluids as prescribed.
- Compartment syndrome: Assess neurovascular status of extremities hourly (warmth, capillary refill, sensation, and movement); report any extremity pain, loss of peripheral pulses or sensation; remove blood pressure cuff after each reading; elevate burned extremities; prepare to assist with escharotomies.
- Paralytic ileus: Insert nasogastric tube and maintain on low intermittent suction until bowel sounds resume; assess abdomen regularly for distention and bowel sounds; begin oral feedings as soon as possible when ileus is resolved.
- Curling's ulcer: Assess gastric aspirate for blood and pH; assess stools for occult blood; administer antacids and histamine blockers (eg, ranitidine [Zantac]) as prescribed.

B

NURSING PROCESS: Acute and Intermediate Phase

The acute or intermediate phase begins 42 to 72 hours after the burn injury. Burn wound care and pain control are priorities at this stage.

Assessment

- Focus on hemodynamic changes, wound healing, pain and psychosocial responses, and early detection of complications.
- Measure vital signs frequently; respiratory and fluid status remains highest priority.
- Assess peripheral pulses frequently for first few days after the burn for restricted blood flow.
- Observe electrocardiogram for dysrhythmias resulting from potassium imbalance, preexisting cardiac disease, or effects of electrical injury or burn shock.
- Assess residual gastric volumes and pH in patients with nasogastric tubes (for clues to early sepsis or need for antacid therapy).
- Note and report blood in gastric fluid or stool.
- Assess wound: size, color, odor, eschar, exudate, abscess formation under the eschar, epithelial buds, bleeding, granulation tissue appearance, progress of graft and donor sites, and quality of surrounding skin. Report significant wound changes to physician.
- Focus on pain and psychosocial responses, daily body weight, caloric intake, general hydration, and serum electrolyte, hemoglobin, and hematocrit levels.
- Assess for excessive bleeding adjacent to areas of surgical exploration and débridement.

Diagnosis

Nursing Diagnoses

- Excess fluid volume related to resumption of capillary integrity and fluid shift from interstitial to intravascular compartment

- Risk for infection related to loss of skin barrier and impaired immune response
- Imbalanced nutrition: Less than body requirements related to hypermetabolism and wound healing needs
- Impaired skin integrity related to open burn wounds
- Acute pain related to exposed nerves, wound healing, and treatments
- Impaired physical mobility related to burn wound edema, pain, and joint contractures
- Ineffective coping related to fear and anxiety, grieving, and forced dependence on health care providers
- Interrupted family processes related to burn injury
- Deficient knowledge about the burn treatment

Collaborative Problems/Potential Complications
- Heart failure and pulmonary edema
- Sepsis
- Acute respiratory failure
- Acute respiratory distress syndrome (ARDS)
- Visceral damage (electrical burns)

Planning and Goals

The major goals include normal fluid balance, absence of infection, anabolic state and normal weight, improved skin integrity, reduction of pain and discomfort, optimal physical mobility, adequate patient and family coping, adequate patient and family knowledge of burn treatment, and absence of complications. Achieving these goals requires a collaborative, interdisciplinary approach to patient management.

Nursing Interventions

Restoring Fluid Balance
- Monitor intravenous and oral fluid intake; use intravenous infusion pumps or rate controllers.
- Measure intake and output and daily weight.

B

- Report changes in hemodynamics (pulmonary arterial, wedge, and central venous pressures, blood pressure, pulse rate) and urine output (less than 30 mL/h) to physician.
- Administer low-dose dopamine as prescribed to increase renal perfusion and diuretics to promote increased urine output; monitor response.

Preventing Infection

- Provide a clean and safe environment; protect patient from sources of cross-contamination (eg, visitors, other patients, staff, equipment).
- Caution patient to avoid touching wounds or dressings; bathe unburned areas and change linens regularly.
- Practice aseptic technique for wound care and invasive procedures. Use meticulous handwashing technique before and after contact with patient.
- Closely scrutinize wound to detect early signs of infection. Monitor culture results and white blood cell counts.

Maintaining Adequate Nutrition

- Initiate oral fluids slowly when bowel sounds resume.
- Collaborate with dietitian to plan a protein- and calorie-rich diet acceptable to patient. Encourage family to bring nutritious favorite foods. Provide nutritional and vitamin and mineral supplements.
- Document caloric intake. Insert feeding tube if caloric goals cannot be met by oral feeding (for continuous or bolus feedings); note residual volumes. Total parenteral nutrition (TPN) may be required.
- Weigh patient daily and graph weights.
- Encourage patient with anorexia to increase food intake: provide pleasant surroundings at mealtime, cater to food preferences, and offer high-protein, high-vitamin snacks.

Promoting Skin Integrity

- Assess wound status.
- Support patient during distressing and painful wound care.
- Coordinate complex aspects of wound care and dressing changes.

- Assess and record any changes and progress in wound healing; inform all members of the health care team of changes in the wound or treatment.
- Assist, instruct, support, and encourage patient and family to take part in dressing changes and wound care.
- Early on, assess strengths of patient and family in preparing for discharge and home care.

Relieving Pain and Discomfort

- Teach patient relaxation techniques. Give some control over wound care and analgesia. Provide frequent reassurance.
- Use guided imagery to alter patient's perceptions and responses to pain; distraction, hypnosis, biofeedback, and behavioral modification are also useful.
- Administer minor antianxiety medications and analgesic agents before pain becomes too severe. Assess and document patient's response to medication. Assess frequently for pain and discomfort.
- Work quickly to complete treatments and dressing changes. Encourage patient to use analgesic medications before painful procedures.
- Promote comfort during healing phase with the following: oral antipruritic agents, a cool environment, lubrication of the skin, exercise and splinting to prevent skin contracture, and diversional activities.

Promoting Mobility

- Prevent complications of immobility (atelectasis, pneumonia, edema, pressure ulcers, and contractures) by deep breathing, turning, and proper repositioning.
- Modify interventions to meet patient's needs. Encourage early sitting and ambulation. When legs are involved, apply elastic pressure bandages before assisting patient to upright position.
- Make aggressive efforts to prevent contractures and hypertrophic scarring of the wound area after wound closure for a year or more.
- Initiate passive and active range-of-motion exercises from admission until after grafting, within prescribed limitations.

- Apply splints or functional devices to extremities for contracture control; monitor for signs of vascular insufficiency and nerve compression.

Strengthening Coping Strategies

- Assist patient to develop effective coping strategies: Set specific expectations for behavior, promote truthful communication to build trust, help patient practice coping strategies, and give positive reinforcement when appropriate.
- Demonstrate acceptance of patient. Enlist a noninvolved person for patient to vent feelings without fear of retaliation.
- Include patient in decisions regarding care. Encourage patient to assert individuality and preferences. Set realistic expectations for self-care.

Supporting Patient and Family Processes

- Support and address patient's and family's verbal and nonverbal concerns.
- Instruct family in ways to support patient.
- Make psychological or social work referrals as needed.
- Provide information about burn care and expected course of treatment.
- Initiate patient and family education during burn management. Assess and consider preferred learning styles; assess ability to grasp and cope with the information; determine barriers to learning when planning and executing teaching.

Monitoring and Managing Potential Complications

- Heart failure: Assess for decreased cardiac output, oliguria, jugular vein distention, edema, or onset of S3 or S4 heart sounds.
- Pulmonary edema: Assess for increasing central venous pressure (CVP), pulmonary artery and wedge pressures, and crackles; report promptly. Position comfortably with head elevated unless contraindicated. Administer medications and oxygen as ordered and assess response.

- Sepsis: Assess for increased temperature, increased pulse, widened pulse pressure, and flushed, dry skin in unburned areas (early signs), and note trends in the data. Perform wound and blood cultures as prescribed. Give scheduled antibiotics on time.
- Acute respiratory failure and ARDS: Monitor respiratory status for dyspnea, change in respiratory pattern, and onset of adventitious sounds. Assess for decrease in tidal volume and lung compliance in patients on mechanical ventilation. The hallmark of onset of ARDS is hypoxemia on 100% oxygen, decreased lung compliance, and significant shunting; notify physician of deteriorating respiratory status.
- Visceral damage (from electrical burns): Monitor ECG and report dysrhythmias; pay attention to pain related to deep muscle ischemia and report. Early detection may minimize severity of this complication. Fasciotomies may be necessary to relieve swelling and ischemia in the muscles and fascia; monitor patient for excessive blood loss and hypovolemia after fasciotomy.

Promoting Home and Community-Based Care

- Recognize that family roles are disrupted when patients are transferred to burn centers; many centers are far from home, compounding role disruption.
- Give patient and family thorough information about burn care and treatment course.
- Assess patient's and family's abilities to process the educational content; do not provide information before they can cope with it.

Evaluation

Expected Patient Outcomes

- Achieves optimal fluid balance
- Experiences no localized or systemic infection
- Demonstrates anabolic nutritional status
- Demonstrates improved skin integrity
- Experiences minimal pain

B

- Demonstrates optimal mobility
- Uses appropriate coping strategies to deal with postburn problems
- Relates appropriately in patient and family processes
- Verbalizes understanding of treatment course
- Experiences no complications

NURSING PROCESS: Rehabilitation and Long-Term Phase

Rehabilitation should begin immediately after the burn has occurred. Wound healing, psychosocial support, and restoring maximum functional activity remain priorities. Maintaining fluid and electrolyte balance and improving nutrition status continue to be important.

Assessment

- In early assessment, obtain information about patient's educational level, occupation, leisure activities, cultural background, religion, and family interactions.
- Assess self-concept, mental status, emotional response to injury and hospitalization, level of intellectual functioning, previous hospitalizations, response to pain and pain relief measures, and sleep pattern.
- Perform ongoing assessments relative to rehabilitation goals, including range of motion of affected joints, functional abilities in activities of daily living (ADLs), early signs of skin breakdown from splints or positioning devices, evidence of neuropathies, activity tolerance, and condition of healing skin.
- Document participation and self-care abilities in wound care, ambulation, and feeding.
- Maintain comprehensive and continuous assessment for early detection of complications, with specific assessments as needed for specific treatments, such as postoperative assessment of patient undergoing primary excision.

Diagnosis

Nursing Diagnoses

- Activity intolerance related to pain on exercise, limited joint mobility, muscle wasting, and limited endurance
- Disturbed body image related to altered appearance and self-concept
- Deficient knowledge of postdischarge home care and follow-up needs

Collaborative Problems/Potential Complications

- Contractures
- Inadequate psychological adaptation to burn injury

Planning and Goals

Goals include increased participation in ADLs; increased understanding of the injury, treatment, and planned follow-up care; adaptation and adjustment to changes in body image, self-concept, and lifestyle; and absence of complications.

Nursing Interventions

Promoting Activity Tolerance

- Schedule care to allow periods of uninterrupted sleep. Administer hypnotic agents, as prescribed, to promote sleep.
- Communicate plan of care to family and other caregivers.
- Reduce metabolic stress by relieving pain, preventing chilling or fever, and promoting integrity of all body systems to help conserve energy. Monitor fatigue, pain, and fever to determine amount of activity to be encouraged daily.
- Incorporate physical therapy exercises to prevent muscular atrophy and maintain mobility required for daily activities.
- Support positive outlook, and increase tolerance for activity by scheduling diversion activities in periods of increasing duration.

Improving Body Image and Self-Concept

- Refer patient to a support group to develop coping strategies to deal with losses.
- Assess patient's psychosocial reactions; provide support and develop a plan to help the patient handle feelings. Promote a healthy body image and self-concept by helping patient practice responses to people who stare or ask about the injury.
- Support patient through small gestures such as providing a birthday cake, combing patient's hair before visitors, and sharing information on cosmetic resources to enhance appearance.
- Teach patient ways to direct attention away from a disfigured body to the self within.
- Coordinate communications of consultants, such as psychologists, social workers, vocational counselors, and teachers, during rehabilitation.

Monitoring and Managing Potential Complications

- Contractures: Provide early and aggressive physical and occupational therapy; support patient if surgery is needed to achieve full range of motion.
- Impaired psychological adaptation to the burn injury: Obtain psychological or psychiatric referral as soon as evidence of major coping problems appears.

Promoting Home and Community-Based Care

Teaching Patients Self-Care

- Throughout the phases of burn care, make efforts to prepare patient and family for the care they will perform at home. Instruct them about measures and procedures.
- Provide verbal and written instructions about wound care, prevention of complications, pain management, and nutrition.
- Include family members in planning and carrying out care according to their interest and ability and patient's needs. Encourage and support follow-up wound care.

- Refer patient with inadequate support system to home care resources for assistance with wound care and exercises.
- Inform and review with patient specific exercises and use of elastic pressure garments and splints; provide written instructions.
- Evaluate patient status periodically for modification of home care instructions and/or planning for reconstructive surgery.

Evaluation

Expected Patient Outcomes

- Demonstrates activity tolerance required for desired daily activities
- Adapts to altered body image
- Demonstrates knowledge of required self-care and follow-up care
- Exhibits no complications

For more information, see Chapter 57 in Smeltzer and Bare: *Brunner and Suddarth's Textbook of Medical-Surgical Nursing*, 11th edition. Philadelphia: Lippincott Williams & Wilkins, 2008.

C

Cancer

Cancer is a disease process that begins when an abnormal cell is transformed by the genetic mutation of the cellular DNA.

Pathophysiology

The mutant cell forms a clone and begins to proliferate abnormally, ignoring growth-regulating signals in the environment surrounding the cell. The cells acquire invasive characteristics, and changes occur in surrounding tissues. The cells infiltrate these tissues and gain access to lymph and blood vessels, which carry the cells to other areas of the body. This phenomenon is called metastasis (cancer spread to other parts of the body).

Cancer cells are described as malignant neoplasms and are classified and named by tissue of origin. The failure of the immune system to promptly destroy abnormal cells permits these cells to grow too large to be managed by normal immune mechanisms. Certain categories of agents or factors implicated in carcinogenesis (malignant transformation) include viruses, physical agents, chemical agents, genetic or familial factors, dietary factors, and hormonal agents.

Cancer is the second leading cause of death in the United States, with most cancers occurring in men and in people older than age 65. Cancer also has a higher incidence in industrialized sectors and nations.

Clinical Manifestations

- Cancerous cells spread from one organ or body part to another by invasion and metastasis; therefore, manifestations are related to the system affected and degree of disruption (see the specific type of cancer).

C

- Generally, cancer causes anemia, weakness, weight loss (dysphagia, anorexia, blockage), and pain (often in late stages).
- Symptoms are from tissue destruction and replacement with nonfunctional cancer tissue or overproductive cancer tissue (eg, bone marrow disruption and anemia or excess adrenal steroid production); pressure on surrounding structures; increased metabolic demands; and disruption of production of blood cells.

Assessment and Diagnostic Methods

Screening to detect early cancer usually focuses on cancers with the highest incidence or those that have improved survival rates if diagnosed early. Examples of these cancers include breast, colorectal, cervical, endometrial, testicular, skin, and oropharyngeal cancers. Patients with suspected cancer undergo extensive testing for the following reasons:

- To determine the presence of tumor and its extent
- To identify possible spread (metastasis) of disease or invasion of other body tissues
- To evaluate the function of involved and uninvolved body systems and organs
- To obtain tissue and cells for analysis, including tumor stage (tumor size, degree of metastasis, and grade [classification, eg, TNM stage])

Diagnostic tests may include imaging (magnetic resonance imaging [MRI], computed tomography [CT] scan, endoscopy, fluoroscopy, positron emission tomography [PET] scan, radioimmunoconjugates, ultrasonography) and biopsy.

TNM Classification System

Staging

Tumors are staged depending on size, lymph node involvement, and metastasis. Staging is also expressed in TNM symbols: T indicates primary tumor; N, lymph node involvement; and M, metastasis (see Box C-1 for a summary of tumor stages).

C

> ## BOX C–1   Stages of Tumors
>
> **Stage I:** tumor less than 2 cm, negative lymph node involvement, no detectable metastases
>
> **Stage II:** tumor greater than 2 cm but less than 5 cm, negative or positive unfixed lymph node involvement, no detectable metastases
>
> **Stage III:** large tumor greater than 5 cm, or a tumor of any size with invasion of the skin or chest wall or positive fixed lymph node involvement in the clavicular area without evidence of metastases
>
> **Stage IV:** tumor of any size, positive or negative lymph node involvement, and distant metastases

Laboratory Values

- Tumor marker identification may be beneficial for some cancers.
- Complete blood count, electrolytes, hormone levels, liver enzyme studies, as well as other chemistry studies may help to identify secondary effects of tumor (eg, anemia, neutropenia).

Medical Management

The range of possible treatment goals may include complete eradication of malignant disease (cure), prolonged survival and containment of cancer cell growth (control), or relief of symptoms associated with the disease (palliation).

- A variety of therapies may be used, including surgery (eg, video-assisted endoscopic surgery, salvage surgery, electrosurgery, cryosurgery, chemosurgery, or laser surgery). Surgery could be for prophylactic, palliative, or reconstructive purposes. The goal of surgery is to remove the tumor or as much as is feasible.
- Radiation therapy and chemotherapy may be used individually or in combination.

• Biologic response modifier (BRM) therapy may be used at various times throughout treatment.

NURSING PROCESS: The Patient with Cancer

Assessment

Infection

• Assess patient for secondary problems, such as infection, reduced white blood cell (WBC) count, bleeding, skin problems, nutritional problems, pain, fatigue, and psychological stress.
• Assess factors that can promote infection, such as impaired skin; chemotherapy, radiation, and other therapy; malignancy; medications; age; chronic illness; intravenous line; urinary catheter; and other invasive procedures.
• Monitor laboratory studies (eg, WBC count for leukopenia or neutropenia).
• Frequently assess common sites of infection (eg, pharynx, skin, perianal area, urinary tract, respiratory tract) for signs of infection (fever, swelling, redness, drainage, pain).
• Monitor patient for sepsis, particularly if invasive catheters or infusion lines are in place.

Bleeding

• Assess patient for factors that may contribute to bleeding (eg, bone marrow suppression from radiation, chemotherapy, and medications such as aspirin, dipyridamole [Persantine], heparin, or warfarin [Coumadin]).
• Monitor common bleeding sites (eg, skin, mucous membranes; intestinal, urinary, and respiratory tracts; brain).
• Monitor and report gross hemorrhage as well as blood in the stools, urine, sputum, or vomitus (melena, hematuria, hemoptysis, hematemesis), oozing at injection sites,

bruising (ecchymosis), petechiae, and changes in mental status.

Skin Breakdown

- Assess patient for risk factors for decreased skin integrity (eg, therapy effects, invasive diagnostic procedures, nutritional deficits, bowel and bladder incontinence, immobility, immunosuppression, and changes related to aging).
- Note skin lesions or ulcerations secondary to the tumor or therapy, particularly alterations throughout the gastrointestinal tract (eg, oral mucous membranes), as well as their effects on the patient's nutritional status and comfort level.
- Note any alopecia (hair loss) and assess the psychological impact of this side effect on the patient and family.

Nutritional Status

- Assess patient's nutritional status (weight, caloric intake and diet history, anorexia, changes in appetite) and cachexia (wasting, emaciation). Impaired nutritional status may contribute to disease progression and a multitude of complications.
- Assess situations and foods that aggravate or relieve anorexia.
- Review patient's medication history.
- Determine difficulty in chewing or swallowing and nausea, vomiting, or diarrhea.
- Assess clinical and laboratory data related to nutritional status (eg, anthropometric measurements [triceps skin fold and middle-upper arm circumference], serum protein levels [albumin and transferrin], lymphocyte count, skin response to intradermal injection of antigens, hemoglobin levels, hematocrit, urinary creatinine levels, and serum iron levels).

Pain, Fatigue, and Attitude

- Assess the level (pain assessment scale), source, and site of pain and factors that increase the patient's perception of

pain (eg, fear and apprehension, fatigue, anger, and social isolation).
- Assess for feelings of weariness, weakness, lack of energy, inability to carry out necessary and valued daily functions, lack of motivation, and inability to concentrate.
- Assess physiologic and psychological stressors that can contribute to fatigue, including pain, nausea, dyspnea, fear, and anxiety or constipation.
- Assess patient's mood and emotional reaction to the results of diagnostic testing and prognosis.
- Assess patient's progress through the stages of grief and ability to talk about the diagnosis and prognosis with family.
- Identify potential threats to self-concept and body image, and assess patient's ability to cope with these changes.

Diagnosis

Nursing Diagnoses

Based on the assessment data, nursing diagnoses of the patient with cancer may include the following:

- Impaired tissue integrity (oral mucous membranes, alopecia, malignant skin lesions) related to the effects of treatment and the disease
- Imbalanced nutrition: Less than body requirements related to anorexia, malabsorption, and cachexia
- Pain or chronic pain related to disease and treatment effects
- Fatigue related to physical and psychological stressors
- Disturbed body image related to changes in appearance and role functions
- Anticipatory grieving related to expected loss and altered role function

Collaborative Problems/Potential Complications

Based on the assessment data, potential complications that may develop include the following:

- Infection and sepsis
- Hemorrhage
- Superior vena cava syndrome

- Spinal cord compression
- Hypercalcemia
- Pericardial effusion
- Disseminated intravascular coagulation
- Syndrome of inappropriate secretion of antidiuretic hormone
- Tumor lysis syndrome

Planning and Goals

The major goals for the patient may include maintenance of tissue integrity, management of stomatitis, maintenance of nutrition, relief of pain, relief of fatigue, improved body image, progression through the grieving process, and absence of complications.

Nursing Interventions

Maintaining Tissue Integrity

Some of the most frequently encountered disturbances include skin and tissue reactions to radiation therapy, mucositis, stomatitis, alopecia, and metastatic skin lesions.

- Provide careful skin care to prevent further skin irritation, drying, and damage. Handle skin over the affected area gently; avoid rubbing and use of hot or cold water, soaps, powders, lotions, and cosmetics.
- Instruct patient to wear loose-fitting clothes and avoid clothes that constrict, irritate, or rub the affected area.
- Provide aseptic wound care (moisture, vapor-permeable dressing, and topical antibiotics, as ordered) on area of moist desquamation (painful, red, moist skin).

 NURSING ALERT Take care not to disrupt any blisters present to reduce the risk of introducing bacteria.

Managing Stomatitis

- Instruct patient on, and assist patient with, good oral hygiene (brushing with soft-bristled toothbrush and nonabrasive toothpaste).

- Use oral swabs with spongelike applicators in place of a toothbrush for painful oral tissues, or oral rinses with saline solution or tap water.
- Assist patient with flossing, unless it causes pain or unless platelet levels are below 40,000/mm^3.
- Avoid products or foods that irritate or traumatize oral tissues or impair healing, such as alcohol-based mouth rinses and food that is difficult to chew or too hot or spicy.
- Lubricate patient's lips to keep the tissues from becoming dry and cracked. Use a topical anti-inflammatory agent and anesthetic agents if prescribed. Products that coat or protect oral mucosa are used to facilitate comfort and to promote healing and minimize discomfort. Give systemic analgesics as required.
- Encourage adequate fluid and food intake; administer parenteral hydration and nutrition as ordered.
- Administer topical or systemic antifungal and antibiotic drugs or other medications, such as IV palifermin, to promote replacement of cells in the mouth and GI tract, as prescribed to treat local or systemic infections.

Addressing Alopecia

- Provide information about alopecia (include that hair usually begins to regrow after completing therapy, although the color and texture of the new hair may be different), and support the patient and family in coping with disturbing effects of therapy.
- Encourage patient to acquire a wig or hairpiece before hair loss occurs so that the replacement matches patient's own hair. Suggest that the use of attractive scarves and hats may make the patient feel less conspicuous.
- Refer patients to supportive programs, such as Look Good, Feel Better, offered by the American Cancer Society.

Managing Malignant Skin Lesions

- Carefully assess and cleanse the skin, reducing superficial bacteria, controlling bleeding, reducing odor, and protecting skin from pain and further trauma.

- Assist and guide the patient and family regarding care for these skin lesions at home; refer for home care as indicated.

Promoting Nutrition

- Assist in selecting foods that patient might eat despite altered sense of taste and smell and decreased appetite.
- Explain how to prepare foods so they look and taste appealing; also discuss ways to avoid unpleasant smells.
- Include family members in the plan of care to encourage adequate food intake.
- Consider patient's preferences as well as physiologic and metabolic requirements in selecting foods.
- Provide and encourage patient to eat small, frequent meals with supplements between meals.
- Offer oral hygiene and pain relief measures before mealtime to make meals more pleasant.
- Use additional strategies as indicated (eg, changing the feeding schedule, using simple diets, and relieving diarrhea).
- Administer enzyme and vitamin replacement if ordered for malabsorption; administer parenteral nutrition (PN) if ordered for severe malabsorption.
- Teach patient and family how to care for venous access devices and how to administer PN; refer for home care nurses to assist with or supervise PN in the home, as needed.
- Before invasive nutritional strategies are instituted, assess patient carefully and discuss the options with patient and family (creative dietary therapies, enteral [tube] feedings, or PN).
- Direct nursing care toward preventing trauma, infection, and other complications that increase metabolic demands.

Relieving Pain

- Use a multidisciplinary team approach to determine optimal management of pain for optimal quality of life.
- Help patient and family play an active role in managing pain.

- Provide education and support to correct fears and misconceptions about opioid use.

Decreasing Fatigue

- Help patient and family to understand that fatigue is usually an expected and temporary side effect of the cancer process and treatments.
- Help patient to identify sources of fatigue and develop ways to conserve energy.
- Help patient plan daily activities, alternating periods of rest and activity.
- Encourage regular, light exercise, which may decrease fatigue and facilitate coping.
- Encourage patient to maintain as normal a lifestyle as possible by continuing with activities he or she values and enjoys.
- Encourage patient and family to plan to reallocate responsibilities, such as child care, cleaning, and preparing meals. A patient who is employed full-time may need to reduce the number of hours worked each week.
- Assist patient and family in coping with these changing roles and responsibilities.
- Address factors that contribute to fatigue and implement pharmacologic and nonpharmacologic strategies to manage pain.
- Provide nutrition counseling to patients who are not eating enough calories or protein; small, frequent meals require less energy for digestion.
- Monitor serum hemoglobin and hematocrit levels for deficiencies, and administer blood products as prescribed.
- Monitor patient for alterations in oxygenation and electrolyte balances.
- Arrange for physical therapy and assistive devices if patient has impaired mobility.

Improving Body Image and Self-Esteem

A positive approach is essential when caring for the patient with a disturbed body image. To help the patient retain control and a sense of self-worth, encourage independence and continued participation in self-care and decision making.

- Assist patient to assume tasks and participate in activities that are valuable to him or her.
- Encourage patient to express any negative feelings or threats to body image.
- Serve as a listener and counselor to patient and family.
- Refer patient and family to a support group for additional assistance in coping with the changes resulting from cancer or its treatment.
- Consult with a cosmetologist, who might provide ideas about hair or wig styling, make-up, and the use of scarves and turbans to help with body image concerns.
- Encourage patients who are experiencing disturbances in sexuality and sexual function to share and discuss concerns openly with their partner. Explore alternative forms of sexual expression with patient and partner to promote self-worth and acceptance.
- Assist patient and partner in seeking further counseling if serious physiologic, psychological, or communication difficulties related to sexuality or sexual function are identified.

Assisting in Grieving

- Answer questions and clarify information provided by the physician.
- Assess response of patient and family to the diagnosis and planned treatment, and assist them in framing their questions and concerns.
- Identify resources and support people (eg, clergy, counselor, and other support available through hospitals and various community organizations).
- Assist patient and family with communicating and sharing their concerns with each other. Encourage patient and family to express their feelings in an atmosphere of trust and support.
- If patient enters the terminal phase of disease, assist patient and family to come to grips with their reactions and feelings

(physical support, such as holding the patient's hand or just being with the patient at home or at the bedside).
- Maintain contact with the surviving family members after death of the patient. This may help them to work through their feelings of loss and grief.

Monitoring and Managing Potential Complications

- Use strict asepsis when handling intravenous lines, catheters, and other invasive equipment.
- Avoid exposing the patient to others with an active infection and to crowds.
- Place patients with profound immunosuppression, such as recipients of bone marrow transplants, in a protective environment in which the room and its contents are sterilized and the air is filtered.
- Provide immunosuppressed patients with low-bacteria diets. Avoid fresh fruits and vegetables.
- Avoid invasive procedures, such as injections, vaginal or rectal examinations, rectal temperatures, and surgery.
- Encourage patient to do coughing and deep-breathing exercises frequently to prevent respiratory problems.
- Teach patient and family to recognize signs and symptoms of infection to report, to perform effective hand washing, to use antipyretic agents, to maintain skin integrity, and to self-administer hematopoietic growth factors when indicated.

Managing Septic Shock

- Assess frequently for infection and inflammation throughout the course of the disease.
- Prevent septicemia and septic shock, or detect and report for prompt treatment.
- Monitor for signs and symptoms of septic shock (altered mental status, either subnormal or elevated temperature, cool and clammy skin, decreased urine output, hypotension, dysrhythmias, electrolyte imbalances, and abnormal arterial blood gas values).

C

- Instruct patient and family about signs of septicemia, methods for preventing infection, and actions to take if infection or septicemia occurs (see Septic Shock).

Managing Bleeding and Hemorrhage

- Monitor laboratory values, and continue to assess patient for bleeding.
- Prevent trauma and minimize the risk of bleeding by encouraging the patient to use a soft (not stiff) toothbrush and an electric (not straight-edged) razor.
- Avoid unnecessary invasive procedures (eg, rectal temperatures, intramuscular injections, and catheterization).
- Assist patient and family to identify and remove environmental hazards that may lead to falls or other trauma.
- Provide soft foods, increased fluid intake, and stool softeners, if prescribed, to reduce trauma to the gastrointestinal tract.
- Handle and move the joints and extremities gently to minimize the risk for spontaneous bleeding.
- Monitor serum hemoglobin and hematocrit carefully for changes indicating blood loss.
- Test all urine, stool, and emesis for occult blood.
- Perform neurologic assessments to detect changes in orientation and behavior.
- Administer fluids and blood products as prescribed to replace any losses and vasopressor drugs and supplemental oxygen as prescribed to maintain blood pressure and ensure tissue oxygenation.

Promoting Home and Community-Based Care
Teaching Patients Self-Care

- Provide information needed by patient and family to address the most immediate care needs likely to be encountered at home.

- Verbally review, and reinforce with written information, the side effects of treatments and changes in the patient's status that should be reported.
- Discuss strategies to deal with side effects of treatment with patient and family.
- Identify learning needs based on the priorities identified by patient and family as well as on the complexity of home care.
- Instruct patient and family and provide ongoing support that allows them to feel comfortable and proficient in managing treatments at home.
- Refer for home care nursing to provide care and support for patients receiving advanced technical care.
- Provide follow-up visits and phone calls to patient and family, and evaluate patient progress and ongoing needs.

Continuing Care

- Refer patient for home care (assessment of the home environment, suggestions for modifications to assist patient and family in addressing patient's physical needs, care, and ongoing assessment of the psychological and emotional effects of the illness on patient and the family).
- Assess adequacy of pain management and the effectiveness of other strategies to prevent or manage side effects of treatment.
- Help coordinate patient care by maintaining close communication with all health care providers involved in the patient's care.
- Make referrals and coordinate available community resources (eg, local office of the American Cancer Society, home aides, church groups, and support groups) to assist patients and caregivers.

Evaluation

Expected Patient Outcomes

- Maintains adequate tissue (skin and mucous membrane) integrity
- Maintains adequate nutritional status

- Achieves relief of pain and discomfort
- Demonstrates increased activity tolerance and decreased fatigue
- Progresses through grieving process
- Exhibits improved body image and self-esteem
- Experiences no complications, such as inflammation, infection, or sepsis, and no episodes of bleeding or hemorrhage

NURSING MANAGEMENT: Cancer Surgery

- Complete a thorough preoperative assessment for all factors that may affect patients undergoing surgery.
- Assist patient and family in dealing with the possible changes and outcomes resulting from surgery; provide education and emotional support by assessing patient and family needs and exploring with them their fears and coping mechanisms. Encourage them to take an active role in decision making when possible.
- Explain and clarify information the physician has provided about the results of diagnostic testing and surgical procedures, if asked.
- Communicate frequently with the physician and other health care team members to ensure that the information provided is consistent.
- After surgery, assess patient's responses to the surgery and monitor for complications such as infection, bleeding, thrombophlebitis, wound dehiscence, fluid and electrolyte imbalance, and organ dysfunction.
- Provide for patient comfort.
- Provide postoperative teaching that addresses wound care, activity, nutrition, and medications.
- Initiate plans for discharge, follow-up care, and treatment as early as possible to ensure continuity of care.
- Encourage patient and family to use community resources such as the American Cancer Society or Make Today Count for support and information.

NURSING MANAGEMENT:
Radiation Therapy

C

- Answer questions and allay fears of patient and family about the effects of radiation on others, on the tumor, and on normal tissues and organs.
- Explain the procedure for delivering radiation. Describe the equipment, the duration of the procedure (often minutes), the possible need for immobilizing the patient during the procedure, and the absence of new sensations, including pain, during the procedure.
- If a radioactive implant is used, inform patient about the restrictions placed on visitors and health care personnel and other radiation precautions as well as the patient's own role before, during, and after the procedure.
- Maintain bed rest for patient with an intracavitary delivery device. Use the log-roll maneuver when positioning patient to prevent displacing the intracavitary device. Provide a low-residue diet and antidiarrheal agents to prevent bowel movements during therapy to prevent the radioisotopes from being displaced. Maintain an indwelling urinary catheter to ensure that the bladder empties.
- Assess patient's skin, nutritional status, and general feeling of well-being.
- Assess skin and oral mucosa frequently for changes (particularly if radiation therapy is directed to these areas). Protect the skin from irritation, and instruct patient to avoid using ointments, lotions, or powders on the area.
- Assist the weak or fatigued patient with activities of daily living and personal hygiene, including gentle oral hygiene to remove debris, prevent irritation, and promote healing.
- Reassure the patient by explaining that these symptoms are a result of the treatment and do not represent deterioration or progression of the disease.
- Follow the instructions provided by the radiation safety officer from the radiology department, which identify the maximum time a health care provider can spend safely in the patient's room, the shielding equipment to be used, and

C

special precautions and actions to be taken if the implant is dislodged. Explain the rationale for these precautions to patient.

> **!** **NURSING ALERT** For safety in brachytherapy, assign the patient to a private room, and post appropriate notices about radiation safety precautions. Have staff members wear dosimeter badges. Make sure that pregnant staff members are not assigned to this patient's care. Prohibit visits by children or pregnant women and limit visits from others to 30 minutes daily. Instruct and monitor visitors to ensure they maintain a 6-foot distance from the radiation source.

NURSING MANAGEMENT: Chemotherapy

- Assess patient's nutritional and fluid and electrolyte status frequently. Use creative ways to encourage adequate fluid and dietary intake.
- Due to increased risk of anemia, infection, and bleeding disorders, focus nursing assessment and care on identifying and modifying factors that further increase the risk.
- Use aseptic technique and gentle handling to prevent infection and trauma.
- Closely monitor laboratory test results (blood cell counts), and promptly report untoward changes and signs of infection or bleeding.
- Carefully select peripheral veins and perform venipuncture, and carefully administer drugs. Monitor for indications of extravasation during drug administration (eg, absence of blood return from the intravenous catheter, resistance to flow of intravenous fluid, or swelling, pain, or redness at the site).
- Assist patient with delayed nausea and vomiting (occurring later than 48 to 72 hours after chemotherapy) by teaching the patient to take antiemetic medications as necessary for the first week at home after chemotherapy and by teaching

relaxation techniques and imagery, which can help to
decrease stimuli contributing to symptoms.

- Advise patient to eat small, frequent meals, bland foods,
  and comfort foods, which may reduce the frequency or
  severity of these symptoms.
- Monitor blood cell counts frequently, note and report
  neutropenia, and protect the patient from infection and
  injury, particularly while blood cell counts are depressed.
- Monitor blood urea nitrogen (BUN), serum creatinine,
  creatinine clearance, and serum electrolyte levels, and
  report any findings that indicate decreasing renal
  function.
- Provide adequate hydration and alkalinization of the urine
  to prevent formation of uric acid crystals, and administer
  allopurinol as ordered to prevent renal damage.
- Monitor closely for signs of heart failure and for pulmonary
  fibrosis (eg, pulmonary function test results).
- Inform patient and partner about potential changes in
  reproductive ability resulting from chemotherapy and
  options. (Banking of sperm is recommended for men before
  treatments.) Advise patient and partner to use reliable birth
  control while receiving chemotherapy because sterility is
  not certain.
- Inform patient that the taxanes and plant alkaloids,
  especially vincristine, can cause peripheral neuropathies,
  loss of deep tendon reflexes, and paralytic ileus; these side
  effects are usually reversible and disappear after completion
  of chemotherapy.
- Help patient and family plan strategies to combat fatigue.
- Use precautions developed by the Occupational Safety and
  Health Administration (OSHA), Oncology Nursing Society
  (ONS), hospitals, and other health care agencies to protect
  health care personnel who handle chemotherapeutic
  agents.

 NURSING ALERT If extravasation is suspected, stop the
drug administration immediately and apply ice to the site
(unless the extravasated vesicant is a vinca alkaloid).

C

NURSING MANAGEMENT: Bone Marrow Transplantation

- Before bone marrow transplantation (BMT), perform nutritional assessments and extensive physical examinations and ensure that organ function tests, as well as psychological evaluations, are completed as ordered.
- Ensure that patient's social support systems and other resources are evaluated.
- Reinforce information for informed consent.
- Provide patient teaching about the procedure and pretransplantation and posttransplantation care.
- During the treatment phase, closely monitor for signs of acute toxicities (eg, nausea, diarrhea, mucositis, and hemorrhagic cystitis), and give constant attention to patient.
- During the bone marrow or stem cell infusions, monitor vital signs and blood oxygen saturation, assess for adverse effects (eg, fever, chills, shortness of breath, chest pain, cutaneous reactions, nausea, vomiting, hypotension or hypertension, tachycardia, anxiety, and taste changes), and provide ongoing support and patient teaching.
- Because of the high risk for dying from sepsis and bleeding, support patient with blood products and hemopoietic growth factors and protect from infection.
- Assess for early graft-versus-host disease (GVHD) effects on the skin, liver, and gastrointestinal tract as well as gastrointestinal complications (eg, fluid retention, jaundice, abdominal pain, ascites, tender and enlarged liver, and encephalopathy).
- Monitor for pulmonary complications, such as pulmonary edema, and interstitial and other pneumonias, which often complicate recovery after BMT.
- Provide for ongoing nursing assessments in follow-up visits to detect late effects (100 days or later) after BMT, such as infections (eg, varicella zoster), restrictive pulmonary abnormalities, and recurrent pneumonias, as well as chronic GVHD involving the skin, liver, intestine, esophagus, eye,

lungs, joints, and vaginal mucosa. Cataracts may develop after total-body irradiation.

- Provide ongoing psychosocial patient assessment, including the stressors affecting patients at each phase of the transplantation experience.
- Assess and address the psychosocial needs of marrow donors and family members. Educate and support donor and family members to reduce anxiety and promote coping. Assist family members to maintain realistic expectations of themselves as well as of the patient.

NURSING MANAGEMENT: Hyperthermia

Explain to patient and family about the procedure, its goals, and its effects. Assess the patient for adverse effects, and make efforts to reduce their occurrence and severity. Provide local skin care at the site of the implanted hyperthermic probes.

NURSING MANAGEMENT: Biologic Response Modifiers

- Assess the need for education, support, and guidance for both patient and family (often the same needs as patients having other treatment approaches, but biologic response modifiers [BRMs] may be perceived as a last-chance effort by patients who have not responded to standard treatments).
- Monitor therapeutic and adverse effects (eg, fever, myalgia, nausea, and vomiting, as seen with interferon therapy) and life-threatening side effects (eg, capillary leak syndrome, pulmonary edema, and hypotension).
- Assess the impact of adverse and side effects on patient's quality of life.
- Work closely with physicians in assessing and managing potential toxicities of BRM therapy.

- Use accurate observations and careful documentation with administration of investigational agents for data collection.
- Teach patients and families, as needed, how to administer BRM agents through subcutaneous injections.
- Arrange for home care nurses to monitor patient's responses to treatment, and provide teaching and continued care.

NURSING MANAGEMENT: Photodynamic Therapy

- Teach patients that the major side effect of therapy is photosensitivity for 4 to 6 weeks after treatment.
- Instruct patients to protect themselves from direct and indirect sunlight to prevent skin burns.
- Observe for and teach patients to observe for local reactions in the area treated.
- Monitor liver and renal function for transient abnormalities.
- Educate, assist, and provide emotional support to patient and family.

For more information, see Chapter 16 in Smeltzer and Bare: *Brunner and Suddarth's Textbook of Medical-Surgical Nursing*, 11th edition. Philadelphia: Lippincott Williams & Wilkins, 2008.

Cancer of the Bladder

Cancer of the urinary bladder is seen more frequently in people aged 50 to 70 years and affects men more often than women (4:1). There are two forms of bladder cancer: superficial (which tends to recur) and invasive. Tumors usually arise at the base of the bladder and involve the ureteral orifices and bladder neck. The predominant cause is cigarette smoking. Chronic schistosomiasis (parasitic infection that irritates the bladder) is also a risk factor. Cancers arising from the prostate, colon, and rectum in men and from the lower gynecologic tract in women may metastasize to the bladder.

Clinical Manifestations

- Gross painless hematuria is the most common symptom.
- Infection of the urinary tract is common and produces frequency, urgency, and dysuria.
- Any alteration in voiding or change in the urine is indicative.
- Pelvic or back pain may occur with metastasis.

Assessment and Diagnostic Methods

Biopsies of the tumor and adjacent mucosa are definitive, but the following procedures are also used:

- Cystoscopy, biopsy of tumor and adjacent mucosa
- Excretory urography
- Computed tomography (CT) scan
- Ultrasonography
- Bimanual examination under anesthesia
- Cytologic examination of fresh urine and saline bladder washings

Molecular assays, bladder tumor antigens, adhesion molecules and others are being studied.

Medical Management

Treatment of bladder cancer depends on the grade of tumor, the stage of tumor growth, and the multicentricity of the tumor. Age and physical, mental, and emotional status are considered in determining treatment.

Surgical Management

- Transurethral resection (TUR) or fulguration for simple papillomas with intravesical bacille Calmette-Guérin (BCG) is the treatment of choice.
- Monitoring of benign papillomas with cytology and cystoscopy periodically for the rest of patient's life

- Simple cystectomy or radical cystectomy for invasive or multifocal bladder cancer
- Trimodal therapy (TUR, radiation, and chemotherapy) to avoid cystectomy remains investigational in the USA.

Pharmacologic Therapy

- Chemotherapy with a combination of methotrexate, 5-fluorouracil (5-FU), vinblastine, doxorubicin (Adriamycin), and cisplatin (M-VAC) and new agents gemcitabine and taxanes, possibly by topical chemotherapy applied directly to the bladder wall
- Intravesical BCG (effective with superficial transitional cell carcinoma)
- Cytotoxic agent infusions through the arterial supply of the involved organ
- Formalin, phenol, or silver nitrate instillations to achieve relief of hematuria and strangury (slow and painful discharge of urine) in some patients

Radiation Therapy

- Radiation of tumor preoperatively to reduce microextension and viability
- Radiation therapy in combination with surgery to control inoperable tumors
- Hydrostatic therapy: for advanced bladder cancer or patients with intractable hematuria (after radiation therapy)

Nursing Management

See Nursing Management for the patient undergoing cancer surgery, radiation, and chemotherapy under Cancer for additional information.

For more information, see Chapter 45 in Smeltzer and Bare: *Brunner and Suddarth's Textbook of Medical-Surgical Nursing*, 11th edition. Philadelphia: Lippincott Williams & Wilkins, 2008.

Cancer of the Breast

Carcinoma of the breast is a pathologic entity that starts with a genetic alteration in a single cell and may take 2 years to become palpable. The most common type of breast cancer is infiltrating ductal carcinoma (75% of cases), which has a poorer prognosis than other types of breast cancer. Infiltrating lobular carcinoma accounts for 5% to 10% of cases. These tumors occur in an area of ill-defined thickening and are multicentric tumors. Infiltrating ductal and lobular carcinomas usually spread to bone, lung, liver, adrenals, pleura, skin, or brain. Several less common invasive cancers, such as medullary carcinoma (5% of cases), mucinous cancer (3% of cases), and tubular ductal cancer (2% of cases) have very favorable prognoses. Inflammatory carcinoma and Paget disease are less common forms of breast cancer. There is no one specific cause; rather, a combination of genetic, hormonal, and possibly environmental events may contribute to its development. If lymph nodes are unaffected, the prognosis is better. The key to improved cure rates is early diagnosis, before metastasis.

Risk Factors

- Gender (female) and increasing age
- Previous breast cancer: the risk of developing cancer in the other breast increases 1% each year
- Genetic alterations (BRCA1 or BRCA2), which may be inherited or acquired, indicate risk.
- Prolonged exposure to hormonal stimulation—that is, early menarche (before 12 years of age), nulliparity, first birth after 30 years of age, and late menopause (after 55 years of age)—breast implants, oral contraceptives, hormone replacement therapy, cigarette smoking, alcohol consumption, and high-fat diet are weakly associated factors.

Protective Factors

Protective factors may include regular vigorous exercise (decreased body fat), pregnancy before age 30, and breastfeeding.

Prevention Strategies

C   Patients at high risk for breast cancer may consult with specialists regarding possible or appropriate prevention strategies such as:

- Long-term surveillance consisting of twice-yearly clinical breast exams starting at age 25, yearly mammography, and possibly MRI (in BRCA-1 and BRCA-2 carriers)
- Chemoprevention to prevent disease before it starts, using tamoxifen (Nolvadex) and possibly raloxifene (Evista)
- Prophylactic mastectomy ("risk-reducing" mastectomy) for patients with strong family history of breast cancer, a diagnosis of LCIS or atypical hyperplasia, a BRCA gene mutation, an extreme fear of cancer ("cancer phobia"), or previous cancer in one breast

Clinical Manifestations

- Symptoms are insidious; generally, lesions are nontender, fixed, and hard with irregular borders; most occur in the upper outer quadrant, more often on the left breast.
- Pain is usually absent except in later stages.
- Some women have no symptoms and no palpable lump but have an abnormal mammogram.
- Without detection and treatment, the following may occur: dimpling or peau d'orange (orange-peel skin), asymmetry and elevation of the affected breast, nipple retraction, lesions fixed to the chest wall, ulceration, and metastasis.

Assessment and Diagnostic Methods

- Chest x-rays, bone scans, liver function tests
- Fine-needle aspiration
- Biopsy (eg, excisional, core, stereotactic) and histologic examination of cancer cells

Staging of Breast Cancer

Classifying tumors as stage 0, I, or IV is fairly straightforward. Stage II and III tumors represent a wide spectrum of breast cancers and are subdivided into stage IIA, IIB, IIIA, IIIB, and IIIC. Factors determining stages include number and characteristics of axillary lymph nodes, status of other regional lymph nodes, and involvement of the skin or underlying muscle. See Staging of Cancer under Cancer.

Medical Management

Various management options are available. The patient and physician may decide on surgery, chemotherapy, radiation therapy, or hormonal therapy or a combination of therapies.

- Modified radical mastectomy involves removal of the entire breast tissue along with axillary lymph nodes.
- Breast-conserving surgery: lumpectomy, segmental mastectomy, or quadrantectomy, and axillary node dissection followed by radiation therapy to residual microscopic disease
- Lymphatic mapping and sentinel node biopsy, possibly sparing the patient unnecessary node dissection
- A course of external-beam radiation therapy to the tumor mass to decrease chances of recurrence and eradicate residual cancer
- Chemotherapy to eradicate micrometastatic spread of the disease: cyclophosphamide (Cytoxan) (C), methotrexate (M), fluorouracil (F), doxorubicin (Adriamycin) (A), and paclitaxel (Taxol) (T)
- CMF or CAF regimen common, or ACT may be used.
- Autologous bone marrow transplant (ABMT) is an increasingly used therapy; current use of growth factors to stimulate the bone marrow has led to an overall decline in mortality.
- Hormonal therapy based on the index of estrogen and progesterone receptors: tamoxifen (Taxol) is the primary hormonal agent used to suppress hormonal-dependent tumors; others are anastrazole (Arimidex), megestrol (Megace), diethylstilbestrol (DES), fluoxymesterone (Halotestin), and aminoglutethimide (Cytadren).
- Investigational therapy (photodynamic techniques) may be an option if chemotherapy or immunotherapy fails.

- Elective reconstructive surgery provides considerable psychological benefit but is contraindicated if cancer is locally advanced, metastatic, or inflammatory.

Nursing Management

See Nursing Process: The Patient With Cancer under Cancer for additional information.

Assessment
Preoperative

- Assess patient's reaction to the diagnosis and ability to cope with it.
- Take a complete health and gynecologic history.
- Ask about coping skills, support systems, knowledge deficit, and presence of discomfort.
- Perform a complete physical assessment, with particular attention to breasts and related mass signs and symptoms.

Postoperative

- Monitor pulse and blood pressure for signs of shock and hemorrhage.
- Avoid performing blood pressure readings, injections, intravenous lines, and venipunctures on the operative side to prevent infection and compromised circulation.
- Inspect dressings for bleeding on a regular basis.
- Monitor drainage.
- Turn and encourage deep breathing.
- Assess graft areas for unusual redness, pain, swelling, or drainage.

Diagnosis
Nursing Diagnoses

- Anxiety related to cancer diagnosis

- Risk for ineffective coping (individual or family) related to the diagnosis of breast cancer and treatment options
- Deficient knowledge about breast cancer and treatment options
- Fear related to specific treatments, body image changes, or possible death
- Decisional conflict related to treatment options
- Pain and discomfort related to surgical procedure
- Impaired skin integrity due to surgical incision
- Risk for infection related to surgical incision and presence of surgical drains
- Deficient knowledge about breast cancer, treatment options, drain management, and arm exercise (if surgery involved radical mastectomy)
- Risk for sexual dysfunction related to loss of body part, change in self-image, and fear of partner's responses
- Self-care deficit related to partial immobility of upper extremity on operative side
- Disturbed body image related to loss or alteration of the breast due to surgical procedure
- Disturbed sensory perception (kinesthetic) related to nerve irritation in affected arm, breast, or chest wall

Collaborative Problems/Potential Complications

- Lymphedema
- Infection
- Hematoma/seroma formation

Planning and Goals

The major goals of the patient may include increased knowledge about the disease and its treatment; reduced preoperative and postoperative fear, emotional stress, and anxiety; improved decision-making ability; pain management; skin integrity; improved self-concept; active participation in self-care activities; improved sexual function; and the absence of complications.

Nursing Interventions

Reducing Stress and Improving Coping Skills

- Preoperatively, give patient time to absorb significance of diagnosis, and give information to help evaluate treatment options.
- Promote the best preoperative physical, psychological, and nutritional conditions possible.
- Arrange for patient to discuss concerns with those who will be administering care and, if desired, a breast cancer survivor.
- Use careful guidance and supportive counseling to assist the patient who cannot make a decision about treatment.
- Avoid forcing patient to look at incision site if not ready.
- Elicit assistance from supportive family or friends to promote acceptance of body alteration.
- Recognize that spouse or partner is often in need of guidance, support, and education to cope with the crisis.

Increasing Knowledge

With consideration for timing and amount of information provided, discuss uses of medications, goals, extent and duration of treatment, side-effect management, and possible reactions after treatment, as well as issues such as prostheses and plastic surgery chosen by the patient. Be aware of and reinforce information given by the physician (eg, diagnosis and treatment options).

Maintaining Skin Integrity

- Maintain patency of surgical drain to prevent fluid from accumulating under the chest wall incision; monitor dressing and drains frequently.
- Inform patient that there will be decreased sensation in the operative area because of nerve disruption; teach signs of infection or irritation.

- Patient usually may shower on second day and wash incision; dressing is applied for 7 days. After incision is healed, lotions or creams may be applied to area to increase skin elasticity.
- Use dressing changes as an opportunity to discuss incision with patient.

Relieving Pain and Discomfort

- Encourage patient to use analgesics before (30 minutes) exercise or bedtime and to take a warm shower to relieve referred muscle pain.
- Elevate the involved extremity moderately.

Promoting Self-Care

- Provide information about postoperative surgical edema and strategies to prevent it; cuts, bruises, and infections on the operative side are dangerous precursors to problems.
- Encourage ambulation when patient is free of postanesthesia nausea and is tolerating fluids.
- Initiate full range-of-motion exercises and hand exercises (3 times/day for 20 minutes) to promote circulation and muscle strength and to prevent stiffness.
- If skin graft or tight surgical incision is present, see prescribed exercises.
- Promote self-care, exercise of both arms (eg, brushing teeth, combing hair), and good posture.
- Encourage patient to perform usual household and work-related arm activities but to avoid heavy lifting (eg, arm movements when walking, cleanliness of operative site).
- Avoid injury to operative side; check with physician before introducing strenuous activity.

Maintaining Sexual Function

- Discuss how patient perceives self and possible decreased libido related to fatigue, nausea, or anxiety.

- Clarify misconceptions (eg, that cancer can be transmitted sexually).
- Encourage couple to discuss fears, needs, and desires.
- Suggest variations in time of day for sexual activity (when least tired) or positions that are most comfortable, and alternatives for sexual activity (eg, hugging, kissing, manual stimulation).
- Refer to psychosocial resources (eg, psychologist, psychiatric clinical nurse specialist, social worker, or sex therapist) if indicated or desired.

Managing Potential Complications

- Promote collateral or auxiliary lymph drainage by encouraging movement and exercise (eg, hand pumps) through postoperative education.
- Elevate arm on pillow so that hand and elbow are higher than shoulder.
- Obtain referral for patient to therapist for custom-made elastic sleeves, exercises, manual lymph drainage, or special pump to decrease swelling.
- Teach patient proper incision care and signs and symptoms of infection and when to contact surgeon or nurse.
- Monitor surgical site for gross swelling or drainage output, and notify surgeon promptly; maintain a calm demeanor with the patient.
- If ordered, apply an elastic bandage wrap and ice pack to the surgical site.

Promoting Home and Community-Based Care

Teaching Patients Self-Care

- Assess patient's readiness to assume self-care. Focus on teaching incision care, signs to report (infection, hematoma/seroma, arm swelling), pain management, arm exercises, hand and arm care, and drainage management. Include family member.

- Provide follow-up with telephone calls to discuss concerns about incision, pain management, and patient and family adjustment.
- Teach patient how to empty drainage reservoir and measure drainage if discharged with a drain in place.

Continuing Care

- Reinforce earlier teaching as needed.
- Teach or reinforce breast self-examination, and encourage patient to perform monthly.
- Refer patient for home care as indicated or desired by patient.
- Reinforce need for follow-up visits to the physician (every 3 months for 2 years, then every 6 months for up to 5 years, then annually).

Evaluation

Expected Patient Outcomes

- Exhibits knowledge about diagnosis and treatment options
- Verbalizes willingness to deal with anxiety and fears
- Demonstrates ability to cope with diagnosis and treatment
- Demonstrates ability to make decisions regarding treatment options in a timely manner
- Exhibits clean, dry, and intact surgical incision without signs of inflammation or infection
- Reports pain has decreased and states pain management strategies
- Lists signs and symptoms of infection to be reported
- Verbalizes feelings regarding change in body image
- Participates actively in self-care activities
- Experiences no complications

For more information, see Chapter 48 in Smeltzer and Bare: *Brunner and Suddarth's Textbook of Medical-Surgical Nursing*, 11th edition. Philadelphia: Lippincott Williams and Wilkins, 2008.

Cancer of the Cervix

C

Cancer of the cervix is predominantly (90%) squamous cell cancer and also includes adenocarcinomas. It is less common than it once was because of early detection by the Pap test, but it remains the third most common reproductive cancer in women. It occurs most commonly between the ages of 30 and 45 years but can occur in women as young as 18 years. Risk factors vary from multiple sex partners to smoking to chronic cervical infection (exposure to HPV virus).

Clinical Manifestations

- Cervical cancer is most often asymptomatic. When discharge, irregular bleeding, or bleeding after sexual intercourse occurs, the disease may be advanced.
- Vaginal discharge gradually increases in amount, becomes watery, and finally is dark and foul-smelling because of necrosis and infection of the tumor mass.
- Bleeding occurs at irregular intervals between periods or after menopause, may be slight (enough to spot undergarments), and is usually noted after mild trauma (intercourse, douching, or defecation). As disease continues, bleeding may persist and increase.
- Nerve involvement, producing excruciating pain in the back and legs, occurs as cancer advances and tissues outside the cervix are invaded, including the fundus and lymph glands anterior to the sacrum.
- Extreme emaciation and anemia, often with fever due to secondary infection and abscesses in the ulcerating mass, and fistula formation may occur in the final stage.

Assessment and Diagnostic Findings

- Pap smear and biopsy results show severe dysplasia, HGSIL, or carcinoma in situ.
- Abnormal Pap test may be followed by biopsy, dilation and curettage (D & C), computed tomography (CT), magnetic

resonance imaging (MRI), intravenous urography (IVU), cystogram, and barium radiographs.

Medical Management

Disease may be staged based on the International Classification staging system or TNM classification to determine treatment as well as progress of the cancer.

- Conservative treatments include cryotherapy (freezing with nitrous oxide), laser therapy, loop electrosurgical excision procedure (LEEP), or conization (removing a cone-shaped portion of cervix).
- Simple hysterectomy if invasion is less than 3 mm. Radical trachelectomy is an alternative to hysterectomy.
- For invasive cancer, radical hysterectomy, radiation (external-beam or brachytherapy), or chemotherapy (cisplatin, carboplatin, and paclitaxel [Taxol]) or a combination of these approaches may be used.
- For recurrent cancer, pelvic exenteration is considered.

NURSING PROCESS: The Patient Undergoing Hysterectomy

See Nursing Process: The Patient With Cancer under Cancer for additional care measures and nursing care of patients with varied treatment regimens.

Assessment

- Obtain a health history.
- Perform a physical and pelvic examination and laboratory studies.
- Gather data about the patient's psychosocial supports and responses.

Diagnosis

Nursing Diagnoses

- Anxiety related to the diagnosis of cancer, fear of pain, perceived loss of femininity, and disfigurement

- Disturbed body image related to altered fertility, fears about sexuality, and relationships with partner and family
- Pain related to surgery and other adjuvant therapy
- Deficient knowledge of perioperative aspects of hysterectomy and self-care

Collaborative Problems/Potential Complications

- Hemorrhage
- Deep vein thrombosis
- Bladder dysfunction

Planning and Goals

The major goals of the patient may include relief of anxiety, self-acceptance after loss of the uterus, absence of pain or discomfort, increased knowledge of self-care requirements, and absence of complications.

Nursing Interventions

Relieving Anxiety

Determine how this experience affects the patient and allow the patient to verbalize feelings and identify strengths. Explain all pre- and postoperative and recovery period preparations and procedures.

Improving Body Image

- Assess how patient feels about undergoing a hysterectomy related to the nature of diagnosis, significant others, religious beliefs, and prognosis.
- Acknowledge patient's concerns about ability to have children, loss of femininity, impact on sexual relations.
- Educate patient about sexual relations: sexual satisfaction, orgasm arises from clitoral stimulation, sexual feeling or comfort related to shortened vagina.
- Explain that depression and heightened emotional sensitivity are expected because of upset hormonal balances.
- Exhibit interest, concern, and willingness to listen to fears.

Relieving Pain

- Administer analgesics to relieve pain and promote movement and ambulation.
- Maintain patency of nasogastric tube (if tube is present).
- Encourage patient to resume intake of food and fluids gradually when peristalsis is auscultated (1 to 2 days). Encourage early ambulation.
- Apply heat to abdomen or insert a rectal tube if prescribed for abdominal distention.

Monitoring and Managing Complications

- Hemorrhage: count perineal pads used and assess extent of saturation; monitor vital signs; check abdominal dressings for drainage; give guidelines for restricting activity to promote healing and prevent bleeding
- Deep vein thrombosis: apply elastic compression stockings; encourage and assist in changing positions frequently; assist with early ambulation and leg exercises; monitor leg pain and positive Homans' sign; instruct patient to avoid prolonged pressure at the knees (sitting) and immobility
- Bladder dysfunction: monitor urinary output and assess for abdominal distention after catheter is removed; initiate measures to encourage voiding

Promoting Home and Community-Based Care

Teaching Patients Self-Care

- Tailor information according to patient's needs: no menstrual cycles, need for hormones.
- Instruct patient to resume activities gradually; no sitting for long periods; postoperative fatigue should gradually decrease.
- Instruct patient to check surgical incision daily and report redness, purulent drainage or discharge.
- Stress the importance of adequate oral intake and maintaining bowel and urinary tract function.
- Teach that showers are preferable to tub baths to reduce risk for infection and injury getting in and out of tub.

- Avoid lifting, straining, sexual intercourse, or driving until advised by physician.
- Report vaginal discharge, foul odor, excessive bleeding, leg redness or pain, or elevated temperature to health care professional promptly.

Continuing Care

- Make follow-up telephone contact with patient to address concerns and determine progress.
- Remind patient to discuss hormone replacement therapy with primary physician, if ovaries were removed.
- Reinforce information regarding resumption of sexual intercourse.
- Reinforce importance of keeping follow-up appointments.

Evaluation

Expected Patient Outcomes

- Experiences decreased anxiety
- Has improved body image
- Experiences minimal pain and discomfort
- Verbalizes knowledge and understanding of self-care
- Experiences no complications

For more information, see Chapter 47 in Smeltzer and Bare: *Brunner and Suddarth's Textbook of Medical-Surgical Nursing*, 11th edition. Philadelphia: Lippincott Williams & Wilkins, 2008.

Cancer of the Colon and Rectum (Colorectal Cancer)

Colorectal cancer is predominantly (95%) adenocarcinoma, with colon cancer affecting more than twice as many people as rectal cancer. It may start as a benign polyp and become malignant and spread (most often to the liver). Risk factors include age greater than 85 years, family history of colon cancer or polyps, history of inflammatory bowel disease, and a diet high in fat, protein, and beef and low in fiber. Almost three out of four patients could be saved by early diagnosis and prompt treatment; the low 5-year survival rate is due primarily to late diagnosis.

Clinical Manifestations

- Changes in bowel habits (most common presenting symptom), passage of blood in the stools (second most common symptom)
- Many patients are asymptomatic for long periods and seek medical help only when the above are noted.
- Unexplained anemia, anorexia, weight loss, and fatigue
- Right-sided lesions are possibly accompanied by dull abdominal pain and melena (black tarry stools).
- Left-sided lesions are associated with obstruction (abdominal pain and cramping, narrowing stools, constipation, and distention) and bright-red blood in stool.
- Rectal lesions are associated with tenesmus (ineffective painful straining at stool), rectal pain, feeling of incomplete evacuation after a bowel movement, alternating constipation and diarrhea, and bloody stool.
- Signs of complications: partial or complete bowel obstruction, and tumor extension and ulceration into the surrounding blood vessels (perforation, abscess formation, peritonitis, sepsis, or shock)

Assessment and Diagnostic Methods

- Abdominal and rectal examination, fecal occult blood testing, barium enema, proctosigmoidoscopy, and colonoscopy, biopsy, or cytology smears
- Carcinoembryonic antigen (CEA) studies should return to normal within 48 hours of tumor excision (reliable in predicting prognosis and recurrence).

🌿 Gerontologic Considerations

Except for prostate and lung cancer in men, colon and rectal cancers are considered the most common malignancies in old age.

Symptoms are often insidious; fatigue is almost always present, due primarily to iron deficiency anemia. Other commonly reported symptoms are abdominal pain, obstruction, tenesmus, and rectal bleeding.

Colon cancer in the elderly has been closely associated with dietary carcinogens, lack of fiber, and excess fat. After surgery, the elderly patient may experience decreased vision and hearing as well as difficulty with skills that require fine motor coordination, which may require the patient to have help in handling ostomy equipment and peristomal care. Most elderly patients require 6 months before they feel comfortable with their ostomy care. In some cases, age-related arteriosclerosis causes decreased blood flow to the wound and stoma site; as a result, healing time may be prolonged. Some patients experience delayed elimination after irrigation because of decreased peristalsis and mucus production.

Medical Management

Treatment of cancer depends on the stage of disease and related complications. Obstruction is treated with intravenous fluids and nasogastric suction and with blood therapy if bleeding is significant. Supportive therapy and adjuvant therapy (eg, chemotherapy, radiation therapy, immunotherapy) are included.

Surgical Management

- Surgery is the primary treatment for most colon and rectal cancers; the type of surgery depends on the location and size of tumor, and it may be curative or palliative.
- Cancers limited to one site can be removed through a colonoscope.
- Laparoscopic colotomy with polypectomy
- Neodymium-yttrium-aluminum-garnet (Nd:YAG) laser is effective in some lesions.
- Bowel resection with anastomosis and possible temporary or permanent colostomy or ileostomy (less than one third of patients) or coloanal reservoir (colonic J pouch)

NURSING PROCESS: The Patient with Colorectal Cancer

Assessment

- Obtain a health history (inflammatory bowel disease or polyps), noting symptoms as stated previously (eg, fatigue, elimination pattern, diet, history of weight loss).
- Note presence and character of abdominal or rectal pain; current drug therapy; past medical history; color, odor, consistency of stool and presence of blood or mucus; weight loss.
- Auscultate abdomen for bowel sounds; palpate for areas of tenderness, distention, solid masses; inspect stool for blood.

Diagnosis

Nursing Diagnoses

- Imbalanced nutrition: Less than body requirements related to nausea and anorexia
- Risk for deficient fluid volume related to vomiting and dehydration
- Anxiety related to impending surgery and diagnosis of cancer
- Risk for ineffective therapeutic regimen management related to deficient knowledge concerning the diagnosis, surgical procedure, and self-care after discharge
- Impaired skin integrity related to surgical incisions, stoma, and fecal contamination of peristomal skin
- Disturbed body image related to colostomy
- Ineffective sexuality patterns related to ostomy and self-concept

Collaborative Problems/Potential Complications

- Intraperitoneal infection
- Complete large bowel obstruction
- Gastrointestinal bleeding and hemorrhage
- Bowel perforation
- Peritonitis, abscess, sepsis

Planning and Goals

The major goals of the patient may include optimal level of nutrition and fluid and electrolyte balance; reduced anxiety; elimination of body waste products; protection of peristomal skin; knowledge of diagnosis, treatment, and surgical procedure and self-care after discharge; optimal tissue healing and skin (ostomy) integrity; exploring and verbalizing feelings and concerns about colostomy and impact on self; and absence of complications.

Nursing Interventions

Preparing Patient for Surgery

- Physically prepare patient for surgery (diet high in calories, protein, and carbohydrates and low in residue; full liquid diet 24 to 48 hours before surgery or parenteral nutrition [PN] if prescribed).
- Administer antibiotics, laxatives, enemas, or colonic irrigations as ordered.
- Perform intake and output measurement of hospitalized patient (include vomitus); nasogastric tube, and intravenous fluid management.
- Monitor hydration status (eg, skin turgor, mucous membranes).
- Monitor for signs of obstruction or perforation (increased abdominal distention, loss of bowel sounds, pain, or rigidity).
- Reinforce and supplement patient's knowledge about diagnosis, prognosis, surgical procedure, and expected level of function postoperatively. Include information about postoperative wound and ostomy care, dietary restrictions, pain control, and medical management.
- See Nursing Management under Cancer for additional information.

Maintaining Optimal Nutrition

- Provide a diet high in calories, protein, and carbohydrates and low in residue.
- Provide a full liquid diet 24 to 48 hours before surgery, if prescribed.

- Administer PN for hospitalized patient.
- Monitor intake and output; administer and monitor intravenous fluids and electrolytes as ordered.
- Insert and monitor nasogastric tube, note drainage.

Maintaining Fluid and Electrolyte Balance

- Administer antiemetics and restrict fluids and food to prevent vomiting; monitor abdomen for distention, loss of bowel sounds, or pain or rigidity (signs of obstruction or perforation).
- Record intake and output, and restrict fluids and oral food to prevent vomiting.
- Monitor serum electrolytes to detect hypokalemia and hyponatremia.
- Assess vital signs to detect signs of hypovolemia: tachycardia, hypotension, and decreased pulse volume.
- Assess hydration status and report decreased skin turgor, dry mucous membranes, concentrated urine.

Providing Emotional Support

- Assess patient's level of anxiety and coping mechanisms used to deal with stress.
- Provide privacy, if desired; suggest and instruct in relaxation exercises and visualization; listen to patient who wishes to express feelings.
- Arrange meetings with a member of the clergy, if desired.
- Provide meetings for patient and family with physicians and nurses to discuss treatment and prognosis; a meeting with an enterostomal therapist may be useful.
- Promote patient comfort by maintaining a relaxed, professional, and empathetic attitude.
- Explain all tests and procedures in language the patient understands; repeat as needed.

Supporting a Positive Body Image

- Encourage patient to verbalize feelings and concerns.
- Provide a supportive environment and attitude to promote adaptation to lifestyle changes related to stoma care.
- Listen to the patient's concerns about sexuality and function (eg, mutilation, fear of importence, leakage during sex).

Offer support and, if appropriate, referral to an enterostomal therapist, sex counselor or therapist, or advanced practice nurse.

Monitoring and Managing Complications

- Before and after surgery, observe for symptoms of complications; report; and institute necessary care.
- Administer antibiotics as ordered to reduce intestinal bacteria in preparation for bowel surgery.
- Postoperatively, examine wound dressing frequently during first 24 hours, checking for infection, dehiscence, hemorrhage, and excessive edema.

Promoting Home and Community-Based Care

Teaching Patients Self-Care

- Assess patient's need and desire for information, and provide information to patient and family (see Providing Emotional Support earlier under Nursing Interventions).
- Provide patients being discharged with specific information relevant to their needs.
- If patient has an ostomy, include information about ostomy care and complications to observe for, including obstruction, infection, stoma stenosis, retraction or prolapse, and peristomal skin irritation.
- Provide dietary instructions to help patient identify and eliminate foods that can cause diarrhea or constipation.
- Provide patient with a list of prescribed medications, with information on action, purpose, and possible side effects.
- Demonstrate and review treatments and dressing changes, stoma care, and ostomy irrigations, and encourage family to participate.
- Provide patient with specific directions about when to call the physician and what complications require prompt attention (eg, bleeding, abdominal distention and rigidity, diarrhea, dumping syndrome).
- Review side effects of radiation therapy (anorexia, vomiting, diarrhea, and exhaustion) if necessary.
- Refer patient for home nursing care as indicated.

Evaluation

Expected Patient Outcomes

- Balanced nutrition and hydration
- Experiences reduced anxiety
- Learns about diagnosis, surgical procedure, preoperative preparation, and self-care after discharge
- Maintains clean incision, stoma, and perineal wound
- Verbalizes feelings and concerns about self
- Recovers without complications

For more information, see Chapter 38 in Smeltzer and Bare: *Brunner and Suddarth's Textbook of Medical-Surgical Nursing*, 11th edition. Philadelphia: Lippincott Williams & Wilkins, 2008.

Cancer of the Endometrium

Cancer of the uterine endometrium (fundus or corpus) is most often adenocarcinoma originating in the lining of the uterus. This cancer is the fourth most common in women and the most common pelvic neoplasm. Risk factors include advanced age and obesity. Women receiving hormone replacement therapy (HRT) without progesterone are at particular risk. Tamoxifen use may also pose a risk. Other risk factors include nulliparity, early menarche, anovulation, diabetes, hypertension, gallbladder disease, and late menopause.

Clinical Manifestations

Irregular bleeding and postmenopausal bleeding raise suspicion of endometrial cancer.

Assessment and Diagnostic Methods

- Annual checkups and gynecologic examination
- Endometrial aspiration or biopsy is performed with perimenopausal or menopausal bleeding.
- Ultrasonography

Medical Management

Treatment is based on the stage, type, differentiation, and invasiveness of the disease. Mainly, treatment consists of total hysterectomy and bilateral salpingo-oophorectomy and node sampling. Intracavitary irradiation or external pelvic irradiation may be part of the preoperative and postoperative treatments. Hormonal therapy or chemotherapy may be used to treat recurrent lesions beyond the vagina. Recurrent vaginal lesions are treated with surgery and radiation.

Nursing Management

See Nursing Management under Cancer of the Cervix for additional information.

_____

For more information, see Chapter 47 in Smeltzer and Bare: *Brunner and Suddarth's Textbook of Medical-Surgical Nursing*, 11th edition. Philadelphia: Lippincott Williams & Wilkins, 2008.

Cancer of the Esophagus

Carcinoma of the esophagus is usually of the squamous cell epidermoid type; the incidence of adenocarcinoma of the esophagus is increasing in the United States. Tumor cells may involve the esophageal mucosa and muscle layers and can spread to the lymphatics; in later stages, they may obstruct the esophagus, perforate the mediastinum, or erode into the great vessels.

Risk Factors

- Gender (male)
- Race (African American)
- Age (greater risk in fifth decade of life)
- Geographic locale (much higher incidence in China and northern Iran). In other parts of the world, there has been

an association with use of opium pipes, ingestion of exceptionally hot beverages or foods, and nutritional deficiencies.
- Chronic esophageal irritation
- Use of alcohol and tobacco
- Gastroesophageal reflux disease (GERD)

Clinical Manifestations

- Patient usually presents with an advanced ulcerated lesion of the esophagus.
- Dysphagia, first with solid foods and eventually liquids
- Feeling of a lump in the throat and painful swallowing
- Substernal pain or fullness; regurgitation of undigested food with foul breath and hiccups later
- Hemorrhage; progressive loss of weight and strength due to starvation

Assessment and Diagnostic Methods

Esophagogastroduodenoscopy (EGD) with biopsy and brushings confirms the diagnosis in 95% of cases. Other studies include CT, PET, endoscopic ultrasound, bronchoscopy, and mediastinoscopy.

Medical Management

Treatment of esophageal cancer is directed toward cure if cancer is in early stage; in late stages, palliation is the goal of therapy. Each patient is approached in a way that appears best for him or her.

- Surgery, radiation, chemotherapy, or a combination of these modalities, depending on extent of disease
- Palliative treatment to maintain esophageal patency: dilation of the esophagus, laser therapy, radiation, and chemotherapy
- Esophagectomy through thorax or abdomen or free jejunal graft transfer

C

NURSING PROCESS: The Patient with Esophageal Cancer

See Nursing Process: The Patient With Cancer under Cancer for additional information.

Assessment

- Obtain a complete health history (appetite, discomfort in swallowing, food associated with pain).
- Ask about past or present causative factors of esophageal discomfort (eg, alcohol or tobacco use).

Diagnosis

Nursing Diagnoses

- Imbalanced nutrition: Less than body requirement related to difficulty swallowing
- Risk for aspiration due to difficulty swallowing and/or tube feeding
- Pain related to difficulty swallowing
- Deficient knowledge of esophageal cancer, diagnostic studies, management, and rehabilitation

Planning and Goals

Goals of care include improved nutritional and physical condition in preparation for surgery, radiation therapy, or chemotherapy; absence of respiratory compromise; relief of pain; increased knowledge level; and absence of postoperative complications.

Nursing Interventions

- Observe carefully for regurgitation, dyspnea, and aspiration postoperatively.
- Monitor for signs of infection or leakage through the anastomosis; monitor temperature.

Preparing Patient for Surgery

Educate patient about the postoperative equipment that will be used (eg, chest drainage, nasogastric suction, parenteral fluid therapy, and gastric intubation).

Caring for Patient After Surgery

- To decrease the risk for aspiration and to prevent reflux of gastric secretions, place patient in semi-Fowler's, and later Fowler's, position.
- Explain the use of oral suction.

Promoting Wound Healing

- If grafting was done, check graft viability hourly for the first 12 hours.
- Assess graft color and use Doppler ultrasound device to assess for presence of pulse at graft site.

> **!** **NURSING ALERT** If an endoprosthesis has been inserted or an anastomosis performed, do not manipulate the nasogastric tube. Mark the tube position immediately after surgery and notify physician if displacement occurs.

Promoting Adequate Nutrition

- Guide patient through a weight-gain program based on a high-calorie and high-protein diet in liquid or soft form, with small, frequent feedings.
- Initiate and monitor parenteral nutrition, if needed.
- Monitor nutrition status continually.
- Encourage small sips of water, and later puréed, small feedings after feeding begins.
- Involve family: home-cooked food may be preferred.
- Prepare foods in an appealing manner.
- Administer antacids for gastric distress; liquid supplements may be more easily tolerated.
- Discontinue parenteral fluids when food intake is sufficient; instruct patient to eat slowly and chew food thoroughly.
- Keep patient upright for at least 2 hours after each meal to assist in movement of food.

- If patient drools, place a wick-type piece of gauze at corner of the mouth to direct secretions to dressing or emesis basin. Provide oral suction as needed.
- Assess for aspiration of saliva into the tracheobronchial tree (danger of pneumonia).

Promoting Home and Community-Based Care

Teaching Patients Self-Care

- Help patient plan for needed physical and psychological adjustment and for follow-up care, if an ongoing condition exists.
- Provide special equipment, if required, and teach patient and family how to use the equipment.
- Help patient in planning meals, using medications as prescribed, and resuming activity.
- Educate patient about nutritional requirements and how to measure the adequacy of nutrition.
- Educate and assist elderly and debilitated patients, in particular, in ways to adjust to their limitations and resume important activities.
- Instruct patient and family in ways to promote nutrition, such as food preparation (six small meals).
- Teach patient and family what to observe for and how to handle signs of complications.
- Assist patient to adjust the medication schedule to allow daily activities as much as possible.
- Instruct patient about management of equipment and treatments.
- Teach patient how to keep comfortable and how to obtain needed physical and emotional support.
- Refer for home health care as indicated.

Evaluation

Expected Patient Outcomes

- Achieves adequate nutritional intake
- Does not aspirate or develop pneumonia
- Is free of pain or able to control pain within a tolerable level

- Increases knowledge level of esophageal condition, treatment, and prognosis

For more information, see Chapter 35 in Smeltzer and Bare: *Brunner and Suddarth's Textbook of Medical-Surgical Nursing*, 11th edition. Philadelphia: Lippincott Williams & Wilkins, 2007.

Cancer of the Kidneys (Renal Tumors)

The most common type of renal tumor (85%) is renal cell or renal adenocarcinoma. Risk factors include gender (male), tobacco use, occupational exposure to industrial chemicals, obesity, and dialysis. These tumors may metastasize early to the lungs, bones, liver, brain, and contralateral kidney. One fourth of patients have metastatic disease at the time of diagnosis.

Clinical Manifestations

- Many tumors are without symptoms and are discovered as a palpable abdominal mass on routine examination.
- The classic triad, occurring in only 10% of patients, is hematuria, pain, and a mass in the flank.
- The sign that usually first calls attention to the tumor is painless hematuria, either intermittent and microscopic or continuous and gross.
- Dull pain occurs in the back from pressure due to compression of the ureter, extension of the tumor, or hemorrhage into the kidney tissue.
- Colicky pains occur if a clot or mass of tumor cells passes down the ureter.
- Symptoms from metastasis may be the first manifestation of renal tumor, including unexplained weight loss, increasing weakness, and anemia.

Assessment and Diagnostic Methods

- Intravenous urography
- Cystoscopic examination
- Nephrotomograms, renal angiograms
- Ultrasonography
- Computed tomography (CT) scan

Medical Management

The goal of management is to eradicate the tumor before metastasis occurs.

- Radical nephrectomy is the preferred treatment, including removal of the kidney, adrenal gland, and surrounding fat, fascia, and lymph nodes; partial nephrectomy may be used for some patients.
- Radiation therapy, hormonal therapy, or chemotherapy may be used with surgery.
- Immunotherapy may be helpful.
- Nephron-sparing surgery for solid renal lesions
- Renal artery embolization may be used in metastasis to occlude the blood supply to the tumor and kill the tumor cells. Postinfarction syndrome of flank and abdominal pain, elevated temperature, and gastrointestinal complaints is treated with parenteral analgesics, antiemetics, restricted oral intake, and intravenous fluids.
- Biologic therapy includes interleukin-2 (IL-2), lymphokine-activated killer (LAK) cells, or possibly interferon.

Nursing Management

See Nursing Process: The Patient With Cancer under Cancer for additional information.

- Assist patient physiologically and psychologically in preparation for extensive diagnostic and therapeutic procedures. Monitor carefully for signs of dehydration and exhaustion.

- After surgery, give frequent analgesia for pain and muscle soreness.
- Provide assistance with turning; encourage patient to turn, cough, and take deep breaths to prevent atelectasis and other pulmonary complications.
- Support patient and family in coping with diagnosis and uncertainties about outcome and prognosis.
- Teach patient to inspect and care for the incision and perform other general postoperative care.
- Inform patient of limitations on activities, lifting, and driving.
- Teach patient about correct use of pain medications.
- Provide instructions about follow-up care and need to notify physician about fever, breathing difficulty, wound drainage, blood in urine, pain, or swelling of the legs.
- Instruct patient and family in need for follow-up care to detect signs of metastases; evaluate all subsequent symptoms with possible metastases in mind.
- Emphasize that a yearly physical examination and chest radiograph throughout life are required for patients who have had surgery for renal carcinoma.
- With follow-up chemotherapy, educate patient and family thoroughly, including treatment plan or chemotherapy protocol, what to expect with visits, and how to notify the physician. Explain the need for periodic evaluation of renal function (creatinine clearance, blood urea nitrogen [BUN], and creatinine).
- Reassure patient and family about patient's well-being.
- Refer to home care nurse as needed to monitor and support patient and coordinate services and resources needed.

For more information, see Chapter 44 in Smeltzer and Bare: *Brunner and Suddarth's Textbook of Medical-Surgical Nursing*, 11th edition. Philadelphia: Lippincott Williams & Wilkins, 2008.

Cancer of the Larynx

Cancer of the larynx is most often squamous cell and may occur in the glottic area: vocal cords (two thirds of cases), supraglottic area, and subglottis. This cancer is potentially curable if detected early. Risk factors include male gender, age 50 to 70 years, tobacco use (including smokeless), alcohol use, vocal straining, chronic laryngitis, industrial exposure to carcinogens, nutritional deficiencies (riboflavin), and family predisposition.

Clinical Manifestations

- Hoarseness, noted early with cancer in glottic area; harsh, low-pitched voice
- Pain and burning in the throat when drinking hot liquids and citrus juices
- Lump felt in the neck
- Late symptoms: dysphagia, dyspnea, unilateral nasal obstruction or discharge, persistent hoarseness or ulceration, and foul breath
- Enlarged cervical nodes, weight loss, general debility, and pain radiating to the ear are suggestive of metastasis.

Assessment and Diagnostic Methods

- Indirect laryngoscopy
- Direct laryngoscopic examination under general anesthesia
- Biopsy of suspicious tissue with staging using the TNM classification developed by the American Joint Committee on Cancer
- Other tests: computed tomography (CT) scan, magnetic resonance imaging (MRI) to assess adenopathy, positron emission tomography (PET) to detect recurrence of tumor after treatment

Medical Management

Treatment varies with the extent of malignancy; options include radiation therapy, chemotherapy, and surgery, or combinations.

- Complete dental examination to rule out oral disease. Dental problems should be resolved before scheduling surgery if possible.
- Radiation therapy provides excellent results in early-stage glottic tumors, when only one cord is affected and mobile; may be used preoperatively to reduce tumor size or as a palliative measure.
- Endoscopic and CO_2 laser surgery for smaller tumors
- Partial laryngectomy is recommended in early stages of glottic cancer with only one vocal cord involved; high cure rate.
- Supraglottic (horizontal) laryngectomy is used in early supraglottic tumors; true cords and trachea remain intact; radical neck dissection is performed on involved side; voice is preserved.
- Hemilaryngectomy (vertical partial laryngectomy) is performed when the tumor extends beyond the vocal cord but is less than 1 cm and is only in the subglottic area.
- Total laryngectomy with permanent tracheal stoma is performed for cancer that extends beyond the vocal cords or for recurrent or persistent cancer; radical neck dissection is recommended; loss of voice but normal swallowing.
- Speech therapy when indicated: esophageal speech, electrolarynx, or tracheoesophageal puncture

NURSING PROCESS: The Patient Undergoing Laryngectomy

See Nursing Process: The Patient With Cancer under Cancer for additional nursing care related to other treatment regimens.

Assessment

- Assess for hoarseness, sore throat, dyspnea, dysphagia, or pain and burning in the throat.
- Palpate the neck for swelling.
- Assess patient's ability to hear, see, read, and write; evaluation by speech therapist if indicated.
- Determine nature of surgery; assess patient's psychological status; evaluate patient's and family's coping methods preoperatively and postoperatively; give effective support.

Diagnosis

Nursing Diagnoses

Based on all the assessment data, major nursing diagnoses may include the following:

- Deficient knowledge about the surgical procedure and postoperative course
- Anxiety and depression related to the diagnosis of cancer and impending surgery
- Ineffective airway clearance related to surgical alterations in the airway
- Impaired verbal communication related to removal of the larynx and to edema
- Imbalanced nutrition: Less than body requirements related to inability to ingest food and swallowing difficulties
- Disturbed body image, self-concept, and self-esteem related to major neck surgery
- Self-care deficit related to postoperative care

Collaborative Problems/Potential Complications

Based on assessment data, potential complications that may develop include the following:

- Respiratory distress (hypoxia, airway obstruction, tracheal edema)
- Hemorrhage
- Infection
- Wound breakdown and aspiration

Planning and Goals

The major goals of the patient may include knowledge about treatment, reduced anxiety, patent airway, improved communication, optimal levels of nutrition and hydration, positive body image and self-esteem, management of self-care, adherence to rehabilitative program, home maintenance management, and absence of complications.

Nursing Interventions

Providing Patient Education

- Clarify any misconceptions, and give patient and family educational materials about surgery (written and audiovisual) for review and reinforcement.
- Explain to patient that natural voice will be lost if complete laryngectomy is planned.
- Assure patient that much can be done through training in a rehabilitation program.
- Review equipment and treatments that will be part of postoperative care.
- Teach coughing and deep-breathing exercises; provide for return demonstration.

Reducing Anxiety and Depression

- Assess patient's psychological preparation, and give patient and family opportunity to verbalize feelings and share perceptions; give patient and family complete, concise answers to questions.
- Arrange a visit from a postlaryngectomy patient to help patient cope with situation and know that rehabilitation is possible.

Maintaining a Patent Airway

- Position patient in semi-Fowler's or Fowler's position after recovery from anesthesia.
- Encourage patient to turn and deep breathe; suction if necessary; encourage early ambulation.

C

- Observe for signs and symptoms of respiratory distress and hypoxia: restlessness, irritation, agitation, confusion, tachypnea, tachycardia, use of accessory muscles, and decreased oxygen saturation.
- Rule out obstruction immediately by suctioning and having patient cough and take deep breaths.
- Contact physician immediately if nursing measures do not improve respiratory status.
- Use medications that depress respirations with caution; monitor for respiratory depression.
- Care for the laryngectomy tube the same way as a tracheostomy tube; maintain humidification.
- Keep stoma clean by cleansing daily as prescribed, and wipe opening clean as needed after coughing.

Promoting Communication and Speech Rehabilitation

- Implement a system of communication such as "magic slate" or hand signals.
- Use nonwriting arm for intravenous infusions.
- If patient cannot write, use alternate system such as hand signals or a picture-word-phrase board.
- Work with patient, speech therapist, and family to find least frustrating system of communication.
- Inform patient of alternative communication methods; most common are esophageal speech, the electrolarynx, and tracheoesophageal puncture.

Promoting Adequate Nutrition and Hydration

- Maintain patient NPO for several days, and provide alternative sources of nutrition as ordered: intravenous fluids, enteral feedings, and parenteral nutrition (PN); explain nutritional plan to patient and family.
- Start oral feedings with thick fluids for easy swallowing; instruct patient to avoid sweet foods, which increase salivation and suppress appetite; introduce solid foods as tolerated.
- Instruct patient to rinse mouth with warm water or mouthwash and brush teeth frequently.

- Observe patient for difficulty swallowing (particularly with eating); report occurrence to physician.
- Monitor weight and laboratory data, skin turgor, and vital signs to maintain hydration.

Improving Self-Concept

- Encourage patient to express feelings about changes from surgery (fear, anger, depression, and isolation); be a good listener and a support to patient and family.
- Use a positive approach; promote participation in self-care activities as soon as possible.
- Refer to a support group, such as A Lost Chord or A New Voice, and I Can Cope.

Monitoring and Managing Potential Postoperative Complications

Complications after laryngectomy include respiratory distress (hypoxia, airway obstruction, tracheal edema), bleeding, infection, and wound breakdown.

- See Maintaining a Patent Airway, earlier, for respiratory distress.
- Note pale, cold, clammy skin, which may indicate active bleeding.
- Monitor for signs of respiratory distress and any changes in respiratory status (hypoxia, cyanosis, obstruction).
- Observe wound drainage; measure and record.
- Contact physician immediately if any active bleeding occurs.
- Monitor vital signs for changes: increase in pulse, decrease in blood pressure, or rapid, deep respirations.
- Observe for early signs and symptoms of infection: change in type of wound drainage, increased areas of redness or tenderness at surgical site, purulent drainage, odor, and increase in wound drainage.
- Observe stoma area for wound breakdown, hematoma, and bleeding, and report significant changes to the surgeon.
- Monitor patient carefully, particularly for carotid hemorrhage.

- Monitor for possible reflux and aspiration. Keep suction equipment handy.

> **! NURSING ALERT** Postoperatively, be alert for the possible serious complications of rupture of the carotid artery. Should this occur, apply direct pressure over the artery, summon assistance, and provide psychological support until the vessel can be ligated.

Promoting Home and Community-Based Care

Teaching Patients Self-Care

- Provide discharge instructions as soon as patient is able to participate; assess readiness to learn.
- Assess knowledge about self-care management; reassure patient and family that strategies can be mastered.
- Give specific information about tracheostomy and stomal care, wound care, and oral hygiene, including suctioning and emergency measures.
- Keep orifice clean and clear of mucus; wash skin around stoma at least twice daily; if crusting occurs, lubricate stoma with a non-oil-based ointment.
- Instruct patient to provide adequate humidification of the environment, minimize air-conditioning, and drink fluids.
- Inform patient to expect a diminished sense of taste and smell after surgery.
- Teach patient to take precautions when showering to prevent water from getting into the stoma.
- Discourage swimming, because the patient with a laryngectomy can drown.
- Recommend that patient avoid getting hairspray, loose hair, and powder into stoma.
- Stress that activity should be undertaken in moderation; when tired, the patient has more difficulty speaking with new voice.

Continuing Care

- Encourage patient to visit physician regularly for physical examinations and advice.

- Recommend that patient keep proper identification to alert first-aid provider about special requirements for cardiopulmonary resuscitation.
- Teach family mouth-to-stoma ventilation and to keep prerecorded emergency messages for police, fire department, and other rescue services for patient to use at home.
- Refer to home care agency for patient and family assistance, follow-up assessment, and teaching.

Evaluation

Expected Patient Outcomes

- Acquires an adequate level of knowledge, verbalizing an understanding of the surgical procedure and performing self-care adequately
- Demonstrates less anxiety and depression
- Maintains a clear airway
- Demonstrates practical, safe, and correct technique involved in cleaning and changing the laryngectomy tube
- Acquires effective communication techniques
- Maintains balanced nutrition and adequate fluid intake
- Exhibits improved body image, self-esteem, and self-concept
- Exhibits no complications
- Adheres to rehabilitation and home care program

For more information, see Chapter 22 in Smeltzer and Bare: *Brunner and Suddarth's Textbook of Medical-Surgical Nursing*, 11th edition. Philadelphia: Lippincott Williams & Wilkins, 2008.

Cancer of the Liver

Few cancers originate in the liver. Primary tumors ordinarily occur in patients with chronic liver disease (cirrhosis). Hepatocellular carcinoma (HCC), the most common type of primary liver tumor, usually cannot be resected because of rapid growth and metastasis elsewhere. Other types include cholangiocellular carcinoma (CCC) and combined HCC and CCC. If found early, resection may be possible; however, early detection is rare.

Cirrhosis, hepatitis B and C, and exposure to certain chemical toxins have been implicated in the etiology of HCC. Cigarette smoking, especially when combined with alcohol use, has also been identified as a risk factor. Other substances that have been implicated include aflatoxins and other similar toxic molds. Half of all advanced liver cancer cases represent metastases from other primary sites.

Clinical Manifestations

- Early manifestations include pain (dull ache in upper right quadrant, epigastrium, or back), recent weight loss, loss of strength, anorexia, and anemia.
- Liver enlargement and irregular surface may be noted on palpation.
- Jaundice is present only if larger bile ducts are occluded.
- Ascites occurs if portal veins are obstructed or tumor tissue is seeded in the peritoneal cavity.

Assessment and Diagnostic Findings

Diagnosis is made on the basis of clinical signs and symptoms, history and physical examination, and results of laboratory and radiographic studies, positron emission tomograms (PET scans), liver scans, computed tomography (CT) scans, ultrasound, magnetic resonance imaging (MRI), arteriography, laparoscopy, or biopsy.

Leukocytosis (increased white blood cells), erythrocytosis (increased red blood cells), hypercalcemia, hypoglycemia, and hypocholesterolemia may be seen on laboratory assessment.

Elevated levels of serum alpha-fetoprotein (AFP)

Medical Management

Radiation Therapy

- Intravenous injection of antibodies tagged with radioactive isotopes that specifically attack tumor-associated antigens
- Percutaneous placement of a high-intensity source for interstitial radiation therapy

Chemotherapy

- Systemic chemotherapy and regional infusion are used to administer antineoplastic agents.
- An implantable pump is used to deliver high-concentration chemotherapy to the liver through the hepatic artery.

Percutaneous Biliary Drainage

- Percutaneous biliary drainage is used to bypass biliary ducts obstructed by the liver, pancreatic, or bile ducts in patients with inoperable tumors or those who are poor surgical risks.
- Complications include sepsis, leakage of bile, hemorrhage, and reobstruction of the biliary system.
- Observe patient for fever and chills, bile drainage around the catheter, changes in vital signs, and evidence of biliary obstruction, including increased pain or pressure, pruritus, and recurrence of jaundice.

Other Nonsurgical Treatment Modalities

- Hyperthermia: heat by laser or radiofrequency energy is directed to tumors to cause necrosis of the tumors while sparing normal tissue
- Cryosurgery is a newer treatment modality.
- Embolization of arterial blood flow to the tumor; effective in small tumors; injection of small particulate embolic or chemotherapeutic agents may be used to cause tumor necrosis

- Immunotherapy: lymphocytes with antitumor reactivity are administered

Surgical Management

Hepatic lobectomy can be performed when the primary hepatic tumor is localized or when the primary site can be completely excised and the metastasis is limited. Capitalizing on the regenerative capacity of the liver cells, 90% of the liver has been successfully removed. The presence of cirrhosis limits the ability of the liver to regenerate.

Preoperative Evaluation and Preparation

- Evaluate and optimize patient's nutritional, fluid, psychological, and physical state before surgery.
- Prepare intestinal tract with cathartics, colonic irrigation, and intestinal antibiotics.

Liver Transplantation to Treat Liver Tumors

Removal of the liver and replacement with a healthy donor organ has been successful, but recurrence rate of primary liver malignancy after transplantation is 70% to 85%.

NURSING MANAGEMENT: Postoperative

See Nursing Management under Cancer for additional information.

- Assess for problems related to cardiopulmonary involvement, vascular complications, and respiratory and liver dysfunction.
- Give careful attention to metabolic abnormalities (glucose, protein, and lipids).
- Provide close monitoring and care for the first 2 or 3 days.

C

- Encourage early ambulation, and initiate other postoperative care measures.
- Closely monitor the patient undergoing cryosurgery for hypothermia, hemorrhage, bile leak, and myoglobinuria.
- Instruct family to assess and report complications and side effects of chemotherapy.
- Instruct patient about the importance of follow-up visits to permit frequent checks on the response of patient and tumor to chemotherapy, condition of the implanted pump site, and any toxic effects.
- Encourage patient to resume activities as soon as possible, but caution patient to avoid activities that may damage the pump.
- Teach patient about signs of complications, and encourage patient to notify nurse or physician if problems or questions occur.
- Provide reassurance and instructions to patient and family to reduce fear that the percutaneous biliary drainage catheter will fall out.
- Provide verbal and written instructions as well as demonstration of biliary catheter care to patient and family; instruct in techniques to keep catheter site clean and dry, to assess the catheter and its insertion site, and to irrigate the catheter to prevent debris and promote patency.
- Refer patient for home care.
- Collaborate with the health care team, patient, and family to identify and implement pain management strategies and approaches to management of other problems: weakness, pruritus, inadequate dietary intake, jaundice, and symptoms associated with metastasis.
- Assist patient and family in making decisions about hospice care, and initiate referrals. Encourage patient to discuss end-of-life care.

For more information, see Chapter 39 in Smeltzer and Bare: *Brunner and Suddarth's Textbook of Medical-Surgical Nursing*, 11th edition. Philadelphia: Lippincott Williams & Wilkins, 2008.

Cancer of the Lung (Bronchogenic Carcinoma)

C

Lung cancers arise from a transformed epithelial cell in tracheo-bronchial airways. A carcinogen (cigarette smoke, radon gas, other occupational and environmental agents) damages the cell, causing abnormal growth and development into a malignant tumor. The survival rate is low because of spread to regional lymphatics (in 70% of patients) by the time of diagnosis. There are four major cell types of lung cancer. Epidermoid or squamous cell carcinoma (30% of patients) is more centrally located, adenocarcinoma (31% to 34%) presents as peripheral masses and often metastasizes, large cell carcinoma (10% to 16%) is a fast-growing tumor that often arises peripherally, and small cell (oat cell) carcinoma (20% to 25% of cases) usually arises in the major bronchi.

Risk factors include tobacco smoke, second-hand smoke, environmental (air) pollution, occupational exposure, and radon. Other risk factors may include dietary factors (vitamin A and beta-carotene deficiency from low fruit and vegetable intake), genetic predisposition, and other underlying respiratory diseases, such as chronic obstructive pulmonary disease and tuberculosis.

Clinical Manifestations

- Lung cancer begins insidiously over several decades and is often asymptomatic until late in its course.
- Signs and symptoms depend on location, tumor size, degree of obstruction, and existence of metastases.
- Most common symptom is a persistent and nonproductive cough, which later becomes productive of thick, purulent sputum.
- Wheezing occurs when the bronchus becomes partially obstructed; expectoration of blood-tinged sputum occurs.
- A recurring fever exists in some patients.
- Chest pain or shoulder pain may indicate chest wall or pleural involvement. Pain is a late symptom and may be related to bone metastasis.

- Chest pain, tightness, hoarseness, dysphagia, head and neck edema, and symptoms of pleural or pericardial infusion exist if the tumor spreads to adjacent structures and lymph nodes.
- Common sites of metastases are lymph nodes, bone, brain, contralateral lung, adrenal glands, and liver.
- Weakness, anorexia, and weight loss appear late.

 NURSING ALERT A cough that changes in character should arouse suspicion of lung cancer.

Assessment and Diagnostic Methods

- Chest films, sputum examinations, endoscopy or bronchoscopy, mediastinoscopy, fine-needle aspiration (FNA), biopsy
- Various computed tomography (CT) and magnetic resonance imaging (MRI) scans
- Pulmonary function tests, arterial blood gas analysis, ventilation-perfusion scans, and exercise testing
- Staging of the tumor refers to the anatomic extent of the tumor, spread to the regional lymph nodes, and metastatic spread. (See Diagnostic Evaluation and Staging of Cancer under Cancer for additional information.)

Medical Management

See Medical Management under Cancer for additional information. The objective of management is to provide the maximum likelihood of cure. Treatment depends on cell type, stage of the disease, and physiologic status.

- Treatment may involve lung resection (preferred unless contraindicated) and/or radiation therapy, chemotherapy, and immunotherapy, used separately or in combination.
- Immunotherapy (minimal success in the past) is still investigational.
- Newer therapies (gene, tumor antigens) are under study.

Nursing Management

See Nursing Management under Cancer for additional information.

Managing Symptoms

Instruct patient and family about the side effects of specific treatments and strategies to manage them.

Relieving Breathing Problems

- Maintain airway patency; remove secretions.
- Encourage deep breathing, aerosol therapy, oxygen therapy; mechanical ventilation may be necessary.
- Encourage patient to assume positions that promote lung expansion.
- Teach breathing exercises, relaxation techniques, and energy conservation.
- Refer for pulmonary rehabilitation as indicated.

Reducing Fatigue

- Assess level of fatigue; identify potentially treatable causes.
- Educate patient in energy conservation techniques and guided exercise as appropriate.
- Refer to physical or occupational therapist as indicated.

Providing Psychological Support

- Help patient and family deal with poor prognosis and progression of the disease (when indicated).
- Assess psychological aspects and assist patient to cope.
- Assist patient and family with informed decision making regarding treatment options.
- Support patient and family in end-of-life decisions and treatment options.

For more information, see Chapter 23 in Smeltzer and Bare: *Brunner and Suddarth's Textbook of Medical-Surgical Nursing*, 11th edition. Philadelphia: Lippincott Williams & Wilkins, 2008.

Cancer of the Oral Cavity

Cancer of the oral cavity can occur in any part of the mouth (lips, lateral tongue, floor of mouth most common) or throat and is highly curable if discovered early. It is associated with use of alcohol and tobacco. Risk factors also include age older than 40 years (but the disease is being seen increasingly in patients under age 30 years), male gender, smokeless tobacco use (buccal mucosa and gingiva), dietary deficiency, and intake of smoked meats, as well as chronic irritation by a warm pipe stem or prolonged exposure to sun and wind (lip cancer). Malignancies of the oral cavity are usually squamous cell cancers.

Clinical Manifestations

- Few or no symptoms; most commonly a painless sore or mass that will not heal
- Typical lesion is a painful indurated ulcer with raised edges.
- As the cancer progresses, patient may complain of tenderness; difficulty in chewing, swallowing, and speaking; coughing blood-tinged sputum; or enlarged cervical lymph nodes.

Assessment and Diagnostic Methods

Oral examination, assessment of cervical lymph nodes, and biopsies of suspicious lesions (not healed within 2 weeks)

Medical Management

Management varies with the nature of the lesion, preference of the physician, and patient choice. Resectional surgery, radiation therapy, chemotherapy, or a combination may be effective.

- Lip cancer: small lesions are excised liberally; larger lesions may be treated by radiation therapy

C

- Tongue cancer: treated aggressively, recurrence rate is high. Radiation and surgery (total resection or hemiglossectomy) are performed.
- Radical neck dissection for metastases of oral cancer to lymphatic channel in the neck region with reconstructive surgery

NURSING PROCESS: The Patient with Oral Cancer

See Nursing Management under Cancer for additional information.

Assessment

- Assess patient's history to determine teaching and learning needs and symptoms requiring medical evaluation. Include questions related to oral cavity: oral and dental hygiene; dentures or partial plate; alcohol and tobacco use (also smokeless chewing tobacco); lesions or irritated areas in the mouth, tongue, or throat; recent history of sore throat or bloody sputum; discomfort caused by certain foods.
- Perform physical examination: inspect and palpate internal and external structures of the mouth and throat; examine for moisture, color, texture, symmetry, and presence of lesions; examine neck for enlarged lymph nodes. Use bright light and gloves to examine oral cavity.
- Inspect lips for moisture, hydration, color, texture, symmetry, and presence of ulcerations or fissures.
- Inspect gums for inflammation, bleeding, retraction, and discoloration, and the hard palate for color and shape. Also note breath odor.
- Inspect tongue for texture, color, and lesions, and the frenulum (superficial veins on the undersurface of the tongue) for location, size, color, and pain.
- Examine neck for enlarged lymph nodes (adenopathy).

Diagnosis

Nursing Diagnoses

- Impaired oral mucous membrane related to pathologic condition, infection, or chemical or mechanical trauma (eg, medications, ill-fitting dentures)
- Imbalanced nutrition: Less than body requirements related to inability to ingest adequate nutrients secondary to oral or dental conditions
- Disturbed body image related to a change in appearance resulting from disease or treatment
- Fear of pain and social isolation related to disease or change in appearance
- Pain related to oral lesion or treatment
- Impaired verbal communication related to treatment
- Risk for infection related to disease or treatment
- Deficient knowledge about disease or treatment

Planning and Goals

The major goals of the patient may include improved condition of the oral mucous membrane, improved nutritional intake, positive self-image, comfort, ability to use alternative communication methods, freedom from infection, and understanding of the disease and treatment.

Nursing Interventions

Promoting Mouth Care

- Identify patients at risk for oral complications, and assist with methods to decrease complications. Encourage or assist with oral care.
- Instruct patient in techniques of preventive mouth care: soft toothbrush, floss, or irrigating solution such as 1 tsp baking soda in 8 oz water, half-strength hydrogen peroxide, or normal saline.

Combating Xerostomia (Dry Mouth)

- Advise patient to avoid dry, bulky, and irritating foods and fluids, alcohol, and tobacco.

C

- Encourage patient to increase fluids and to use a humidifier during sleep.
- Provide synthetic saliva, moisturizing gel, or saliva production stimulant for patient, if needed.

Relieving Stomatitis or Mucositis

Start prophylactic mouth care as soon as chemotherapy or radiation therapy begins; if poor dentition·is present, tooth extraction or fluoride treatment may be needed.

Ensuring Adequate Food and Fluid Intake

- Perform dietary assessment with calorie count, and recommend changes in consistency of foods and frequency of eating based on disease and patient preferences. Dietitian consult may be beneficial.
- Help patient attain and maintain desirable body weight and level of activity.
- Promote the healing of tissue.

Supporting a Positive Self-Image

- Encourage patient to verbalize perceived change in appearance; realistically discuss actual changes or losses.
- Offer support while patient verbalizes fears and negative feelings (withdrawal, depression, anger).
- Reinforce strengths, achievements, and positive attributes. Refer for support from groups, social worker, clergy, or others as appropriate.
- Note signs of grieving, and record emotional changes and progress toward positive self-esteem.

Minimizing Discomfort and Pain

- Provide an analgesic agent such as viscous lidocaine (Xylocaine viscous 2%).
- Advise patient to avoid foods that are spicy, hot, or hard.
- Instruct patient about mouth care and pain control methods.

Promoting Effective Communication

- Assess patient's ability to communicate in writing preoperatively.
- Provide a "magic slate" or pen and paper for postoperative communication.
- Provide a communication board if patient cannot write; involve a speech therapist postoperatively.

Promoting Infection Control

- Evaluate laboratory results frequently (leukopenia may be noted).
- Check temperature every 4 to 8 hours for elevation, which may indicate infection.
- Monitor for signs of infection such as redness, swelling, drainage, or tenderness.
- Prohibit visitors who may transmit microorganisms.
- Avoid trauma to sensitive skin tissues; use strict aseptic technique when changing dressings.
- Provide instruction about antibiotics.

Promoting Home and Community-Based Care

Teaching Patients Self-Care

- Assess patient's needs and instruct patient regarding mouth care, nutrition, infection prevention, and signs and symptoms of complications. Refer to home care nurse for physical care, assessment, and further teaching.
- Prepare an individualized plan of care. If prostheses are used, teach patient in the use and care of these and the importance of clean dressings and strict oral hygiene.
- Determine what equipment is needed (eg, suction or tracheostomy tube, prostheses) and where items can be obtained.
- Give consideration to humidification and aeration of patient's room and measures to control odors.
- Encourage the use of commercial baby foods if patient is unable/unwilling to prepare liquid and soft diets.
- Instruct patient and family in use of enteral or parenteral feedings (if unable to take foods orally).

- Provide caregivers with information regarding signs of obstruction, hemorrhage, infection, depression, and withdrawal.
- Work with patient, family (or the person responsible for home care), and other health care professionals (eg, speech therapist, nutritionist, psychologist) to prepare an individual plan of care.
- Instruct patient in the importance of keeping follow-up visits to monitor condition and to receive directions about modifications in treatment or general care. Reinforce instructions to promote self-care and comfort.

Evaluation

Expected Patient Outcomes

- Learns about course of treatment
- Shows evidence of intact oral mucous membranes
- Attains and maintains desirable body weight and adequate intake of foods and fluids
- Demonstrates good respiratory exchange
- Is free of infection
- Demonstrates ability to cope, decreased fear of pain and isolation, and positive body image
- Attains an acceptable level of comfort
- Experiences no complications

For more information, see Chapter 35 in Smeltzer and Bare: *Brunner and Suddarth's Textbook of Medical-Surgical Nursing*, 11th edition. Philadelphia: Lippincott Williams & Wilkins, 2008.

Cancer of the Ovary

Ovarian cancer is most distressing because it is usually (75% of cases) diagnosed in an advanced stage. The peak incidence is in the fifth decade of life. No definitive causative factors have been determined, but oral contraceptives appear to provide a protective effect. Serous adenocarcinoma is the most common type of tumor. Risk factors include a high-fat diet; smoking; alcohol; use of talcum powder on the perineal area; a history of breast, colon, or endometrial cancer; and a family history of breast or ovarian cancer. Nulliparity, infertility, and anovulation are additional risks.

Clinical Manifestations

- Flatulence, fullness after a light meal, and increasing abdominal girth
- Irregular menses, increasing premenstrual tension, menorrhagia with breast tenderness, early menopause, abdominal discomfort, dyspepsia, pelvic pressure, and urinary urgency
- A combination of a long history of ovarian dysfunction and vague gastrointestinal symptoms or a palpable ovary in a postmenopausal woman

Assessment and Diagnostic Methods

- No screening mechanism exists; tumor markers are being explored. Biannual pelvic exams are recommended for at-risk women.
- Any enlarged ovary must be investigated; pelvic examination does not detect early ovarian cancer.
- Transvaginal ultrasound and CA-125 antigen testing are helpful for high-risk women.

Medical Management

- Surgical removal is the treatment of choice.
- Preoperative workup can include barium enema, proctosigmoidoscopy, upper gastrointestinal series, chest radiograph, intravenous pyelogram (IVP), CT scan, and intravenous urography.
- Staging of the tumor is done to direct treatment.
- Total abdominal hysterectomy with bilateral salpingo-oophorectomy and omentectomy for early disease

C

- Radiation therapy and intraperitoneal isotopes are sometimes used.
- Gene therapy is a future possibility.
- Chemotherapy, including liposomal and intraperitoneal delivery, is the most common form of treatment for advanced disease (eg, cisplatin, paclitaxel [Taxol]).
- Bone marrow transplantation and peripheral blood stem cell support may be used with chemotherapy.

Nursing Management

- Monitor for complications of therapy and abdominal surgery; report manifestations of complications to physician.
- Determine patient's emotional needs, including desire for childbearing. Provide emotional support by giving comfort, showing attentiveness and caring. Allow patient to express feelings about condition and risk for death.
- Perform nursing measures, including treatments related to surgery, radiation, chemotherapy, and palliation. See Nursing Interventions under Cancer and under Preoperative and Postoperative Nursing Management.

For more information, see Chapter 47 in Smeltzer and Bare: *Brunner and Suddarth's Textbook of Medical-Surgical Nursing*, 11th edition. Philadelphia: Lippincott Williams & Wilkins, 2008.

Cancer of the Pancreas

Cancer of the pancreas may arise in any portion of the pancreas. Symptoms vary depending on the location of the lesion and whether functioning insulin-secreting pancreatic islet cells are involved. It occurs most frequently in the fifth to seventh decades of life. Risk factors include exposure to industrial chemicals or toxins in the environment; a diet high in fat, meat, or both; and cigarette smoking. Pancreatic cancer is also associated with hereditary pancreatitis, diabetes mellitus, and chronic pancreatitis. Tumors that originate in the head of the pancreas are the most common and obstruct the common bile duct; functioning islet cell tumors are responsible for the syndrome of hyperinsulinism, particularly in islet cell tumors. The pancreas can also be the site of metastasis from other tumors. Pancreatic carcinoma has a 4% survival rate at 5 years, regardless of the stage of disease at diagnosis.

Clinical Manifestations

- Abdominal pain, jaundice, or both are present in 90% of patients. Weight loss is considered a classic sign but often appears only when the disease is far advanced.
- Rapid, profound, and progressive weight loss
- Malabsorption of nutrients and fat-soluble vitamins, anorexia and malaise, and clay-colored stools and dark urine are common with tumors in the head of the pancreas.
- Vague upper or mid-abdominal pain or discomfort unrelated to any gastrointestinal function; radiates as a boring pain in the midback and is more severe at night and when lying supine; pain is often progressive and severe. Ascites is common.
- Meals often aggravate epigastric pain.
- Symptoms of insulin deficiency (diabetes: glucosuria, hyperglycemia, and abnormal glucose tolerance) may be an early sign of carcinoma.
- Gastrointestinal x-rays may show deformities in adjacent viscera related to pancreatic mass.

Assessment and Diagnostic Methods

- MRI, ultrasound, spiral computed tomography (CT), endoscopic retrograde cholangiopancreatography (ERCP) with cell analysis, percutaneous fine-needle biopsy, percutaneous transhepatic cholangiography (PTC), angiography, laparoscopy or duodenography
- Glucose tolerance test to diagnose a pancreatic islet tumor
- Tumor markers are useful indicators of disease progression.

Medical Management

- Surgical procedure is extensive to remove resectable localized tumors (eg, pancreatectomy, Whipple resection).
- Diet high in protein with pancreatic enzymes, adequate hydration, vitamin K, and treatment of anemia with blood components and total parenteral nutrition (PN) may be instituted before surgery when indicated.
- Treatment is often limited to palliative measures owing to widespread metastases, especially to liver, lungs, and bones.
- Radiation and chemotherapy may be used; intraoperative radiation therapy (IORT) or interstitial implantation of radioactive sources may be used for pain relief.
- A biliary stent may be used to relieve jaundice.

Nursing Management

See Preoperative and Postoperative Nursing Management for additional information.

- Provide pain management and attention to nutrition. Be alert for hypoglycemia in patient with pancreatic islet tumor.
- Assist patient to explore all aspects and effects of radiation therapy, chemotherapy, or surgery on an individual basis.
- Provide skin care and measures to relieve pain and discomfort associated with jaundice, anorexia, and profound weight loss.
- Monitor patient postoperatively: vital signs, arterial blood gases and pressures, pulse oximetry, laboratory values, and urine output.
- Provide emotional support to patient and family before, during, and after treatment.
- Discuss patient-controlled analgesia (PCA) for severe, escalating pain.
- If chemotherapy is elected, focus teaching on prevention of side effects and complications of agents used.
- If surgery was performed, teach patient about managing the drainage system and monitoring for complications.

- Teach patient and family strategies to prevent skin breakdown and relieve pain, pruritus, and anorexia, including instruction about PCA, TPN, and diet modification with pancreatic enzymes if indicated because of malabsorption and hyperglycemia. Monitor serum glucose levels if patient had a pancreatic islet tumor.
- Discuss palliative care with patient and family to relieve discomfort, assist with care, and comply with end-of-life decisions.
- Instruct family about changes in patient's status that should be reported to the physician.
- Refer patient for home care for help dealing with problems, discomforts, and psychological effects. Discharge to a long-term care setting with communication to staff about prior teaching.

For more information, see Chapter 40 in Smeltzer and Bare: *Brunner and Suddarth's Textbook of Medical-Surgical Nursing*, 11th edition. Philadelphia: Lippincott Williams & Wilkins, 2008.

Cancer of the Prostate

Cancer of the prostate is the most common cancer in men, the second most common cause of cancer deaths in American men older than 55, and the most prevalent cancer overall in African American men. About 1 in 5 men in the United States develop prostate cancer. Risk factors include increasing age and possibly a high-fat diet.

Clinical Manifestations

- Usually asymptomatic in early stage
- Nodule felt within the substance of the gland or extensive hardening in the posterior lobe

Advanced Stage

C

- Lesion is stony hard and fixed.
- Obstructive symptoms occur late in the disease: difficulty and frequency of urination, urinary retention, decreased size and force of urinary stream.
- Blood in urine or semen; painful ejaculation
- Cancer metastasizes to bone, lymph nodes, brain, and lungs.
- Symptoms of metastases include backache, hip pain, perineal and rectal discomfort, anemia, weight loss, weakness, nausea, and oliguria; hematuria may result from urethral or bladder invasion.
- Sexual dysfunction

Assessment and Diagnostic Methods

- To promote early detection, all men over 50 years of age should have a digital rectal examination (DRE) as part of their regular health checkup. This is the key to a higher cure rate.
- The diagnosis is confirmed by histologic examination of tissue, transurethral resection, open prostatectomy, and fine-needle aspiration.
- Prostate-specific antigen (PSA) level, transrectal ultrasound, bone scan, radiographs, excretory urography, renal function tests, computed tomography (CT) scans, lymphangiography, or monoclonal antibody-based imaging may also be used.

Medical Management

Treatment is based on the stage of the disease and patient's age and symptoms. PSA concentration is used to monitor patient's response to cancer therapy and to detect local progression and early recurrence.

Radical Prostatectomy

- Removal of the prostate and seminal vesicles through suprapubic approach (greater blood loss), perineal

approach (easily contaminated, incontinence, impotence, and rectal injury common), or retropubic approach (infection can readily start).
- This procedure is performed in patients who have potentially curable disease and life expectancy of 10 years of more.
- Sexual impotency and various degrees of urinary incontinence follow radical prostatectomy.

Radiation Therapy

- If cancer is in the early stage, treatment may be curative.
- For locally advanced cancer, hormonal treatments are given before and after radiation.
- Side effects, usually transitory, include inflammation of the rectum, bowel, and bladder.
- There is better preservation of sexual potency, and young patients may prefer this treatment.

Hormone Therapy

- Method of control rather than cure
- Accomplished by either orchiectomy or administration of estrogens
- Diethylstilbestrol (DES) is the most widely used estrogen.
- Luteinizing hormone–releasing hormone (LHRH) agonists and antiandrogen drugs such as flutamide and cyproterone are newer hormonal therapies.

Other Therapies

- Transurethral resection of the prostate (TUR or TURP) or transurethral incision of the prostate (TUIP) for benign condition
- Cryosurgery for those who cannot physically tolerate surgery or for recurrence
- Chemotherapy (doxorubicin, cisplatin, and cyclophosphamide)

- Repeated TUR to keep urethra patent; suprapubic or transurethral catheter drainage when repeat TUR is impractical
- Opioid or nonopioid medications (antiandrogen, prednisone, and mitoxantrone) to control pain with metastasis to bone
- Blood transfusions to maintain adequate hemoglobin levels
- Prosthetic penile implants or other options to create a penile erection for the patient with impotence
- Laparoscopic radical prostatectomy (LAP): a new method, not widespread

NURSING PROCESS: The Patient Undergoing Prostatectomy

Assessment

- Take a complete history, with emphasis on urinary function and the effect of the underlying disorder on patient's lifestyle.
- Note reports of urgency, frequency, nocturia, dysuria, urinary retention, hematuria, or decreased ability to initiate voiding.
- Note family history of cancer, heart disease, or kidney disease, including hypertension.

Diagnosis

Preoperative Nursing Diagnoses

- Anxiety related to inability to void
- Acute pain related to bladder distention
- Deficient knowledge of the problem and treatment protocol

Postoperative Nursing Diagnoses

- Acute pain related to surgical incision, catheter placement, and bladder spasms
- Deficient knowledge about postoperative care

Collaborative Problems/Potential Complications

- Hemorrhage and shock
- Infection
- Deep vein thrombosis
- Catheter obstruction
- Sexual dysfunction

Planning and Goals

The major preoperative goals of the patient may include reduced anxiety and increased knowledge about the prostate problem and the perioperative experience. The major postoperative goals may include correction of fluid volume disturbances, relief of pain and discomfort, ability to perform self-care activities, and absence of complications.

Preoperative Nursing Interventions

Reducing Anxiety

- Provide privacy, and establish a trusting and professional relationship.
- Encourage patient to discuss feelings and concerns.
- Clarify the nature of the surgery and expected postoperative outcomes.

Preparing Patient for Treatment

- Explain diagnostic tests, surgery procedure, and drainage system.
- Answer questions and provide support.
- Establish a private time for patient to review the anatomy and function of affected parts.
- Explain rationale for use of preoperative compression stockings.
- Administer enema, if ordered.

Postoperative Nursing Interventions

Relieving Discomfort

- While patient is on bed rest, administer analgesic agents; initiate measures to relieve anxiety.
- Monitor voiding patterns; watch for bladder distention.
- Insert indwelling catheter if urinary retention is present or if laboratory test results indicate azotemia.
- Prepare patient for a cystostomy if urinary catheter is not tolerated.

See Preoperative and Postoperative Nursing Management for additional information.

Caring for Patient After Treatment

- Distinguish cause and location of pain, including bladder spasms.
- Give analgesic agents for incisional pain and smooth muscle relaxants for bladder spasm.
- Monitor drainage tubing and irrigate drainage system to correct any obstruction.
- Secure catheter to leg or abdomen.
- Monitor dressings, and adjust to ensure they are not too snug or not too saturated or are improperly placed.
- Provide stool softener, prune juice, or an enema, if prescribed.
- Monitor for electrolyte imbalances (eg, hyponatremia).

Monitoring and Managing Complications

- Hemorrhage: observe catheter drainage, note bright-red bleeding with increased viscosity and clots; monitor intake and output and vital signs; administer medications, intravenous fluids, and blood as prescribed. Provide explanations and reassurance to patient and family.
- Infection: assess for urinary tract infection and epididymitis; administer antibiotics as prescribed. Provide sitz bath and heat lamps to promote healing after sutures are removed. Use aseptic technique with dressing changes; avoid rectal thermometers, tubes, and enemas.

- Thrombosis: assess for deep vein thrombosis and pulmonary embolism; apply compression stockings. Assist patient to progress from dangling the day of surgery to ambulating the next morning; encourage patient to walk but not sit for long periods of time. Monitor the patient receiving heparin for excessive bleeding.
- Obstructed catheter: observe lower abdomen for bladder distention. Provide for patent drainage system; perform gentle irrigation as prescribed to remove blood clots.
- Sexual dysfunction: erectile dysfunction, decreased libido, and fatigue may be a concern soon or months after surgery. Medications, surgically placed implants, or negative-pressure devices may help restore function. Reassurance that libido usually returns and fatigue diminishes after recuperation may help. Providing privacy, confidentiality, and time to discuss issues of sexuality is important. Referral to a sex therapist may be indicated.

> **!** **NURSING ALERT** Urine leakage around the wound may be noted after catheter removal.

Promoting Home and Community-Based Care

Teaching Patients Self-Care

- Teach patient and family how to manage drainage system, monitor urinary output, perform wound care, and use strategies to prevent complications.
- Inform patient about signs and symptoms that should be reported to the physician (eg, blood in the urine, decreased urine output, fever, change in wound drainage, or calf tenderness).
- Teach perineal exercises to help regain urinary control.
- As indicated, discuss possible sexual dysfunction (provide a private environment) and refer for counseling.
- Instruct patient not to perform Valsalva maneuver for 6 to 8 weeks because it increases venous pressure and may produce hematuria.
- Urge patient to avoid long car trips and strenuous exercise, which increases tendency to bleed.

C

- Inform patient that spicy foods, alcohol, and coffee can cause bladder discomfort.
- Encourage fluids to avoid dehydration and clot formation.

Continuing Care

- Refer for home care as indicated.
- Remind patient that return of bladder control may take time.

Evaluation

Expected Preoperative Patient Outcomes

- Demonstrates reduced anxiety
- States pain and discomfort are decreased
- Relates understanding of surgical procedure and postoperative care (perineal muscle exercises and bladder control techniques)

Expected Postoperative Patient Outcomes

- Relates relief of discomfort
- Performs self-care measures
- Remains free of complications
- Exhibits fluid and electrolyte balance
- Reports understanding of changes in sexual function

For more information, see Chapter 49 in Smeltzer and Bare: *Brunner and Suddarth's Textbook of Medical-Surgical Nursing*, 11th edition. Philadelphia: Lippincott Williams & Wilkins, 2008.

Cancer of the Skin (Malignant Melanoma)

A malignant melanoma is a malignant neoplasm in which atypical melanocytes (pigment cells) are present in both the epidermis and the dermis (and sometimes the subcutaneous cells). It is the most lethal of all skin cancers. It can occur in one of several forms: superficial spreading melanoma, lentigo-maligna melanoma, nodular melanoma, and acral-lentiginous melanoma.

Most melanomas are derived from cutaneous epidermal melanocytes; some appear in preexisting nevi (moles) in the skin or develop in the uveal tract of the eye. Melanomas occasionally appear simultaneously with cancer of other organs. The incidence and mortality rates of malignant melanoma are increasing, probably related to increased recreational sun exposure and better early detection. Prognosis is related to the depth of dermal invasion and the thickness of the lesion. Malignant melanoma can spread through both the bloodstream and lymphatic system and can metastasize to the bones, liver, lungs, spleen, central nervous system, and lymph nodes.

Risk Factors

The etiology of malignant melanoma is unknown, but ultraviolet rays are strongly suspected. Risk factors include the following:

- Fair complexion, blue eyes, red or blond hair, and freckles
- Celtic or Scandinavian origin
- Tendency to burn and not tan
- Older age; residence in the southwestern United States
- Family history of melanoma, the absence of a gene on chromosome 9P, presence of giant congenital nevi, or significant history of severe sunburn
- Dysplastic nevus syndrome

Clinical Manifestations
Superficial Spreading Melanoma

- Most common form; usually affects middle-aged people, occurs most frequently on trunk and lower extremities
- Circular lesions with irregular outer portions
- Margins of lesion flat or elevated and palpable
- May appear in combination of colors, with hues of tan, brown, and black mixed with gray, bluish-black, or white;

sometimes a dull, pink-rose color is noted in a small area within the lesion

Nodular Melanoma

- Second most common type; spherical, blueberry-like nodule with relatively smooth surface and uniform blue-black color
- May be dome-shaped or have other shadings of red, gray, or purple
- May appear as irregularly shaped plaques
- May be described as a blood blister that fails to resolve
- Invades directly into adjacent dermis (vertical growth); poor prognosis

Lentigo-Maligna Melanoma

- Slowly evolving pigmented lesion
- Occurs on exposed skin areas; head and neck in elderly people
- First appears as tan, flat lesion, which in time undergoes changes in size and color

Acral-Lentiginous Melanoma

- Occurs in areas not excessively exposed to sunlight
- Found on the palms of the hands, soles, in nail beds, and mucous membranes in dark-skinned people
- Appears as an irregular pigmented macule that develops nodules
- Becomes invasive early

Assessment and Diagnostic Methods

- Excisional biopsy specimen, sentinel node biopsy may be performed.
- Chest radiograph, complete blood count, liver function tests, radionuclide or computed tomography (CT) scans are ordered for staging once melanoma is confirmed.

Medical Management

- The therapeutic approach to malignant melanoma depends on the level of invasion and the depth of the lesion. Chemotherapy may be used; hyperthermia may be induced to enhance treatment.
- Immunotherapy (interferon, monoclonal antibodies) may be used, or investigational treatments.
- Laboratory assay of tyrosinase is under investigation for treatment.

Surgical Management

- Surgical excision is the treatment of choice for small superficial lesions.
- Deeper lesions require wide local excision and skin graft.
- A regional lymph node dissection may be performed to rule out metastasis, although newer approaches call for sentenal node biopsy to avoid problems from extensive lymph node removal.
- Debulking the tumor or other palliative procedures may be performed.

NURSING PROCESS: The Patient with Malignant Melanoma

Assessment

Question patient with a lesion specifically about pruritus, tenderness, and pain, which are not features of a benign nevus. Also investigate changes in preexisting moles or development of new pigmented lesions. Assess persons at risk carefully, focusing on the skin:

- Use a magnifying lens to examine for irregularity and changes in the mole.
- Signs that suggest malignant changes include variegated color, irregular border, asymmetry (irregular surface), and large diameter.

- Pay attention to common sites of melanoma (eg, back, legs, between toes, face, feet and scalp, fingernails and backs of hands).
- Measure diameter of mole; melanomas are often larger than 6 mm.

Diagnosis

Nursing Diagnoses

- Acute pain related to surgical incision and grafting
- Anxiety and depression related to possible life-threatening consequences of melanoma and disfigurement
- Deficient knowledge about early signs of melanoma

Collaborative Problems/Potential Complications

- Metastasis
- Infection of surgical site

Planning and Goals

The major goals of the patient may include relief of pain and discomfort, reduced anxiety, knowledge of early signs of melanoma, and absence of complications.

Nursing Interventions

Relieving Pain and Discomfort

Anticipate need for and administer appropriate analgesic agents.

Reducing Anxiety

- Give support, and allow patient to express feelings.
- Convey understanding of anger and depression.
- Answer questions and clarify information during the diagnostic workup and staging of the tumor.
- Point out resources, past effective coping mechanisms, and support systems to help the patient cope with diagnosis and treatment.
- Include immediate family in all discussions to clarify information and provide emotional support.

Teaching Preventive Measures

- Teach patient to recognize early signs of melanoma.
- Instruct patient to examine skin and scalp monthly in an orderly manner using a full-length mirror and a small hand mirror. Have patient determine locations of present moles and birthmarks. Show patient how to inspect moles and other pigmented lesions and immediately report to physician or other care provider moles that change colors, enlarge, become raised or thicker, itch, or bleed.
- Inform patient who has had a malignant melanoma to have lifelong follow-up; these persons are at higher risk for developing a second one.
- Teach patient and family to avoid exposure to sunlight.

Monitoring and Managing Potential Complications: Metastasis

- Educate patient about treatment and deliver supportive care; provide and clarify information: present treatment is largely unsuccessful, and cure is generally not possible; surgical intervention may be performed to debulk the tumor or to remove part of the organ involved; more extensive surgery is for relief of symptoms, not for cure; chemotherapy may be effective in controlling metastasis.
- Provide time for patient to express fears and concerns about the future.
- Arrange for hospice and palliative care services.
- Encourage patient to have hope in the therapy while being realistic.
- Offer information about support groups and contact people.
- See Cancer overview for additional nursing care measures.

Evaluation

Expected Patient Outcomes

- Experiences relief of pain and discomfort
- Achieves reduced anxiety

- Demonstrates understanding of disease and melanoma detection methods

C

- Experiences absence of complications

For more information, see Chapter 56 in Smeltzer and Bare: *Brunner and Suddarth's Textbook of Medical-Surgical Nursing*, 11th edition. Philadelphia: Lippincott Williams & Wilkins, 2008.

Cancer of the Stomach (Gastric Cancer)

Cancer of the stomach is usually adenocarcinoma. It typically occurs in males and people older than age 40 (occasionally in younger people). Most stomach cancers occur in the lesser curvature or antrum of the stomach and infiltrate surrounding mucosa, stomach wall, adjacent organs, and structures. The incidence of gastric cancer is much greater in Japan. Diet appears to be a significant factor (ie, high in smoked foods and lacking in fruits and vegetables). Other factors related to the incidence of stomach cancer include chronic inflammation of the stomach, pernicious anemia, achlorhydria, gastric ulcers, *Helicobacter pylori* bacteria, and heredity. Prognosis is poor because most patients have metastases (liver, pancreas, and esophagus or duodenum) at the time of diagnosis.

Clinical Manifestations

- Early stages: symptoms may be absent or may resemble those of patients with benign ulcers (eg, pain relieved with antacids)
- Progressive disease: symptoms include indigestion, anorexia, dyspepsia, weight loss, abdominal pain (usually a late symptom), constipation, anemia, nausea and vomiting, and ascites (with metastasis to liver)

Assessment and Diagnostic Methods

- Radiography of upper gastrointestinal system with barium
- Endoscopy for biopsy and cytologic washings
- Computed tomography (CT) scan, bone scan, and liver scan to determine extent of metastasis
- Complete radiographic examination of the gastrointestinal tract if dyspepsia of more than 4 weeks' duration in any person older than 40 years of age

Medical Management

- Removal of gastric carcinoma; curative if tumor can be removed while still localized to the stomach
- Effective palliation (to prevent symptoms such as obstruction) by resection of the tumor; radical subtotal gastrectomy; total gastrectomy with anastomosis of esophagus and jejunum
- Chemotherapy for further disease control or for palliation (5-fluorouracil, doxorubicin [Adriamycin], mitomycin C)
- Radiation for palliation
- Tumor marker assessment to determine treatment effectiveness

NURSING PROCESS: The Patient with Stomach Cancer

Assessment

- Elicit history of dietary intake (intake of smoked or cured foods and of fruits and vegetables).
- Identify weight loss, including time frame and amount; assess appetite and eating habits; include pain assessment.
- Obtain cigarette smoking history: how many a day, how long has patient been smoking, any stomach discomfort during or after smoking?
- Obtain history of alcohol intake: how much?

- Obtain family history of cancer (first- or second-degree relatives).
- Assess psychosocial support (marital status, coping skills, emotional and financial resources).
- Perform complete physical examination (palpate and percuss abdomen for tenderness, masses, or ascites).

Diagnosis

Nursing Diagnoses

- Anxiety related to disease and anticipated treatment
- Imbalanced nutrition: Less than body requirements related to anorexia
- Pain related to abnormal epithelial cells
- Anticipatory grieving related to diagnosis of cancer
- Deficient knowledge regarding self-care activities

Planning and Goals

The major goals of the patient include reduced anxiety, optimal nutrition, relief of pain, and adjustment to the diagnosis and to anticipated lifestyle changes.

Nursing Interventions

Reducing Anxiety

- Provide a relaxed, nonthreatening atmosphere (helps patient express fears, concerns, and anger).
- Encourage family in efforts to support the patient, offering assurance and supporting positive coping measures.
- Advise about any procedures and treatments.
- Suggest that patient discuss feelings with support person (eg, spiritual advisor), if desired.

Promoting Optimal Nutrition

- Encourage small, frequent feedings of nonirritating foods to decrease gastric irritation.
- Facilitate tissue repair by ensuring food supplements are high in calories and vitamins A and C and iron.

- Administer parenteral vitamin B_{12} indefinitely if a total gastrectomy is performed.
- Monitor rate and frequency of intravenous therapy.
- Record intake, output, and daily weights.
- Assess signs of dehydration (thirst, dry mucous membranes, poor skin turgor, tachycardia, decreased urine output).
- Review results of daily laboratory studies to note any metabolic abnormalities (sodium, potassium, glucose, blood urea nitrogen).
- Administer antiemetic agents as prescribed.

Relieving Pain

- Administer analgesic agents as prescribed (continuous infusion of an opioid).
- Assess frequency, intensity, and duration of pain to determine effectiveness of analgesic agent.
- Work with patient to help manage pain (eg, position changes, decreased environmental stimuli, restricted visiting).
- Suggest nonpharmacologic methods for pain relief (eg, imagery, distraction, relaxation tapes, back rubs, and massage).
- Encourage periods of rest and relaxation.

Providing Psychosocial Support

- Help patient express fears and concerns about diagnosis.
- Allow patient freedom to grieve; answer patient's questions honestly.
- Encourage patient to participate in treatment decisions.
- Support patient's disbelief and time needed to accept diagnosis.
- Offer emotional support, and involve family members and significant others whenever possible; reassure that emotional responses are normal and expected.
- Be aware of mood swings and defense mechanisms (denial, rationalization, displacement, regression).
- Provide professional services as necessary (eg, clergy, psychiatric clinical nurse specialists, psychologists, social workers, and psychiatrists).

C

- Assist patient and family with decisions regarding end-of-life care.

Promoting Home and Community-Based Care

See Nursing Management under Cancer for additional information.

Teaching Patients Self-Care

- Teach self-care activities specific to treatment regimen.
- Include information about diet and nutrition, treatment regimens, activity and lifestyle changes, pain management, and complications for which to observe.
- Explain that the possibility of dumping syndrome exists with any enteral feeding, and teach ways to manage it.
- Explain need for daily rest periods and frequent visits to physician after discharge.
- Refer for home care; nurse can supervise any enteral or parenteral feeding and teach patient and family members how to use equipment and formulas as well as how to detect complications.
- Teach patient to record daily intake and output and weight.
- Teach patient how to cope with pain, nausea, vomiting, and bloating.
- Teach patient to recognize and report complications that require medical attention, such as bleeding (overt or covert hematemesis, melena), obstruction, perforation, or any symptoms that become consistently worse.
- Teach patient how to care for incision and how to examine the wound for signs of infection.
- Explain chemotherapy or radiation regimen and the care needed during and after treatment.

For more information, see Chapter 37 in Smeltzer and Bare: *Brunner and Suddarth's Textbook of Medical-Surgical Nursing*, 11th edition. Philadelphia: Lippincott Williams & Wilkins, 2008.

Cancer of the Testis

Testicular cancer is the most common cancer in men 15 to 35 years of age and the second most common cancer in men aged 35 to 39 years. Testicular cancer is classified as germinal or nongerminal. Most neoplasms are germinal (90%), arising from the germinal cells of the testes. Germinal tumors may be further classified as seminomas (remain localized) and fast-growing nonseminomas (teratocarcinomas, choriocarcinomas, yolk sac carcinomas, and embryonal carcinomas). Secondary testicular tumors (lymphoma) metastasize from other organs. Nongerminal tumors arise from the epithelium. The cause of testicular tumors is unknown, but cryptorchidism, infections, and genetic and endocrine factors appear to play a part in their development. Testicular tumors are usually malignant and tend to metastasize early, spreading from the testicles to the lymph nodes in the retroperitoneum and to the lungs.

Clinical Manifestations

- Symptoms appear gradually, with a mass or lump on the testicle.
- Painless enlargement of the testis occurs; patient may complain of heaviness in the scrotum, inguinal area, or lower abdomen.
- Backache, pain in the abdomen, loss of weight, and general weakness may result from metastasis.

Assessment and Diagnostic Methods

- Testicular self-examination (TSE) is an effective early detection method.
- Elevated alpha-fetoprotein and human chorionic gonadotropin levels are used as tumor markers.
- Tumor marker levels are used for diagnosis, staging, and monitoring the response to treatment.

- Intravenous urography, lymphangiography, ultrasound, computed tomography scan, MRI, PET scan, and surgical biopsy

Medical Management

The goals of management are to eradicate the disease and achieve a cure. Treatment is based on cell type and the anatomic extent of the disease.

- Orchiectomy and retroperitoneal lymph node dissection (RPLND)
- Sperm banking before surgery is suggested.
- Postoperative irradiation of the lymph nodes from the iliac region to the diaphragm to treat seminomas
- Chemotherapy
- Good results may be obtained by combining different types of treatments, including surgery, radiation therapy, and chemotherapy.

Nursing Management

See Nursing Management under Cancer for additional information.

- Address issues related to body image and sexuality.
- Encourage patient to maintain a positive attitude during therapy.
- Inform patient that radiation therapy will not necessarily cause infertility, nor does unilateral excision of a tumor necessarily decrease virility.
- Encourage follow-up evaluation studies and continual TSE (a patient with a history of one tumor of the testis has a greater chance of developing subsequent tumors).

For more information, see Chapter 49 in Smeltzer and Bare: *Brunner and Suddarth's Textbook of Medical-Surgical Nursing*, 11th edition. Philadelphia: Lippincott Williams & Wilkins, 2008.

Cancer of the Thyroid

Cancer of the thyroid is less prevalent than other forms of cancer. The most common type, papillary adenocarcinoma, accounts for more than half of thyroid malignancies; it starts in childhood or early adult life, remains localized, and eventually metastasizes. When papillary adenocarcinoma occurs in an elderly patient, it is more aggressive. Risk factors include female gender and external irradiation of the head, neck, or chest in infancy and childhood. Follicular adenocarcinoma usually appears in patients older than 40 years of age.

Clinical Manifestations

Lesions that are single, hard, and fixed on palpation or that are associated with cervical lymphadenopathy suggest malignancy.

Assessment and Diagnostic Methods

- Needle biopsy or aspiration biopsy of thyroid gland
- Thyroid function tests
- Ultrasound, magnetic resonance imaging (MRI), computed tomography (CT), thyroid scans, radioactive iodine uptake studies, and thyroid suppression tests

Medical Management

- Treatment of choice is surgical removal (total or near-total thyroidectomy).
- Modified or extensive radical neck dissection is done if lymph nodes are involved.
- Radioactive iodine (^{131}I) is used to eradicate residual thyroid tissue.
- Thyroid hormone is administered in suppressive doses after surgery to lower the levels of thyroid-stimulating hormone (TSH) to a euthyroid state.
- Lifelong thyroxine (T_4) is required if remaining thyroid tissue is inadequate to produce sufficient hormone.

- Radiation therapy is administered by several routes.
- Chemotherapy is used only occasionally.

Nursing Management

See Nursing Management under Cancer for additional information.

- Encourage follow-up for recurrence of cancer: total-body scans are done 2 to 4 months and 1 year after surgery. If measurements are stable, a final scan is obtained in 3 to 5 years.
- Before planned total body scans, stop thyroid hormones for 6 weeks.
- Monitor FT_4, TSH, serum calcium, and phosphorus levels to determine if thyroid supplementation is adequate, and maintain calcium balance.
- Provide instructions about the need to take exogenous thyroid hormone.
- Reinforce that surgery combined with radioiodine produces a higher survival rate than surgery alone.
- Instruct in assessment and management of side effects of radiation therapy.

For more information, see Chapter 42 in Smeltzer and Bare: *Brunner and Suddarth's Textbook of Medical-Surgical Nursing*, 11th edition. Philadelphia: Lippincott Williams & Wilkins, 2008.

Cancer of the Vagina

Cancer of the vagina usually results from metastasized choriocarcinoma or from cancer of the cervix or adjacent organs, such as the uterus, vulva, bladder, or rectum. Primary cancer of the vagina is squamous in origin. Risk factors include cervical cancer, in utero exposure to diethylstilbestrol (DES), previous vaginal or vulvar cancer, previous radiation therapy, and a history of human papillomavirus (HPV) or of pessary use.

Clinical Manifestations

- Often asymptomatic, but slight bleeding after intercourse may be reported.
- Spontaneous bleeding, vaginal discharge, pain, urinary or rectal symptoms

Assessment and Diagnostic Methods

- Colposcopy for women exposed to DES in utero
- Pap smear of the vagina

Medical Management

- Laser treatment, chemotherapeutic cream, and radiation therapy, depending on the extent of the disease
- Surgery: radical node dissection (local excision) followed by radiation therapy

Nursing Management

- Encourage close follow-up by health care providers.
- Provide emotional support.
- Teach specific vaginal dilating procedures for women who have had vaginal reconstructive surgery.
- Inform patient that water-soluble lubricants are helpful in reducing dyspareunia.

For more information, see Chapter 47 in Smeltzer and Bare: *Brunner and Suddarth's Textbook of Medical-Surgical Nursing*, 11th edition. Philadelphia: Lippincott Williams & Wilkins, 2008.

Cancer of the Vulva

Primary cancer of the vulva is seen mostly in postmenopausal women, but its incidence in younger women is rising. More whites than nonwhites are affected. Squamous cell carcinoma accounts for most primary vulvar tumors. The median age for cancer limited to the vulva is 44 years; the median age for invasive vulvar cancer is 61 years. Little is known about what causes this disease; however, smoking, HPV and HIV infections, immunosuppression, and chronic vulvar irritation may contribute.

Clinical Manifestations

- Long-standing pruritus and soreness are the most common symptoms; itching occurs in half of all patients.
- Bleeding, foul-smelling discharge, and pain are signs of advanced disease.
- Early lesions appear as chronic dermatitis; later, a lump that continues to grow and becomes a hard, ulcerated, cauliflower-like growth.

Assessment and Diagnostic Methods

- Vulvar examination
- Biopsy

Medical Management

- Preinvasive (vulvar carcinoma in situ): local excision, laser vaporization (ablation), chemotherapeutic creams (fluorouracil), or cryosurgery
- Invasive: wide excision or vulvectomy (primary treatment), radiation (unresectable tumors), radical vulvectomy with bilateral groin dissection

NURSING PROCESS: The Patient Undergoing a Vulvectomy

Assessment

- Develop a rapport with patient; ascertain her health habits and receptivity for learning.
- Give preoperative preparation and psychological encouragement.

Diagnosis

Nursing Diagnoses

- Anxiety related to diagnosis and surgery
- Impaired skin integrity related to wound and drainage
- Acute pain related to surgical incision and subsequent wound care
- Sexual dysfunction related to change in body part
- Self-care deficit related to lack of understanding of perineal care and general health status.

Collaborative Problems/Potential Complications

- Wound infection and sepsis
- Deep vein thrombosis
- Hemorrhage

Planning and Goals

Goals for the patient may include acceptance of and preparation for surgical intervention, recovery of optimal sexual function, ability to perform adequate and appropriate self-care, and absence of complications.

Nursing Interventions: Preoperative

Relieving Anxiety

- Allow patient time to talk and ask questions.
- Advise patient that the possibility of having sexual relations is good and that pregnancy is possible after a wide excision.
- Reinforce information about the surgery, and address patient's questions and concerns.

Nursing Interventions: Postoperative

Relieving Pain and Discomfort

- Administer analgesic agents prophylactically.
- Position patient to relieve tension on incision (pillow under knees or low Fowler's position), and give soothing back rubs.

Improving Skin Integrity

- Provide pressure-reducing mattress.
- Install over-bed trapeze.
- Protect intact skin from drainage and moisture.
- Monitor for accumulation of purulent material (suppuration) under graft.
- Assist patient to keep perineal area clean and dry (warm saline or antiseptic irrigation).
- Assess and document surgical site characteristics and drainage.

Supporting Positive Sexuality and Sexual Function

- Establish a trusting relationship with patient.
- Encourage patient to share and discuss concerns with sexual partner.
- Consult with surgeon to clarify expected changes.
- Refer patient and partner to a sex counselor, as indicated.

Monitoring and Managing Potential Complications

- Monitor closely for local and systemic signs and symptoms of infection: purulent drainage, redness, increased pain, fever, increased white blood cell count.
- Assist in obtaining tissue specimens for culture.
- Administer antibiotics as prescribed.
- Avoid cross-contamination; carefully handle catheters, drains, and dressings; handwashing is crucial.
- Provide a low-residue diet to prevent straining on defecation and wound contamination.
- Discourage sitz baths because of risk for infection.
- Assess for signs and symptoms of deep vein thrombosis and pulmonary embolism; apply elastic compression stockings; encourage ankle exercises.
- Encourage and assist in frequent position changes, avoiding pressure behind the knees.
- Monitor closely for signs of hemorrhage and hypovolemic shock.

Promoting Home and Community-Based Care
Teaching Patients Self-Care

- Encourage patient to share concerns as she recovers.
- Encourage participation in dressing changes and self-care.
- Give complete instructions to family member or other who will provide posthospital care regarding wound care, urinary catheterization, and possible complications.

Continuing Care

- Encourage communication with home care nurse to ensure continuity of care.
- Reinforce teaching with follow-up call between home visits.

Evaluation

Expected Patient Outcomes

- Adjusts to the trauma of the surgical experience
- Obtains pain relief
- Maintains skin integrity
- Exhibits positive outlook about sexuality and sexual functioning
- Increases participation in self-care activities
- Experiences no complications

For more information, see Chapter 47 in Smeltzer and Bare: *Brunner and Suddarth's Textbook of Medical-Surgical Nursing*, 11th edition. Philadelphia: Lippincott Williams & Wilkins, 2008.

Cardiac Arrest

Cardiac arrest occurs when the heart suddenly ceases to produce an effective pulse and circulate blood. All heart action may stop (asystole), asynchronized muscle twitchings (tachycardia or ventricular fibrillation) may occur, or a slow heart rate (bradycardia or AV block) may occur. Cardiac arrest may also result when electrical activity is present but there is ineffective cardiac contraction or circulating volume. This is called pulseless electrical activity (PEA).

With arrest comes immediate loss of consciousness and absence of pulses, audible heart sounds, and blood pressure. Dilation of the pupils begins within 45 seconds. Ineffective respiratory gasping may occur. Seizures may or may not occur.

Clinical Manifestations

An interval of about 4 minutes occurs between cessation of circulation and development of irreversible brain damage. The interval varies with the age of the patient. During this period, the diagnosis of cardiac arrest must be made and circulation restored. The most reliable sign of arrest is the absence of a carotid pulse.

> **NURSING ALERT** In the adult and the child, the carotid pulse is assessed. In an infant, the brachial pulse is assessed. Do not waste valuable time taking the blood pressure, listening for the heartbeat, or checking proper contact of electrodes.

Management

- Initiate immediate cardiopulmonary resuscitation (CPR).
- Institute follow-up monitoring once patient is resuscitated.

For more information, see Chapter 30 in Smeltzer and Bare: *Brunner and Suddarth's Textbook of Medical-Surgical Nursing*, 11th edition. Philadelphia: Lippincott Williams & Wilkins, 2008.

Cardiomyopathies

The cardiomyopathies are a group of diseases that affect the structure and function of the myocardium. The types of cardiomyopathies are classified according to the structural and functional abnormalities of the heart muscle: (1) dilated or congestive cardiomyopathy (most common); (2) hypertrophic cardiomyopathy (obstructive or nonobstructive); (3) restrictive cardiomyopathy (rarest); (4) arrhythmogenic right ventricular cardiomyopathy (ARVC); and (5) unclassified cardiomyopathy. These diseases lead to severe heart failure, significant dysrhythmias, and often death. Ischemic cardiomyopathy is a term frequently used to describe an enlarged heart caused by coronary artery disease, which is usually accompanied by heart failure. The condition may occur at any age and affects both men and women

Pathophysiology

Cardiomyopathy is a series of progressive events that culminate in impaired pumping of the left ventricle, which enlarges to accommodate the demands of increased systemic vascular resistance and eventually fails. Failure of the right ventricle usually accompanies this process.

Clinical Manifestations

- Presents initially with signs and symptoms of heart failure (shortness of breath on exertion, paroxysmal nocturnal dyspnea [PND], cough, chest pain, palpitations, fatigue, dizziness, and syncope)
- Systemic venous congestion, jugular vein distention, pitting edema of dependent body parts, hepatic engorgement, and tachycardia on physical examination

Assessment and Diagnostic Methods

- Patient history; rule out other causes of failure
- Electrocardiogram (ECG), chest radiograph, echocardiogram, cardiac catheterization, and possibly an endomyocardial biopsy

Medical Management

- Medical management is directed toward determining and managing possible underlying or precipitating causes,

C

correcting the heart failure with medications, and controlling dysrhythmias, possibly with an implanted defibrillator or pacemaker.
- Surgical intervention, including a myectomy, or heart transplantation (an orthotopic transplant is the most common) is considered when heart failure has progressed beyond being medically responsive.
- In some cases, ventricular assist devices (eg, a left ventricular assist device [LVAD]) are necessary to support the failing heart until a suitable donor becomes available.

NURSING PROCESS: The Patient with a Cardiac Myopathy

Assessment

- Take detailed history of presenting signs and symptoms and possible etiologic factors.
- Careful psychosocial history: identify family support system and involve family in patient management
- Physical assessment directed toward signs and symptoms of heart failure. Evaluate fluid volume status, vital signs (pulse pressure), pulmonary auscultation for crackles, auscultation for a systolic murmur and S_3 and S_4 heart sounds, and palpation for a shift to the left of the point of maximum impulse.
- Use cardiac monitor if dysrhythmia is a significant problem.

Diagnosis

Nursing Diagnoses

- Decreased cardiac output related to structural disorders secondary to cardiomyopathy or dysrhythmia
- Ineffective tissue perfusion related to decreased peripheral blood flow
- Impaired gas exchange related to pulmonary congestion secondary to myocardial failure
- Activity intolerance related to excessive fluid volume

- Anxiety related to disease process
- Powerlessness related to disease process
- Noncompliance with self-care program

Collaborative Problems/Potential Complications

- Cardiac failure
- Ventricular and atrial dysrhythmias
- Cardiac conduction defects
- Pulmonary or cerebral embolism
- Valvular dysfunction

Planning and Goals

Major goals of the patient include improved or maintained cardiac output, increased activity tolerance, reduced anxiety, adherence to the self-care program, increased sense of power with decision making, and absence of complications.

Nursing Interventions

Improving Cardiac Output and Relieving Respiratory Difficulties

- Assist patient into a resting position (usually sitting with legs down) during a symptomatic episode.
- Administer oxygen if indicated.
- Note and document patient's response (daily weight, oxygen saturation); correlate interventions with patient's response.
- Administer prescribed medications on time.
- Assist patient to rest at the bedside in a chair for most comfort.
- Keep patient warm, and change positions frequently to stimulate circulation and reduce skin breakdown.
- Promote low-sodium meals and adequate fluid intake.

Increasing Activity Tolerance

- Plan nursing care so that activities occur in cycles, alternating rest with activity.
- Help patient learn to conserve energy.

Reducing Anxiety

- Provide patient with appropriate information about signs and symptoms.
- Provide an atmosphere in which the patient feels free to verbalize fears.
- Assist patient to accomplish a goal, no matter how small, to enhance a sense of well-being.
- Provide time for the patient to discuss concerns if facing death or awaiting transplantation.
- Give spiritual, psychological, and emotional support.
- Establish trust with patient, and provide realistic hope to reduce anxiety while awaiting a donor heart.

Reducing Sense of Powerlessness

- Assist patient in identifying things he or she has lost (eg, foods enjoyed).
- Assist patient in identifying emotional responses to the loss (eg, anger and depression).
- Assist patient in identifying the amount of control that he or she still has (eg, selecting food choices).

Promoting Home and Community-Based Care

Teaching Patients Self-Care

- Teach patient what self-care activities are necessary and how to perform them at home.
- Maintain attention to a medication program and dietary restrictions to prevent cardiac failure.
- Allow patient and significant others the freedom to begin the grieving process when they can no longer be helped by any therapeutic technique.

Continuing Care

- Refer patient for home care and support.
- Teach patient about medication regimen and dietary and fluid restrictions.
- Assist in review of lifestyle, and suggest strategies to incorporate therapeutic activities to balance lifestyle and work.

- Teach patient and family symptoms that should be reported to the physician.
- Establish trust with patient, and provide support during end-of-life decision making.

Evaluation

Expected Patient Outcomes

- Demonstrates improved cardiac function
- Increases activity tolerance
- Experiences reduction of anxiety
- Complies with self-care program

For more information, see Chapter 29 in Smeltzer and Bare: *Brunner and Suddarth's Textbook of Medical-Surgical Nursing*, 11th edition. Philadelphia: Lippincott Williams & Wilkins, 2008.

Cataract

A cataract is an opacity of the eye's normally clear, transparent crystalline lens. It is commonly associated with aging (senile cataracts) but can develop at any age. It may also be associated with blunt or penetrating trauma, long-term corticosteroid use, systemic disease such as diabetes mellitus, hypoparathyroidism, radiation exposure, exposure to long hours of bright sunlight (ultraviolet light), or other eye disorders. Vision impairment depends on the size, density, and location in the lens.

Clinical Manifestations

- Diminished visual acuity, disabling sensitivity to glare, painless, dimmed or blurred vision with distortion of images, poor night vision. Other effects include myopic shift, astigmatism, monocular diplopia (double vision), color shift (aging lens becomes progressively more absorbent at the blue end of the spectrum), brunescence (color values shift to yellow brown), and reduced light transmission.

- Yellowish, gray, or white pupil
- Develops gradually over a period of years; as the cataract worsens, stronger glasses no longer improve sight
- May develop in both eyes, although one is more compromised than the other

Assessment and Diagnostic Methods

- Degree of visual acuity is directly proportionate to density of the cataract.
- Snellen visual acuity test
- Ophthalmoscopy
- Slit-lamp biomicroscopic examination
- A-scan ultrasonography

Medical Management

There is no medical treatment for cataracts, although use of vitamins C and E and beta-carotene is being investigated. Glasses or contact, bifocal, or magnifying lenses may improve vision. Mydriatics can be used short term, but glare is increased.

Surgical Management

Two surgical techniques are available: intracapsular cataract extraction (ICCE) and extracapsular cataract extraction (ECCE) including phacoemulsification. Less than 15% of people with cataracts require surgery.

Indications for surgery are loss of vision that interferes with normal activities or a cataract that is causing glaucoma. Cataracts are removed under local anesthesia on an outpatient basis. Lens replacement may involve aphakic eyeglasses, contact lens, and intraocular lens (IOL) implants. When both eyes have cataracts, one eye is surgically treated at a time.

Nursing Management

- Because surgery is performed on an outpatient basis, instruct patient to make arrangements for transportation home, care that evening, and a follow-up visit to the surgeon the next day.
- Withhold any anticoagulants the patient is receiving, if medically appropriate. In some cases, anticoagulant therapy may continue.
- Administer dilating drops every 10 minutes for four doses at least 1 hour before surgery. Antibiotic, corticosteroid, and NSAID drops may be administered prophylactically to prevent postoperative infection and inflammation.
- Instruct patient to wear a protective eye shield for 24 hours after surgery to prevent accidental rubbing or poking of the eye. After 24 hours, eyeglasses (sunglasses in bright light) should be worn during the day and a metal shield worn at night for 1 to 4 weeks.
- Provide postoperative discharge teaching concerning eye medications, cleansing and protection, activity level and restrictions, diet, pain control, positioning, office appointments, expected postoperative course, and symptoms to report immediately to the surgeon.
- Instruct patient to restrict bending and lifting heavy objects.
- Caution patient that vision may blur for several days to weeks.
- Inform patient that vision gradually improves as the eye heals; IOL implants improve vision faster than glasses or contact lenses.
- Reinforce that vision correction is usually needed for remaining visual acuity deficit.

For more information, see Chapter 58 in Smeltzer and Bare: *Brunner and Suddarth's Textbook of Medical-Surgical Nursing*, 11th edition. Philadelphia: Lippincott Williams & Wilkins, 2008.

Cerebral Vascular Accident (Ischemic Stroke)

A cerebrovascular accident (CVA), an ischemic stroke or "brain attack," is a sudden loss of brain function resulting from a disruption of the blood supply to a part of the brain. It is usually the result of long-standing cerebrovascular disease. Stroke is the primary neurologic problem in the United States and in the world. Strokes are usually hemorrhagic (15%) or ischemic/nonhemorrhagic (85%). Ischemic strokes are categorized according to their cause: large artery thrombosis (20%), small penetrating artery thrombosis (25%), cardiogenic embolic stroke, cryptogenic (30%), and others (5%). Cryptogenic strokes have no known cause, and other strokes result from causes such as cocaine use, coagulopathies, migraine, and spontaneous dissection of the carotid or vertebral arteries. The result is an interruption in the blood supply to the brain, causing temporary or permanent loss of movement, thought, memory, speech, or sensation.

Strokes are also classified by time course as follows: (1) transient ischemic attack, (2) reversible ischemic neurologic deficit, (3) stroke in evolution, and (4) completed stroke.

Risk Factors

- Hemorrhagic strokes are caused by arteriovenous malformations (AVMs), aneurysm ruptures, certain drugs, uncontrolled hypertension, hemangioblastomas, and trauma. These strokes can occur in epidural, subarachnoid, or intracerebral hemorrhage.
- Ischemic strokes can be caused by cardiovascular disease (cerebral embolism may originate in the heart) and dysrhythmia (atrial fibrillation); risk factors for coronary artery disease apply to stroke as well. Ischemic stroke can also be caused by vasospasm, migraines, and coagulopathies (eg, high hematocrit).

- General cerebral ischemia may be caused by excessive or prolonged drop in blood pressure.
- Drug abuse (cocaine) can cause stroke, particularly in adolescents and young adults.
- Alcohol consumption may also be a risk factor.

Clinical Manifestations

General signs and symptoms include numbness or weakness of face, arm, or leg; confusion or change in mental status; trouble speaking or understanding speech; visual disturbances, loss of balance, dizziness, difficulty walking, or sudden severe headache.

Motor Loss

- Hemiplegia, hemiparesis
- Flaccid paralysis and loss of or decrease in the deep tendon reflexes (initial clinical feature) followed by (after 48 hours) abnormally increased muscle tone (spasticity)

Communication Loss

- Dysarthria (difficulty speaking)
- Dysphasia or aphasia (defective speech or loss of speech)
- Apraxia (inability to perform a previously learned action)

Perceptual Disturbances and Sensory Loss

- Visual perceptual dysfunctions (homonymous hemianopia [loss of half of the visual field])
- Disturbances in visuospatial relationships (perceiving the relation of two or more objects in spatial areas), frequently seen in patients with left hemispheric damage
- Sensory losses: slight impairment of touch or more severe with loss of proprioception, difficulty in interrupting visual, tactile, and auditory stimuli

Impaired Cognitive and Psychological Effects

- Frontal lobe damage: learning capacity, memory, or other higher cortical intellectual functions may be impaired. Such dysfunction may be reflected in a limited attention span, difficulties in comprehension, forgetfulness, and lack of motivation.
- Depression, other psychological problems: emotional lability, hostility, frustration, resentment, and lack of cooperation

Bladder Dysfunction

- Transient urinary incontinence
- Persistent urinary incontinence or urinary retention (may be symptomatic of bilateral brain damage)
- Continuing bladder and bowel incontinence (may reflect extensive neurologic damage)

Assessment and Diagnostic Methods

- Complete physical and neurologic examination
- Noncontrast computed tomography (CT) or magnetic resonance imaging (MRI) scan, transthoracic or transesophageal echocardiogram, SPECT scan
- Carotid ultrasonography
- Cerebral angiography
- Transcranial Doppler flow studies
- Electrocardiography
- Echocardiography

Prevention

- Help patients alter risk factors for stroke.
- Prepare and support patient through carotid endarterectomy.
- Administer anticoagulant agents as ordered (eg, low-dose aspirin therapy).

Medical Management

- Recombinant tissue plasminogen activator (t-PA), unless contraindicated; monitor for bleeding
- Management of increased intracranial pressure: osmotic diuretics, maintain $PaCO_2$ at 30 to 35 mm Hg, avoid hypoxia, elevate head of bed (to promote venous drainage and to lower increased ICP), pulmonary toilet with supplemental oxygen, airway patency
- Intubation with an endotracheal tube to establish a patent airway, if necessary
- Maintain cardiac output at 4 to 8 L/min.
- Anticoagulation therapy
- Carotid endarterectomy (for managing transient ischemic attacks and small stroke)

Management of Complications

- Cerebral hypoxia: administer supplemental oxygen, maintain hemoglobin and hematocrit at acceptable levels
- Decreased cerebral blood flow and extension of the area of injury: adequate hydration, avoid hypertension or hypotension, maintain patent airway, administer oxygen
- Monitor for urinary tract infections, cardiac dysrhythmias, immobility.

NURSING PROCESS: The Patient with CVA

Assessment

Weigh patient (used to determine medication dosages), and maintain a neurologic flow sheet to reflect the following nursing assessment parameters:

- Change in level of responsiveness, ability to speak, and orientation

C

- Presence or absence of voluntary or involuntary movements of the extremities: muscle tone, body posture, and head position
- Stiffness or flaccidity of the neck
- Eye opening, comparative size of pupils and pupillary reactions to light, and ocular position
- Color of face and extremities; temperature and moisture of skin
- Quality and rates of pulse and respiration; arterial blood gases, body temperature, and arterial pressure
- Volume of fluids ingested or administered and volume of urine excreted per 24 hours
- Signs of bleeding
- Blood pressure maintained within normal limits

Assessment After t-PA Therapy

Obtain vital signs every 15 minutes for the first 2 hours, every 30 minutes for the next 6 hours, then every hour for 16 hours. Blood pressure should be maintained with the systolic pressure less than 180 mm Hg and the diastolic pressure less than 100 mm Hg to prevent bleeding.

Acute Phase (24 to 72 Hours)

- Maintain airway and adequate ventilation.
- Maintain a neurologic flow sheet assessing level of consciousness, responsiveness, ability to speak, orientation, eye opening, pupillary response, voluntary/involuntary movement, muscle tone, body posture, neck stiffness or flaccidity, color of face and extremities; temperature and moisture of skin.
- Assess quality and rates of pulse and respiration; arterial blood gas values as indicated, body temperature, and arterial pressure.
- Monitor volume of fluids ingested or administered, volume of urine excreted each 24 hours.
- Note any bleeding.
- Elevate head of bed.

- Maintain endotracheal intubation and mechanical ventilation.
- Monitor for pulmonary complications (aspiration, atelectasis, pneumonia).
- Examine heart for abnormalities in size and rhythm and signs of heart failure.

Postacute Phase

Assess the following functions:

- Mental status (memory, attention span, perception, orientation, affect, speech and language)
- Sensation and perception (usually patient has decreased awareness of pain and temperature)
- Motor control (upper and lower extremity movement); swallowing ability, nutritional and hydration status, skin integrity, activity tolerance, and bowel and bladder function
- Continue focusing nursing assessment on impairment of function in patient's daily activities (baseline with an instrument such as the functional independence measure [FIM]).

Diagnosis

Nursing Diagnoses

- Impaired physical mobility related to hemiparesis, loss of balance and coordination, spasticity, and brain injury
- Acute pain related to hemiplegia and disuse
- Deficient self-care (hygiene, toileting, transfers, feeding) related to stroke sequelae
- Disturbed sensory perception
- Impaired swallowing
- Total urinary incontinence related to flaccid bladder, detrusor instability, confusion, difficulty in communicating
- Disturbed thought processes related to brain damage, confusion, inability to follow instructions
- Impaired verbal communication related to brain damage, confusion, inability to follow instructions
- Risk for impaired skin integrity related to hemiparesis or hemiplegia, decreased mobility

- Interrupted family processes related to catastrophic illness and caregiving burdens
- Sexual dysfunction related to neurologic deficits or fear of failure

Collaborative Problems/Potential Complications

Pneumonia; decreased cerebral blood flow due to increased intracranial pressure; inadequate oxygen delivery to the brain

Planning and Goals

Main patient goals may include improved mobility, avoidance of shoulder pain, achievement of self-care, continence, improved thought processes, relief of sensory/perceptual deprivation, achievement of a form of communication, skin integrity, restored family functioning, improved sexual function and absence of complications. Goals are affected by knowledge of what the patient was like before the stroke.

Nursing Interventions

Monitoring and Managing Potential Complications

- Assess vital signs and oxygenation status for adequate blood flow to the brain and tissues.
- Improve respiratory gas exchange with supplemental oxygen, suctioning, and chest physiotherapy.
- Maintain adequate cardiac output by medications and fluid administration.

Improving Mobility and Preventing Deformities

- Position to prevent contractures; use measures to relieve pressure, assist in maintaining good body alignment, and prevent compressive neuropathies.
- Prevent foot drop and heel cords from shortening by using a foot board at intervals during the flaccid period.
- Apply a posterior splint at night to prevent flexion of affected extremity.
- Prevent external rotation of hip joint with a trochanter roll.

- Prevent adduction of the affected shoulder with a pillow placed in the axilla.
- Elevate affected arm to prevent edema and fibrosis.
- Position fingers so that they are barely flexed; place hand in slight supination. If upper extremity spasticity is noted, do not use a hand roll.
- Use a volar resting splint to support wrist and hand.
- Change position every 2 hours; place patient in a prone position for 15 to 30 minutes several times a day.

Establishing an Exercise Program

- Provide full range of motion four or five times a day to maintain joint mobility, regain motor control, and prevent contracture development; prevent further deterioration of the neuromuscular system; enhance circulation; and exercise to prevent venous stasis. If tightness occurs in any area, perform range-of-motion exercises more frequently.
- Observe for signs of pulmonary embolus or excessive cardiac workload during exercise period (eg, shortness of breath, chest pain, cyanosis, and increasing pulse rate).
- Supervise and support patient during exercises; plan frequent short periods of exercise, not longer periods; encourage patient to exercise unaffected side at intervals throughout the day.

Preparing for Ambulation

- Start an active rehabilitation program when consciousness returns (and all evidence of bleeding is gone, when indicated).
- Teach patient to maintain balance in a sitting position, then to balance while standing (use a tilt table if needed).
- Begin walking as soon as standing balance is achieved (use parallel bars and have wheelchair available in anticipation of possible dizziness).
- Keep training periods for ambulation brief and frequent.

 NURSING ALERT Initiate a full rehabilitation program even for elderly patients.

C

Preventing Shoulder Pain

- Never lift patient by the flaccid shoulder or pull on the affected arm or shoulder.
- Use proper patient movement and positioning (eg, flaccid arm on a table or pillows when patient is seated, use of sling when ambulating).
- Range-of-motion exercises are beneficial, but avoid overstrenuous arm movements.
- Elevate arm and hand to prevent dependent edema of the hand; administer analgesic agents as indicated.

Enhancing Self-Care

- Encourage patient to assist in personal hygiene; select suitable self-care activities that can be carried out with one hand.
- Help patient to set realistic goals; add a new task daily.
- As possible, encourage patient to carry out all self-care activities on the unaffected side as the first step.
- Make sure patient does not neglect affected side; provide assistive devices as indicated.
- Improve morale by making sure patient is fully dressed during ambulatory activities.
- Assist with dressing activities (eg, clothing with Velcro closures; put garment on the affected side first); keep environment uncluttered and organized.
- Provide emotional support and encouragement to prevent fatigue and discouragement.

Managing Sensory-Perceptual Difficulties

- Approach patient with a decreased field of vision on the side where visual perception is intact; place all visual stimuli on this side.
- Teach patient to turn and look in the direction of the defective visual field to compensate for the loss; make eye contact with patient, and draw attention to affected side.
- Increase natural or artificial lighting in the room; provide eyeglasses to improve vision.

- Remind patient with hemianopsia of the other side of the body; place extremities so that patient can see them.

Managing Dysphagia

- Observe patient for paroxysms of coughing, food dribbling out or pooling in one side of the mouth, food retained for long periods in the mouth, or nasal regurgitation when swallowing liquids.
- Consult with speech therapist to evaluate gag reflexes; assist in teaching alternate swallowing techniques, advise patient to take smaller boluses of food, and inform patient of foods that are easier to swallow; provide thicker liquids or puréed diet as indicated.
- Have patient sit upright, preferably in chair, when eating and drinking; advance diet as tolerated.
- Prepare for gastrointestinal feedings through a tube if indicated; elevate head of bed during feedings, check tube position before feeding, administer feeding slowly, and ensure that cuff of tracheostomy tube is inflated (if applicable); monitor and report excessive retained or residual feeding.

Attaining Bowel and Bladder Control

- Perform intermittent sterile catheterization during period of loss of sphincter control.
- Analyze voiding pattern and offer urinal or bedpan on this schedule.
- Assist the male patient to an upright posture for voiding.
- Provide high-fiber diet and adequate fluid intake (2 to 3 L/day), unless contraindicated.
- Establish a regular time (after breakfast) for toileting.

Improving Thought Processes

- Reinforce structured training program using cognitive-perceptual retraining, visual imagery, reality orientation, and cueing procedures to compensate for losses.
- Support patient: observe performance and progress, give positive feedback, convey an attitude of confidence and

C

hopefulness; provide other interventions as used for
improving cognitive function after a head injury.

Achieving Communication

- Reinforce the individually tailored program.
- Jointly establish goals, with patient taking an active part.
- Make the atmosphere conducive to communication,
  remaining sensitive to patient's reactions and needs and
  responding to them in an appropriate manner; treat patient
  as an adult.
- Lend strong moral support and understanding to allay
  anxiety; avoid completing patient's sentences.
- Be consistent in schedule, routines, and repetitions. A
  written schedule, checklists, and audiotapes may help with
  memory and concentration; a communication board may be
  used.
- Talk to aphasic patients when providing care activities to
  provide social contact.
- Maintain patient's attention when talking with patient,
  speak slowly, and give one instruction at a time; allow
  patient time to process.

Maintaining Skin Integrity

- Frequently assess skin for signs of breakdown, with
  emphasis on bony areas and dependent body parts.
- Employ pressure-relieving devices; continue regular turning
  and positioning (every 2 hours minimally), minimize shear
  and friction when positioning.
- Keep skin clean and dry, gently massage healthy dry skin,
  and maintain adequate nutrition.

Improving Family Coping Through Health Teaching

- Provide counseling and support to family.
- Ease the burden of the family in providing continuous
  24-hour care with respite care or adult day care center.
  Provide information and encourage caregiver to arrange for
  assistance.

- Involve others in patient's care; teach stress management techniques and maintenance of personal health for family coping.
- Give family information about the expected outcome of the stroke, and counsel them to avoid doing things for patient that he or she can do.
- Develop attainable goals for patient at home by involving the total health care team, patient, and family.
- Encourage everyone to approach patient with a supportive and optimistic attitude, focusing on abilities that remain; explain to family that emotional lability usually improves with time.

Regaining Sexual Function

- Perform in-depth assessment to determine sexual history before and after the stroke.
- Interventions for patient and partner focus on providing relevant information, education, reassurance, medication adjustments, counseling regarding coping skills, and suggestions for alternative positions and means of sexual expression and satisfaction.
- Encourage sexual counseling about alternative approaches to sexual expression.

Promoting Home and Community-Based Care

- Teach patient to resume as much self-care as possible; provide assistive devices as indicated.
- Have occupational therapist make a home assessment and recommendations to help patient become more independent.
- Coordinate care provided by numerous health care professionals; help family plan aspects of care.
- Make referral for home speech therapy. Encourage family involvement. Provide family with practical instructions to help patient between speech therapy sessions.
- Advise family that patient may tire easily, become irritable and upset by small events, and show less interest in daily events.

- Discuss patient's depression with physician for possible antidepressant therapy.
- Encourage family to support patient and give positive reinforcement.
- Remind spouse and family to attend to personal health and well-being.
- Encourage patient to attend community-based stroke clubs to give a feeling of belonging and fellowship with others.
- Encourage patient to continue with hobbies, recreational and leisure interests, and contact with friends to prevent social isolation.

Evaluation

Expected Patient Outcomes

- Achieves improved mobility
- Has no complaints of pain
- Achieves self-care
- Turns head to see people or objects
- Demonstrates improved swallowing ability
- Achieves normal bowel and bladder elimination
- Has no skin breakdown
- Demonstrates improved communication
- Family members demonstrate a positive attitude and coping mechanisms.
- Has positive attitude regarding alternative approaches to sexual expression

---

For more information, see Chapter 62 in Smeltzer and Bare: *Brunner and Suddarth's Textbook of Medical-Surgical Nursing*, 11th edition. Philadelphia: Lippincott Williams & Wilkins, 2008.

Cholelithiasis (and Cholecystitis)

In cholelithiasis calculi (gallstones) usually form in the gallbladder from solid constituents of bile and vary greatly in size, shape, and composition. There are two major types of gallstones:

pigment stones, which contain an excess of unconjugated pigments in the bile, and cholesterol stones (the more common form), which result from bile supersaturated with cholesterol due to increased synthesis of cholesterol and decreased synthesis of bile acids that dissolve cholesterol. Risk factors for pigment stones include cirrhosis, hemolysis, and infections of the biliary tree. These stones cannot be dissolved and must be removed surgically. Risk factors for cholesterol stones include gender (women have a four times higher incidence than men); use of oral contraceptives, estrogens, and clofibrate; age (usually older than 40 years); multiparous status; and obesity. There is also an increased risk related to diabetes, gastrointestinal disease, T-tube fistula, and ileal resection or bypass.

Cholecystitis, an acute complication of cholelithiasis, is an acute infection of the gallbladder. Most patients with cholecystitis have gallstones (calculous cholecystitis). A gallstone obstructs bile outflow and bile in the gallbladder initiates a chemical reaction, resulting in edema, compromise of the vascular supply, and gangrene. In the absence of gallstones, cholecystitis (acalculous) may occur after surgery, severe trauma, or burns, or with torsion cystic duct obstruction, multiple blood transfusions, and primary bacterial infections of the gallbladder. Infection causes pain, tenderness, and rigidity of the upper right abdomen and is associated with nausea and vomiting and the usual signs of inflammation. Purulent fluid inside the gallbladder indicates an empyema of the gallbladder. See Nursing Process for additional information.

Clinical Manifestations

- May be silent, producing no pain and only mild gastrointestinal symptoms
- May be acute or chronic with epigastric distress (fullness, abdominal distention, and vague upper right quadrant pain) after a high-fat meal
- If the cystic duct is obstructed, the gallbladder becomes distended and eventually infected; fever and palpable abdominal mass; biliary colic with excruciating upper right abdominal pain, radiating to back or right shoulder with

nausea and vomiting several hours after a heavy meal; restlessness and constant or colicky pain
- Jaundice, accompanied by marked itching, with obstruction of the common bile duct, in a small percentage of patients
- Very dark urine; clay-colored stool
- Deficiencies of vitamin A, D, E, and K (fat-soluble vitamins)
- Abscess, necrosis, and perforation with peritonitis if the gallstone continues to obstruct the duct

Assessment and Diagnostic Methods

- Abdominal radiograph, ultrasonography or cholecystography, radionuclide imaging, or cholescintigraphy
- Endoscopic retrograde cholangiopancreatography (ERCP)
- Percutaneous transhepatic cholangiography (PTC)

🌿 Gerontologic Considerations

- Surgical intervention for disease of the biliary tract is the most common operation performed in the elderly.
- Biliary disease may be accompanied or preceded by symptoms of septic shock: oliguria, hypotension, mental changes, tachycardia, and tachypnea.
- Mortality from serious complications is high. Risk of complications and shorter hospital stays make it essential that older patients and their family members receive specific information about signs and symptoms of complications and measures to prevent them.
- Cholecystectomy is usually well tolerated and carries a low risk if expert assessment and care are provided before, during, and after surgery.

Medical Management

Major objectives of medical therapy are to reduce the incidence of acute episodes of gallbladder pain and cholecystitis by supportive and dietary management and, if possible, to remove the cause by pharmacotherapy, endoscopic procedures, or surgical intervention.

- Infusion of a solvent into the gallbladder to dissolve gallstones
- Stone removal using an instrument with a basket or by ERCP endoscope
- Extracorporeal shock-wave lithotripsy (repeated shock waves directed at the gallbladder or common bile duct to fragment the stones), intracorporeal shock-wave lithotripsy (fragmentation by ultrasound, pulsed laser, or hydraulic lithotripsy applied through an endoscope directly to the stones)

Supportive and Dietary Management

- Achieve remission with rest, intravenous fluids, nasogastric suction, analgesia, and antibiotics
- Diet immediately after an episode is usually low-fat liquids with high protein and carbohydrates followed by solid soft foods as tolerated, avoiding eggs, fatty rich foods, gas-forming vegetables, and alcohol.

Pharmacologic Therapy

- Analgesic agents such as meperidine may be required; avoid morphine because it increases spasm of the sphincter of Oddi.
- Ursodeoxycholic acid and chenodeoxycholic acid (chenodiol, or CDCA) are effective in dissolving primarily cholesterol stones.
- Long-term follow-up and monitoring of liver enzymes

Surgical Management

Goal of surgery is to relieve persistent symptoms, remove the cause of colic, and treat acute cholecystitis.

- Laparoscopic cholecystectomy: performed through a small incision or puncture made through the abdominal wall in the umbilicus
- Cholecystectomy: gallbladder removed after ligation of the cystic duct and artery
- Mini-cholecystectomy: gallbladder removed through a 3- to 4-cm incision
- Choledochostomy: incision into the common duct for stone removal
- Cholecystostomy (surgical or percutaneous): gallbladder is opened and the stone, bile, or purulent drainage is removed

NURSING PROCESS: The Patient Undergoing Cholecystectomy

Assessment

- Assess health history: note history of smoking or prior respiratory problems.
- Assess respiratory status: note shallow respirations, persistent cough, or ineffective or adventitious breath sounds.
- Evaluate nutritional status (dietary history, general examination, and laboratory study results).

Diagnosis

Nursing Diagnoses

- Acute pain and discomfort related to surgical incision
- Impaired gas exchange related to high abdominal surgical incision
- Impaired skin integrity related to altered biliary drainage after surgical incision
- Imbalanced nutrition related to inadequate bile secretion
- Deficient knowledge about self-care activities related to incisional care, dietary modifications (if needed),

medications, reportable signs or symptoms (fever, bleeding, vomiting)

Collaborative Problems/Potential Complications

- Bleeding
- Gastrointestinal symptoms

Planning and Goals

Goals include relief of pain, adequate ventilation, intact skin and improved biliary drainage, optimal nutritional intake, understanding of self-care routines, and absence of complications.

Nursing Interventions: Postoperative

- Place patient in low Fowler's position.
- Provide intravenous fluids and nasogastric suction.
- Provide water and other fluids and soft diet, after bowel sounds return.

Relieving Pain

- Instruct patient to use a pillow to splint incision.
- Administer analgesic agents as ordered.

Improving Respiratory Status

- Remind patient to expand lungs fully and to cough hourly to prevent atelectasis; promote early ambulation.
- Monitor elderly and obese patients most closely for respiratory problems.

Improving Nutritional Status

Advise patient at time of discharge to maintain a nutritious diet and avoid excessive fats; fat restriction is usually lifted in 4 to 6 weeks.

Promoting Skin Care and Biliary Drainage

- Connect tubes to drainage receptacle and secure tubing to avoid kinking (elevate above abdomen).
- Place drainage bag in patient's pocket when ambulating.

- Observe for indications of infection, leakage of bile, obstruction of bile drainage, clay-colored stool, and change in vital signs.
- Observe for jaundice (check the sclera).
- Note and report right upper quadrant pain, nausea, and vomiting.
- Change dressing frequently, using ointment to protect skin from irritation.
- Keep careful record of intake and output.
- Measure bile collected every 24 hours; document amount, color, and character of drainage.

Monitoring and Managing Complications

- Bleeding: assess periodically for increased tenderness and rigidity of abdomen and report; instruct patient and family to report change in color of stools. Monitor vital signs closely. Inspect incision for bleeding.
- Gastrointestinal symptoms: assess for loss of appetite, vomiting, pain, distention of abdomen, and temperature elevation; report promptly and instruct patient and family to report symptoms promptly; provide written reinforcement of verbal instructions.

Promoting Home and Community-Based Care

Teaching Patients Self-Care

- Instruct patient, verbally and in writing, about care of drainage tubes and to report to physician promptly changes in amount or characteristics of drainage.
- Teach about medications and their actions.
- Instruct patient to report to physician symptoms of jaundice, dark urine, pale stools, pruritus, or signs of inflammation and infection (eg, pain or fever after laparoscopy).
- Provide written and verbal instructions to patient and family about management of postoperative pain and about signs and symptoms of intra-abdominal complications that should be reported (loss of appetite, vomiting, pain, distention of abdomen, and temperature elevation).

- Refer for home care during the first 24 to 48 hours because of drowsiness.
- Emphasize importance of keeping follow-up appointments.

Evaluation

Expected Patient Outcomes

- Reports decrease in pain
- Demonstrates appropriate respiratory function
- Exhibits normal skin integrity around biliary drainage sites
- Obtains relief of dietary intolerance
- Is free of complications

For more information, see Chapter 40 in Smeltzer and Bare: *Brunner and Suddarth's Textbook of Medical-Surgical Nursing*, 11th edition. Philadelphia: Lippincott Williams & Wilkins, 2008.

Chronic Obstructive Pulmonary Disease (COPD)

Chronic obstructive pulmonary disease (COPD) is a disease characterized by airflow limitation that is not fully reversible. The airflow obstruction is usually progressive and associated with airway hyperreactivity, resulting in narrowing of peripheral airways, airflow limitation, and changes in the pulmonary vasculature. Asthma is now considered a separate disorder, although symptoms overlap with symptoms of COPD. Cigarette smoking, air pollution, and occupational exposure (coal, cotton, grain) are important risk factors that contribute to COPD development, which may occur over a 20- to 30-year span. Complications of COPD vary but include respiratory insufficiency and failure (major complications) as well as pneumonia, atelectasis, and pneumothorax.

Clinical Manifestations

C

- COPD is characterized by chronic cough, sputum production, and increased work of breathing as well as dyspnea on exertion.
- Weight loss is common.
- Symptoms are specific to the disease.

See Clinical Manifestations under Asthma, Bronchiectasis, Bronchitis, and Emphysema.

❧ Gerontologic Considerations

COPD accentuates many of the physiologic changes associated with aging and is manifested in airway obstruction (in bronchitis) and excessive loss of elastic lung recoil (in emphysema). Additional changes in ventilation-perfusion ratios occur.

Medical Management

- Smoking cessation, if appropriate
- Bronchodilators, corticosteroids, and other drugs
- Oxygen therapy, including nighttime oxygen
- Varied treatments specific to disease. See Medical Management under Asthma, Bronchiectasis, Bronchitis, and Emphysema.
- Surgery: bullectomy to reduce dyspnea; lung volume reduction to improve lobar elasticity and function; lung transplantation

NURSING PROCESS: The Patient with COPD

Assessment

Determining Risk Factors

Assess for risk factors such as cigarette, pipe, cigar or other kinds of smoking or the passive inhalation of these products.

Obtaining Health History

Obtain a history about current symptoms and previous disease manifestations:

- Duration of respiratory difficulty
- Dyspnea, shortness of breath, wheezing, exercise tolerance, fatigue
- Effect on eating and sleeping habits

Performing Physical Examination

Complete a thorough physical examination to obtain baseline data:

- Pulse, respiratory rate, and rhythm
- Contraction of abdominal muscles during inspiration
- Use of accessory muscles to breathe; prolonged expiration
- Cyanosis, neck vein engorgement
- Peripheral edema
- Cough; color, amount and consistency of sputum
- Status of sensorium, increasing stupor, apprehension

Diagnosis

Nursing Diagnoses

- Impaired gas exchange related to ventilation-perfusion inequality or inhalation of toxins
- Ineffective airway clearance related to bronchoconstriction, increased mucus production, ineffective cough, and bronchopulmonary infection
- Ineffective breathing pattern related to shortness of breath, mucus, bronchoconstriction, and airway irritants
- Self-care deficit related to fatigue secondary to increased work of breathing and insufficient ventilation and oxygenation
- Activity intolerance due to fatigue, hypoxemia, and ineffective breathing patterns
- Ineffective coping related to less socialization, anxiety, depression, lower activity level, and inability to work
- Deficient knowledge of self-care stretegies to use at home

Collaborative Problems/Potential Complications

- Respiratory insufficiency or failure
- Atelectasis
- Pneumonia and other pulmonary infection
- Pneumothorax
- Pulmonary hypertension

Planning and Goals

Major goals of the patient include improved gas exchange, smoking cessation, improved breathing pattern, maximal self-management, improved activity tolerance, achievement of airway clearance, improved coping ability, improved health-related quality of life, and adherence to the therapeutic program and home care.

Nursing Interventions

Improving Gas Exchange

- Monitor dyspnea and hypoxia.
- Administer medications, and be alert for potential side effects.
- Assess relief of bronchospasm through patient report of less dyspnea.
- Monitor prescribed oxygen effectiveness with pulse oximetry or arterial blood gas (ABG) analysis.

NURSING ALERT Because hypoxemia is a stimulus for respiration in the patient with COPD, avoid depressing the respiratory drive when administering oxygen to correct hypoxemia.

Achieving Airway Clearance

- Encourage high fluid intake to liquefy secretions.
- Instruct patient in directed or controlled coughing.
- Provide chest physiotherapy with postural drainage and intermittent positive-pressure breathing (IPPB), when ordered.

- Eliminate pulmonary irritants.
- Instruct patient in effective breathing techniques.
- Measure expiratory flow rates.
- Teach breathing techniques to reduce respiratory rate and expel maximal air.

Preventing Bronchopulmonary Infections

- Instruct patient to report signs of infection (eg, fever; change in sputum color, character, consistency, or amount), and report any worsening of symptoms.
- Advise patient to avoid outdoor exposure during high pollen counts or significant air pollution because these may increase bronchospasm. Also advise patient to avoid high temperatures and humidity as much as possible.
- Encourage immunization against *Haemophilus influenzae* and *Streptococcus pneumoniae*. Also encourage yearly flu vaccination and pneumococcal vaccine every 5 to 7 years.

Improving Activity Tolerance

- Recommend the patient adopt a lifestyle of moderate activity, ideally in a climate with minimal shifts in temperature and humidity.
- Encourage patient to avoid emotional disturbances and stressful situations.
- Recommend strategies for smoking cessation, and review progress with patient.

Promoting Home and Community-Based Care

- Refer patient for home care as appropriate.
- Demonstrate and supervise patient and family in performing all aspects of treatment regimen (eg, metered-dose inhaler [MDI], IPPB, chest physiotherapy, and postural drainage), with return demonstration from patient before discharge.

Teaching About Pulmonary Rehabilitation and Self-Care

- Identify candidates for rehabilitation, and reinforce material learned in rehabilitation program.

C

- Plan actions with patient to restore highest level of independent function and to improve quality of life; attend to both physiologic and emotional needs; help patient to accept realistic short-term and long-range goals.
- Reinforce breathing exercises and retraining and exercise programs, and teach patient methods to alleviate symptoms. Instruct patient in activity pacing (avoiding activities requiring arm lifting and movement until after patient has been up and moving around for an hour or more).
- If prescribed, assist patient in learning inspiratory muscle training: breathing against resistance for 10 to 15 minutes every day, and increasing the resistance gradually. Then teach patient ways to coordinate diaphragmatic breathing with activities such as walking, bathing, bending, and climbing stairs.
- Encourage patient to begin gradually to bathe, dress, and take short walks, resting as needed to avoid fatigue and excessive dyspnea, and to keep fluids readily available.
- Educate patient about normal anatomy and physiology of the lung, pathophysiology and changes with COPD, medications and home oxygen therapy, nutrition, respiratory therapy treatments, symptom alleviation, smoking cessation, sexuality, coping with chronic disease, communicating with the health care team, and planning for the future (advance directives, living wills, informed decisions about health care alternatives).
- Assess nutritional and caloric needs and counsel patient about meal planning and nutritional supplementation.
- If ordered, assist patient to adhere to the oxygen prescription by explaining the proper flow rate and required number of hours for oxygen use as well as the dangers of arbitrary changes in flow rates or duration of therapy. Reassure patient that oxygen is not "addictive," and explain the need to have regular evaluations of blood oxygenation by pulse oximetry or ABG analysis.
- Inform patient that smoking with or near oxygen is extremely dangerous.
- Teach proper use of bronchodilators, inhalers.

- Teach coping measures (eg, remaining active up to level of symptom tolerance; how to control symptoms to increase self-esteem, sense of mastery, and well-being; and use of support groups).
- Arrange specific services for patient (eg, respiratory therapy education, physical therapy for exercise and breathing retraining, and occupational therapy for conservation of energy during activities of daily living).
- Inform patient and family of resources such as American Lung Association, American Association of Cardiovascular and Pulmonary Rehabilitation, American Association of Respiratory Therapy.

Monitoring and Managing Complications

- Assess patient for complications (respiratory insufficiency and failure, respiratory infection, and atelectasis). Teach proper use of bronchodilator medications to help prevent complications.
- Monitor for cognitive changes, increasing dyspnea, tachypnea, and tachycardia.
- Monitor pulse oximetry values and administer oxygen as prescribed.
- Instruct patient and family about signs and symptoms of infection or other complications and to report changes in physical or cognitive status.
- Emphasize that if condition worsens to the point of acute respiratory failure, intubation and mechanical ventilation will be necessary.

Evaluation

Expected Patient Outcomes

- Demonstrates improved gas exchange
- Achieves maximal airway clearance
- Improves breathing pattern
- Maintains maximal level of self-care and physical functioning
- Achieves activity tolerance, and exercises and performs activities with less shortness of breath

C

- Develops effective coping mechanisms, and participates in a pulmonary rehabilitation program
- Adheres to the therapeutic program

For more information, see Chapter 24 in Smeltzer and Bare: *Brunner and Suddarth's Textbook of Medical-Surgical Nursing*, 11th edition. Philadelphia: Lippincott Williams & Wilkins, 2008.

Cirrhosis, Hepatic

Cirrhosis is a chronic disease characterized by replacement of normal liver tissue with diffuse fibrosis that disrupts the structure and function of the liver. Cirrhosis, or scarring of the liver, is divided into three types: alcoholic, most frequently due to chronic alcoholism and the most common type of cirrhosis; postnecrotic, a late result of a previous acute viral hepatitis; and biliary, a result of chronic biliary obstruction and infection (least common type of cirrhosis).

Clinical Manifestations

- Compensated cirrhosis: usually found secondary to routine physical examination; vague symptoms
- Decompensated cirrhosis: symptoms of decreased proteins, clotting factors, and other substances and of portal hypertension
- Liver enlargement early in the course (fatty liver); later in course, liver size decreases from scar tissue
- Portal obstruction and ascites: chronic dyspepsia, constipation or diarrhea, splenomegaly; spider telangiectases may be observed
- Gastrointestinal varices: distended abdominal blood vessels; varices or hemorrhoids; hematemesis; profuse hemorrhage from the stomach; and esophageal varices in about 25% of patients
- Edema, jaundice, fever
- Vitamin deficiency (A, C, and K) and anemia

- Mental deterioration with impending hepatic encephalopathy and hepatic coma

Assessment and Diagnostic Methods

- Liver function tests (eg, serum alkaline phosphatase, AST [SGOT], ALT [SGPT], GGT, and bilirubin), prothrombin time, ABGs, laparoscopy, in conjunction with biopsy
- Ultrasound scanning
- Computed tomography (CT) scan
- Magnetic resonance imaging (MRI)
- Radioisotopic liver scans

Medical Management

Medical management is based on presenting symptoms.

- Treatment includes antacids, vitamins, balanced diet, and nutritional supplements; potassium-sparing diuretics (for ascites); avoidance of alcohol.
- Colchicine may increase the length of survival in patients with mild to moderate cirrhosis.

NURSING PROCESS: The Patient with Hepatic Cirrhosis

Assessment

- Focus on dietary intake, nutritional status, onset of symptoms, history of precipitating factors, including long-term alcohol abuse, exposure to toxic agents, medications.
- Assess mental status through interview and interaction with patient; note orientation to time, place, person.
- Note relationships with family, friends, and coworkers regarding incapacitation secondary to alcohol abuse and cirrhosis.
- Note abdominal distention and bloating, gastrointestinal bleeding, bruising, and weight changes.

- Document exposure to toxic agents, such as hepatotoxic medications or illicit drugs.

Diagnosis

Nursing Diagnoses

- Activity intolerance related to fatigue, general debility, muscle wasting, and discomfort
- Imbalanced nutrition: Less than body requirements, related to chronic gastritis, decreased gastrointestinal motility, and anorexia
- Impaired skin integrity related to compromised immunologic status, edema, and poor nutrition
- Risk for injury and bleeding related to altered clotting mechanisms

Collaborative Problems/Potential Complications

- Bleeding and hemorrhage
- Hepatic encephalopathy
- Fluid volume excess

Planning and Goals

Goals may include independence in activities, improved nutritional status, improved skin integrity, decreased potential for injury, improved mental status, and absence of complications.

Nursing Interventions

Providing Rest

- Position bed for maximal respiratory efficiency; provide oxygen if needed.
- Initiate efforts to prevent respiratory, circulatory, and vascular disturbances.
- Encourage patient to increase activity gradually and plan rest with activity and mild exercise.

Improving Nutritional Status

- Provide a nutritious, high-protein diet supplemented by B-complex vitamins and others, including A, C, and K and folic acid if there is no indication of impending coma.
- Provide small, frequent meals, consider patient preferences, and encourage patient to eat; provide protein supplements, if indicated.
- Provide nutrients by feeding tube or total parenteral nutrition (PN).
- Provide patients who have fatty stools (steatorrhea) with water-soluble forms of fat-soluble vitamins A, D, and E, and give folic acid and iron to prevent anemia.
- Provide a low-protein diet temporarily if patient shows signs of impending or advancing coma; restore protein intake to moderate (1 to 1.5/Kg) when patient's condition permits.

Providing Skin Care

- Change position frequently.
- Avoid using irritating soaps and adhesive tape.
- Provide lotion to soothe irritated skin; take measures to prevent patient from scratching the skin.

Reducing Risk of Injury

- Use padded side rails if patient becomes agitated or restless.
- Orient to time, place, and procedures to minimize agitation.
- Instruct patient to ask for assistance to get out of bed.
- Provide safety measures to prevent injury or cuts (electric razor, soft toothbrush).
- Apply pressure to venipuncture sites to minimize bleeding.

Monitoring and Managing Complications

Preventing bleeding due to decreased production of prothrombin and monitoring for hepatic encephalopathy are the primary concerns.

- Observe for melena, and check stools for blood.
- Take precautionary measures (eg, use padded side rails, apply pressure to injection site for long period of time, and avoid sharp objects).

- Use appropriate dietary modification and stool softeners to prevent straining during defecation.
- Monitor closely for gastrointestinal bleeding.
- Keep equipment to treat hemorrhage from esophageal varices readily available: intravenous fluids, medications, Sengstaken-Blakemore tube.
- Monitor closely to identify early evidence of condition.
- Explain event and treatment if complication noted. Patient may need to be treated in ICU.

See Nursing Management under Hepatic Encephalopathy for additional information.

Promoting Home and Community-Based Care

Prepare for discharge by providing dietary instruction, including exclusion of alcohol.

- Refer to Alcoholics Anonymous if indicated.
- Continue sodium restriction; stress avoidance of raw shellfish.
- Provide written instructions, teaching, support, and reinforcement to patient and family.
- Encourage rest and probably a change in lifestyle (adequate, well-balanced diet and elimination of alcohol).
- Instruct family about symptoms of impending encephalopathy and possibility of bleeding tendencies and infection.
- Refer patient to home care nurse, and assist in transition from hospital to home.

Evaluation

Expected Patient Outcomes

- Demonstrates ability to participate in activities
- Increases nutritional intake; avoids skin breakdown and other injuries

For more information, see Chapter 39 in Smeltzer and Bare: *Brunner and Suddarth's Textbook of Medical-Surgical Nursing*, 11th edition. Philadelphia: Lippincott Williams & Wilkins, 2008.

Constipation

Constipation refers to an abnormal infrequency or irregularity of defecation, abnormal hardening of stools that makes their passage difficult and sometimes painful, decrease in stool volume, or prolonged retention of stool in the rectum. This type is referred to as colonic constipation. It can be caused by certain medications; rectal or anal disorders; obstruction; metabolic, neurologic, and neuromuscular conditions; endocrine disorders; lead poisoning; connective tissue disorders; and a variety of disease conditions. Other causative factors include weakness, immobility, debility, fatigue, and inability to increase intra-abdominal pressure to pass stools. Constipation develops when people do not take the time to defecate or as the result of dietary habits (low consumption of fiber and inadequate fluid intake), lack of regular exercise, and a stress-filled life. Perceived constipation is a subjective problem that occurs when an individual's bowel elimination pattern is not consistent with what he or she perceives as normal. Chronic laxative use contributes to this problem, particularly in elderly people.

Clinical Manifestations

- Abdominal distention, borborygmus (intestinal rumbling), pain, and pressure
- Decreased appetite, headache, fatigue, indigestion, sensation of incomplete emptying
- Straining at stool; elimination of small volume of hard, dry stool; fewer than three bowel movements per week
- Complications such as hypertension, hemorrhoids and fissures, fecal impaction, and megacolon

Assessment and Diagnostic Methods

Diagnosis is based on history, physical examination, possibly a barium enema, sigmoidoscopy, stool for occult blood, anorectal manometry (pressure studies), defecography, and bowel transit studies.

Medical Management

Treatment should be aimed at the underlying cause of constipation.

- Discontinue laxative abuse; increase fluid intake; include fiber in diet; try biofeedback, exercise routine to strengthen abdominal muscles.
- If laxative is necessary, use bulk-forming agents, saline and osmotic agents, lubricants, stimulants, or fecal softeners.
- Specific medication therapy to increase intrinsic motor function (eg, cholinergies or cholinesterase inhibitors)

Nursing Management

Assessment

Use tact and respect with patient when talking about bowel habits and obtaining health history. Note the following:

- Onset and duration of constipation, current and past elimination patterns, patient's expectation of normal bowel elimination, food and fluid intake, lifestyle, stress level, and occupation
- Current medications, history of laxative or enema use, and past medical and surgical history
- Report of any of the following: rectal pressure or fullness, abdominal pain, straining at defecation, and flatulence

Diagnosis

Nursing Diagnoses

- Colonic constipation or fecal impaction related to health habits or effect of immobility on peristalsis
- Deficient knowledge about health maintenance practices to prevent constipation

Planning and Goals

Major goals of the patient may include a regular pattern of bowel elimination, adequate intake of fluids and high-fiber foods, knowledge of methods to avoid constipation, relief of anxiety about bowel elimination patterns, and absence of complications.

C

Promoting Home and Community-Based Care

Teaching Patients Self-Care

- Teach patient to assume normal position for defecation (semisquatting) when possible (assist patient to a bedside commode).
- Explain the physiology of defecation, and emphasize heeding the urge to defecate.
- Discuss normal variations in patterns of defecation.
- Teach patient how to establish a bowel routine (eg, after breakfast).
- Provide dietary information; suggest eating high-residue, high-fiber food, adding bran daily (introduce gradually), and increasing fluid intake (unless contraindicated).
- Detail the benefits of an exercise regimen, increased ambulation, and abdominal muscle toning.
- Describe abdominal toning exercises: contracting abdomen muscles four times daily and leg to chest lifts 10 to 20 times daily.
- Encourage patient confined to bed to perform range-of-motion exercises, turn frequently from side-to-side, and lie prone (if not contraindicated) for 30 minutes every 4 hours.

For more information, see Chapter 38 in Smeltzer and Bare: *Brunner and Suddarth's Textbook of Medical-Surgical Nursing*, 11th edition. Philadelphia: Lippincott Williams & Wilkins, 2008.

Contact Dermatitis

Contact dermatitis is an inflammatory reaction of the skin to physical, chemical, or biologic agents. It may be of the primary irritant type, or it may be allergic. The epidermis is damaged by repeated physical and chemical irritation. Common causes of irritant dermatitis are soaps, detergents, scouring compounds, and industrial chemicals. Predisposing factors include extremes of heat and cold, frequent use of soap and water, and a preexisting skin disease.

Clinical Manifestations

- Eruptions when the causative agent contacts the skin
- Itching, burning, and erythema are followed by edema, papules, vesicles, and oozing or weeping as first reactions.
- In the subacute phase, the vesicular changes are less marked and alternate with crusting, drying, fissuring, and peeling.
- If repeated reactions occur or the patient continually scratches the skin, lichenification and pigmentation occur; secondary bacterial invasion may follow.

Medical Management

- Rest involved skin and protect it from further damage.
- Determine the distribution pattern of the reaction to differentiate between allergic type and irritant type.
- Identify and remove the offending irritant; soap is generally not used on site until healed.
- Use bland, unmedicated lotions for small patches of erythema; apply cool wet dressings over small areas of vesicular dermatitis; a corticosteroid ointment may be used.
- Medicated baths at room temperature are prescribed for larger areas of dermatitis.
- In widespread conditions, a short course of systemic steroids may be prescribed.

Nursing Management

Instruct patient to adhere to the following instructions for at least 4 months, until the skin appears completely healed:

- Think about what may have caused the problem.
- Avoid contact with the irritants, or wash skin thoroughly immediately after exposure to the irritants.

- Avoid heat, soap, and rubbing the skin.
- Avoid topical medications, lotions, or ointments, except when prescribed.
- Choose bath soaps, detergents, and cosmetics that do not contain fragrance; avoid using a fabric softener dryer sheet.
- Wear cotton-lined gloves for washing dishes, but not more than 15 to 20 minutes at a time.
- Use cool wet dressings to clear lesions, followed by corticosteroid ointment, as ordered.

For more information, see Chapter 56 in Smeltzer and Bare: *Brunner and Suddarth's Textbook of Medical-Surgical Nursing*, 11th edition. Philadelphia: Lippincott Williams & Wilkins, 2008.

Coronary Atherosclerosis and Coronary Artery Disease

Coronary atherosclerosis is characterized by an abnormal accumulation of lipid or fatty substances and fibrous tissue in the vessel wall. These substances block or narrow the vessel, reducing blood flow to the myocardium and resulting in coronary heart disease (CHD). Recent studies indicate that atherosclerosis involves repeated inflammatory responses to artery wall injury and alteration in the biophysical and biochemical properties of the arterial walls. Atherosclerosis is a progressive disease but can be curtailed and in some cases reversed.

Risk Factors
Modifiable

- Cigarette smoking
- Elevated blood pressure
- High blood cholesterol (hyperlipidemia)
- Hyperglycemia (diabetes mellitus)
- Obesity

C

- Physical inactivity
- Use of oral contraceptives
- Infection (eg, gingivitis): possibly associated
- Behavior patterns (stress, aggressiveness, hostility)
- Geography: higher incidence in industrialized regions

Not Modifiable

- Positive family history (a first-degree relative with cardiovascular disease at age 55 or less for males and at age 65 or less for females)
- Age (more than 45 years for men, more than 55 years for women)
- Gender: occurs three times more often in men than in women
- Race: higher incidence in African Americans than in Caucasians

Clinical Manifestations

Clinical features result from narrowing of the arterial lumen and obstruction of blood flow to myocardium. Symptoms include:

- Chest pain: angina pectoris (may not be noted if patient is older, diabetic, or has heart failure)
- Atypical symptoms of myocardial ischemia (shortness of breath, nausea, and unusual fatigue)
- Myocardial infarction
- Electrocardiogram (ECG) changes, ventricular aneurysms
- Dysrhythmias, sudden death

Assessment and Diagnostic Methods

Identification of risk factors for CHD primarily involves taking a thorough history, including family history, physical examination (note blood pressure and weight), and laboratory work (eg, cholesterol levels [LDL to HDL], glucose).

Prevention

The major management goal is prevention of CHD. Primary prevention (taken before CHD develops) and secondary prevention are aimed at reducing risk factors, particularly cholesterol abnormalities, cigarette smoking, hypertension, and diabetes mellitus. (ATP III is the current standard for cholesterol management.)

🌿 Gerontologic Considerations

Aging produces changes in the integrity of the lining of the walls of arteries (arteriosclerosis), impeding blood flow and tissue nutrition. These changes are often sufficient to diminish oxygenation and increase myocardial oxygen consumption (MVO_2). The result can be debilitating angina pectoris and eventually heart failure.

Medical Management

See Medical Management under Angina and Myocardial Infarction for additional information.

Nursing Management

See Nursing Management under Angina and Myocardial Infarction for additional information.

- Identify at-risk patients, and teach lifestyle modifications to prevent development of coronary artery disease.
- Teach patient to control cholesterol levels through dietary reduction of cholesterol intake, exercise, smoking cessation, and, if needed, medications.
- Note and report findings from history, physical examination, and laboratory results that indicate hypertension or diabetes, and teach patient to control blood pressure and blood glucose by adhering to treatment regimen.
- Encourage and help patient learn to change behaviors and responses to stress-triggering events; teach cognitive restructuring and relaxation techniques.

C

- Prepare and support patient and family if patient develops symptoms of CHD or complications and requires diagnostic or treatment procedures (eg, nitroglycerin, thrombolytic therapy, angiography, percutaneous transluminal coronary angioplasty [PTCA], coronary artery stent, atherectomy, transmyocardial revascularization, or coronary artery bypass).

For more information, see Chapter 28 in Smeltzer and Bare: *Brunner and Suddarth's Textbook of Medical-Surgical Nursing*, 11th edition. Philadelphia: Lippincott Williams & Wilkins, 2008.

Cushing's Syndrome

Cushing's syndrome results from excessive adrenocortical activity. It may result from excessive administration of corticosteroids or adrenocorticotropic hormone (ACTH) or from hyperplasia of the adrenal cortex. It may be caused by several mechanisms, including a tumor of the pituitary gland or less commonly an ectopic malignancy that produces ACTH. Regardless of the cause, the normal feedback mechanisms that control the function of the adrenal cortex become ineffective, resulting in oversecretion of glucocorticoids, androgens, and possibly mineralocorticoid. Cushing's syndrome occurs five times more often in women ages 20 to 40 years than in men.

Clinical Manifestations

- Arrested growth, weight gain and obesity, musculoskeletal changes, and glucose intolerance
- Classic features: central-type obesity, with a fatty "buffalo hump" in the neck and supraclavicular areas, a heavy trunk, and relatively thin extremities; skin is thin, fragile, easily traumatized, with ecchymoses and striae
- Weakness and lassitude; sleep is disturbed because of altered diurnal secretion of cortisol

- Excessive protein catabolism with muscle wasting and osteoporosis; kyphosis, backache, and compression fractures of the vertebrae are possible
- Retention of sodium and water, producing hypertension and heart failure
- "Moon-faced" appearance, oiliness of skin and acne
- Increased susceptibility to infection; slow healing of minor cuts and bruises
- Hyperglycemia or overt diabetes
- Virilization in females (due to excess androgens) with appearance of masculine traits and recession of feminine traits (eg, excessive hair on face, breasts atrophy, menses cease, clitoris enlarges, and voice deepens); libido is lost in males and females
- Changes occur in mood and mental activity; psychosis may develop and distress and depression are common.
- If Cushing's syndrome is the result of a pituitary tumor, visual disturbances are possible because of pressure on the optic chiasm.

Assessment and Diagnostic Findings

- Overnight dexamethasone suppression test to measure plasma cortisol level (stress, obesity, depression, and medications may falsely elevate results)
- Computed tomography (CT) or magnetic resonance imaging (MRI) scan or ultrasound may localize adrenal tissue and detect adrenal tumors.

Medical Management

Treatment is usually directed at the pituitary gland because most cases are due to pituitary tumors rather than tumors of the adrenal cortex.

- Surgical removal of the tumor (transsphenoidal hypophysectomy) is the treatment of choice (90% success rate).
- Radiation of the pituitary gland is successful but takes several months for symptom control.

C

- Adrenalectomy is performed in patients with primary adrenal hypertrophy.
- Postoperatively, temporary replacement therapy with hydrocortisone may be necessary until the adrenal glands begin to respond normally (may be several months).
- If bilateral adrenalectomy was performed, lifetime replacement of adrenal cortex hormones is necessary.
- Adrenal enzyme inhibitors (eg, metyrapone or mitotane) may be used with ectopic ACTH-secreting tumors that cannot be totally removed; monitor closely for inadequate adrenal function and side effects.
- If Cushing's syndrome results from exogenous corticosteroids, taper the drug to the minimum level or use alternate-day therapy to treat the underlying disease.

NURSING PROCESS: The Patient with Cushing's Syndrome

Assessment

- Focus on the effects on the body of high concentrations of adrenal cortex hormones.
- Assess patient's level of activity and ability to carry out routine and self-care activities.
- Observe skin for trauma, infection, breakdown, bruising, and edema.
- Note changes in appearance and patient's responses to these changes; family is good source of information about patient's emotional status and changes in appearance.
- Assess patient's mental function, including mood, response to questions, depression, and awareness of environment.

Diagnosis

Nursing Diagnoses

- Risk for injury related to weakness
- Risk for infection related to altered protein metabolism and inflammatory response

- Self-care deficits related to weakness, fatigue, muscle wasting, and altered sleep patterns
- Impaired skin integrity related to edema, impaired healing, and thin and fragile skin
- Disturbed body image related to altered appearance, impaired sexual functioning, and decreased activity level
- Disturbed thought processes related to mood swings, irritability, and depression

Collaborative Problems/Potential Complications

- Addisonian crisis
- Adverse effects of adrenocortical activity

Planning and Goals

Major goals include decreased risk for injury, decreased risk for infection, increased ability to carry out self-care activities, improved skin integrity, improved body image, improved mental function, and absence of complications.

Nursing Interventions

Decreasing Risk for Injury

- Provide a protective environment to prevent falls, fractures, and other injuries to bones and soft tissues.
- Assist the patient who is weak in ambulating to prevent falls or colliding into furniture.
- Recommend foods high in protein, calcium, and vitamin D to minimize muscle wasting and osteoporosis; refer to dietitian for assistance.

Decreasing Risk for Infection

- Avoid unnecessary exposure to people with infections.
- Assess frequently for subtle signs of infections (corticosteroids mask signs of inflammation and infection).

Promoting Skin Care

- Use meticulous skin care to avoid traumatizing fragile skin.
- Avoid adhesive tape, which can tear and irritate the skin.

C

- Assess skin and bony prominences frequently.
- Encourage and assist patient to change positions frequently.

Improving Body Image

- Discuss the impact that changes have had on patient's self-concept and relationships with others. Major physical changes will disappear in time if the cause of Cushing's syndrome can be treated.
- Weight gain and edema may be modified by a low-carbohydrate, low-sodium diet; a high-protein intake can reduce some bothersome symptoms.

Improving Thought Processes

- Explain to patient and family the cause of emotional instability, and help them cope with mood swings, irritability, and depression.
- Report any psychotic behavior.
- Encourage patient and family members to verbalize feelings.

Encouraging Rest and Activity

- Encourage moderate activity to prevent complications of immobility and promote self-esteem.
- Plan rest periods throughout the day and promote a relaxing, quiet environment for rest and sleep.

Preparing Patient for Surgery

Monitor blood glucose levels, and assess stools for blood because diabetes mellitus and peptic ulcer are common problems (see also Preoperative Preparation under Preoperative and Postoperative Nursing Management).

Monitoring and Managing Complications

- Adrenal hypofunction and addisonian crisis: monitor for hypotension; rapid, weak pulse; rapid respiratory rate; pallor; and extreme weakness. Note factors that may have led to crisis (eg, stress, trauma, surgery).
- Administer intravenous fluids and electrolytes and corticosteroids before, during, and after surgery or treatment as indicated.

- Monitor for circulatory collapse and shock present in addisonian crisis; treat promptly.
- Assess fluid and electrolyte status by monitoring laboratory values and daily weight.
- Monitor blood glucose level, and report elevations to physician.

Teaching Patients Self-Care

- Present information about Cushing's syndrome verbally and in writing to patient and family.
- If indicated, stress to patient and family that stopping corticosteroid use abruptly and without medical supervision can result in adrenal insufficiency and reappearance of symptoms.
- Emphasize the need to keep an adequate supply of the corticosteroid to prevent running out or skipping a dose, because this could result in addisonian crisis.
- Stress the need for dietary modifications to ensure adequate calcium intake without increasing risk for hypertension, hyperglycemia, and weight gain.
- Teach patient and family to monitor blood pressure, blood glucose levels, and weight.
- Stress the importance of wearing a medical alert bracelet and notifying other health professionals (eg, dentist) that he or she has Cushing's syndrome.
- Refer for home care as indicated to ensure safe environment with minimal stress and risk for falls and other side effects.
- Emphasize importance of regular medical follow-up, and ensure patient is aware of side and toxic effects of medications.

Evaluation

Expected Patient Outcomes

- Has decreased risk of injury
- Has decreased risk of infection
- Increases participation in self-care activities
- Attains or maintains skin integrity
- Achieves improved body image

C

- Exhibits improved mental functioning
- Experiences no complications

For more information, see Chapter 42 in Smeltzer and Bare: *Brunner and Suddarth's Textbook of Medical-Surgical Nursing*, 11th edition. Philadelphia: Lippincott Williams & Wilkins, 2008.

Cystitis (Lower Urinary Tract Infection)

Cystitis is an inflammation of the urinary bladder. The most common route of infection is transurethral, often from fecal contamination, ureterovesical reflux, or the use of a catheter or cystoscope. Bacteria may enter the urinary tract through the blood (hematogenous spread) from a distant site of infection or through direct extension by way of a fistula from the gut. *Escherichia coli* accounted for 54% of urinary tract infections (UTIs) in a large-scale study. Cystitis occurs more often in women, particularly sexually active women. Cystitis in men is secondary to some other factor (eg, infected prostate, epididymitis, or bladder stones).

Clinical Manifestations

- Urgency, frequency, burning, and pain on urination
- Nocturia, incontinence, and back, suprapubic, or pelvic pain
- Pyuria, bacteriuria, and hematuria
- With complicated UTIs (eg, patients with indwelling catheters), symptoms can range from asymptomatic bacteriuria to a gram-negative sepsis with shock.

Assessment and Diagnostic Methods

- Urinalysis, leukocyte esterase test, and nitrites (Griess nitrate reduction test)
- Urine culture, colony counts, cellular studies

- Tests for sexually transmitted diseases (STDs)
- Computed tomography (CT) scans and transrectal ultrasonography

🌿 Gerontologic Considerations

Elderly patients often lack the typical symptoms of UTI and sepsis. Nonspecific symptoms, such as altered sensorium, lethargy, anorexia, new incontinence, hyperventilation, and low-grade fever may be the only clues to cystitis in these patients.

Medical Management

- Drug therapy and patient education are the key treatment measures. UTIs may require 7 to 10 days of medication, or a short course (3 to 4 days) may be effective; antibiotic use in the treatment of asymptomatic bacteriuria in the institutionalized elderly patient is controversial.

Pharmacologic Therapy

- Ideal treatment is an antibacterial agent that eradicates bacteria from the urinary tract with minimal effects on fecal and vaginal flora.
- Medications may include sulfisoxazole (Gantrisin); co-trimoxazole (trimethoprim-sulfamethoxazole [Bactrim, Septra]), the drug of choice; or nitrofurantoin (Macrodantin). Levofloxacin (Levaquin) may be used for short-course therapy.
- Occasionally, ampicillin or amoxicillin (but *E. coli* has developed resistance to these agents)

Management of Recurrent Cystitis

- About 20% of women treated for uncomplicated UTIs experience a recurrence.
- Repeated infections at close intervals suggest a cause for referral to a urologist to investigate and correct abnormalities.

C

- Recurrence in men is usually due to persistence of the same organism; further evaluation and treatment are indicated. Reinfection of women with new bacteria is more common than persistence of the initial bacteria.
- If diagnostic evaluation reveals no structural abnormalities, patient may be instructed to begin treatment on own, testing urine with a dipstick whenever symptoms occur, and to contact health care provider only with persistence of symptoms, at the occurrence of fever, or if the number of treatment episodes exceeds four in a 6-month period.
- Long-term use of antimicrobial agents decreases risk of reinfection.

NURSING PROCESS: The Patient with Cystitis

Assessment

- Take careful history of urinary signs and symptoms.
- Assess for pain and urinary frequency, urgency, and hesitancy and changes in urine.
- Determine usual pattern of voiding to detect factors that may predispose patient to infection.
- Assess for infrequent emptying of the bladder, association of symptoms of UTIs with sexual intercourse, contraceptive practices, and personal hygiene.
- Check urine for volume, color, concentration, cloudiness, and odor.

Diagnosis

Nursing Diagnoses

- Acute pain related to inflammation and infection of the urethra, bladder, and other urinary tract structures
- Deficient knowledge related to factors predisposing to infection and recurrence, detection and prevention of recurrence, and pharmacologic therapy

Collaborative Problems/Potential Complications

- Renal failure due to extensive damage of kidney
- Sepsis

C

Planning and Goals

Goals of the patient may include relief of pain and discomfort, increased knowledge of preventive measures and treatment modalities, and absence of complications.

Nursing Interventions

Relieving Pain

- Use antispasmodic drugs to relieve bladder irritability and pain.
- Relieve pain and spasm with aspirin and heat to the perineum (hot tub baths).
- Encourage patient to drink liberal amounts of fluid (water is best); provide adequate hydration to patients at risk for dehydration (surgical patients, patients having diagnostic tests).
- Instruct patient to avoid urinary tract irritants (eg, coffee, tea, citrus, spices, alcohol).
- Encourage frequent voiding (every 2 to 3 hours).

Monitoring and Managing Complications

- Recognize and teach patient to recognize the signs and symptoms of UTIs early; initiate prompt treatment.
- Manage UTIs with appropriate antimicrobial therapy, liberal fluids, frequent voiding, and hygiene measures.
- Notify physician if fatigue, nausea, vomiting, or pruritus occurs.
- Provide for periodic monitoring of renal function.
- Avoid indwelling catheters if possible; remove at earliest opportunity. Use strict aseptic technique if an indwelling catheter is necessary.
- Check vital signs and level of consciousness for impending sepsis.

- Report positive blood cultures and elevated white blood cell counts.

Promoting Home and Community-Based Care
Teaching Patients Self-Care

- Teach patient to reduce concentrations of pathogens of the vaginal opening by hygiene measures: cleanse around perineum and urethral meatus after bowel movement with front-to-back motion.
- Advise drinking liberal amounts of fluid (not coffee, tea, colas, or alcohol) during the day to flush out bacteria.
- Recommend voiding every 2 to 3 hours during the day, completely emptying the bladder.
- If sexual intercourse is the initiating event for development of bacteriuria, void immediately after sexual intercourse and take prescribed single-dose oral antimicrobial agent.
- Instruct patient to take medication after emptying bladder before going to bed to ensure adequate concentration of the drug during the night.
- Instruct patient to monitor and test urine for bacteria with dip slides (Microstix).
- Emphasize importance of seeing health care provider regularly for follow-up, recurrence of symptoms, and infection that is nonresponsive to treatment.

Evaluation

Expected Patient Outcomes

- Experiences relief of pain
- Understands UTIs and their treatment
- Experiences no complications

For more information, see Chapter 45 in Smeltzer and Bare: *Brunner and Suddarth's Textbook of Medical-Surgical Nursing*, 11th edition. Philadelphia: Lippincott Williams & Wilkins, 2008.

Diabetes Insipidus

Diabetes insipidus is a disorder of the posterior lobe of the pituitary gland due to a deficiency of vasopressin, the antidiuretic hormone (ADH). It is characterized by polydipsia and polyuria. Diabetes insipidus may be (1) secondary, related to head trauma, brain tumor, or surgical ablation or irradiation of the pituitary gland or to infections of the central nervous system or metastatic tumors (lung or breast); (2) nephrogenic (failure of the renal tubules to respond to ADH), possibly related to hypokalemia, hypercalcemia, and a variety of medications (eg, lithium, demeclocycline); or (3) primary (hereditary), with symptoms possibly beginning at birth (defect in pituitary gland).

The disease cannot be controlled by limiting the intake of fluids because loss of high volumes of urine continues even without fluid replacement. Attempts to restrict fluids cause the patient to experience an insatiable craving for fluid and to develop hypernatremia and severe dehydration.

Clinical Manifestations

- Polyuria: enormous daily output of very dilute urine (specific gravity 1.001 to 1.005). Primary diabetes insipidus may have an abrupt onset or an insidious onset in adults.
- Polydipsia: patient experiences intense thirst, drinking 2 to 20 liters of fluid daily, with a special craving for cold water.
- Polyuria continues even without fluid replacement.

Assessment and Diagnostic Findings

- Fluid deprivation test: fluids are withheld for 8 to 12 hours until 3% to 5% of the body weight is lost. Inability to

increase specific gravity and osmolality of the urine during test is characteristic of diabetes insipidus.
- Urine specific gravity, serum osmolality, and serum sodium levels may be obtained.

Medical Management

Objectives of therapy are to ensure adequate fluid replacement, to replace vasopressin, and to search for and correct the underlying intracranial pathology. Treatment for diabetes insipidus of nephrogenic origin involves using thiazide diuretics, mild salt depletion, and prostaglandin inhibitors (eg, ibuprofen, indomethacin, and aspirin).

Vasopressin Replacement

- Desmopressin (DDAVP), administered intranasally, 1 or 2 administrations daily to control symptoms
- Lypressin (Diapid), absorbed through nasal mucosa into blood; duration may be short for patients with severe disease
- Intramuscular administration of ADH (vasopressin tannate in oil) every 24 to 96 hours to reduce urinary volume (shake vigorously or warm; administer in the evening; rotate injection sites to prevent lipodystrophy)

Fluid Conservation

- Clofibrate, a hypolipidemic agent, has an antidiuretic effect on patients who have some residual hypothalamic vasopressin.
- Chlorpropamide (Diabinese) and thiazide diuretics are used in mild forms to potentiate the action of vasopressin; may cause hypoglycemic reactions.

Nursing Management

- Encourage and support patient undergoing studies for possible cranial lesion.

- Instruct patient and family members about follow-up care and emergency measures.
- Advise patient to wear a medical identification bracelet and to carry medication information about this disorder at all times.
- Use caution with administration of vasopressin if coronary artery disease is present because of vasoconstrictive action of this drug.

For more information, see Chapter 42 in Smeltzer and Bare: *Brunner and Suddarth's Textbook of Medical-Surgical Nursing*, 11th edition. Philadelphia: Lippincott Williams & Wilkins, 2008.

Diabetes Mellitus

Diabetes mellitus is a group of metabolic disorders characterized by elevated levels of blood glucose (hyperglycemia) resulting from defects in insulin production and secretion, decreased cellular response to insulin, or both. Hyperglycemia may lead to acute metabolic complications, such as diabetic ketoacidosis (DKA) and hyperglycemic hyperosmolar nonketotic syndrome (HHNS). Long-term hyperglycemia may contribute to chronic microvascular complications (kidney and eye disease) and neuropathic complications. Diabetes is also associated with an increased occurrence of macrovascular diseases, including coronary artery disease (myocardial infarction), cerebrovascular disease (stroke), and peripheral vascular disease.

Types of Diabetes

Type 1 (Formerly Insulin-Dependent Diabetes Mellitus)

- About 5% to 10% of diabetic patients have type 1 diabetes. Beta cells of the pancreas that normally produce insulin are

destroyed by an autoimmune process. Insulin injections are needed to control the blood glucose levels.
- Type 1 diabetes has a sudden onset, usually before the age of 30 years.

Type 2 (Formerly Non-Insulin-Dependent Diabetes Mellitus)

- About 90% to 95% of diabetics have type 2 diabetes. It results from a decreased sensitivity to insulin (insulin resistance) or from a decreased amount of insulin production.
- Type 2 diabetes is first treated with diet and exercise, then oral hypoglycemic agents as needed.
- Type 2 diabetes occurs most frequently in patients older than 30 years of age and in obese patients.

Gestational Diabetes Mellitus

- Gestational diabetes is characterized by any degree of glucose intolerance with onset during pregnancy (second or third trimester).
- It occurs in women 25 years of age or older, women younger than 25 years of age who are obese, women with a family history of diabetes in first-degree relatives, or members of certain ethnic racial groups (eg, Hispanic American, Native American, Asian American, African American, or Pacific Islander). It increases their risk for hypertensive disorders of pregnancy.

Clinical Manifestations

- Polyuria, polydipsia, and polyphagia
- Fatigue and weakness, sudden vision changes, tingling or numbness in hands or feet, dry skin, sores that heal slowly and recurrent infections

- Onset of type 1 diabetes may be associated with nausea, vomiting, or stomach pains.
- Type 2 diabetes results from a slow (over years), progressive glucose intolerance and results in long-term complications if diabetes goes undetected for many years (eg, eye disease, peripheral neuropathy, peripheral vascular disease). Complications may have developed before the actual diagnosis is made.
- Signs and symptoms of DKA include abdominal pain, nausea, vomiting, hyperventilation, and a fruity breath odor. Untreated DKA may result in altered level of consciousness, coma, and death.

Assessment and Diagnostic Methods

- High blood glucose levels: fasting plasma glucose levels 126 mg/dL or more, or random plasma glucose levels more than 200 mg/dL on more than one occasion
- Evaluation for complications

Prevention

For obese patients (especially those with type 2 diabetes): weight loss is the key to treatment and the major preventive factor for the development of diabetes.

Complications of Diabetes

Complications associated with both types of diabetes are classi-fied as acute or chronic. Acute complications occur from short-term imbalances in blood glucose and include:

- Hypoglycemia
- DKA
- HHNS
  Chronic complications generally occur 10 to 15 years after the onset of diabetes mellitus. They include:

D

- Macrovascular (large vessel) disease: affects coronary, peripheral vascular, and cerebral vascular circulations
- Microvascular (small vessel) disease: affects the eyes (retinopathy) and kidneys (nephropathy); control blood glucose levels to delay or avoid onset of both microvascular and macrovascular complications
- Neuropathic disease: affects sensory motor and autonomic nerves and contributes to such problems as impotence and foot ulcers

🌿 Gerontologic Considerations

Because the incidence of elevated blood glucose levels increases with advancing age, elderly adults should be advised that physical activity that is consistent and realistic is beneficial to those with diabetes. Advantages of exercise include a decrease in hyperglycemia, a general sense of well-being, metabolism of ingested calories, and weight reduction. Consider physical impairment from other chronic diseases when planning an exercise regimen for elderly diabetic patients.

Medical Management

The main goal of treatment is to normalize insulin activity and blood glucose levels to reduce the development of vascular and neuropathic complications. The therapeutic goal within each type of diabetes is to achieve normal blood glucose levels (euglycemia) without hypoglycemia and without seriously disrupting the patient's usual activities. There are five components of management for diabetes: nutrition, exercise, monitoring, pharmacologic therapy, and education.

- Primary treatment of type 1 diabetes is insulin.
- Primary treatment of type 2 diabetes is weight loss.
- Exercise is important in enhancing the effectiveness of insulin.
- Use oral hypoglycemic agents if diet and exercise are not successful in controlling blood glucose levels. Insulin injections may be used in acute situations.

- Because treatment varies throughout course because of changes in lifestyle and physical and emotional status as well as advances in therapy, continuously assess and modify treatment plan as well as daily adjustments in therapy. Education is needed for both patient and family.

D

Nutritional Management

- Meal plan should be based on patient's usual eating habits and lifestyle and should provide all essential food constituents (eg, vitamins, minerals).
- Goals are to achieve and maintain ideal weight, meet energy needs, prevent wide daily fluctuations in blood glucose levels (keep as close to normal as is safe and practical), and decrease blood lipid levels, if elevated.
- For patients who require insulin to help control blood glucose levels, consistency is required in maintaining calories and carbohydrates consumed at different meals.
- Consult dietitian for diabetes management planning to gradually increase or add fiber in meal plan (grains, vegetables).

Caloric Requirements

- Determine basic caloric requirements, taking into consideration age, gender, body weight, and height and factoring in degree of activity (Harris-Benedict formula for basal energy expenditure).
- Long-term weight reduction can be achieved (1- to 2-pound loss per week) by reducing basic caloric intake by 500 to 1,000 calories from calculated basic caloric requirements.
- The American Diabetes and American Dietetic Associations recommend that for all levels of caloric intake, 50% to 60% of calories be derived from carbohydrates, 20% to 30% from fat, and the remaining 10% to 20% from protein. Using food combinations to lower the glycemic response (glycemic index) can be useful. Carbohydrate counting and the food guide pyramid can be useful tools.

NURSING PROCESS: The Patient with Newly Diagnosed Diabetes Mellitus

Assessment

- Focus on signs and symptoms of prolonged hyperglycemia and physical, social, and emotional factors that affect ability to learn and perform diabetes self-care activities.
- Ask for a description of symptoms that preceded the diagnosis: polyuria, polydipsia, polyphagia, skin dryness, blurred vision, weight loss, vaginal itching, and nonhealing ulcers.
- Assess for signs of DKA, including ketonuria, Kussmaul respirations, orthostatic hypotension, and lethargy.
- Question regarding DKA symptoms of nausea, vomiting, and abdominal pain.
- Monitor laboratory signs for metabolic acidosis (decreased pH, decreased bicarbonate) and electrolyte imbalance.
- Assess patients with type 2 diabetes for signs of HHNS: hypotension, altered sensorium, seizures, decreased skin turgor, hyperosmolarity, and electrolyte imbalance.
- Assess physical factors that impair ability to learn or perform self-care skills: visual defects, motor coordination defects, neurologic defects.
- Evaluate patient's social situation for factors that influence diabetic treatment and education plan (literacy, financial resources, health insurance, family support); evaluate typical daily schedule (eg, work, meals, exercise, travel plans).
- Assess emotional status through observation of general demeanor (eg, withdrawn, anxious, body language).
- Assess coping skills by asking how patient has dealt with difficult situations in the past.

Diagnosis

Nursing Diagnoses

- Risk for fluid volume deficit related to polyuria and dehydration

- Imbalanced nutrition related to imbalance of insulin, food, and physical activity
- Deficient knowledge about diabetes self-care skills and information
- Potential self-care deficit related to physical impairments or social factors
- Anxiety related to loss of control, fear of inability to manage diabetes, misinformation related to diabetes, and fear of diabetes complications
- Risk for complications

Collaborative Problems/Potential Complications

- Fluid overload, pulmonary edema, congestive heart failure
- Hypokalemia
- Hyperglycemia and DKA
- Hypoglycemia
- Cerebral edema

Planning and Goals

The major goals of the patient may include attainment of fluid and electrolyte balance, optimal control of blood glucose, regaining weight lost, ability to perform basic (survival) diabetes skills and self-care activities, reduction in anxiety, and absence of complications.

Nursing Interventions

Maintaining Fluid and Electrolyte Balance

- Measure intake and output.
- Administer intravenous fluids and electrolytes as ordered.
- Encourage fluid intake.
- Measure serum electrolytes (sodium, potassium), and monitor closely.
- Monitor vital signs to detect dehydration: tachycardia, orthostatic hypotension.

Improving Nutritional Intake

- Plan the diet with glucose control as the primary goal.
- Take into consideration patient's lifestyle, cultural background, activity level, and food preferences.
- Encourage patient to eat full meals and snacks as per diabetic diet.
- Make arrangements for extra snacks before increased physical activity.
- Ensure that insulin orders are altered as needed for delays in eating due to diagnostic and other procedures.

Reducing Anxiety

- Provide emotional support; set aside time to talk with patient.
- Clear up misconceptions patient or family may have regarding diabetes.
- Assist patient and family to focus on learning self-care behaviors.
- Encourage patient to perform the skills feared most: self-injection or finger stick for glucose monitoring.
- Give positive reinforcement for self-care behaviors attempted.

Monitoring and Managing Potential Complications

- Fluid overload: measure vital signs and monitor central venous pressure (CVP) and total hemodynamic status at frequent intervals; assess cardiac rate and rhythm, breath sounds, venous distention, skin turgor, and urine output; monitor intravenous fluid and other fluid intake.
- Hypokalemia: replace potassium cautiously, ensure that kidneys are functioning before administration; monitor cardiac rate, rhythm, electrocardiogram (ECG), and serum potassium levels.
- Hyperglycemia and DKA: monitor blood glucose levels and urine ketones; administer medications (insulin, oral hypoglycemic agents); monitor for signs and symptoms of impending hyperglycemia and DKA, administering insulin and intravenous fluids to correct.

- Hypoglycemia: treat with juice or glucose tablets; encourage patient to eat full meals or snacks as prescribed; review signs and symptoms, possible causes, and measures to prevent or treat.
- Cerebral edema: prevent by gradual reduction in blood glucose level; monitor blood glucose level, serum electrolyte levels, urine output, mental status, and neurologic signs; minimize activities that increase intracranial pressure.

Teaching Patients About Self-Care

- Teach preventive behaviors for long-term diabetic complications and patient survival skills. Cover simple pathophysiology, treatment modalities, recognition and prevention of acute complications, and pragmatic information (where to obtain supplies, when to call physician).
- Provide special equipment for instruction on diabetic survival skills (eg, magnifying glass for insulin preparation or injection aid device for insulin injection).
- Tailor information according to patient's ability to understand.
- Instruct family so that they may assist in diabetes management.
- Recommend follow-up education with outpatient diabetic specialist regarding optimal equipment for patients with physical impairment; recommend and arrange for home care nurse, as indicated.
- Assist in identifying community resources for education and supplies, giving consideration to financial and physical limitations.

Nutrition

- Initial education addresses the importance of consistency in eating habits, the relationship of food and insulin, and provision of individualized meal plan.
- Follow-up education focuses on more in-depth management skills, such as restaurant eating, food labels, and adjusting meals for exercise, illness, and special occasions.

- Determine whether patient can learn and use the exchange system.
- Simplify information, and provide many opportunities for practice and repetition.
- Teach patients to read labels of "health" foods because they often contain sugar products (eg, honey, brown sugar, and corn syrup) and may contain saturated vegetable fats, hydrogenated vegetable fats, or animal fats that may be contraindicated with elevated blood lipids.

Exercise

Exercise is extremely important because of its effects on lowering blood glucose levels and reducing cardiovascular risk factors. Exercise is useful in losing weight, easing stress, and maintaining a feeling of well-being. Exercise alters blood lipids, increasing levels of high-density lipoproteins (HDL) and decreasing total cholesterol and triglyceride levels.

- Teach patient with blood glucose levels of more than 250 mg/dL not to begin exercising until the urine ketone test is negative and blood glucose levels are closer to normal. (High blood glucose levels stimulate secretion of glucagon, growth hormone, and catecholamines, resulting in release of more glucose from the liver and an increase in blood glucose.)
- Encourage patient to eat a 15-g carbohydrate snack (fruit exchange) or a snack of complex carbohydrates with protein before moderate exercise to prevent hypoglycemia.
- Warn patient about postexercise hypoglycemia, which occurs many hours after exercise.
- Discuss testing blood glucose before, during, and after exercise and eating carbohydrate snacks as needed to maintain blood glucose. Advise patient to reduce dosage of insulin that peaks at the time of exercise if necessary.
- Explain that exercise and dietary management improve glucose metabolism and enhance loss of body fat in people with type 2 diabetes. Also explain that exercise, coupled with weight loss, improves insulin sensitivity and may decrease need for insulin or oral agents in type 2 diabetes.

- Encourage regular daily exercise rather than sporadic exercise.
- Advise all patients with diabetes to discuss an exercise program with their physician.

Self-Monitoring of Blood Glucose Levels

Self-monitoring of blood glucose (SMBG) allows adjustment in the treatment regimen for optimal blood glucose levels and motivates patients to continue treatment.

- Provide initial training in SMBG techniques.
- Evaluate the techniques of patients experienced in SMBG.
- Discourage patient from purchasing SMBG products from stores or catalogs that do not provide direct education.
- Ensure that the method used by patients is matched to their skill level, visual acuity, fine-motor coordination, cognitive ability, comfort with technology, willingness, and financial resources.
- Instruct patient to keep a record of blood glucose test results.

Assessing Glycosylated Hemoglobin

If the patient's glycosylated hemoglobin level (A_1C) is high but blood glucose levels test normal, a special blood test that reflects average blood glucose levels over a period of about 2 to 3 months is performed (normal values, 4% to 8%). Depending on the results, determine the presence of errors in methods of SMBG.

Testing Urine for Ketones (Acetone)

Urine testing is for patients who cannot or will not perform blood glucose testing. Provide instruction in the urine testing procedure for the patient with type 1 diabetes who has glucosuria or unexplained elevated blood glucose levels (more than 250 mg/dL) and for patients who are ill or pregnant.

Administering Insulin Therapy

Insulin preparations vary according to four main characteristics: time course of action, concentration, species (source), and manufacturer.

- Time course: insulins may be grouped into three categories based on onset, peak, and duration of action. Rapid-acting insulins (eg, insulin lispro) have an effect of shorter duration than regular insulin (onset 5–15 min; peak 60–90 min; duration 2–4 h). Short-acting insulin includes regular insulin (marked "R" on the bottle), also known as crystalline zinc insulin (CZI); it is clear in appearance. Onset of regular insulin is 30 minutes to 1 hour; peak, 2 to 4 hours; duration, 6 to 8 hours. Intermediate-acting insulins include NPH insulin and Lente ("L") insulin and are white and milky in appearance. Onset of intermediate-acting insulins is 3 to 4 hours; peak, 4 to 12 hours; duration, 16 to 20 hours. Long-acting insulin includes Ultralente ("UL") insulin, which has a long, slow, sustained action with an onset of 6 to 8 hours; peak, 12 to 16 hours; duration, 20 to 30 hours.
- Peakless basal insulin (insulin glargine) is absorbed over 24 hours and can be given once a day.
- U-100 is the most common concentration of insulin in the United States (100 units of insulin per 1 cubic centimeter).
- Common sources of insulin include that obtained from the pancreas of cows and pigs. Human insulins are now produced by recombinant DNA technology.
- Alternate methods of insulin delivery include insulin pens, jet injectors, insulin pumps, and implantable and inhalant insulin. Transplantation of a whole or partial pancreas may be performed.

Recognizing Problems with Insulin

- Local allergic reactions may occur in the form of redness, swelling, tenderness, and induration up to 1 to 2 hours after the injection is given.
- Systemic allergic reactions are rare and occasionally associated with generalized edema or anaphylaxis.

- Insulin lipodystrophy is a localized disturbance of fat metabolism, prevented by rotating injection sites and avoiding injecting insulin into hypertrophied areas.
- Clinical insulin resistance may occur because immune antibodies develop and bind the insulin, decreasing availability for use. It is treated by administering a purer insulin preparation and occasionally prednisone to block the production of antibodies.
- Morning hyperglycemia may be noted. This includes the dawn phenomenon (glucose level rises after 3 AM), which occurs as insulin is waning, causing a progressive increase in glucose, and the Somogyi effect (nocturnal hypoglycemia followed by rebound hyperglycemia). Instruct patient with insulin waning to move the evening dose of NPH insulin to bedtime (from before dinner). Instruct patient and family to test blood glucose levels at bedtime, at 3 AM, and on awakening.

Teaching About Oral Hypoglycemic Agents

Oral hypoglycemic agents may be effective for patients with type 2 diabetes who cannot be treated by diet and exercise. A functioning pancreas is necessary for these agents to be effective, and they cannot be used in the treatment of type 1 diabetes, in patients prone to DKA, or during pregnancy.

- Explain that hypoglycemia may occur when an excessive dose of an oral hypoglycemic is used, meals are omitted, or food intake is decreased.
- Advise patient to avoid ingestion of alcohol, because a disulfiram (Antabuse) type of reaction may occur.
- If hyperglycemia develops due to infection, trauma, or surgery, tell the patient that oral hypoglycemic drugs may be discontinued temporarily when insulin is needed. Oral hypoglycemics include sulfonylureas, biguanides, alpha-glucosidase inhibitors, thiazolidinediones, and meglitinides.

> **NURSING ALERT**   Avoid using scare tactics (citing future
> blindness or amputation) if patient does not comply with
> the treatment plan. Do not judge the patient; it only
> promotes feelings of guilt and low self-esteem.
> Distinguish among problems of compliance, deficient
> knowledge, and self-care deficit, and do not assume that
> problems with diabetes are related to noncompliance.

Promoting Compliance

- Recognize that physical (eg, visual acuity) and emotional
  factors may impair the patient's ability to perform self-care
  skills.
- Assess for signs of infection or emotional stress that lead to
  elevated glucose levels despite adherence to treatment
  regimen.

For more information, see Chapter 41 in Smeltzer and Bare: *Brunner and Suddarth's Textbook of Medical-Surgical Nursing*, 11th edition. Philadelphia: Lippincott Williams & Wilkins, 2008.

Diabetic Ketoacidosis

Diabetic ketoacidosis (DKA) is caused by an absence or inadequate amount of insulin. This results in disorders in the metabolism of carbohydrates, protein, and fat. The three main clinical features of DKA are (1) hyperglycemia, due to decreased use of glucose by the cells and increased production of glucose by the liver; (2) dehydration and electrolyte loss, resulting from polyuria, with a loss of up to 6.5 liters of water and up to 400 to 500 mEq each of sodium, potassium, and chloride over 24 hours; and (3) acidosis, due to an excess breakdown of fat to fatty acids and production of ketone bodies, which are also acids. Three main causes of DKA are decreased or missed dose of insulin, illness or infection, and initial manifestation of undiagnosed or untreated diabetes.

Clinical Manifestations

- Polyuria and polydipsia (increased thirst)
- Blurred vision, weakness, and headache
- Orthostatic hypotension in patients with volume depletion
- Weak, rapid pulse
- Gastrointestinal symptoms, such as anorexia, nausea/vomiting, and abdominal pain (may be severe)
- Acetone breath (fruity odor)
- Kussmaul respirations: hyperventilation with very deep, but not labored, respirations
- Mental status changes, which vary widely from patient to patient (alert to lethargic or comatose)

Assessment and Diagnostic Findings

- Blood glucose level: 300 to 800 mg/dL (may be lower or higher)
- Low serum bicarbonate level: 0 to 15 mEq/L
- Low pH: 6.8 to 7.3
- Low pCO_2: 10 to 30 mm Hg
- Sodium and potassium levels may be low, normal, or high depending on amount of water loss (dehydration).
- Elevated creatinine, blood urea nitrogen (BUN), hemoglobin, and hematocrit values may be seen with dehydration. After rehydration, continued elevation in the serum creatinine and BUN levels will be present in the patient with underlying renal insufficiency.

Medical Management

Treatment of DKA is aimed at correcting hyperglycemia, dehydration, electrolyte loss, and acidosis.

Management of Dehydration

Patients may need 6 to 10 liters of intravenous fluid (0.9% normal saline is administered at a high rate of 0.5 to 1 L/h for 2 to 3 hours) to replace fluid loss caused by polyuria, hyperventilation, diarrhea, and vomiting. Hypotonic (0.45%) normal saline solution may be used for hypertension or hypernatremia or congestive heart failure. This is the fluid of choice (200 to 500 mL/h for several additional hours) after the first few hours provided blood pressure is stable and sodium level is not low. Plasma expanders may be used to correct severe hypotension that does not respond to intravenous fluid treatment.

Management of Electrolyte Loss

Potassium is the main electrolyte of concern in treating DKA. Cautious replacement of potassium is vital for avoiding severe cardiac dysrhythmias that occur with hypokalemia.

Management of Acidosis

Acidosis of DKA is reversed with insulin, which inhibits the breakdown of fat. Insulin (regular insulin only) is infused at a slow, continuous rate (eg, 5 units per hour). Dextrose is added to intravenous fluids (D5W) when blood glucose reaches 300 mg/dL or less to avoid too rapid a drop in the blood glucose level. Intravenous insulin must be infused continuously until subcutaneous administration of insulin can be resumed. However, intravenous insulin must be continued until the serum bicarbonate level improves and patient can eat. Normalized blood glucose levels are *not* an indication that acidosis has resolved.

Nursing Management
Promoting Fluid Balance

- Administer fluids as ordered, and monitor infusion carefully.
- Monitor fluid volume status (including checking for orthostatic changes of blood pressure and heart rate), lung assessment, and intake and output (initial urine output will lag behind intravenous fluid intake until dehydration is corrected).
- Monitor urine output to ensure adequate renal function.

- Monitor for signs of fluid overload in elderly patients and those at risk for congestive heart failure.

 NURSING ALERT Monitor carefully for hypokalemia due to rehydration and insulin treatment.

 D

Promoting Electrolyte and Acid-Base Balance

Observe frequently for signs of hyperkalemia (ie, tall, peaked T waves on the ECG) and obtain frequent (every 2 to 4 hours) potassium values during first 8 hours of treatment.

 NURSING ALERT Withhold potassium only if hyperkalemia is present and patient is not urinating; notify physician.

NURSING ALERT Administer continuous insulin drip as ordered, and monitor blood glucose values hourly.

Teaching Patients Self-Care

Teach patient about "sick-day rules," which are strategies to help prevent diabetic complications.

- Do not eliminate insulin doses when nausea and vomiting occur.
- Take usual insulin dose or previously prescribed sick-day doses, and attempt to consume frequent small portions of carbohydrates.
- Drink fluids (including broth) every hour to avoid dehydration.
- Check blood glucose level every 3 to 4 hours.
- Notify physician if unable to take fluids without vomiting or if elevated glucose level persists.
- Make sure patient knows how to contact the physician 24 hours a day. Teach self-management skills, including careful insulin administration and blood glucose and urine ketone

testing. Assess patient's skills to prevent accidental errors in insulin administration or blood glucose testing.

Recommend psychological counseling for patient and family if intentional alteration in insulin dosing was the cause of DKA.

For more information, see Chapter 41 in Smeltzer and Bare: *Brunner and Suddarth's Textbook of Medical-Surgical Nursing*, 11th edition. Philadelphia: Lippincott Williams & Wilkins, 2008.

Diarrhea

Diarrhea is a condition defined by an increased frequency of bowel movements (more than three per day), increased amount of stool (more than 200 g per day), and altered consistency (liquid stool). It is usually associated with urgency, perianal discomfort, incontinence, or a combination of these factors. Diarrhea can result from any condition that causes increased intestinal secretions, decreased mucosal absorption, or altered (increased) motility.

Types of diarrhea include secretory, osmotic, or mixed diarrhea. It can be acute (self-limiting and often associated with infection) or chronic (persists for a long period and may return sporadically). It is classified as secretory (high volume), osmotic (nonabsorbed particles), or mixed (includes inflammatory bowel disease). It can be caused by certain medications, tube feedings, metabolic and endocrine disorders, and viral and bacterial infections. Other causes are nutritional and malabsorptive disorders, anal sphincter deficit, Zollinger-Ellison syndrome, paralytic ileus, acquired immunodeficiency syndrome (AIDS), and intestinal obstruction.

Clinical Manifestations

- Increased frequency and fluid content of stool
- Abdominal cramps, distention, intestinal rumbling (borborygmus), anorexia, and thirst

• Painful spasmodic contractions of the anus and ineffectual straining (tenesmus) with each defecation

Other symptoms, depending on the cause and severity and related to dehydration and fluid and electrolyte imbalances, include:

• Watery stools, which may indicate small bowel disease
• Loose, semisolid stools, which are associated with disorders of the colon
• Voluminous greasy stools, which suggest intestinal malabsorption
• Mucus and pus in the stools, which denote inflammatory enteritis or colitis
• Oil droplets on the toilet water, which are diagnostic of pancreatic insufficiency
• Nocturnal diarrhea, which may be a manifestation of diabetic neuropathy

Complications

Complications of diarrhea include cardiac dysrhythmias due to fluid and electrolyte (potassium) imbalance, urinary output less than 30 mL/h, muscle weakness, paresthesia, hypotension, anorexia, drowsiness (report if potassium level is less than 3 mEq/L [SI 3 mmol/L]), and death if imbalances become severe.

Assessment and Diagnostic Findings

When cause is unknown: stool examination for infectious or parasitic organisms, bacterial toxins, blood, fat, and electrolytes, complete blood count, chemical profile, endoscopy, or barium enema

Medical Management

• Primary medical management is directed at controlling symptoms, preventing complications, and eliminating or treating the underlying disease.

- Certain medications (eg, antibiotics, anti-inflammatory agents) may reduce the severity of diarrhea and the disease.
- Increase oral fluids; oral glucose and electrolyte solution may be prescribed.
- Antidiarrheals, such as diphenoxylate (Lomotil) and loperamide (Imodium), may be prescribed to decrease motility from a noninfectious source.
- Antimicrobials are prescribed when the infectious agent has been identified or diarrhea is severe.
- Intravenous therapy is used for rapid hydration in very young or elderly patients.

NURSING PROCESS: The Patient with Diarrhea

Assessment

- Elicit a complete health history to identify character and pattern of diarrhea, and the following: any related signs and symptoms, current medication therapy, daily dietary patterns and intake, past related medical and surgical history, and recent exposure to an acute illness or travel to another geographic area.
- Perform a complete physical assessment, paying special attention to auscultation (characteristic bowel sounds), palpation for abdominal tenderness, inspection of stool (obtain a sample for testing).
- Inspect mucous membranes and skin to determine hydration status, and assess blood pressure (postural hypotension).
- Inspect perianal skin for irritation.
- Note intake and output and weight.

Diagnosis

Nursing Diagnoses

- Diarrhea related to infection, ingestion of irritating foods, or disorder of the bowel

- Risk for deficient fluid volume related to frequent passage of stools and insufficient fluid intake
- Anxiety related to frequent, uncontrolled elimination
- Risk for impaired skin integrity related to frequent, loose stools

Collaborative Problems/Potential Complications
- Dehydration
- Fluid and electrolyte imbalance
- Cardiac dysrhythmias

Planning and Goals

Major goals include regaining normal bowel patterns, avoidance of fluid and electrolyte deficit, reduction of anxiety, maintenance of perianal skin integrity, and absence of complications.

Nursing Interventions

Controlling Diarrhea
- Encourage bed rest, liquids, and foods low in bulk until acute period subsides.
- Recommend bland diet (semisolids to solids) when food intake is tolerated.
- Encourage patient to limit intake of caffeine and carbonated beverages, and avoid very hot and cold foods because these increase intestinal motility.
- Advise patient to restrict intake of milk products, fat, whole grain products, fresh fruits, and vegetables for several days.
- Administer antidiarrheal drugs as prescribed.

Maintaining Fluid and Electrolyte Balance
- Assess for dehydration (decreased skin turgor, tachycardia, decreased pulse volume, decreased serum sodium, thirst).
- Administer intravenous fluids if ordered for rapid rehydration (in elderly patients or those with preexisting gastrointestinal disturbance).
- Encourage oral fluid replacement in the form of water, juices, bouillon, and commercial preparations, such as Gatorade; give parenteral fluids as ordered.

- Monitor serum electrolyte levels closely.
- Report evidence of dysrhythmias or change in level of consciousness immediately.

> **NURSING ALERT** Older people can quickly become dehydrated and suffer from low potassium levels (hypokalemia) as a result of diarrhea. Teach the older patient taking digitalis about how quickly dehydration and hypokalemia can occur with diarrhea. Instruct the patient to recognize the signs of hypokalemia (which intensifies the action of digitalis, leading to digitalis toxicity).

Reducing Anxiety

- Provide opportunity for patient to express fears or worry about being embarrassed by lack of control over bowel elimination.
- Assist to identify any factors that precipitate diarrhea. Teach patient to be sensitive to body clues, use absorbent underwear, and take prescribed antianxiety medications.

Providing Skin Care

- Instruct patient to follow a perianal care routine, such as wiping or patting the area dry after defecation, cleansing with mild soap and warm water, and patting dry.
- Apply lotion or ointment as a skin barrier; a skin sealant may be used.
- Treat all patients with diarrhea as potentially infectious; use gloves and standard precautions, as with all patients.

> **NURSING ALERT** Skin in elderly patients is sensitive to rapid perianal excoriation because of decreased turgor and reduced subcutaneous fat layers.

For more information, see Chapter 38 in Smeltzer and Bare: *Brunner and Suddarth's Textbook of Medical-Surgical Nursing*, 11th edition. Philadelphia: Lippincott Williams & Wilkins, 2008.

Disseminated Intravascular Coagulopathy

Disseminated intravascular coagulopathy (DIC) is a potentially life-threatening sign (not a disease itself) of a serious underlying disease mechanism.

Pathophysiology

In DIC, the normal hemostatic mechanisms are altered so that tiny clots form within the microcirculation of the body. These clots consume platelets and clotting factors, eventually causing coagulation to fail and bleeding to result. This bleeding disorder is characterized by low fibrinogen levels; prolonged prothrombin time (PT), partial thromboplastin time (PTT), and thrombin time; low platelet counts (thrombocytopenia); and elevated fibrin degradation products (D-dimers). Many serious illnesses may predispose a patient to DIC, including septicemia, premature separation of the placenta, metastatic malignancies, hemolytic transfusion reactions, massive tissue trauma, and shock.

Clinical Manifestations

Clinical manifestations of DIC are reflected in the organs affected either by excessive clot formation (with resultant ischemia to that organ or part of organ) or bleeding.

- Patient may bleed from mucous membranes, venipuncture sites, and gastrointestinal and urinary tracts.
- Bleeding can range from minimal occult internal bleeding to profuse hemorrhage from all orifices.
- Patient may also develop organ dysfunction, such as renal failure and pulmonary and multifocal central nervous system infarctions due to microthrombosis, macrothrombosis, or hemorrhage.
- Initially, the only manifestation is a progressive decrease in the platelet count; then, progressively, the patient exhibits

signs and symptoms of thrombosis in the organs involved. Eventually bleeding occurs (at first subtle, advancing to frank hemorrhage). Signs depend on the organs involved.

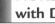

Medical Management

The most important management issue is treating the underlying cause of DIC. A second goal is to correct the secondary effects of tissue ischemia by improving oxygenation, replacing fluids, and administering vasopressor medications. If serious hemorrhage occurs, the depleted coagulation factors and platelets may be replaced (cryoprecipitate to replace fibrinogen and factors V and VII; fresh-frozen plasma to replace other coagulation factors).

A heparin infusion, which is a controversial management method, may be used to interrupt the thrombosis process. An even more controversial management method involves administering fibrinolytic inhibitors such as aminocaproic acid (Amicar), which reduces fibrin degradation products by decreasing the lysis of microthrombi. Other therapies include recombinant activated protein C and antithrombin infusions.

NURSING PROCESS: The Patient with DIC

Assessment

- Be aware of patients at risk for DIC (sepsis and acute promyelocytic leukemia are the most common causes).
- Assess patients thoroughly and frequently for signs and symptoms of thrombi or bleeding, and monitor for any progression of these signs.

Diagnosis

Nursing Diagnoses

- Risk for deficient fluid volume related to bleeding
- Risk for impaired skin integrity related to ischemia or bleeding

- Risk for imbalanced fluid volume related to excessive blood/factor component replacement
- Ineffective tissue perfusion related to microthrombi
- Death anxiety

Collaborative Problems/Potential Complications

- Renal failure
- Gangrene
- Pulmonary embolism or hemorrhage
- Altered level of consciousness
- Acute respiratory distress syndrome
- Stroke

Planning and Goals

The major goals for the patient include maintaining hemodynamic status, intact skin and oral mucosa, fluid balance and tissue perfusion; enhancing coping; and preventing complications.

Nursing Interventions

Maintaining Hemodynamic Status

- Avoid procedures and activities that can increase intracranial pressure, such as coughing and straining.
- Closely monitor vital signs, including neurologic checks, and assess for amount of external bleeding.
- Avoid medications that interfere with platelet function, if possible (eg, beta-lactam antibiotics, acetylsalicylic acid, nonsteroidal anti-inflammatory drugs).
- Avoid rectal probes and rectal or intramuscular injection medications.
- Use low pressure with any suctioning.
- Administer oral hygiene carefully: use sponge-tipped swabs, salt or soda mouth rinses; avoid lemon-glycerine swabs, hydrogen peroxide, commercial mouthwashes.
- Avoid dislodging any clots, including those around intravenous sites, injection sites, and so forth.

D

Maintaining Skin Integrity

- Assess skin, with particular attention to bony prominences and skin folds.
- Reposition carefully; use pressure-reducing mattress and lamb's wool between digits and around ears and soft absorbent material in skin folds, as needed.
- Perform skin care every 2 hours; administer oral hygiene carefully (see earlier).
- Use prolonged pressure (5 minutes minimum) after essential injections.

Monitoring for Imbalanced Fluid Volume

- Auscultate breath sounds every 2 to 4 hours.
- Monitor extent of edema.
- Monitor volume of intravenous medications and blood products; decrease volume of intravenous medications if possible.
- Administer diuretics as prescribed.

Assessing for Ineffective Tissue Perfusion Related to Microthrombi

- Assess neurologic, pulmonary, and skin systems.
- Monitor response to heparin therapy; monitor fibrinogen levels.
- Assess extent of bleeding.
- Stop epsilon-aminocaproic acid if symptoms of thrombosis occur.

Reducing Fear and Anxiety

- Identify previous coping mechanisms, if possible; encourage patient to use them as appropriate.
- Explain all procedures and rationale in terms that the patient and family can understand.
- Assist family in supporting patient.
- Use services from behavioral medicine and clergy, if desired.

Monitoring and Managing Potential Complications

- If dialysis is required, place dialysis catheter with extreme caution, and prepare for transfusion of adequate platelets and plasma.
- Monitor for complications; implement measures to address complications as indicated (see specific condition).

Evaluation

Expected Patient Outcomes

- Has stable hemodynamic status and vital signs; remains free of bleeding episodes
- Demonstrates intact skin and oral mucous membranes without evidence of breakdown
- Has no or minimal edema or evidence of thrombosis
- Reports relief of anxiety and fears

For more information, see Chapter 33 in Smeltzer and Bare: *Brunner and Suddarth's Textbook of Medical-Surgical Nursing*, 11th edition. Philadelphia: Lippincott Williams & Wilkins, 2008.

Diverticular Disorders

A diverticulum is a sac-like outpouching or herniation of the lining of the bowel (the mucosa and submucosa) that protrudes through a weak portion of the muscle layer. Diverticula may occur anywhere along the gastrointestinal tract. Diverticulosis exists when multiple diverticula are present without inflammation or symptoms. Diverticulitis results when food and bacteria retained in the diverticulum produce infection and inflammation that can impede draining and lead to perforation or abscess. It may occur in acute attacks or persist as a chronic, smoldering infection. Diverticulitis is more common in the sigmoid colon. A congenital predisposition is likely when the disorder is present in those younger than 40 years of age. Diverticulosis is most common in people older than 60 years of age. A low intake of dietary fiber is considered a major predisposing factor. Complications of diverticulitis include fistulas, obstruction, peritonitis, abscess formation, and bleeding.

D

Clinical Manifestations

Diverticulosis

- Frequently, no problematic symptoms are noted; constipation from spastic colon syndrome often precedes development.
- Bowel irregularity and diarrhea
- Crampy pain in left lower quadrant
- Low-grade fever
- Nausea and anorexia and some bloating or abdominal distention

Diverticulitis

- Narrowing of the large bowel with fibrotic stricture
- Cramps, narrow stools, and increased constipation
- Occult bleeding
- Weakness, fatigue, and anorexia
- Tenderness, a palpable mass, fever, and leukocytes, which may indicate abscess development
- Abdominal pain, a rigid boardlike abdomen, loss of bowel sounds, and signs and symptoms of shock, which may indicate peritonitis
- Septicemia if condition remains untreated

Assessment and Diagnostic Findings

- Computed tomography (CT) scan (procedure of choice)
- Abdominal x-ray and barium enema studies (unless peritoneal irritation is present)
- Colonoscopy

- Complete blood count (white blood cell count and sedimentation rate elevated)

🌿 Gerontologic Considerations

The incidence of diverticular disease increases with age because of degeneration and structural changes in the circular muscle layers of the colon and cellular hypertrophy. Symptoms are less pronounced among elderly patients, who may not experience abdominal pain until infection occurs. They delay reporting symptoms because they fear surgery or cancer. Blood in stool may frequently be overlooked because of failure to examine the stool or inability to see changes because of impaired vision.

Medical Management

Management of Mild Diverticulosis

A high-fiber diet is prescribed to prevent constipation.

Management of Mild to Moderate Diverticulitis

The patient is instructed to ingest clear liquids until inflammation subsides, then a high-fiber, low-fat diet. Antibiotics are prescribed for 7 to 10 days and a bulk-forming laxative is also prescribed.

Management of Severe Problems

- Patients with significant symptoms and often those who are elderly, immunocompromised, or on steroidal therapy are hospitalized. The bowel is rested by withholding oral intake, administering intravenous fluids, and instituting nasogastric suctioning.
- Broad-spectrum antibiotics and analgesics are prescribed. Oral intake is increased as symptoms subside. A low-fiber diet may be necessary until signs of infection decrease.

D

- For spastic pain, antispasmodics are taken before meals and at bedtime; sedatives and tranquilizers and bowel antimicrobials may be required.
- Normal stools can be achieved by administering bulk preparations (Metamucil), stool softeners, warm oil enemas, and evacuant suppositories.

Surgical Management

Surgery (resection) is usually necessary only if perforation, peritonitis, abscess formation, hemorrhage, or obstruction occurs; recurrence of diverticula is common. Type of surgery performed varies according to the extent of complications (one-stage resections or multistaged procedures). In some cases fecal diversion (colostomy) may be performed.

NURSING PROCESS: The Patient with Diverticulitis

Assessment

- Assess health history, including onset and duration of pain, dietary habits (fiber intake), and past and present elimination patterns (straining at stool, constipation with diarrhea, tenesmus [spasm of the anal sphincter with pain and persistent urge to defecate]).
- Auscultate for presence and character of bowel sounds; palpate for tenderness, pain, or firm mass over left lower quadrant; inspect stool for pus, mucus, or blood. Monitor blood pressure, temperature, and pulse for abnormal variations.

Diagnosis

Nursing Diagnoses

- Constipation related to narrowing of the colon secondary to thickened muscular segments and strictures
- Acute pain related to inflammation and infection

Collaborative Problems/Potential Complications

- Peritonitis
- Abscess formation
- Bleeding

D

Planning and Goals

The major goals of the patient may include attainment and maintenance of normal elimination, reduction in pain, improvement in gastrointestinal tissue perfusion, and absence of potential complications.

Nursing Interventions

Maintaining Normal Elimination Patterns

- Increase fluid intake to 2 L/day within limits of patient's cardiac and renal reserve.
- Promote foods that are soft but have increased fiber content.
- Encourage individualized exercise program to improve abdominal muscle tone.
- Review patient's routine to establish a set time for meals and defecation.
- Encourage daily intake of bulk laxatives (eg, Metamucil, stool softeners, or oil-retention enemas).

Relieving Pain

- Administer analgesic agents (usually opioid analgesics) for pain and antispasmodic medications.
- Record and monitor intensity, duration, and location of pain.

Monitoring and Managing Potential Complications

- Identify patients at risk.
- Assess for indicators of perforation: tender, rigid abdomen; elevated white blood cell count; elevated sedimentation rate; increased temperature; tachycardia and hypotension.
- Perforation is a surgical emergency: monitor vital signs and urine output, and administer intravenous fluids as ordered.

Evaluation

Expected Patient Outcomes

- Attains a normal pattern of elimination
- Experiences no or decreased pain or discomfort
- Recovers without complications

For more information, see Chapter 38 in Smeltzer and Bare: *Brunner and Suddarth's Textbook of Medical-Surgical Nursing*, 11th edition. Philadelphia: Lippincott Williams & Wilkins, 2008.

Emphysema, Pulmonary

Pulmonary emphysema is defined as a nonuniform pattern of abnormal, permanent distention of the air spaces with destruction of the alveolar walls and eventually a reduced pulmonary capillary bed. It appears to be the end stage of a process that has progressed slowly for many years. Smoking is the major cause. In a few patients, there is a familial predisposition associated with a plasma protein abnormality (deficiency of alpha-1-antitrypsin), making the person sensitive to environmental factors (air pollution, infectious agents, allergens). Emphysema manifests commonly in the fifth decade of life and is classified as follows:

- Panlobular (panacinar): characterized by destruction of the respiratory bronchiole, alveolar duct, and alveoli; air spaces within the lobule are enlarged, with little inflammatory disease
- Centrilobular (centriacinar): causes pathologic changes in the center of the secondary lobule, producing chronic hypoxemia, hypercapnia, polycythemia, and episodes of right-sided heart failure.

Both types of emphysema can occur together.

Clinical Manifestations

- Dyspnea with insidious onset progressing to severe dyspnea with slight exertion (major symptom)
- Chronic cough, sputum production, wheezing, dyspnea, fatigue, and tachypnea
- On inspection, hyperinflated "barrel chest" due to air trapping, muscle wasting, and pursed-lip breathing

- On auscultation, diminished breath sounds with crackles, wheezes, rhonchi, and prolonged expiration
- Hyperresonance with percussion and a decrease in fremitus
- Anorexia, weight loss, weakness, and inactivity
- Hypoxemia and hypercapnia, morning headaches in advanced stages
- Inflammatory reactions and infections from pooled secretions

Assessment and Diagnostic Methods

Evaluation entails primarily chest x-rays, chest computed tomography (CT) scans, pulmonary function tests, pulse oximetry, blood gases, and complete blood count.

Complications

Right-sided heart failure (cor pulmonale) leading to central cyanosis and respiratory failure

Medical Management

The major goals of medical management are to improve quality of life, slow progression of the disease, and treat obstructed airways to relieve hypoxia. Treatment is directed at improving ventilation, decreasing work of breathing and preventing infection.

- Smoking cessation
- Physical therapy to conserve and increase pulmonary ventilation
- Maintenance of proper environmental conditions to facilitate breathing
- Psychological support
- Ongoing program of patient education and rehabilitation
- Bronchodilators and metered-dose inhalers (aerosol therapy, dispensing particles in fine mist)
- Treatment of infection (antimicrobial therapy at the first sign of respiratory infection)
- Oxygenation in low concentrations for severe hypoxemia

See Nursing Management under Chronic Obstructive Pulmonary Disease for additional information.

For more information, see Chapter 24 in Smeltzer and Bare: *Brunner and Suddarth's Textbook of Medical-Surgical Nursing*, 11th edition. Philadelphia: Lippincott Williams & Wilkins, 2008.

Empyema

Empyema is a collection of purulent (infected) liquid or pus in the pleural cavity. At first the pleural fluid is thin, but it progresses to a fibropurulent stage and then to a stage at which it encloses the lung with a thick exudative membrane (loculated empyema).

Clinical Manifestations

- Fever, night sweats, pleural pain, cough, dyspnea, anorexia, and weight loss
- Decreased or absence of breath sounds; dullness on chest percussion; decreased fremitus
- Symptoms vague (immunocompromised patient) or less obvious if patient has received antimicrobial therapy

Assessment and Diagnostic Methods

- Chest auscultation, which demonstrates decreased or absent breath sounds over the affected area; dullness on chest percussion; decreased fremitus
- Chest radiographs, chest CT, and thoracentesis

Medical Management

Objectives of management are to drain the pleural cavity and to achieve full expansion of the lung. This is accomplished by adequate drainage, antibiotics (large doses), streptokinase, or a combination of these. Drainage of the pleural fluid depends on the stage of the disease and is accomplished as follows:

- Needle aspiration (thoracentesis) if fluid is not too thick
- Tube thoracostomy water-seal chest drainage, with fibrinolytic agents instilled through chest tube when indicated
- Open chest drainage to remove thickened pleura, pus, and debris and to remove the underlying diseased pulmonary tissue
- Decortication, surgical removal, if inflammation has been long-standing

Nursing Management

- Provide care specific to method of drainage of pleural fluid.
- Help patient cope with condition; instruct in lung expansion breathing exercises (pursed-lip and diaphragmatic breathing). See Perioperative Nursing Management for additional information.
- Instruct patient and family about care of drainage system and drain site and measurement and observation of drainage.
- Teach patient and family signs and symptoms of infection and how and when to contact the health care provider.

For more information, see Chapter 23 in Smeltzer and Bare: *Brunner and Suddarth's Textbook of Medical-Surgical Nursing*, 11th edition. Philadelphia: Lippincott Williams & Wilkins, 2008.

Endocarditis, Infective

Infective endocarditis (bacterial endocarditis) is an infection of the valves and the endothelial surface of the heart. It is caused by direct invasion of bacteria or other organisms, leading to deformity of the valve leaflets. Causative organisms include many bacteria (eg, streptococci, pneumococci, staphylococci), fungi, and rickettsiae.

Risk Factors

- Valvular heart disease, rheumatic heart disease, mitral valve prolapse, and prosthetic valve surgery
- Age: Infective endocarditis is more common in older people because of their decreased immunologic response, the metabolic changes of aging, and increased invasive diagnostic procedures.
- Intravenous drug use: There is a high incidence of staphylococcal endocarditis among intravenous drug users.
- Hospitalization: Hospital-acquired endocarditis occurs most often in patients with debilitating disease or indwelling catheters and in those receiving prolonged intravenous or antibiotic therapy.
- Immunosuppression: Patients taking immunosuppressive medications or steroids may develop fungal endocarditis.

Clinical Manifestations

- Insidious onset; signs and symptoms develop from toxicity of infection, destruction of heart valves, and embolization of fragments of vegetative growths on the heart.
- General manifestations include vague complaints of malaise, anorexia, weight loss, and back and joint pain.
- Fever is intermittent; may be absent in patients who are receiving antibiotics or corticosteroids, elderly patients, and patients with heart failure or renal failure.
- Splinter hemorrhages under fingernails and toenails and petechiae in conjunctiva and mucous membranes
- Hemorrhages with pale centers (Roth's spots) in fundi of eyes
- Small painful nodules (Osler's nodes) in pads of fingers or toes
- Cardiac manifestations: heart enlargement, heart failure, and heart murmurs (may be absent initially); progressively changing murmurs indicate valvular damage.
- Central nervous system manifestations: headache, transient cerebral ischemia, focal neurologic lesions, stroke
- Emboli involving other organ systems manifest in the lung (recurrent pneumonia, pulmonary abscesses), kidney

E

(hematuria, renal failure), spleen (left upper quadrant pain), heart (myocardial infarction), brain (stroke), and peripheral vessels.

Assessment and Diagnostic Methods

E

A diagnosis of acute infective endocarditis is made when the onset of infection and resulting valvular destruction are rapid, occurring within days to weeks.

- Blood cultures
- Doppler or transesophageal echocardiography

Complications

Heart failure, cerebral vascular complications, valve stenosis or regurgitation, myocardial damage, mycotic aneurysms

Medical Management

Objectives of treatment are to eradicate the invading organism through adequate doses of an appropriate antimicrobial agent (continuous intravenous infusion for 2 to 6 weeks at home). Treatment measures include:

- Isolating causative organism through serial blood cultures. Blood cultures are taken to monitor the course of therapy.
- Monitoring patient's temperature for treatment effectiveness.
- After recovery from the infectious process, seriously damaged valves may require débridement or replacement. For example, surgical valve replacement is required if heart failure develops, if patient has more than one serious systemic embolic episode, if infection cannot be controlled or is recurrent, or if infection is caused by a fungus.

Nursing Management

- Provide psychosocial support while patient is confined to hospital or home with restrictive intravenous therapy.

- Assess heart sounds for new or worsening murmur.
- If patient received surgical treatment, provide postsurgical care and instruction.
- After surgery, monitor patient's temperature; a fever may be present for weeks.
- Monitor for signs and symptoms of systemic embolization, or, for patients with right heart endocarditis, signs and symptoms of pulmonary infarction and infiltrates.
- Assess for signs and symptoms of organ damage such as stroke (CVA, brain attack), meningitis, heart failure, myocardial infarction, glomerulonephritis, and splenomegaly.
- Instruct patient and family about activity restrictions, medications, and signs and symptoms of infection.
- Reinforce that antibiotic prophylaxis is recommended for patients who have had infective endocarditis and who are undergoing invasive procedures.
- Refer to home care nurse to supervise and monitor intravenous antibiotic therapy in the home. For additional nursing interventions, see Preoperative and Postoperative Nursing Management.

For more information, see Chapter 29 in Smeltzer and Bare: *Brunner and Suddarth's Textbook of Medical-Surgical Nursing*, 11th edition. Philadelphia: Lippincott Williams & Wilkins, 2008.

Endocarditis, Rheumatic

Rheumatic endocarditis is associated with rheumatic fever caused by group A beta-hemolytic streptococcal infection.

Pathophysiology

The infectious agent does not invade the tissues but causes a sensitivity phenomenon or reaction in response to hemolytic streptococci. Rheumatic fever affects all bony joints, producing a polyarthritis. The most serious damage occurs in the heart. Rheumatic endocarditis manifests as tiny, translucent vegetations that resemble beads about the size of a pinhead, arranged in a row along the free margins of the valve flaps. The flaps gradually become shorter and thicker than normal, which prevents them from closing the valve orifice completely. The result is valvular regurgitation (leakage); most common is mitral regurgitation. Valvular stenosis may also occur. A few patients become critically ill with intractable heart failure, serious dysrhythmias, and rheumatic pneumonia. The myocardium can compensate for these valvular defects very well for a time. Sooner or later, however, decompensation occurs and is manifested by heart failure.

Clinical Manifestations

- Eventually, the heart murmurs characteristic of valvular stenosis, regurgitation, or both become audible on auscultation; "thrills" may be detected on palpation.
- Cardiac symptoms depend on which side of the heart is involved. Severity of symptoms depends on size and location of the lesion.
- The mitral valve is most often affected, producing symptoms of left-sided heart failure: shortness of breath, crackles, and wheezes.

Assessment and Diagnostic Methods

A throat culture for accurate diagnosis of streptococcal infection of the throat should be performed.

Medical Management

Objectives of medical management are aggressive eradication of the causative organism and prevention of additional complications, such as a thromboembolic event. Prevention is achieved through early and adequate treatment of streptococcal infection in all patients. Long-term antibiotic therapy is the treatment of choice. Parenteral penicillin remains the medication of choice.

If valve dysfunction is mild and the disease is quiet, no therapy is required as long as the heart pumps effectively.

Nursing Management

A key nursing role in rheumatic endocarditis is teaching patients about the disease, its treatment, and the steps needed to avoid complications.

- Educate patient and community regarding recognition of streptococcal infections and the need to treat them adequately and to control community epidemics.
- Teach susceptible patients that they may require long-term oral antibiotic therapy and may be required to take prophylactic antibiotics before procedures, such as dental checkups. They will also need routine cardiac evaluations.
- Emphasize that less common diagnostic procedures, such as cystoscopy, also require prophylactic antibiotic therapy.

For more information, see Chapter 29 in Smeltzer and Bare: *Brunner and Suddarth's Textbook of Medical-Surgical Nursing*, 11th edition. Philadelphia: Lippincott Williams & Wilkins, 2008.

Endometriosis

Endometriosis is a benign lesion with cells similar to those lining the uterus, growing aberrantly in the pelvic cavity outside the uterus. During menstruation, the lesion bleeds (pseudocyst), mostly in areas without outlet, resulting in adhesions, cysts, scar tissue, pain, and infertility. Endometrial tissue can also be spread by lymphatic or venous channels. There is a high incidence among patients who bear children later and have fewer children. It is usually found in young, nulliparous woman aged 25 to 35 years. There appears to be a familial predisposition to endometriosis. It is a major cause of infertility.

E

Clinical Manifestations

- Symptoms vary with the location of endometrial tissue. The chief symptom is a type of dysmenorrhea: pelvic discomfort or pain (deep-seated aching in the lower abdomen, vagina, posterior pelvis, and back), occurring 1 or 2 days before the menstrual cycle and lasting 2 or 3 days.
- Some patients have no pain.
- Abnormal uterine bleeding and dyspareunia (painful intercourse) can occur.
- Nausea and diarrhea may be reported, as may depression, loss of work due to pain, and relationship difficulties.

Assessment and Diagnostic Methods

Laparoscopy confirms the diagnosis and helps to stage the disease.

Medical Management

Treatment depends on symptoms, desire for pregnancy, and extent of the disease. In asymptomatic cases, routine examination may be all that is required. Other therapies include palliative measures (eg, analgesic agents, hormone administration, prostaglandin inhibitors, and surgery). Pregnancy alleviates symptoms because no ovulation or menstruation occurs.

Pharmacologic Therapy

- Oral contraceptives are used to suppress menstruation and relieve menstrual pain.
- Synthetic androgen, danazol (Danocrine), causes atrophy of the endometrium and subsequent amenorrhea. (Danazol is expensive and may cause troublesome side effects such as fatigue, depression, weight gain, oily skin, decreased breast size, mild acne, hot flashes, and vaginal atrophy.)
- Gonadotropin-releasing hormone (GnRH) agonist or GnRH blocker (nafarelin acetate [Synarel]) results in decreased estrogen production and subsequent amenorrhea. This

agent is administered by nasal spray twice a day for 6 months. Side effects are related to low estrogen levels.

Surgical Management

- Laparoscopy to fulgurate endometrial implants and to lyse (release) adhesions
- Laser surgery to vaporize endometrial implants or to coagulate the implant and destroy the endometriosis
- Other surgical procedures may include laparotomy, laser therapy, endo- and electrocoagulation, uterine suspension, abdominal hysterectomy, oophorectomy, bilateral salpingo-oophorectomy, and appendectomy. Hysterectomy may be an option for some women.

Nursing Management

- Obtain health history and physical examination, concentrating on identifying when and how long specific symptoms have been bothersome and on defining the woman's reproductive desires.
- Assess for pain, and evaluate techniques and prescribed medications that provide relief.
- Explain various diagnostic procedures to alleviate anxiety.
- Provide emotional support to the woman and her partner who wish to have children.
- Respect and address psychosocial impact of realization that pregnancy is not easily possible. Discuss alternatives, such as in vitro fertilization (IVF) or adoption.
- Encourage patient to seek care of dysmenorrhea or abnormal bleeding patterns.
- Direct patient to the Endometriosis Association for more information and support.

For more information, see Chapter 47 in Smeltzer and Bare: *Brunner and Suddarth's Textbook of Medical-Surgical Nursing*, 11th edition. Philadelphia: Lippincott Williams & Wilkins, 2008.

Epididymitis

Epididymitis is an infection of the epididymis that usually results from an infected prostate or urinary tract. It may also develop as a complication of gonorrhea. In men younger than 35 years of age, the major cause is *Chlamydia trachomatis* infection. In boys the major cause is *Escherichia coli*.

Clinical Manifestations

- Unilateral pain and soreness in the inguinal canal along the course of the vas deferens
- Pain and swelling in the scrotum and groin
- Extremely painful and swollen epididymis; temperature elevated
- Pyuria and bacteriuria with resulting chills and fever

Medical Management

- If seen within first 24 hours after onset of pain, patient's spermatic cord may be infiltrated with a local anesthetic agent for relief.
- If infection is chlamydial in origin, patient and patient's sexual partners must be treated with antibiotics.
- Observe for abscess formation.
- If no improvement within 2 weeks, consider underlying testicular tumor.
- Epididymectomy (excision of the epididymis from the testes) is done for recurrent, incapacitating episodes or chronic, painful conditions.

Nursing Management

- Place patient on bed rest with scrotum elevated with a scrotal bridge or folded towel to prevent traction on spermatic cord, to improve venous drainage, and to relieve pain.

- Give antimicrobial medications as prescribed.
- Provide intermittent cold compresses to scrotum to help ease pain; later, local heat or sitz baths may hasten resolution of inflammatory process.
- Give analgesic agents as prescribed for pain relief.
- Instruct patient to avoid straining, lifting, and sexual stimulation until infection is under control.
- Instruct patient to continue with analgesic and antibiotic medications as prescribed and to use ice packs as necessary for discomfort.
- Explain that it may take 4 weeks or longer for the epididymis to return to normal.

For more information, see Chapter 49 in Smeltzer and Bare: *Brunner and Suddarth's Textbook of Medical-Surgical Nursing*, 11th edition. Philadelphia: Lippincott Williams & Wilkins, 2008.

Epilepsies

The epilepsies are a symptom complex of several disorders of brain function characterized by recurring seizures. There may be associated loss of consciousness, excess movement, or loss of muscle tone or movement and disturbances of behavior, mood, sensation, and perception. The basic problem is an electrical disturbance (dysrhythmia) in the nerve cells in one section of the brain, causing them to emit abnormal, recurring, uncontrolled electrical discharges. The characteristic epileptic seizure is a manifestation of this excessive neuronal discharge. In most cases, the cause is unknown (idiopathic). Susceptibility to some types may be inherited. Epilepsies often follow many medical disorders, traumas, and drug or alcohol intoxication. They are also associated with brain tumors, abscesses, and congenital malformations. Epilepsy begins before 20 years of age in more than 75% of patients. Epilepsy is not synonymous with mental retardation or illness; it is not associated with intellectual level.

Clinical Manifestations

Seizures range from simple staring episodes to prolonged convulsive movements with loss of consciousness. Seizures are classified as partial, generalized, and unclassified according to the area of brain involved. Aura, a premonitory or warning sensation, occurs before seizure (eg, seeing a flashing light, hearing a sound).

Simple Partial Seizures

Only a finger or hand may shake; the mouth may jerk uncontrollably; the patient may talk unintelligibly, may be dizzy, or may experience unusual or unpleasant sights, sounds, odors, or taste—all without loss of consciousness.

Complex Partial Seizures

The patient remains motionless or moves automatically but inappropriately for time and place; may experience excessive emotions of fear, anger, elation, or irritability; does not remember episode when it is over.

Generalized Seizures (Grand Mal Seizures)

Grand mal seizures involve both hemispheres of the brain. There is intense rigidity of the entire body, followed by jerky alternations of muscle relaxation and contraction (generalized tonic-clonic contraction).

- Simultaneous contractions of diaphragm and chest muscles produce characteristic epileptic cry.
- Tongue is chewed; patient is incontinent of urine and stool.
- Convulsive movements last 1 or 2 minutes.
- The patient then relaxes and lies in a deep coma, breathing noisily.

Postictal State

After the seizure, patients are often confused and hard to arouse and may sleep for hours. Many complain of headache or sore muscles.

E

Assessment and Diagnostic Methods

- Developmental history and physical and neurologic examinations are done to determine the type, frequency, and severity of seizures. Biochemical, hematologic, and serologic studies are included.
- Computed tomography (CT) imaging or magnetic resonance imaging (MRI) is performed to detect lesions, focal abnormalities, cerebral vascular abnormalities, and cerebral degenerative changes.
- Electroencephalograms (EEG) aid in classifying the type of seizure.

Medical Management

The management of epilepsy and status epilepticus is planned according to immediate and long-range needs and is tailored to meet the patient's needs because some cases arise from brain damage and others are due to altered brain chemistry. The goals of treatment are to stop the seizures as quickly as possible, to ensure adequate cerebral oxygenation, and to maintain a seizure-free state.

An airway and adequate oxygenation (intubate if necessary) are established, as is an intravenous line for administering medications and obtaining blood samples for analysis.

Pharmacologic Therapy

Medications are used to achieve seizure control. The usual treatment is single-drug therapy.

- Intravenous diazepam, lorazepam, or fosphenytoin is administered slowly in an attempt to halt the seizures.

General anesthesia with a short-acting barbiturate may be used if initial treatment is unsuccessful.

- To maintain a seizure-free state, other anticonvulsant medications (carbamazepine, primidone, phenytoin, phenobarbital, ethosuximide, and valproate) are prescribed after the initial seizure is treated.

Surgical Management

- Surgery is indicated when epilepsy results from intracranial tumors, abscess, cysts, or vascular anomalies.
- Surgical removal of the epileptogenic focus is done for seizures that originate in a well-circumscribed area of the brain that can be excised without producing significant neurologic defects.

NURSING PROCESS: The Patient with Epilepsy

Assessment

- Observe and assess neurologic condition during and after a seizure. Assess vital and neurologic signs continuously. Patient may die from cardiac involvement or respiratory depression.
- Obtain a complete seizure history. Ask about factors or events that precipitate the seizures; document alcohol intake.
- Assess EEG to determine the nature of epileptogenic activity.
- Measure serum concentration of the anticonvulsant medication the patient is taking.
- Assess potential for postictal cerebral swelling.
- Assess effects of epilepsy on lifestyle.

Diagnosis

Nursing Diagnoses

- Risk for injury related to seizure activity
- Fear related to the ever-present possibility of having seizures

- Ineffective coping related to stresses imposed by epilepsy
- Deficient knowledge about epilepsy and its control

Collaborative Problems/Potential Complications

Status epilepticus (see Box E-1) and toxicity related to medications

Planning and Goals

Major goals include prevention of injury, control of seizures, satisfactory psychosocial adjustment, knowledge acquisition, understanding of the condition, and absence of complications.

Nursing Interventions

General Care and Injury Prevention

- Perform periodic physical examinations and laboratory tests for patients taking medications known to have toxic hematopoietic, genitourinary, or hepatic effects.
- Provide ongoing assessment and monitoring of respiratory and cardiac function.
- Monitor the seizure type and general condition of patient.
- Turn patient to side-lying position to assist in draining pharyngeal secretions.
- Have suction equipment available if patient aspirates.
- Monitor intravenous line closely for dislodgment during seizures.

BOX E-1 Status Epilepticus

Status epilepticus (acute prolonged seizure activity) is a series of generalized seizures that occur without full recovery of consciousness between attacks. The condition is a medical emergency that is characterized by continuous clinical or electrical seizures lasting at least 30 minutes. Repeated episodes of cerebral anoxia and swelling may lead to irreversible and fatal brain damage. Common factors that precipitate status epilepticus include withdrawal of antiepileptic medication, fever, and intercurrent infection.

- Protect patient from injury during seizures with padded side rails, and keep under constant observation.
- Do not restrain patient's movements during seizure activity. Do not insert anything in patient's mouth.

E

Controlling Fear of Seizures

- Reduce fear that a seizure may occur unexpectedly by encouraging compliance with prescribed treatment.
- Emphasize that prescribed antiepileptic medication must be taken on a continuing basis and is not habit-forming.
- Assess lifestyle and environment to determine factors that precipitate seizures, such as emotional disturbances, environmental stressors, onset of menstruation, or fever. Encourage patient to avoid such stimuli.
- Encourage patient to follow a regular and moderate routine in lifestyle, diet (avoiding excessive stimulants), exercise, and rest (regular sleep patterns).
- Advise patient to avoid photic stimulation (eg, bright flickering lights, television viewing); dark glasses or covering one eye may help.
- Encourage patient to attend classes in stress management.

Improving Coping Mechanisms

- Understand that epilepsy imposes feelings of fear, alienation, depression, discrimination and social isolation, and uncertainty.
- Provide counseling to patient and family to help them understand the condition and limitations imposed.
- Encourage patient to participate in social and recreational activities.
- Instruct patient to avoid over-the-counter medications unless approved by health care provider.
- Provide comprehensive mental health services to patients who exhibit symptoms of schizophrenia or impulsive or irritable behavior.

Promoting Home and Community-Based Care

Teaching Patients Self-Care

- Instruct patient and family about medication side effects and toxicity.
- Prevent or control gingival hyperplasia, a side effect of phenytoin (Dilantin) therapy, by teaching patient to perform thorough oral hygiene and gum massage and seek regular dental care.
- Provide specific guidelines to assess and report signs and symptoms of medication overdose.
- Instruct patient to notify physician if unable to take medications due to illness.
- Teach patient to keep a drug and seizure chart, noting when medications are taken and any seizure activity.
- Instruct patient to take showers rather than tub baths to avoid drowning and never to swim alone.
- Encourage realistic attitude toward the disease; provide facts concerning epilepsy.
- Instruct patient to carry an emergency medical identification card or wear an identification bracelet.
- Advise patient to seek preconception and genetic counseling if desired (inherited transmission of epilepsy has not been proved).

Continuing Care

- Financial considerations: Epilepsy Foundation of America offers a mail-order program for medications at minimum cost and access to life insurance as well as information on vocational rehabilitation and coping with epilepsy.
- Vocational rehabilitation: the state Vocational Rehabilitation Agency, Epilepsy Foundation of America, and federal and state agencies may be of assistance in cases of job discrimination.

Evaluation

Expected Patient Outcomes

- Sustains no injuries from seizure activity
- Maintains control of seizures

- Exhibits adequate psychosocial adjustment and decreased fear
- Exhibits knowledge and understanding of epilepsy
- Experiences no complications of seizures (injury) or complications of status epilepticus

E

For more information, see Chapter 61 in Smeltzer and Bare: *Brunner and Suddarth's Textbook of Medical-Surgical Nursing*, 11th edition. Philadelphia: Lippincott Williams & Wilkins, 2008.

Epistaxis (Nosebleed)

Epistaxis is a hemorrhage from the nose caused by the rupture of tiny, distended vessels in the mucous membrane of any area of the nasal passage. The anterior septum is the most common site. Causes include trauma, infection, drugs, cardiovascular diseases, blood dyscrasias, nasal tumors, low humidity, foreign body, and a deviated nasal septum. Vigorous nose blowing and nose picking are additional causes.

Medical Management

The bleeding site is determined by using a nasal speculum or headlight. The patient sits upright with the head tilted forward to prevent swallowing and aspiration of blood. Then direct pressure is applied to the site by compressing the soft outer portion of the nose against the midline septum for 5 or 10 minutes continuously.

Vessels involved in anterior nosebleeds are cauterized by chemical agents (eg, silver nitrate and Gelfoam) or electrocautery; topical vasoconstrictors, such as adrenaline (1:1,000), cocaine (0.5%), and phenylephrine, are also used.

For posterior nosebleeds, cotton pledgets moistened with vasoconstricting solution are inserted into the nostril to reduce blood flow; suction is used to remove excess blood and clots from the field of inspection.

E

The nose is packed with petrolatum-impregnated gauze when the origin of bleeding cannot be identified. Packing remains in place for 48 hours or up to 5 or 6 days, if necessary, to control bleeding. Antibiotics may be given to manage or prevent infection.

Nursing Management

- Monitor vital signs and assist in control of bleeding.
- Provide tissues and an emesis basin for expectoration of blood.
- Reassure patient that bleeding can be controlled.
- Maintain a calm, efficient manner.
- Teach patient to provide self-care by reviewing ways to prevent epistaxis: avoid forceful nose blowing, straining, high altitudes, and nasal trauma (including nose picking).
- Provide adequate humidification to prevent drying of nasal passages.
- Instruct patient how to apply direct pressure to nose with thumb and index finger for 15 minutes if nosebleed recurs.
- Instruct patient to seek medical attention if recurrent bleeding cannot be stopped.

For more information, see Chapter 22 in Smeltzer and Bare: *Brunner and Suddarth's Textbook of Medical-Surgical Nursing*, 11th edition. Philadelphia: Lippincott Williams & Wilkins, 2008.

Esophageal Varices, Bleeding

Bleeding or hemorrhage from esophageal varices is one of the major causes of death in patients with cirrhosis. Esophageal varices are dilated tortuous veins usually found in the submucosa of the lower esophagus; they may develop higher in the esophagus or extend into the stomach. The condition nearly always is caused by portal hypertension. Risk factors for hemorrhage include muscular strain from heavy lifting; straining at stool, sneezing, coughing, or vomiting; esophagitis or irritation of vessels (rough food or irritating fluids); and salicylates or any drug that erodes the esophageal mucosa.

Clinical Manifestations

- Hematemesis and melena occur, mainly in those who have abused alcohol.
- Dilated veins usually cause no symptoms unless portal pressure increases and mucosa becomes thin; then massive hemorrhage takes place with shock (cool clammy skin, hypotension, tachycardia).

> **!**   **NURSING ALERT** Bleeding esophageal varices can quickly lead to hemorrhagic shock and should be considered an emergency.

Assessment and Diagnostic Methods

- Endoscopy, barium swallow, ultrasound, computed tomography (CT) scan, and angiography
- Neurologic and portal hypertension assessment
- Liver function tests (serum aminotransferase [transaminase], bilirubin, alkaline phosphatase, and serum proteins)
- Splenoportography, hepatoportography, and celiac angiography

> **!**   **NURSING ALERT** Provide support before and during examination by endoscopy to relieve stress. Monitor carefully to detect early signs of cardiac dysrhythmias, perforation, and hemorrhage. Do not allow the patient to drink fluids after the examination until the gag reflex returns. Offer lozenges and gargles to relieve throat discomfort, but withhold any oral intake if patient is actively bleeding. Provide support and explanations regarding care and procedures.

Medical Management

- Aggressive medical care includes evaluation of extent of bleeding and continuous monitoring of vital signs when hematemesis and melena are present.
- Signs of potential hypovolemia are noted; blood volume is monitored with a central venous pressure or arterial catheter.
- Oxygen is administered to prevent hypoxia and to maintain adequate blood oxygenation, and intravenous fluids and volume expanders are administered to restore fluid volume and replace electrolytes.
- Need for blood transfusion is assessed, and intake and output (insert indwelling urinary catheter) are monitored.

Nonsurgical treatment is preferred because of the high mortality associated with emergency surgery to control bleeding from esophageal varices and because of the poor physical condition of most of these patients. Nonsurgical measures include:

- Pharmacologic therapy: somatostatin, octreotide (Sandostatin), vasopressin (Pitressin), beta-blocker (propranolol [Inderal]), and nitrates
- Balloon tamponade, saline lavage, endoscopic sclerotherapy
- Transjugular intrahepatic portosystemic shunting (TIPS)
- Esophageal banding therapy, variceal band ligation
- Endoscopic sclerotherapy

Surgical Management

If necessary, surgery may involve:

- Bypass procedures (eg, portacaval shunts, splenorenal shunt, mesocaval shunt)
- Devascularization and transection

Nursing Management

Provide postoperative care similar to that for any thoracic or abdominal operation. See Preoperative and Postoperative Nursing Management for additional information.

> **!** **NURSING ALERT** The risk for postsurgical
> complications (hypovolemic or hemorrhagic shock,
> hepatic encephalopathy, electrolyte imbalance, metabolic
> and respiratory alkalosis, alcohol withdrawal syndrome,
> and seizures) is high. In addition, bleeding may recur as
> new collateral vessels develop.

- Monitor patient's physical condition and evaluate emotional responses and cognitive status.
- Monitor and record vital signs. Assess nutritional status.
- Perform a neurologic assessment, monitoring for signs of hepatic encephalopathy (findings may range from drowsiness to encephalopathy and coma).
- Treat bleeding by complete rest of the esophagus. Initiate parenteral nutrition (PN) as ordered.
- Assist patient to avoid straining and vomiting. Maintain gastric suction to keep the stomach as empty as possible.
- Provide frequent oral hygiene and moist sponges to the lips to relieve thirst.
- Closely monitor blood pressure.
- Provide vitamin K therapy and multiple blood transfusions as ordered for blood loss.
- Provide a quiet environment and calm reassurance to reduce anxiety and agitation. Provide emotional support and pertinent explanations regarding medical and nursing interventions.
- Monitor closely to detect and manage complications, including hypovolemic or hemorrhagic shock, hepatic encephalopathy, electrolyte imbalance, metabolic and respiratory alkalosis, alcohol withdrawal syndrome, and seizures.
- Monitor closely to prevent accidental removal or displacement of tube, subsequent airway obstruction, and aspiration related to balloon tamponade. Explain procedure to patient briefly to obtain cooperation with insertion and maintenance of esophageal-tamponade tube. Provide frequent oral hygiene. Ensure patency of nasogastric tube to

prevent aspiration. Observe gastric aspirate for blood and cessation of bleeding.
- Report onset of chest pain.
- Observe for aspiration, perforation of esophagus, and recurrence of bleeding related to endoscopic sclerotherapy or variceal banding.

For more information, see Chapter 39 in Smeltzer and Bare: *Brunner and Suddarth's Textbook of Medical-Surgical Nursing*, 11th edition. Philadelphia: Lippincott Williams & Wilkins, 2008.

Exfoliative Dermatitis

Exfoliative dermatitis is a serious condition characterized by progressive inflammation in which erythema and scaling occur in a more or less generalized distribution. This condition starts acutely as either a patchy or a generalized erythematous eruption. Exfoliative dermatitis has a variety of causes. It is considered to be a secondary or reactive process to an underlying skin or systemic disease. It may appear as a part of the lymphoma group of diseases and may precede the appearance of lymphoma. Preexisting skin disorders implicated as a cause include psoriasis, atopic dermatitis, and contact dermatitis. It also appears as a severe medication reaction to penicillin and phenylbutazone. The cause is unknown in about 25% of cases.

Clinical Manifestations

- Chills, fever, prostration, occasional gastrointestinal symptoms, severe toxicity, and an itchy scaling of the skin
- Profound loss of stratum corneum (outermost layer of the skin), capillary leakage, hypoproteinemia, negative nitrogen balance
- Widespread dilation of cutaneous vessels, resulting in large amounts of body heat loss

- Skin color changes from pink to dark red; after a week, exfoliation (scaling) begins in the form of thin flakes that leave the underlying skin smooth and red, with new scales forming as the older ones come off.
- Possible hair loss
- Relapse common
- Systemic effects: high-output heart failure, intestinal disturbances, gynecomastia (breast enlargement), hyperuricemia, temperature disturbances

Medical Management

Goals of management are to maintain fluid and electrolyte balance and to prevent infection. Treatment is individualized and supportive and is started as soon as condition is diagnosed.

- Hospitalize patient and place on bed rest.
- Discontinue all medications that may be implicated.
- Maintain comfortable room temperature because of patient's abnormal thermoregulatory control.
- Maintain fluid and electrolyte balance because of considerable water and protein loss from skin surface.
- Give plasma expanders as indicated.

 NURSING ALERT Observe for signs and symptoms of high-output heart failure due to hyperemia and increased blood flow.

Nursing Management

- Carry out continual nursing assessment to detect infection.
- Administer prescribed antibiotics on the basis of culture and sensitivity test results.
- Assess for hypothermia because of increased skin blood flow coupled with increased heat and water loss through the skin.
- Use topical therapy for symptomatic relief.

- Recommend soothing baths, compresses, and lubrication with emollients to treat extensive dermatitis.
- Administer prescribed oral or parenteral steroids when disease is not controlled by more conservative therapy.
- Advise patient to avoid all irritants, particularly medications.

E

For more information, see Chapter 56 in Smeltzer and Bare: *Brunner and Suddarth's Textbook of Medical-Surgical Nursing*, 11th edition. Philadelphia: Lippincott Williams & Wilkins, 2008.

F

Fractures

A fracture is a break in the continuity of bone. It is defined according to type and extent. Fractures occur when the bone is subjected to stress greater than it can absorb. Fractures can be caused by a direct blow, crushing force, sudden twisting motion, or even extreme muscle contraction. When the bone is broken, adjacent structures are also affected, resulting in soft tissue edema, hemorrhage into the muscles and joints, joint dislocations, ruptured tendons, severed nerves, and damaged blood vessels. Body organs may be injured by the force that caused the fracture or by the fracture fragments.

Types of Fractures

- Complete fracture: a break across the entire cross-section of the bone, which is frequently displaced
- Incomplete fracture, also called greenstick fracture: break occurs through only part of the cross-section of the bone
- Comminuted fractures: a break with several bone fragments
- Closed fracture, or simple fracture: does not produce a break in the skin
- Open fracture, or compound or complex fracture: a break in which the skin or mucous membrane wound extends to the fractured bone. Open fractures are classified as follows: grade I: a clean wound less than 1 cm long; grade II: a larger wound without extensive soft tissue damage; grade III: wound is highly contaminated and has extensive soft tissue damage (most severe type).
- Fractures may also be described according to anatomic placement of fragments, particularly if they are displaced or nondisplaced.

Early complications of fracture include shock, fat embolism, compartment syndrome, thromboembolism (pulmonary embolism), disseminated intravascular coagulopathy (DIC), and infection. Delayed complications include delayed union and nonunion, avascular necrosis of bone, reaction to internal-fixation devices, complex regional pain syndrome, and heterotopic ossification.

F

Clinical Manifestations

Not all of the clinical manifestations are present in every fracture.

- The patient experiences muscle spasm and continuous pain that increases in severity until bone fragments are immobilized.
- Loss of function, deformity, abnormal movement, and shortening of the extremity may be noted.
- Crepitus, local swelling, and discoloration may be seen (avoid testing; see the Nursing Alert).

Manifestations of Complications

- If fat embolism syndrome occurs, with blockage of the small blood vessels that supply the brain, lungs, kidneys, and other organs (sudden onset, usually occurring within 24 to 72 hours but may occur up to a week after injury), the following may be noted: hypoxia, tachypnea, tachycardia, and pyrexia, mental status changes varying from mild agitation and confusion to delirium and coma, dyspnea, crackles, wheezes, precordial chest pain, cough, large amounts of thick white sputum, hypoxia and blood gas values with PaO_2 below 60 mm Hg, with an early respiratory alkalosis and later respiratory acidosis. The chest radiograph exhibits a typical "snowstorm" infiltrate. Eventually, acute pulmonary edema, adult respiratory distress syndrome (ARDS), and heart failure develop.
- With systemic embolization, the patient appears pale. Petechiae appear in the buccal membranes and conjunctival

sacs, on the hard palate, on the fundus of the eye, and over the chest and anterior axillary folds. Fever (temperature above 39.5°C [103.8°F]) develops. Free fat may be found in the urine when emboli reach the kidneys. Kidney failure may develop.

- Compartment syndrome (develops when tissue perfusion in the muscles is less than that required for tissue viability). Acute compartment syndrome may produce deep, throbbing, unrelenting pain not controlled by opioids (can be due to a tight cast or constrictive dressing or an increase in muscle compartment contents because of edema or hemorrhage). Cyanotic (blue-tinged) nail beds and pale or dusky and cold fingers or toes are present; nail bed capillary refill times are prolonged (greater than 3 seconds); pulse may be diminished (Doppler) or absent; motor weakness, paralysis, and paresthesia may occur.

- Manifestations of DIC include ecchymoses, unexpected bleeding after surgery, and bleeding from the mucous membranes, venipuncture sites, and gastrointestinal and urinary tracts.

- Symptoms of infection may include tenderness, pain, redness, swelling, local warmth, elevated temperature, and purulent drainage.

- Nonunion is manifested by persistent discomfort and abnormal movement at the fracture site. Some risk factors include infection at the fracture site, inadequate immobilization or manipulation that disrupts healing, bone gap, and impaired blood supply.

- Manifestations of other complications may be noted (deep vein thrombosis, thromboembolism, pulmonary embolus). See specific disorders for additional information.

> **! NURSING ALERT** Avoid testing for crepitus because testing can cause further tissue damage. Subtle personality changes, restlessness, irritability, or confusion in a patient who has sustained a fracture are indications for immediate blood gas studies.

Assessment and Diagnostic Findings

The diagnosis of a fracture depends on the symptoms, the physical signs, and radiographic examination. Usually, the patient reports an injury to the area.

🌿 Gerontologic Considerations

Hip fractures occur with a high incidence among elderly people, who have brittle bones from osteoporosis (particularly women) and who tend to fall frequently. The patient who has sustained a hip fracture often has a comorbid disease (eg, cardiovascular, pulmonary, renal, or endocrine disorders). Fractures of the neck of the femur may destroy blood vessels, disrupting blood supply to the head and the neck of the femur and resulting in bone death and commonly nonunion or aseptic necrosis.

Hip fractures are a frequent contributor to death after the age of 75 years. The stress and immobility related to the trauma predispose the older adult to pneumonia, sepsis, and reduced ability to cope with other health problems.

Medical Management

Emergency Management

- Immediately after injury, immobilize the body part before the patient is moved. If an injured patient must be moved before splints can be applied, support the extremity above and below the fracture site to prevent rotation or angular motion.
- Splint the fracture, including joints adjacent to the fracture, to prevent damage to the soft tissue.
- Apply temporary, well-padded splints, firmly bandaged over clothing, to immobilize the fracture.
- Assess neurovascular status distal to the injury to determine adequacy of peripheral tissue perfusion and nerve function. Be alert for paresthesia or paralysis (compartment syndrome).

- Cover the wound of an open fracture with a clean (sterile) dressing to prevent contamination of deeper tissues.

Reduction of Fractures

The principles of fracture treatment include reduction, immobilization, and regaining of normal function and strength through rehabilitation.

- The fracture is reduced ("setting" the bone) using a closed method (manipulation and manual traction [eg, splint or cast]) or an open method (surgical placement of internal-fixation devices [eg, pins, wires, screws, plates, nails]) to restore the fracture fragments to anatomic alignment and rotation. The specific method depends on the nature of the fracture.
- After the fracture has been reduced, immobilization holds the bone in correct position and alignment until union occurs. Immobilization is accomplished by external or internal fixation.
- Function is maintained and restored by controlling swelling by elevating the injured extremity and applying ice as prescribed. Restlessness, anxiety, and discomfort are controlled using a variety of approaches (eg, reassurance, position changes, pain relief strategies, including analgesic agents). Isometric and muscle-setting exercises are done to minimize disuse atrophy and to promote circulation. With internal fixation, the surgeon determines the amount of movement and weight-bearing stress the extremity can withstand and prescribes the level of activity.

Management of Complications

- Treatment of shock consists of restoring blood volume and circulation, relieving pain, providing adequate splinting, and protecting the patient from further injury and other complications. See Nursing Management under Hypovolemic Shock for additional information.

- Prevention and management of fat embolism includes immediate immobilization of fractures and adequate support for fractured bones during turning and positioning. Prompt initiation of respiratory support with prevention of respiratory and metabolic acidosis and correction of homeostatic disturbances is essential. Corticosteroids may be given as well as vasoactive medications, fluid replacement therapy, and morphine for pain and anxiety.

- Compartment syndrome is managed by controlling swelling by elevating the extremity to heart level or by releasing restrictive devices (dressings or cast). A fasciotomy (surgical decompression with excision of the fibrous membrane covering and separating muscles) may be needed to relieve the constrictive muscle fascia. The wound remains open and covered with moist sterile saline dressings for 3 to 5 days. The limb is splinted and elevated. Range-of-motion exercises may be performed every 4 to 6 hours.

- Nonunion (failure of the ends of a fractured bone to unite) is treated with internal fixation, bone grafting (osteogenesis, osteoconduction, osteoinduction), electronic bone stimulation, or a combination of these.

- Management of reaction to internal fixation devices involves protection from osteoporosis, altered bone structure, and trauma.

- Management of complex regional pain syndrome involves elevation of the extremity, pain relief, range-of-motion exercises, and helping patients with chronic pain, disuse atrophy, and osteoporosis. Avoid taking blood pressure or performing venipuncture in the affected extremity.

- Other complications are treated as indicated (see specific disorders).

Nursing Management
Promoting Fracture Healing

- Provide pharmacologic and nonpharmacologic measures for pain management.

F

F

- Monitor for signs of infection (if grafts were done, monitor the donor and recipient sites).
- Provide patient education and reinforce information concerning the objectives of the bone graft, immobilization, avoidance of weight bearing, wound care, signs of infection, and follow-up care with the orthopedic surgeon.
- For the patient receiving electrical stimulation for nonunion (prolonged therapy), provide emotional support and encourage compliance with the treatment regimen. Include patient education regarding daily use of the stimulator as prescribed and need for follow-up evaluation by the orthopedist, who will evaluate the progression of bone healing with periodic radiographic studies.

Managing Closed Fractures

- Encourage patients with closed (simple) fractures to return to their usual activities as rapidly as possible, within the limits of the fracture immobilization.
- Teach patients how to control swelling and pain associated with the fracture and soft tissue trauma.
- Teach exercises to maintain the health of unaffected muscles and to strengthen muscles needed for transferring and for using assistive devices (eg, crutches, walker).
- Teach patients how to use assistive devices safely.
- Arrange to help patients modify their home environment as needed and to secure personal assistance if necessary.
- Provide patient teaching, including self-care, medication information, monitoring for potential complications, and the need for continuing health care supervision.

Managing Open Fractures

- The objectives of management are to prevent infection of the wound, soft tissue, and bone and to promote healing of soft tissue and bone. In an open fracture, there is the risk of osteomyelitis, tetanus, and gas gangrene.
- Administer tetanus prophylaxis.

- Perform serial irrigation and dèbridement to remove anaerobic organisms.
- Administer intravenous antibiotics to prevent or treat infection.
- Perform aseptic dressing changes with sterile gauze to permit swelling and wound drainage, with wound irrigation and dèbridement as ordered.
- Provide, or teach patient and family to perform, wound care to flap or skin graft after the wound is closed in 5 to 7 days.
- Elevate, and teach patient and family to elevate, the extremity to minimize edema.
- Assess neurovascular status frequently.
- Take the patient's temperature at regular intervals, and monitor for signs of infection.
- Promote intake of adequate nutrition to promote wound healing.

Managing Fractures at Specific Sites

Maximum functional recovery is the goal of management.

Clavicle

- With a clavicle fracture, head or cervical spine injuries may be present. Caution the patient not to elevate the arm above shoulder level until the ends of the bone have united (about 6 weeks). Encourage the patient to exercise the elbow, wrist, and fingers as soon as possible and, when prescribed, to perform shoulder exercises. Tell the patient that vigorous activity is limited for 3 months.

Humerus

- With humeral neck fractures (seen most frequently in older women after a fall on an outstretched arm), perform neurovascular assessment of the involved extremity to evaluate the extent of injury and possible involvement of the neurovascular bundle (nerves and blood vessels) of the arm. Teach the patient to support the arm and immobilize it

F

by a sling and swathe that secure the supported arm to the trunk. Place a soft pad in the axilla to absorb moisture and avoid skin breakdown. Begin pendulum exercises as soon as tolerated by the patient. Instruct the patient to avoid vigorous activity, such as tennis, for an additional 10 to 14 weeks. Inform the patient that residual stiffness, aching, and some limitation of range of motion may persist for 6 or more months. When a humeral neck fracture is displaced with required fixation, exercises are started only after a prescribed period of immobilization.

- With humeral shaft fractures, the nerves and brachial blood vessels may be injured. Monitor for wrist drop, which indicates radial nerve injury. With an oblique, spiral, or displaced fracture that has resulted in shortening of the humeral shaft, instruct patient in care of a hanging cast, if used. Emphasize that a hanging cast must be dependent (hang free without support) because the weight of the cast provides the continuous traction to the arm. Advise patient to sleep in an upright position so that traction from the weight of the cast is maintained. Teach patient to perform finger exercises as soon as the cast is applied, pendulum-shoulder exercises as prescribed, and isometric exercises. Instruct patient to use a sling after the cast is removed and to begin exercises of the shoulder, elbow, and wrist. For elderly patients who do not tolerate a cast, provide a sling and swathe for comfort and immobilization. If ordered, provide and teach patient about functional bracing. Instruct patient regarding a shoulder spica cast if used for early treatment of an unstable humerus fracture or skeletal traction (eg, over-the-face traction, balanced side-arm traction).

Elbow

- Elbow fractures (distal humerus) may result in injury to the median, radial, or ulnar nerves. Evaluate the patient for paresthesia and signs of compromised circulation in the forearm and hand. Monitor closely for Volkmann's ischemic contracture (a compartment syndrome) as well as for hemarthrosis (blood in the joint). Reinforce information regarding reduction and fixation of the fracture and planned active motion when swelling has subsided and healing has begun. Explain care if the arm is immobilized in a cast or posterior splint with a sling. Encourage active finger exercises. Teach and encourage patient to do gentle range-of-motion exercise of the injured joint about 1 week after internal fixation and after 2 weeks with closed reduction.

- Radial head fractures are usually produced by a fall on the outstretched hand with the elbow extended. Instruct patient in use of a splint for immobilization. If the fracture is displaced, reinforce the need for postoperative immobilization of the arm in a posterior plaster splint and sling. Encourage the patient to carry out a program of active motion of the elbow and forearm when prescribed.

Wrist

- Wrist fractures (distal radius [Colles' fracture]) usually result from a fall. They are frequently seen in elderly women with osteoporotic bones and weak soft tissues that do not dissipate the energy of a fall. Reinforce care of the cast, or with more severe fractures with wire insertion, teach incision care. Instruct patient to keep the wrist and forearm elevated for 48 hours after reduction. Begin active motion of the fingers and shoulder promptly by teaching patient to do the following exercises to reduce swelling and prevent stiffness:
- Hold the hand at the level of the heart.
- Move the fingers from full extension to flexion. Hold and release. Repeat at least 10 times every hour when awake.
- Use the hand in functional activities.
- Actively exercise the shoulder and elbow, including complete range-of-motion exercises of both joints.
- Assess the sensory function of the median nerve by pricking the distal aspect of the index finger, and assess the motor function by testing patient's ability to touch the thumb to the little finger. If diminished circulation and nerve function

is noted, prepare to treat with prompt release of constricting bandages.

Hand and Fingers

- Hand trauma often requires extensive reconstructive surgery. The objective of treatment is always to regain maximum function of the hand. With a nondisplaced fracture, the finger is splinted for 3 to 4 weeks to relieve pain and protect the fingertip from further trauma, but displaced fractures and open fractures may require open reduction with internal fixation, using wires or pins.

  Evaluate the neurovascular status of the injured hand. Teach the patient to control swelling by elevating the hand. Encourage functional use of the uninvolved portions of the hand.

Rib

- Rib fractures occur frequently in adults and usually result in no impairment of function but produce painful respirations. Assist patient to cough and take deep breaths by splinting the chest with hands or pillow during cough. Reassure patient that pain associated with rib fracture diminishes significantly in 3 or 4 days, and the fracture heals within 6 weeks. Monitor for complications, which may include a flail chest, pneumothorax, and hemothorax. (See specific disorders for nursing management.)

Pelvis

- Pelvic fractures may be caused by falls, motor vehicle crashes, or crush injuries. At least two thirds of these patients have significant and multiple injuries.
- Monitor for symptoms, including ecchymosis; tenderness over the symphysis pubis, anterior iliac spines, iliac crest, sacrum, or coccyx; local swelling; numbness or tingling of pubis, genitals, and proximal thighs; and inability to bear weight without discomfort.

- Complete a neurovascular assessment of the lower extremities to detect injury to pelvic blood vessels and nerves. Monitor for hemorrhage and shock, two of the most serious consequences that may occur. Palpate both lower extremities for absence of peripheral pulses, which may indicate a torn iliac artery or one of its branches.

- Assess for injuries to the bladder, rectum, intestines, other abdominal organs, and pelvic vessels and nerves. Examine urine for blood to assess for urinary tract injury. In male patients, do not insert a catheter until the status of the urethra is known. Monitor for abdominal pain and signs of peritonitis as well as signs of a paralytic ileus.

- If patient has a stable pelvic fracture, maintain on bed rest for a few days and provide symptom management until the pain and discomfort are controlled.

- Provide fluids, dietary fiber, ankle and leg exercises, log rolling, coughing and deep breathing, and skin care to reduce the risk for complications and to increase comfort.

- Monitor bowel sounds. If patient has a fracture of the coccyx and experiences pain on sitting and with defecation, assist with sitz baths as prescribed to relieve pain, and administer stool softeners to prevent the need to strain on defecation.

- As pain resolves, instruct patient to resume activity gradually, using ambulatory aids for protected weight bearing. Patients with unstable pelvic fractures may be treated with external fixation or open reduction and internal fixation (ORIF).

- Promote hemodynamic stability and comfort, and encourage early mobilization.

- Teach and encourage patient to perform exercises (leg, respiratory, range-of-motion, and strengthening).

- Apply and encourage use of elastic pressure stockings and elevation of the foot of the bed (without the bed gatched at the knee) to aid venous return and to help diminish the effects of bed rest. When prescribed, assist the patient in mobility with progressive weight bearing, usually with crutches.

F

Femur and Hip

- Femoral shaft fractures are most often seen in young men involved in a motor vehicle crash or a fall from a high place. Frequently, these patients have associated multiple trauma and develop shock from a loss of 2 to 3 units of blood.
- Assess neurovascular status of the extremity, especially circulatory perfusion of the foot (popliteal, posterior tibial, and pedal pulses and toe capillary refill as well as Doppler ultrasound monitoring).
- Note signs of dislocation of the hip and knee, and knee effusion, which may suggest ligament damage and possible instability of the knee joint.
- Apply and maintain skin traction for comfort and immobilization of the fracture or skeletal traction to achieve muscle relaxation and alignment of the fracture fragments before ORIF procedures, and later a cast brace.
- Assist patient in minimal partial weight bearing when indicated and progress to full weight bearing as tolerated.
- Reinforce that the cast brace is worn for 12 to 14 weeks.
- Instruct in and encourage patient to perform exercises of lower leg, foot, and toes on a regular basis. Assist patient in performing active and passive knee exercises as soon as possible, depending on the management approach and the stability of the fracture and knee ligaments.

Tibia and Fibula

- Tibia and fibula fractures (most common fractures below the knee) result from a direct blow, falls with the foot in a flexed position, or a violent twisting motion.
- Provide instruction on care of the long leg walking cast or patellar-tendon-bearing cast.
- Monitor for anterior compartment syndrome (pain unrelieved by medications and increasing with plantar flexion, tense and tender muscle lateral to tibial crest, and paresthesia).
- Instruct patient in and assist with partial weight bearing, usually in 7 to 10 days.

F

- Instruct patient on care of a short leg cast or brace (in 3 to 4 weeks), which allows for knee motion.
- Instruct patient in care of skeletal traction, if applicable. Encourage patient to perform foot and knee exercises within the limits of the immobilizing device.
- Instruct patient to begin weight bearing when prescribed (usually in about 4 to 8 weeks).
- Instruct patient to elevate extremity to control edema.
- Perform continuous neurovascular evaluation.

NURSING PROCESS: The Patient with a Hip Fracture

In many cases, the patient with a hip fracture will be elderly, and many elderly people hospitalized with a hip fracture are confused as a result of the stress of the trauma, unfamiliar surroundings, sleep deprivation, medications, and systemic illness. Preoperative predictors of postoperative delirium include age over 70 years, alcohol abuse, poor cognitive or functional status, and marked electrolyte imbalance.

As with younger patients, treatment includes ORIF with temporary skin traction, or Buck's extension, to reduce muscle spasm, immobilize the extremity, and relieve pain, and applying and maintaining sandbags or a trochanter roll.

Assessment

Assess the elderly patient for chronic conditions that require close monitoring. Examine the legs for edema due to congestive heart failure, and assess for peripheral pulselessness from arteriosclerotic vascular disease.

Diagnosis

Nursing Diagnoses

- Pain related to fracture, soft tissue damage, muscle spasm, and surgery
- Impaired physical mobility related to fractured hip

- Impaired skin integrity related to surgical incision
- Risk for impaired urinary elimination related to immobility
- Risk for disturbed thought process related to age, stress of trauma, unfamiliar surroundings, and drug therapy
- Risk for ineffective coping related to injury, anticipated surgery, and dependence
- Risk for impaired home maintenance related to fractured hip and impaired mobility

Collaborative Problems/Potential Complications

- Hemorrhage
- Pulmonary complications
- Neurovascular compromise
- Deep vein thrombosis
- Pressure ulcers

Planning and Goals

Major goals may include relief of pain, achievement of a functional stable hip, wound healing, maintenance of normal urinary elimination patterns, use of effective coping mechanisms to modify stress, oriented and participating in decision making, ability to care for self at home, and absence of complications.

Nursing Interventions

Postoperatively, after ORIF or replacement of the femoral head with a prosthesis (hemiarthroplasty), provide routine postoperative monitoring and interventions. (See Postoperative Nursing Management for additional information.)

Relieving Pain

- Assess type, degree (pain scale), and location of pain.
- Inform patient of available analgesic agents.
- Handle affected extremity gently, supporting it with hands or pillow.
- Use pain-modifying strategies (eg, modify environment, administer analgesic agents, evaluate response to medications).

- Position for comfort and function, and assist with frequent changes in position.

Promoting Hip Function and Stability

- Maintain neutral positioning of hip.
- Maintain temporary skin traction, or Buck's extension, to reduce muscle spasm, to immobilize the extremity, and to relieve pain. Apply and maintain sandbags or a trochanter roll to control external rotation.
- Place a pillow between the legs to maintain abduction and alignment and to provide needed support when turning.
- Turn the patient on the affected or unaffected extremity as prescribed by the physician.
- Encourage the patient to exercise as much as possible by means of the over-bed trapeze.
- Arrange for physical therapists to work with the patient on transfers, ambulation, and the safe use of walker and crutches.
- Instruct in and supervise safe use of ambulatory aids.

Promoting Wound Healing

- Monitor vital signs.
- Perform aseptic dressing changes.
- Assess wound appearance and character of drainage.
- Assess complaint of pain.
- Administer prescribed intravenous prophylactic antibiotic agents.
- Suspect infection if the patient complains of moderate hip discomfort and has mildly elevated sedimentation rate.

Promoting Skin Integrity

- Apply elastic tape in a vertical fashion to reduce the incidence of tape blisters.
- Provide proper skin care, especially to the heels, back, sacrum, and shoulders.
- Obtain and use a high-density foam, static air, or other special mattress to provide protection and distribute pressure more evenly.

Promoting Normal Urinary Elimination Patterns

- Monitor intake and output.
- Avoid or minimize use of indwelling catheter.
- Monitor clients for loss of bladder control (incontinence) or urinary retention.
- Assess the patient's voiding patterns.
- Encourage liberal fluid intake within the cardiovascular tolerance of the patient.

Promoting Patient Orientation and Participation in Decision Making

- Assess orientation status.
- Interview family regarding patient's orientation and cognitive abilities before injury.
- Assess patient for auditory and visual deficits.
- Orient patient to and stabilize environment.
- Encourage participation in hygiene and nutritional activities.
- Provide for safety (eg, keep side rails up when patient is in bed, keep light on at night, have call bell available).
- Assess mental responses to medications, especially sedative and analgesic agents.

Promoting Effective Coping Mechanisms

- Encourage patient to express concerns and to discuss the possible impact of fractured hip.
- Support use of coping mechanisms. Involve significant others and support services as needed.
- Contact social services, if needed.
- Encourage patient to participate in planning.
- Explain anticipated treatment regimen and routines to facilitate positive attitude in relation to rehabilitation.

Monitoring and Preventing Potential Complications

- Pulmonary complications: Monitor chronic respiratory problems, if present, and encourage coughing and deep-breathing exercises. Monitor elderly patients who are taking cardiac, antihypertensive, or respiratory medications for their response to these medications. Assess breath sounds at least every 4 to 8 hours to detect adventitious or diminished sounds.

- Pressure ulcers and deep vein thrombosis: Monitor and promote treatment of dehydration and poor nutrition by encouraging patient to consume adequate fluids and a balanced diet; monitor urine output. Encourage patient to move all joints (except the involved hip and knee) and to use arms and overhead trapeze for repositioning and to strengthen the arms and shoulders to facilitate walking with assistive devices; promote early mobilization. Encourage foot flexion exercises every 1 to 2 hours. Apply thigh-high elastic compression stockings and pneumatic compression devices to prevent venous stasis. On the first postoperative day, transfer the patient to a chair with assistance and begin assisted ambulation. Assess legs at least every 4 hours for signs of DVT.

Promoting Home and Community-Based Care
Teaching Patients Self-Care

- Arrange for a home environment assessment, and refer patient for home care as needed.
- Assist patient as needed to make modifications in the home to permit safe use of walkers and crutches and for continuing care.
- Teach patient to monitor for neurovascular complications by monitoring the neurovascular status of the affected leg.
- Instruct patient in measures to prevent DVT; encourage fluids and ankle and foot exercises. Encourage use of elastic stockings, sequential compression devices, and prophylactic anticoagulant therapy as prescribed.
- Instruct patient to perform deep-breathing exercises, to change position at least every 2 hours, and to use an incentive spirometer to help prevent respiratory complications.
- Teach patient and family to monitor or prevent delayed complications of hip fractures, including infection, nonunion, avascular necrosis of the femoral head

(particularly with femoral neck fractures), and fixation device problems (eg, protrusion of the fixation device through the acetabulum; loosening of hardware).

Evaluation

Expected Patient Outcomes

- Reports pain relief
- Engages in therapeutic positioning
- Exhibits normal wound healing and intact skin
- Maintains normal urinary elimination pattern
- Remains oriented and participates in decision making
- Demonstrates use of effective coping mechanisms
- Establishes effective communication
- Experiences no complications

For more information, see Chapter 69 in Smeltzer and Bare: *Brunner and Suddarth's Textbook of Medical-Surgical Nursing*, 11th edition. Philadelphia: Lippincott Williams & Wilkins, 2008.

G

Gastritis

Acute gastritis is inflammation of the stomach mucosa lasting several hours to a few days. Dietary indiscretion is the usual cause (eating irritating food that is too highly seasoned or food that is infected). Other causes include excessive alcohol, aspirin, or other nonsteroidal anti-inflammatory drug (NSAID) use, bile reflux, or radiation therapy. A more severe form of acute gastritis is caused by strong acids or alkali, which may cause the mucosa to become gangrenous or to perforate. Gastritis may also be the first sign of acute systemic infection.

Chronic gastritis is a prolonged inflammation of the stomach that may be caused by either benign or malignant ulcers of the stomach or by bacteria such as *Helicobacter pylori*. Chronic gastritis may be associated with autoimmune diseases such as pernicious anemia and with dietary factors such as caffeine, drug use (eg, NSAIDs, bisphosphonates, such as alendronate [Fosamax] or risedronate [Actonel]), alcohol, smoking, or reflux of intestinal contents into the stomach. It occurs in the fundus or body of the stomach. Superficial ulceration may occur and can lead to hemorrhage.

Clinical Manifestations

Acute Gastritis

- Can be asymptomatic
- Abdominal discomfort with headache, lassitude, nausea, anorexia, vomiting, and hiccuping
- Hemorrhage
- Colic and diarrhea resulting from irritating food that is not vomited but reaches the bowel

- Recovery in about 1 day, although appetite may be diminished for 2 to 3 days

Chronic Gastritis

- May be asymptomatic except for symptoms of vitamin B12 deficiency, when present
- Anorexia, heartburn after eating, belching, sour taste in mouth, or nausea and vomiting

G

Assessment and Diagnostic Findings

- Gastritis is associated with achlorhydria or hypochlorhydria (absence or low levels of hydrochloric acid) or with high acid levels.
- Endoscopy, gastroscopy, upper gastrointestinal x-ray series, and biopsy with histologic examination are performed.
- Serologic testing for antibodies to the *H. pylori* antigen and a breath test may be performed.

Medical Management

Acute Gastritis

The patient should refrain from alcohol and eating until symptoms subside. Then the patient can progress to a nonirritating diet. If symptoms persist, intravenous fluids may be necessary. If bleeding is present, management is similar to that of upper gastrointestinal tract hemorrhage.

If gastritis is due to ingestion of strong acids or alkali, dilute and neutralize the acid with common antacids (eg, aluminum hydroxide); neutralize alkali with diluted lemon juice or diluted vinegar. If corrosion is extensive or severe, avoid emetics and lavage because of danger of perforation.

Supportive therapy may include nasogastric intubation, analgesic agents, and sedative medications.

Emergency surgery may be required to remove gangrenous or perforated tissue; gastric resection (gastrojejunostomy) may be necessary to treat pyloric obstruction.

Chronic Gastritis

Diet modification, rest, stress reduction, and pharmacotherapy are key treatment measures. If gastritis is related to *H. pylori* infection, treatment may include antibiotic therapy (eg, tetracycline or amoxicillin) and bismuth salts (Pepto-Bismol).

NURSING PROCESS: The Patient with Gastritis

Assessment

- Ask about presenting signs and symptoms: heartburn, indigestion, nausea, vomiting. When do symptoms occur? Are symptoms related to anxiety, stress, allergies, eating or drinking too much or too quickly? How are symptoms relieved? Explore diet history and 72-hour dietary recall.
- Inquire about whether others in patient's environment have similar symptoms and whether blood has been vomited or any caustic element has been swallowed.
- Perform complete physical assessment. Note abdominal tenderness, dehydration, and evidence of systemic disorder that may be responsible for symptoms.

Diagnosis

Nursing Diagnoses

- Anxiety related to treatment
- Imbalanced nutrition: Less than body requirements related to inadequate intake of nutrients
- Risk for imbalanced fluid volume related to insufficient fluid intake and excessive fluid loss subsequent to vomiting
- Pain related to irritated stomach mucosa
- Deficient knowledge about dietary management and disease process

Collaborative Problems/Potential Complications

- Perforation
- Hemorrhage
- Pyloric obstruction

Planning and Goals

Major goals include reducing anxiety, adequate nutritional intake, maintaining fluid balance, increasing awareness of dietary management, and absent or minimal pain.

Nursing Interventions

Reducing Anxiety

G

- Carry out emergency measures for ingestion of acids or alkalies.
- Offer supportive therapy to patient and family during treatment and after the ingested acid or alkali has been neutralized or diluted.
- Prepare patient for additional diagnostic studies (endoscopy) or surgery.
- Calmly listen to and answer questions as completely as possible; explain all procedures and treatments.

Promoting Optimal Nutrition

- Provide physical and emotional support for patients with acute gastritis.
- Avoid foods and fluids by mouth for hours or days until acute symptoms subside.
- Provide intravenous therapy as necessary and monitor serum electrolyte values daily.
- Offer ice chips and clear liquids when symptoms subside.
- Encourage patient to report any symptoms suggesting a repeat episode of gastritis as food is introduced.
- Discourage caffeinated beverages (caffeine increases gastric activity and pepsin secretion).
- Discourage alcohol and cigarette smoking (nicotine inhibits neutralization of gastric acid in the duodenum). Instruct patient that nicotine increases muscular activity in the bowel, leading to nausea and vomiting (parasympathetic stimulation).
- Refer patient for alcohol counseling and smoking cessation when appropriate.

Providing Adequate Fluid Intake

- Monitor daily intake and output for dehydration (minimal intake of 1.5 L/day and urine output of 30 mL/h). Infuse intravenous fluids if prescribed.
- Assess electrolyte values every 24 hours for fluid imbalance.
- Be alert for indicators of hemorrhagic gastritis (hematemesis, tachycardia, hypotension), and notify physician.

G

Relieving Pain

- Instruct patient to avoid foods and beverages that may be irritating to the gastric mucosa.
- Instruct patient in the use of medications to relieve chronic gastritis.
- Assess pain and attainment of comfort through use of medications and avoidance of irritating substances.

Teaching Patients Self-Care

- Assess knowledge about gastritis and develop an individualized teaching plan that incorporates patient's pattern of eating, daily caloric needs, and food preferences.
- Provide a list of substances to avoid (caffeine, nicotine, spicy foods, irritating or highly seasoned foods, alcohol); consult with nutritionist if indicated.
- Educate about antibiotic agents, antacids, bismuth salts, sedative medications, or anticholinergic agents that may be prescribed.
- Instruct patients with pernicious anemia about need for long-term vitamin B12 injections. Teach self-administration or arrange for patient to receive injections from health care provider.

For more information, see Chapter 37 in Smeltzer and Bare: *Brunner and Suddarth's Textbook of Medical-Surgical Nursing*, 11th edition. Philadelphia: Lippincott Williams & Wilkins, 2008.

Glaucoma

Glaucoma refers to a group of ocular conditions characterized by visual field loss caused by damage to the optic nerve. Damage is related to increased intraocular pressure (IOP), caused by congestion of aqueous humor in the eye. Glaucoma is one of the leading causes of blindness among adults in the United States. When glaucoma is diagnosed early and managed properly, blindness is almost always preventable. Most cases are asymptomatic until extensive and irreversible damage has occurred. Glaucoma affects people of all ages but is more prevalent with increasing age (over 40 years). Others at risk are patients with diabetes, African Americans, those with a family history of glaucoma, and people with previous eye trauma or surgery or those who have had long-term steroid treatment.

Open Angle and Angle Closure Glaucomas

Main categories of glaucoma, based on the mechanism of impaired aqueous humor outflow, are open angle and angle closure. Congenital glaucomas and glaucomas resulting from other conditions are additional forms. The categories are further divided into the following:

- Primary glaucomas: cause unknown; usually bilateral and thought to have a hereditary component
- Secondary glaucomas: cause known; often unilateral

Clinical Manifestations

- Glaucoma is insidious in onset, slowly progressive, and often asymptomatic until late in the disease course. Small areas of peripheral vision loss may go unnoticed.
- One eye frequently is involved earlier and more severely than the other.
- Symptoms include pain (aching or discomfort around eyes and headache), halo vision, blurred vision, difficulty seeing

in low light, redness, and change in the eye's appearance (pallor and cupping of the optic nerve disc).
- As the optic nerve damage increases, visual perception in the area is lost.
- Ocular pain caused by rapid rise in IOP as a result of inflammation or medication-induced side effects, possibly accompanied by nausea, vomiting, sweating, or bradycardia

Assessment and Diagnostic Methods

- Routine eye examinations and screening clinics are vital to detection.
- Ocular and medical history (exposes predisposing factors), tonometry (measures IOP), ophthalmoscopy (to inspect the optic nerve), gonioscopy (to examine the filtration angle of the anterior chamber), and perimetry (visual fields assessment) are major diagnostic tests.

Gerontologic Considerations

Most patients with glaucoma are in the older age group. Often, dimming vision is accepted as part of aging, and medical assistance is not sought. For people older than age 35, tonometry is recommended, with periodic checking of eye pressure thereafter.

> **NURSING ALERT** Help the elderly patient to understand that eyedrops must be continued to keep glaucoma from worsening. Discontinuation of the medication allows glaucoma to continue insidiously until blindness occurs. Elderly patients with glaucoma may have other problems, such as arthritis, depression, and potential for falling and accidents.

Medical Management

Objective of treatment is to prevent optic nerve damage by lowering the IOP to a level consistent with retaining vision. Therapy is almost always lifelong. Treatment also focuses on achieving the greatest benefit at the least risk, cost, and inconvenience to the patient. Treatment varies depending on classification of the disease and response to therapy. Medication, laser surgery, and conventional surgery, or a combination of these, may be used to control progressive damage. First one eye is treated, then the second eye.

Pharmacologic Therapy

Pharmacotherapy is the initial and principal treatment for glaucoma. Acute angle-closure glaucoma is treated with medication (including miotics) to reduce IOP before laser or incisional iridectomy. Commonly used agents include:

- Beta-adrenergic blockers/antagonists are the most widely used hypotensive agents. They are effective in many types of glaucoma.
- Cholinergic agents (topical) are miotics (cause pupillary constriction) and are used in short-term management of glaucoma with pupillary block.
- Alpha-2-adrenergic agonists (topical) reduce IOP by increasing aqueous humor outflow.
- Carbonic anhydrase inhibitors (systemic) and prostaglandins lower IOP by reducing aqueous humor formation.
- Osmotic diuretics reduce IOP by increasing the osmolality of the plasma to draw water from the eye into the vascular circulation.

Surgical Management

- Ophthalmic laser trabeculoplasty or iridotomy is indicated as the primary treatment for glaucoma or is required when medication therapy is poorly tolerated or ineffective in lowering IOP.
- Conventional surgery procedures are performed when laser techniques are unsuccessful or when patient is not a good candidate for laser surgery (eg, patient cannot sit still or follow instructions).

- Filtering procedures: an opening or a fistula in the trabecular meshwork (trabeculectomy) is made to allow drainage, or drainage implant or shunt surgery may be performed.

Nursing Management

- Assess patient's knowledge of glaucoma (even patient with long-standing disease).
- Teach that optimal reduction of IOP and control of glaucoma damage require strict adherence to the medication regimen and regular follow-up examinations.
- Give written instructions that identify names of medications, descriptions of containers, and frequency and times of administration. Check for understanding of the expected action and possible side effects. Verify accuracy of eyedrop instillation, even with experienced patients.
- Advise patient to review all medications with ophthalmologist and mention side effects at each visit.
- Stress importance of making medication administration a part of daily routine so that doses are not missed. Stress that medication is to be continued even when IOP is under control. Patient may ask if generic form of medication is available for cost savings.
- Make patient aware that glaucoma medications may cause focus problems, and advise patient to move with caution.
- Teach patient to note how the eyes look and feel and report unusual changes to the physician: excessive irritation, watering, blurring, cloudy vision, discharge, rainbows around lights at night, flashes of light, and floating objects in the field of vision.
- Inform patient of possible interactions between glaucoma medications and other medications.
- Refer patients with severe impairment for assistive services.
- When patients appear to meet criteria for legal blindness, refer to agencies that assist in obtaining benefits from federally assisted programs.
- Encourage patient to maintain good health and limit stress: proper nutrition, salt restriction, avoiding excessive fluid

intake, maintaining appropriate weight, exercising, and taking time for fun and relaxation.

- Encourage patient to share feelings and concerns with family and friends or talk with other patients with glaucoma; support family caregivers.

For more information, see Chapter 58 in Smeltzer and Bare: *Brunner and Suddarth's Textbook of Medical-Surgical Nursing*, 11th edition. Philadelphia: Lippincott Williams & Wilkins, 2008.

Glomerulonephritis, Acute

Acute glomerulonephritis is a disease of the kidney in which there is an inflammation of the glomerular capillaries. In most cases, the stimulus of the reaction is group A streptococcal infection, which ordinarily precedes the onset of glomerulonephritis by 2 to 3 weeks.

Pathophysiology

Antigen–antibody complexes in the blood are trapped in the glomeruli, stimulating inflammation and producing injury to the kidney. Glomerulonephritis may also follow impetigo and acute viral infections, including upper respiratory infections, mumps, varicella zoster virus infection, Epstein-Barr virus infection, hepatitis B, and human immunodeficiency virus (HIV) infection. It is predominantly a disease of youth.

Clinical Manifestations

- Urine is cola-colored as a result of hematuria and proteinuria. Azotemia (urea and nitrogenous wastes in the blood) is another manifestation.
- In the more severe form of the disease, headache, malaise, facial edema, flank pain, and renal failure with oliguria occur.

- Mild to severe hypertension, some degree of edema (circulatory overload possible in elderly patients), and tenderness of the costovertebral angle are common.
- Elderly patients may have circulatory overload: dyspnea, engorged neck veins, cardiomegaly, and pulmonary edema.

Assessment and Diagnostic Findings

- Primary presenting feature: microscopic or gross (macroscopic) hematuria
- Proteinuria, increased antistreptolysin-O or anti-DNase B titer, elevated blood urea nitrogen (BUN) and serum creatinine levels, and anemia
- Kidney biopsy is performed for definitive diagnosis.

Medical Management

Goals of management are to preserve kidney function and to treat complications promptly. The patient is placed on bed rest during the acute phase until the urine clears and BUN and creatinine levels and blood pressure return to normal.

Pharmacologic Therapy

- Penicillin for residual streptococcal infection
- Diuretics and antihypertensive agents
- Corticosteroids and immunosuppressants for rapidly progressing disease
- Plasma exchange (plasmapheresis) and treatment with immunosuppressants, corticosteroids, and cytotoxic drugs to reduce inflammatory response in rapidly progressive disease
- Dialysis occasionally necessary

Nutritional Management

- Dietary protein restricted with renal insufficiency and elevated BUN

- Sodium restricted with hypertension, edema, and congestive heart failure
- Carbohydrates for energy and to reduce protein catabolism
- Fluids according to fluid losses and daily body weight and intake and output

Nursing Management

- Review fluid and diet restrictions. Measure and record intake and output.
- Instruct patient to schedule follow-up evaluations of blood pressure, urinalysis for protein, and BUN and creatinine studies to determine if disease has worsened.
- Instruct patient to notify physician if infection or symptoms of renal failure occur: fatigue, nausea, vomiting, diminishing urinary output.
- Refer to home care nurse as indicated for assessment and detection of early symptoms and follow-up evaluations.

For more information, see Chapter 45 in Smeltzer and Bare: *Brunner and Suddarth's Textbook of Medical-Surgical Nursing*, 11th edition. Philadelphia: Lippincott Williams & Wilkins, 2008.

Glomerulonephritis, Chronic

Chronic glomerulonephritis may have its onset as acute glomerulonephritis or some other type of antigen–antibody reaction that is overlooked. After repeated occurrences of these reactions, the kidneys are reduced to as little as one fifth of their normal size and consist largely of fibrous tissue. As chronic glomerulonephritis progresses, signs and symptoms of renal insufficiency and chronic renal failure occur. The result is severe glomerular damage that results in end-stage renal disease (ESRD).

Clinical Manifestations

Symptoms are variable. Some patients with severe disease have no symptoms for many years.

Common Signs and Symptoms

- First indications may be sudden, severe nosebleed, stroke, or convulsions/seizures.
- Many patients merely notice that their feet are slightly swollen at night.
- Other symptoms include loss of weight and strength, increasing irritability, and nocturia.
- Headaches, dizziness, and digestive disturbances are common.

Renal Insufficiency and Chronic Renal Failure

- Patient appears poorly nourished with a yellow-gray pigmentation of the skin, periorbital and peripheral edema, and pale mucous membranes.
- Blood pressure is normal or severely elevated.
- Retinal findings include hemorrhage, exudate, narrowed tortuous arterioles, and papilledema.
- Neck veins may be distended from fluid overload.
- Cardiomegaly, gallop rhythm, and other signs of heart failure may be present.
- Crackles in lungs
- Possibly, peripheral neuropathy with diminished deep tendon reflexes
- Neurosensory changes occur late in the illness, resulting in confusion and limited attention span. Other late signs include pericarditis with pericardial friction rub and pulsus paradoxus.

Assessment and Diagnostic Findings

On laboratory analysis, the following abnormalities may be found:

- Urinalysis: fixed specific gravity of 1.010, variable proteinuria, and urinary casts
- Blood studies related to renal failure progression: hyperkalemia, metabolic acidosis, anemia, hypoalbuminemia, decreased serum calcium and increased serum phosphorus, and hypermagnesemia
- Chest x-rays: cardiac enlargement and pulmonary edema
- Electrocardiogram: normal or may reflect left ventricular hypertrophy
- Impaired nerve conduction; mental status changes

Medical Management

The treatment of ambulatory patients is guided by symptoms.

- If hypertension is present, the blood pressure is lowered with sodium and water restriction.
- Proteins of high biologic value are provided to support good nutritional status (dairy products, eggs, meats).
- Urinary tract infections are treated promptly.
- If severe edema develops, patient is placed on bed rest with head of bed elevated to promote comfort and diuresis.
- Weight is monitored daily.
- Diuretics are administered to reduce fluid overload.
- Sodium and fluid intake is adjusted according to the kidneys' ability to excrete water and sodium.
- Dialysis is considered early in the course of disease to keep patient in optimal physical condition, prevent fluid and electrolyte imbalances, and minimize the risk of complications of renal failure.

Nursing Management

- Observe for deteriorating renal function; report changes in fluid and electrolyte status and in cardiac and neurologic status.
- Give emotional support throughout the disease and treatment course by providing opportunities for patient and

family to verbalize concerns. Answer questions and discuss options.

- Educate patient and family about prescribed treatment plan and the risk of noncompliance. Explain about need for follow-up evaluations of blood pressure, urinalysis for protein and casts, blood for BUN, and creatinine. Instruct in recommended diet and fluid modifications, and provide medication teaching.
- Refer to community health or home care nurse for assessment of patient progress and continued education about problems to report to health care provider.
- Give patient and family assistance and support regarding dialysis and long-term implications.

For more information, see Chapter 44 in Smeltzer and Bare: *Brunner and Suddarth's Textbook of Medical-Surgical Nursing*, 11th edition. Philadelphia: Lippincott Williams & Wilkins, 2008.

Gout

Gout is a heterogeneous group of inflammatory conditions related to a genetic defect of purine metabolism and resulting in hyperuricemia.

Pathophysiology

In gout, there is an oversecretion of uric acid or a renal defect resulting in decreased excretion of uric acid, or a combination of both. Primary hyperuricemia may be due to severe dieting or starvation, excessive intake of foods high in purines (shellfish, organ meats), or heredity. In secondary hyperuricemia, the gout is a minor clinical feature secondary to any of a number of genetic or acquired processes, including conditions with an increase in cell turnover (leukemias, multiple myeloma, psoriasis, some anemias) and an increase in cell breakdown.

Clinical Manifestations

Gout is characterized by deposits of uric acid in various joints. Four stages of gout can be identified: asymptomatic hyperuricemia, acute gouty arthritis, intercritical gout, and chronic tophaceous gout.

Acute Gouty Arthritis

- Acute arthritis of gout is the most common early sign.
- The metatarsophalangeal (MTP) joint of the big toe is most commonly affected; the tarsal area, ankle, or knee may also be affected.
- The acute attack may be triggered by trauma, alcohol ingestion, dieting, medication, surgical stress, or illness.
- Abrupt onset occurs at night, causing severe pain, redness, swelling, and warmth over the affected joint.
- Early attacks tend to subside spontaneously over 3 to 10 days without treatment.
- The next attack may not come for months or years; in time, attacks tend to occur more frequently, involve more joints, and last longer.

Hyperuricemia

- Fewer than one in five hyperuricemic people develop clinically apparent urate crystal deposits.
- Subsequent development of gout is directly related to duration and magnitude of hyperuricemia.

Tophi

- Tophi, chalky deposits of sodium urate, are noted an average of 10 years after the onset of gout.
- Tophi are generally associated with frequent and severe inflammatory episodes.
- Higher serum concentrations of uric acid are associated with tophus formation.

- Tophi occur in the synovium, olecranon bursa, subchondral bone, infrapatellar and Achilles' tendons, subcutaneous tissue, and overlying joints.
- Tophi have also been found in aortic walls, heart valves, nasal and ear cartilage, eyelids, cornea, and sclerae.
- Joint enlargement may cause loss of motion.

Risk for Urolithiasis (Kidney Stones)

- Incidence of renal stones is two times higher in patients with secondary gout than in those with primary gout.
- Stone formation is related to increased serum uric acid levels, acidity of urine, and urinary concentration.

Assessment and Diagnostic Methods

- Polarized light microscopy of the synovial fluid of the affected joint

Medical Management

- Hyperuricemia, tophi, joint destruction, and renal problems are treated after the acute inflammatory process has subsided.
- Uricosuric agents, such as probenecid, correct hyperuricemia and dissolve deposited urate.
- Colchicine (oral or parenteral) or a nonsteroidal anti-inflammatory drug (NSAID), such as indomethacin, is used to relieve acute attacks.
- Allopurinol is effective when renal insufficiency or renal calculi are a risk.
- Aspiration and intra-articular corticosteroids are used to treat large-joint acute attacks.

Nursing Management

Encourage patient to restrict consumption of foods high in purines, especially organ meats, and to limit alcohol intake.

Encourage patient to maintain normal body weight. These measures may help to prevent a painful episode of gout.

In an acute episode of gouty arthritis, pain management is essential. Review medications with patient and family. Stress the importance of continuing medications to maintain effectiveness. See Nursing Management under Arthritis for additional information.

For more information, see Chapter 54 in Smeltzer and Bare: *Brunner and Suddarth's Textbook of Medical-Surgical Nursing*, 11th edition. Philadelphia: Lippincott Williams & Wilkins, 2008.

Guillain-Barré Syndrome (Polyradiculoneuritis)

Guillain-Barré syndrome (GBS) results in the acute, rapid, segmental demyelination of nerves, causing an ascending weakness. In most patients, the syndrome is preceded by an infection (respiratory or gastrointestinal) 2 to 3 weeks before the onset of symptoms. In some instances, it has occurred after vaccination, pregnancy, or surgery.

Pathophysiology

GBS results from an autoimmune (cell-mediated and humoral) attack on peripheral nerve myelin proteins (substances speeding conduction of nerve impulses). The Schwann cell (which produces myelin in the peripheral nervous system) is spared in GBS, allowing for remyelination in the recovery phase of the disease.

Clinical Manifestations

Classic clinical features of GBS include areflexia and ascending weakness, although there may be variations in presentation. GBS does not affect cognitive function or level of consciousness.

- Initial neurologic symptoms are muscle weakness of the legs, which may progress to the upper extremities, trunk (quadriplegia), and facial muscles. Hyporeflexia and weakness may be followed quickly by complete paralysis, including paralysis of the diaphragm and intercostal muscles, resulting in respiratory failure.
- Cranial nerves are frequently affected, leading to paralysis of the ocular, facial, and oropharyngeal muscles, causing difficulty in talking, chewing, and swallowing.
- Autonomic dysfunction frequently occurs in the form of overreactivity or underreactivity of the sympathetic or parasympathetic nervous system. It is manifested by disturbances in heart rate and rhythm (tachycardia or bradycardia), blood pressure changes (hypertension or orthostatic hypotension), and a variety of other vasomotor disturbances.
- Patient may report severe, persistent pain in the back and calves.
- In many cases, patients have a loss of positional sense and diminished or absent tendon reflexes.
- Sensory changes are manifested by paresthesias (tingling and numbness).
- Most patients make a full recovery after several months to a year; about 10% have residual disability.

G

Assessment and Diagnostic Findings

- Clinical presentation (upward progression of weakness), history of recent viral infection, and results of laboratory and diagnostic studies provide key information for diagnosis.
- Spinal fluid shows an increased protein concentration with normal cell count.
- Electrophysiologic testing shows marked slowing of nerve conduction velocity.
- Pulmonary function tests: vital capacity and negative inspiratory force changes may indicate impending respiratory failure.

Medical Management

- GBS is considered a medical emergency; patient is managed in an intensive care unit.
- Respiratory problems may require mechanical ventilation.
- Plasmapheresis (plasma exchange) or intravenous immunoglobulin (IVIG) may be used to limit deterioration and demyelination.
- Continuous electrocardiogram (ECG) monitoring: Observe and treat cardiac dysrhythmias and other labile complications of autonomic dysfunction. Tachycardia and hypertension are treated with short-acting medications such as alpha-adrenergic blocking agents. Hypotension is managed by increasing the amount of intravenous fluid administered.

Pharmacologic Therapy

Atropine may be administered to avoid episodes of bradycardia during endotracheal suctioning and physical therapy. Anticoagulants and thigh-high elastic compression stockings or sequential compression boots may be ordered to prevent thrombosis and pulmonary emboli secondary to immobility.

NURSING PROCESS: The Patient with Guillain-Barré Syndrome

Assessment (Ongoing and Critical)

Assess for acute respiratory failure, a life-threatening problem. Assess also for complications, including ECG monitoring for cardiac dysrhythmias, deep vein thrombosis (DVT), and pulmonary embolism. Documentation of disease progression is crucial.

Diagnosis

Nursing Diagnoses

- Ineffective breathing pattern and impaired gas exchange related to rapidly progressive weakness and impending respiratory failure

- Impaired physical mobility related to paralysis
- Imbalanced nutrition: Less than body requirements related to inability to swallow, which is secondary to cranial nerve dysfunction (bulbar paralysis)
- Impaired verbal communication related to cranial nerve dysfunction
- Fear and anxiety related to loss of control and paralysis

Collaborative Problems/Potential Complications

- Respiratory failure
- Autonomic dysfunction

Planning and Goals

Major goals include improved respiratory function, increased mobility, improved nutritional status, effective communication, decreased fear and anxiety, and absence of complications.

Nursing Interventions

Maintaining Respiratory Function

- Assess carefully for difficulty in coughing and swallowing, which may cause aspiration of saliva and precipitate acute respiratory failure.
- Encourage use of incentive spirometry, provide chest physical therapy, and elevate head of bed to facilitate respirations and promote effective coughing.
- Suction to maintain a clear airway.

Monitoring for Complications: Respiratory Failure and Cardiovascular Problems

- Assess for and report difficulty in coughing and swallowing or decreasing vital capacity below 15 mL/kg, PaO_2 below 70 mmHg, progressive bulbar weakness, and an inability to clear secretions, indicating deterioration of respiratory function and need for ventilation.
- Watch for breathlessness while talking, shallow and irregular breathing, increasing pulse rate, use of accessory muscles while breathing, and change in respiratory pattern.

- Address potential need for mechanical ventilation with patient and family on admission to allow time for discussion and psychological preparation.
- Monitor for and report cardiac dysrhythmias (through ECG monitoring), transient hypertension, orthostatic hypotension, DVT, pulmonary embolism, urinary retention.

Enhancing Mobility and Preventing Complications From Immobility

- Monitor for and institute preventive measures related to urinary retention, transient hypertension, orthostatic hypotension, or other threats to the immobilized or paralyzed patient.
- Provide passive range-of-motion exercises at least twice daily; support the paralyzed extremities in functional positions. Change patient's position at least every 2 hours.
- Collaborate with physical therapist to prevent contracture deformities.
- Ensure adequate hydration and nutrition to prevent malnutrition or dehydration, since both of these conditions increase risk for pressure ulcers (see below).
- Administer prescribed anticoagulant regimen to prevent DVT and pulmonary embolism; assist with physical therapy; and use thigh-high elastic compression stockings or sequential compression boots.
- Place padding over bony prominences such as elbows and head of fibula to prevent compression neuropathies of ulnar and peroneal nerves.
- Use principles of nursing management of the unconscious patient.
- When recovery begins, prevent orthostatic hypotension by using a tilt table to help the patient assume an upright posture.

Providing Adequate Hydration and Nutrition

- Evaluate laboratory test results that may indicate malnutrition or dehydration (both of these conditions increase the risk for pressure ulcers).

- Collaborate with physician and dietitian to meet patient's nutritional and hydration needs. Provide adequate nutrition to prevent muscle wasting.
- If patient has paralytic ileus, provide intravenous fluids and parenteral nutrition as prescribed, and monitor for return of bowel sounds.
- Provide gastrostomy tube feedings if patient cannot swallow.
- Resume oral feeding when patient can swallow normally.

Assisting Communication

- Establish communication through lip reading, use of picture cards, or a system of blinking eyes to indicate yes or no if patient is on mechanical ventilation or otherwise unable to speak. Collaborate with speech therapist, as indicated.
- Provide diversions such as television, tapes, and visits to alleviate frustration.

Relieving Fear and Anxiety

- Involve family and friends with selected patient care activities and diversion to reduce sense of isolation.
- Provide patient with information about condition, emphasizing a positive appraisal of coping resources.
- Encourage relaxation exercises and distraction techniques, giving positive feedback.
- Create a positive attitude and atmosphere.
- Give expert nursing care, explanations, and reassurance to help patient gain control over situation.

Promoting Home and Community-Based Care

Teaching Patients Self-Care

- Teach patient and family about the disorder and its generally favorable prognosis.
- During the acute phase, instruct patient and family about strategies they can implement to minimize the effects of immobility and other complications.
- Explain care of patient and roles of patient and family in rehabilitation process.

- Use an interdisciplinary effort for family or caregiver education (nurse, physician, occupational and physical therapists, speech therapist, and respiratory therapist).

Continuing Care

- Provide care in a comprehensive inpatient program or an outpatient program, if patient can travel by car, or encourage a home program of physical and occupational therapy.
- Support patient and family through long recovery phase, and promote involvement for return of former abilities.
- Inform patient and caregivers about support groups.

Evaluation

Expected Patient Outcomes

- Maintains effective respirations and airway clearance
- Shows increasing mobility
- Receives adequate nutrition and hydration
- Demonstrates recovery of speech
- Shows lessening fear and anxiety
- Remains free of complications

For more information, see Chapter 64 in Smeltzer and Bare: *Brunner and Suddarth's Textbook of Medical-Surgical Nursing*, 11th edition. Philadelphia: Lippincott Williams & Wilkins, 2008.

Headache

Headache (cephalgia) is one of the most common of all human physical complaints. Headache is actually a symptom rather than a disease entity and may indicate organic disease (neurologic), a stress response, vasodilation (migraine), skeletal muscle tension (tension headache), or a combination of these factors.

A secondary headache is a symptom associated with organic causes, such as a brain tumor or aneurysm, subarachnoid hemorrhage, stroke, severe hypertension, meningitis, and head injury. Headaches classified as primary headaches include the following:

- Migraine (with and without aura)
- Tension-type headache
- Cluster headache and paroxysmal hemicrania

Headaches are also classified as secondary headaches, such as the following:

- Miscellaneous headaches associated with structural lesions
- Headache associated with head trauma
- Headache associated with vascular disorders (eg, subarachnoid hemorrhage)
- Headache associated with nonvascular intracranial disorders (eg, brain tumor)
- Headache associated with use of chemical substances or their withdrawal
- Headache associated with noncephalic infection
- Headache associated with metabolic disorder (eg, hypoglycemia)
- Headache or facial pain associated with disorder of the head or neck or their structures (eg, acute glaucoma)
- Cranial neuralgias (persistent pain of cranial nerve origin)

Migraine Headache

This symptom complex is characterized by periodic and recurrent attacks of severe headache. The cause of migraine has not been clearly demonstrated, but it is primarily a vascular disturbance that occurs more commonly in women and has strong familial tendencies. Onset typically occurs in puberty, with highest incidence between 20 and 35 years of age.

Clinical Manifestations

H

Headache often begins in early morning (headache on awakening). The classic migraine attack can be divided into four phases: prodrome, aura, headache, and recovery.

Prodrome Phase

- Present in 60% of patients with migraine headache
- Symptoms may occur consistently hours to days before onset of migraine.
- Depression, irritability, feeling cold, food cravings, anorexia, change in activity level, increased urination, diarrhea, or constipation may be noted with each migraine.

Aura Phase

- Occurs in up to 31% of patients and lasts less than 1 hour
- Focal neurologic symptoms, predominantly visual disturbances (light flashes), occur and may be hemianoptic (occurring in half of the visual field).
- Numbness and tingling of lips, face or hands, mild confusion, slight weakness of an extremity, and drowsiness and dizziness may be present.

Headache Phase

This phase, occurring in 60% of patients, involves a unilateral, throbbing headache that intensifies over several hours. Pain is severe and incapacitating, often associated with photophobia, nausea, and vomiting. Duration varies from about 4 to 72 hours.

Recovery Phase (Termination and Postdrome)

- Pain gradually subsides.
- There is a period of muscle contraction in the neck and scalp with associated muscle ache and point (localized) tenderness, exhaustion, and mood changes.
- Any physical exertion exacerbates the headache pain.
- Patient may sleep for an extended period.

Assessment and Diagnostic Methods

- Physical assessment of head and neck
- Neurologic examination
- Detailed health and headache assessment and history
- Cerebral angiography, CT, or MRI if abnormalities on neurologic examination
- Electromyography (EMG) and laboratory tests (complete blood count, electrolytes, glucose, creatinine, erythrocyte sedimentation rate, and thyroid panel)

Medical Management

Therapy is divided into abortive (symptomatic) and preventive approaches. Abortive approach is used for frequent attacks and is aimed at relieving or limiting a headache at onset or while in progress. Preventive approach is used for those who have frequent attacks at regular or predictable intervals and may have medical conditions that preclude abortive therapies.

Management of Acute Attack

Treatment varies greatly; close monitoring is indicated.

- Ergotamine preparations may be effective if taken early. Cafergot is a combination of ergotamine and caffeine. Dihydroergotamine (DHE) is highly effective in attacks lasting more than 72 hours (contraindicated in patients with coronary or peripheral vascular disease). Ergotamine preparations may be taken PO, SC, IM, sublingually, or rectally, or they may be inhaled.

- Patient should lie quietly in a darkened room with head slightly elevated.
- Possibly, 100% oxygen by face mask for 15 minutes
- Drinking black coffee may be helpful.
- Sumatriptan (Imitrex), naratriptan (Amerge), rizatriptan (Maxalt), zolmitriptan (Zomig), and almotriptan are used for acute migraine and cluster headaches; Cafergot is used to relieve moderate to severe migraines.
- Symptomatic therapy includes analgesics, sedatives, antianxiety agents, and antiemetics.

Prevention: Pharmacologic Therapy

- Daily use of medications thought to block the headache attack.
- Beta-blockers such as propranolol (Inderal), most widely used. Also used are amitriptyline (Elavil), divalproex (Valproate), flunarizine, and serotonin antagonists.
- Antidepressants, barbiturates, tranquilizers (use cautiously and on short-term basis)
- Calcium antagonists used frequently (require several weeks until effective); methysergide (Sansert) or anticonvulsants (divalproex sodium [Depakote]) may be used; lidocaine nose drops are effective in treating cluster headaches and migraine.

NURSING PROCESS: The Patient with Headaches

Assessment

- Obtain a detailed history and physical assessment; data obtained for the health history should reflect patient's own

words. Include medications, toxic substance exposure, stress, insomnia, and family history.
- Focus health history on assessment of headache (location, quality, frequency, precipitating factors, time, associated symptoms).

Nursing Diagnoses

Pain related to vascular changes

Planning and Goals

Goals include treating the acute event of the headache and preventing recurrent episodes.

Nursing Interventions

Relieving Pain
- Attempt to abort headache early.
- Provide comfort measures (eg, a quiet, dark environment); elevate head of bed 30 degrees. Administer medications if nonpharmacologic measures are ineffective.
- Provide symptomatic treatment, such as antiemetics, as indicated.

Promoting Home and Community-Based Care
Teaching Patients Self-Care
- Teach that migraine headaches are likely to occur when patient is ill, overtired, or feeling stressed.
- Instruct about the importance of avoiding known triggers and maintaining a proper diet, adequate rest, and coping strategies.
- Help patient identify circumstances that precipitate headache, and assist in development of alternative means of coping.
- Help patients develop insight into their feelings, behaviors, and conflicts to make necessary lifestyle modifications.
- Suggest regular periods of exercise and relaxation and avoidance of offending factors.

- Avoid long intervals between meals.
- Advise patient to awaken at the same time each day; disruption of normal sleeping pattern provokes a migraine in many patients.

Continuing Care

The National Headache Foundation provides a list of clinics in the United States and the names of physicians who are members of the American Association for the Study of Headaches.

H   Evaluation

Expected Patient Outcomes

- Demonstrates relief of pain
- Verbalizes techniques to prevent or minimize headache

Cluster Headache

Cluster headaches, another severe form of vascular headache, are seen most frequently in men. The attacks come in clusters of one to eight daily, with excruciating pain localized in the eye and orbit and radiating to the facial and temporal regions. The pain is accompanied by watering of the eye and nasal congestion lasting from 15 minutes to 3 hours and may have a crescendo-decrescendo pattern. They have been described as penetrating. They may be precipitated by alcohol, nitrites, vasodilators, and histamines.

Cranial Arteritis

Inflammation of the cranial arteries is characterized by a severe headache localized in the region of the temporal artery. The inflammation may be generalized or focal. This is a cause of headache in the older population, particularly those older than age 70. Clinical manifestations include inflammation (eg, heat, redness, swelling, and tenderness or pain over the involved artery). A tender, swollen, or nodular temporal artery may be visible. Visual problems are caused by ischemia of the involved structures. The headache is treated with corticosteroid drugs (do not stop abruptly) and analgesic agents.

Tension Headache (Muscle Contraction Headache)

Emotional or physical stress may cause contraction of the muscles in the neck and scalp, resulting in tension headache. This is characterized by a steady, constant feeling of pressure that usually begins in the forehead, the temple, or the back of the neck. Tension headaches tend to be more chronic than severe and are probably the most common type of headache. Relief may be obtained by local heat, massage, analgesics, antidepressants, and muscle relaxants. Reassure patient that the headache does not indicate a brain tumor, and teach stress reduction techniques (biofeedback, exercise, medication).

H

For more information, see Chapter 61 in Smeltzer and Bare: *Brunner and Suddarth's Textbook of Medical-Surgical Nursing*, 11th edition. Philadelphia: Lippincott Williams & Wilkins, 2008.

Head Injury (Brain Injury)

Injuries to the head involve trauma to the scalp, skull, and brain and represent the most common cause of death from trauma in the United States. Head injuries are among the most common and serious sources of neurologic impairment and have reached epidemic proportions as a result of motor vehicle crashes. Other causes include falls, assaults, and sports injuries. A major risk to a patient who experiences a head injury is traumatic brain injury (TBI), damage to the brain from bleeding or swelling that causes increased intracranial pressure (ICP). Groups at highest risk for TBI are persons 15 to 24 years of age, with an almost 2:1 male-to-female incidence ratio. The very young (under 5) and very old (over age 75) are also at increased risk.

Scalp and Skull Injuries

- Scalp trauma may result in an abrasion (brush wound), contusion, laceration, or hematoma. The scalp bleeds profusely when injured. Scalp wounds are a portal of entry for intracranial infections.
- Fracture of the skull is a break in the continuity of the skull caused by trauma. Fractures may occur with or without damage to the brain. They are classified as linear, comminuted, depressed, or basilar and may be open (dura is torn) or closed (dura is not torn).

Clinical Manifestations

Symptoms, other than local, depend on the severity and distribution of brain injury.

- Persistent, localized pain usually suggests fracture.
- Fractures of the cranial vault may or may not produce swelling in that region.
- Fractures of the base of the skull frequently produce hemorrhage from the nose, pharynx, or ears, and blood may appear under the conjunctiva.
- Ecchymosis may be seen over the mastoid (Battle's sign).
- Drainage of cerebral spinal fluid (CSF) from the ears and the nose suggests basal skull fracture.
- Drainage of CSF may cause serious infection (eg, meningitis) through a tear in the dura mater.
- Bloody spinal fluid suggests brain laceration or contusion.
- Brain injury may have various signs, including altered level of consciousness, pupillary abnormalities, altered or absent gag reflex or corneal reflex, neurologic deficits, change in vital signs (eg, respiration pattern, hypertension, bradycardia), hyperthermia or hypothermia, and sensory, vision, or hearing impairment.
- Signs of a postconcussion syndrome may include headache, dizziness, anxiety, irritability, and lethargy.
- In acute or subacute subdural hematoma, changes in level of consciousness, pupillary signs, hemiparesis, coma,

hypertension, bradycardia, and slowing respiratory rate are signs of expanding mass.

• Chronic subdural hematoma may result in severe headache, alternating focal neurologic signs, personality changes, mental deterioration, and focal seizures.

Assessment and Diagnostic Methods

• Physical examination and evaluation of neurologic status
• Radiographic studies: computed tomography (CT), magnetic resonance imaging (MRI)
• Cerebral angiography, spinal tap

Medical Management

• Nondepressed skull fractures generally do not require surgical treatment but require close observation of patient.
• Depressed skull fractures may be managed conservatively; contaminated or deforming fractures require surgery.
• Antibiotic treatment is instituted with blood component therapy, if indicated.

Concussion (Brain Injury)

A cerebral concussion after head injury is a temporary loss of neurologic function with no apparent structural damage. Concussion generally involves a period of unconsciousness lasting from a few seconds to a few minutes. Jarring of the brain may be so slight as to cause only dizziness and spots before the eyes, or severe enough to cause complete loss of consciousness. If the frontal lobe is affected, patient may exhibit bizarre, irrational behavior. If the temporal lobe is affected, patient may exhibit temporary amnesia or disorientation.

Nursing Management

• Give information, explanations, and encouragement to reduce postconcussion syndrome.

- Instruct family to look for the following signs and notify physician or clinic: difficulty in awakening, difficulty in speaking, confusion, severe headache, vomiting, or weakness of one side of the body.
- Advise patient to resume normal activities slowly.

Contusion

A cerebral contusion is a more severe cerebral injury. The brain is bruised, with possible surface hemorrhage. The patient is unconscious, may exhibit faint pulse, shallow respirations, cool, pale skin, subnormal blood pressure and temperature, and may be incontinent of bowel or bladder. The patient may be aroused with effort but soon slips back into unconsciousness. In general, patients with widespread injury who have abnormal motor function, abnormal eye movements, and elevated ICP have a poor outcome (brain damage, disability, or death). Conversely, these patients may recover consciousness completely, may pass into a stage of cerebral irritability (ie, conscious and easily disturbed by any form of stimulation, such as noise and light), and may become hyperactive. Recovery is often delayed, and residual headache and vertigo are common; impaired mentality or seizures may occur.

Diffuse Axonal Injury

Diffuse axonal injury may occur with mild, moderate, or severe head trauma. The injury involves widespread damage to axons in the cerebral hemispheres, corpus callosum, and brain stem. The patient has no lucid intervals and experiences immediate coma, decorticate and decerebrate posturing, and global cerebral edema. Diagnosis is made by clinical signs and a CT or MRI scan. Recovery depends on the severity of the axonal injury.

Intracranial Hemorrhage

Hematomas that develop within the cranial vault are the most serious results of brain injury. A hematoma may be epidural, subdural, or intracerebral, depending on location. Its main effects are frequently delayed until the hematoma is large enough to cause distortion, increased ICP, and herniation of the brain.

Epidural Hematoma (Extradural Hematoma or Hemorrhage)

Blood collects in the epidural space between the skull and dura mater. The hematoma can result from a skull fracture that causes a rupture or laceration of the middle meningeal artery, the artery that runs between the dura and the skull inferior to a thin portion of temporal bone. Symptoms are caused by the pressure of the expanding hematoma: usually, a momentary loss of consciousness at time of injury followed by an interval of apparent recovery while compensation for the increased volume occurs. When compensation is no longer possible, sudden signs of compression may appear, including deterioration of consciousness and signs of focal neurologic deficits (dilation and fixation of a pupil or paralysis of an extremity); the patient deteriorates rapidly.

Medical Management

This is an extreme emergency because marked neurologic deficit or respiratory arrest may occur within minutes. Bur holes are made to remove the clots, and the bleeding point is controlled (craniotomy, drain insertion).

Subdural Hematoma

Blood collects between the dura and the underlying brain and is more frequently venous in origin. The most common cause is trauma, but it may also be associated with various bleeding tendencies (coagulopathies), and rupture of an aneurysm. Subdural hematoma may be acute (major head injury), subacute (sequelae of less severe contusions), or chronic (minor head injuries in the elderly may be cause; signs and symptoms fluctuate and may be mistaken for neurosis, psychosis, or stroke).

Intracerebral Hemorrhage and Hematoma

Bleeding occurs into the substance of the brain. Hematoma is commonly seen when forces are exerted to the head over a small area (missile injuries or bullet wounds; stab injury). It may also result from systemic hypertension causing degeneration and rupture of a vessel, rupture of a saccular aneurysm; vascular anomalies; intracranial tumors; systemic causes, including bleeding disorders such as leukemia, hemophilia, aplastic anemia, and thrombocytopenia; and complications of anticoagulant therapy. Its onset may be insidious, with neurologic deficits followed by headache.

Medical Management

Presume that a person with a head injury has a cervical spine injury until proven otherwise. From the scene of the injury, the patient is transported on a board, with head and neck maintained in alignment with the axis of the body. Apply a cervical collar and maintain it until cervical spine x-rays have been obtained and the absence of cervical spinal cord injury documented. All therapy is directed toward preserving brain homeostasis and preventing secondary brain injury.

- Management involves supportive care, control of ICP, maintenance of fluid and electrolyte balance, administration of antihypertensive medications, or craniotomy.
- Increased ICP is managed by adequate oxygenation, mannitol administration, ventilatory support, hyperventilation, elevation of the head of the bed, maintenance of fluid and electrolyte balance, nutritional support, pain and anxiety management, or neurosurgery.

See Medical Management and Nursing Management under Increased Intracranial Pressure for additional information.

NURSING PROCESS: The Patient with a Head Injury

Assessment

Obtain health history, including time of injury, cause of injury, direction and force of the blow, loss of consciousness, and condition following injury. Detailed neurologic information (level of consciousness, ability to respond to verbal commands if patient is conscious), response to tactile stimuli (if patient is unconscious), pupillary response to light, corneal and gag reflexes, motor function, and system assessments provide baseline data. The Glasgow Coma Scale serves as a guide for assessing levels of consciousness (LOC) based on three criteria: (1) eye opening, (2) verbal responses, and (3) motor responses to a verbal command or painful stimulus. The Rancho Los Amigos Level of Cognitive Function is another useful evaluation scale.

Monitoring Vital Signs

- Monitor patient at frequent intervals to assess intracranial status.
- Assess for increasing ICP, including slowing of pulse, increasing systolic pressure, and widening pulse pressure. As brain compression increases, vital signs are reversed, pulse and respirations become rapid, and blood pressure may decrease.
- Monitor for rapid rise in body temperature; keep temperature below 38°C (100.4°F) to avoid increased metabolic demands on the brain.
- Keep in mind that tachycardia and hypotension may indicate bleeding elsewhere in the body.

Assessing Motor Function

- Observe spontaneous movements; ask patient to raise and lower extremities; compare strength of hand grasp at periodic intervals.
- Note presence or absence of spontaneous movement of each extremity.

- Assess responses to painful stimuli in absence of spontaneous movement; abnormal response carries a poorer prognosis.
- Determine patient's ability to speak; note quality of speech.

Evaluating Eye Signs

- Evaluate spontaneous eye opening.
- Evaluate size of pupils and reaction to light (unilaterally dilated and poorly responding pupils may indicate developing hematoma). If both pupils are fixed and dilated, it usually indicates overwhelming injury and poor prognosis.

Monitoring for Complications (Cerebral Edema and Herniation)

- Deterioration in condition may be due to expanding intracranial hematoma, progressive brain edema, and herniation of the brain.
- Peak swelling occurs about 72 hours after injury, with resulting elevation of ICP.

Monitoring for Other Complications

- Assess for complications, including systemic infections or neurosurgical infections: wound infection, osteomyelitis, or meningitis.
- After injury, some patients develop focal nerve palsies, such as anosmia (lack of sense of smell) or eye movement abnormalities and focal neurologic defects, such as aphasia, memory defects, and posttraumatic seizures or epilepsy.
- Patients may be left with organic psychosocial deficits and may lack insight into their emotional responses.

Diagnosis

Nursing Diagnoses

- Ineffective airway clearance and ventilation related to hypoxia
- Ineffective cerebral tissue perfusion related to increased ICP and decreased cerebral perfusion pressure

- Deficient fluid volume related to disturbances of consciousness and hormonal dysfunction
- Imbalanced nutrition: Less than body requirements related to metabolic changes, fluid restrictions, and inadequate intake
- Risk for injury (self-directed and directed to others) related to disorientation, restlessness, and brain damage
- Risk for imbalanced body temperature related to damage to temperature-regulating mechanism
- Risk for impaired skin integrity related to bed rest, hemiparesis, hemiplegia, and immobility
- Disturbed thought processes (deficits in intellectual function, communication, memory, information processing) related to results of brain injury
- Disturbed sleep pattern related to head injury and frequent neurologic checks
- Interrupted family processes related to unresponsiveness of patient, unpredictability of outcome, prolonged recovery period, and patient's residual physical and emotional deficits
- Deficient knowledge about rehabilitation process

Collaborative Problems/Potential Complications

- Cerebral edema and herniation
- Decreased cerebral perfusion
- Impaired oxygenation and ventilation
- Impaired fluid, electrolyte, and nutritional balance
- Risk for posttraumatic seizures

Planning and Goals

Goals may include maintenance of a patent airway, adequate cerebral perfusion pressure, fluid and electrolyte balance, and adequate nutritional status; prevention of secondary injury; maintenance of skin integrity and normal body temperature; improved cognitive function; effective family processes; increased knowledge about rehabilitation process; and absence of complications.

Nursing Interventions

Maintaining the Airway

- Position the unconscious patient to facilitate drainage of secretions; elevate head of bed 30 degrees to decrease intracranial venous pressure.
- Establish effective suctioning procedures.
- Guard against aspiration and respiratory insufficiency.
- Monitor arterial blood gases to assess adequacy of ventilation.
- Monitor patient on mechanical ventilation.
- Monitor for pulmonary complications (ARDS and pneumonia).

Maintaining Fluid and Electrolyte Balance

Fluid and electrolyte balance is particularly important in patients receiving osmotic diuretics, those with inappropriate antidiuretic hormone secretion, and those with posttraumatic diabetes insipidus.

- Monitor serum and urine electrolyte levels (including blood glucose and urine acetone), osmolality, and intake and output to evaluate endocrine function.
- Record daily weights (which may indicate fluid loss from diabetes insipidus).

Providing Adequate Nutrition

- Parenteral nutrition (PN) via a central line or enteral feedings administered via a nasogastric or nasojejunal feeding tube may be used.
- Start nasogastric feedings as soon as condition stabilizes unless there is discharge of CSF from the nose; oral feeding tubes may be used. Food intake may resume when swallowing reflex returns and patient can meet caloric requirements orally.
- Give small, frequent feedings to lessen the possibility of vomiting and diarrhea (continuous-drip infusion or controlling pump to regulate the feeding); elevate head of bed, and check residual feeding before feedings.

Preventing Injury

- Observe for restlessness, which may be due to hypoxia, fever, pain, or a full bladder. Restlessness may also be a sign that the unconscious patient is regaining consciousness.
- Avoid bladder distention.
- Protect patient from injury (padded side rails, hands wrapped in mitts).
- Avoid restraints when possible because straining can increase ICP.
- Avoid using narcotics for restlessness because they depress respiration, constrict pupils, and alter level of consciousness.
- Keep environmental stimuli to a minimum.
- Provide adequate lighting to prevent visual hallucinations.
- Do not disrupt sleep/wake cycles.
- Use an external sheath catheter for incontinence because an indwelling catheter may produce infection.

Maintaining Body Temperature

- Monitor temperature every 2 to 4 hours.
- If temperature rises, administer acetaminophen and cooling blankets as prescribed to achieve normothermia.
- Monitor for infection related to fever.

Maintaining Skin Integrity

- Assess all body surfaces, and document skin integrity every 8 hours.
- Turn patient and reposition every 2 to 4 hours.
- Provide skin care every 4 hours; use skin lubricant to prevent irritation due to rubbing against the sheet.
- Assist patient to get out of bed three times a day (when appropriate).

Improving Cognitive Functioning

- Develop patient's ability to devise problem-solving strategies through cognitive rehabilitation over time; use a multidisciplinary approach.

H

- Be aware that there are fluctuations in orientation and memory and that these patients are easily distracted.
- Do not push to a level greater than patient's impaired cortical functioning allows because fatigue, headache, and stress (headache, dizziness) may occur.

Preventing Sleep Pattern Disturbance

- Group nursing activities so that patient is disturbed less frequently.
- Decrease environmental noise, and dim room lights.
- Provide strategies (eg, back rubs) to increase comfort.

Supporting Family Processes

- Provide family with accurate and honest information.
- Encourage family to continue to set well-defined, mutual, short-term goals.
- Encourage family counseling to deal with feelings of loss and helplessness, and provide guidance in the management of inappropriate behaviors.
- Refer family to support groups that provide a forum for networking, sharing problems, and gaining assistance in maintaining realistic expectations and hope. The National Head Injury Foundation provides information and other resources.

Monitoring and Managing Potential Complications

- Monitor for a patent airway, altered breathing pattern, and hypoxemia and pneumonia. Assist with intubation and mechanical ventilation.
- Provide enteral feedings, intravenous fluids and electrolytes, or insulin as prescribed.
- Initiate PN as ordered if patient is unable to eat.
- Monitor for systemic or neurosurgical infection and heterotopic ossification.
- Take measures to control cerebral perfusion pressure: elevate head of bed 30 degrees, maintain head and neck in alignment (no twisting), prevent Valsalva maneuver, use

medications to decrease ICP, maintain normal body temperature, hyperventilate on mechanical ventilation, maintain fluid restriction, avoid noxious stimuli (suctioning), administer sedation to reduce metabolic demands.

- Assess carefully for development of posttraumatic seizures.

Promoting Home and Community-Based Care
Teaching Patients Self-Care

- Reinforce information given to family about patient's condition and prognosis early in the course of head injury.
- As patient's status changes over time, focus teaching on interpretation and explanation of changes in patient's responses.
- Instruct patient and family about limitations that can be expected and complications that may occur if patient is to be discharged.
- Identify and teach the complications that merit contacting the neurosurgeon.
- Teach about self-care management strategies, if patient's status indicates.
- Instruct about side effects of medications and importance of taking them as prescribed.

Continuing Care

- Encourage patient to continue rehabilitation program after discharge. Improvement may take 3 or more years after injury, during which time the family and their coping skills need frequent assessment.
- Inform patient and family that posttraumatic seizures occur frequently and that anticonvulsants may be prescribed for 1 to 2 years after injury.
- Encourage patient to return to normal activities gradually.
- Continue support and teaching for patient and family, with frequent assessment of coping abilities during long-term rehabilitation.

H

Evaluation

Expected Patient Outcomes

- Attains or maintains effective airway clearance, ventilation, and brain oxygenation
- Achieves normal blood gas values and has normal breath sounds
- Achieves satisfactory fluid and electrolyte balance
- Attains adequate nutritional status
- Avoids injury
- Has no fever
- Demonstrates intact skin integrity
- Shows improvement in cognitive function and improved memory
- Demonstrates normal sleep/wake cycle
- Family demonstrates adaptive coping processes.
- Patient and family participate in rehabilitation process as indicated.
- Patient experiences no posttraumatic seizures.
- Demonstrates absence of complications

For more information, see Chapter 63 in Smeltzer and Bare: *Brunner and Suddarth's Textbook of Medical-Surgical Nursing*, 11th edition. Philadelphia: Lippincott Williams & Wilkins, 2008.

Heart Failure (Cor Pulmonale)

Heart failure, sometimes referred to as congestive heart failure, is the inability of the heart to pump sufficient blood to meet the needs of the tissues for oxygen and nutrients. Heart failure is a clinical syndrome characterized by signs and symptoms of fluid overload or inadequate tissue perfusion. The underlying mechanism of heart failure involves impaired contractile properties of the heart (systolic dysfunction) or filling of the heart (diastolic) that leads to a lower-than-normal cardiac output. The low cardiac output can lead to compensatory mechanisms that cause increased workload on the heart and eventual resistance to filling of the heart.

Heart failure is a life-long diagnosis managed with lifestyle changes and medications to prevent acute congestive episodes. Congestive heart failure is usually an acute presentation of heart failure. Common underlying conditions include coronary atherosclerosis (primary cause), valvular disease, cardiomyopathy, inflammatory or degenerative muscle disease, and arterial hypertension. A number of systemic factors can contribute to the development and severity of cardiac failure. Increased metabolic rate (fever, thyrotoxicosis), hypoxia, and anemia require an increased cardiac output to satisfy systemic oxygen demand. Dysrhythmia decreases the efficiency of myocardial function.

Clinical Manifestations

- Symptoms of inadequate tissue perfusion
- Diminished cardiac output with accompanying dizziness, confusion, fatigue, exercise or heat intolerance, cool extremities, and oliguria
- Congestion of tissues
- Increased pulmonary venous pressure (pulmonary edema) manifested by cough and shortness of breath
- Dysrhythmia may indicate heart failure or may be noted as a result of the treatment for heart failure.
- Increased systemic venous pressure, as evidenced by generalized peripheral edema and weight gain

Left-Sided Heart Failure

Most often precedes right-sided cardiac failure

Backward Failure

- Pulmonary congestion; cough; fatigability; tachycardia with an S_3 heart sound; anxiety; restlessness
- Dyspnea on exertion (DOE), orthopnea, paroxysmal nocturnal dyspnea (PND)

- Cough may be dry and nonproductive but is most often moist.
- Bibasilar crackles advancing to crackles in all lung fields
- Large quantities of frothy sputum, which is sometimes pink (blood-tinged)

Forward Failure

Tachycardia, weak, thready pulse, anxiety, oliguria and nocturia, altered digestion, ashen, pale, cool and clammy skin

Right-Sided Heart Failure

- Congestion of the viscera and peripheral tissues
- Edema of lower extremities (dependent edema), usually pitting edema, weight gain, hepatomegaly
- Distended neck veins (jugular vein distention), ascites, anorexia, and nausea
- Nocturia and weakness

Assessment and Diagnostic Methods

- Evaluation of clinical manifestations
- Hemodynamic monitoring
- Cardiac catheterization with radionuclide ventriculography, or invasively, by ventriculogram
- Echocardiogram (ejection fraction)
- Chest radiographs, ECG
- Exercise testing to detect coronary artery disease
- Laboratory studies (blood urea nitrogen [BUN], creatinine, thyroid stimulating hormone, complete blood count [CBC], urinalysis)

Medical Management

Treatment goals are to eliminate or reduce etiologic factors, reduce the workload on the heart, increase the force and efficiency of myocardial contractions with pharmacologic agents, and eliminate the excessive accumulation of body water. Smoking, alcohol, and excess fluid intake are prohibited. Medications and oxygen (including intubation) are prescribed as indicated. Nutritional therapy may include sodium restriction (2 to 3 g/day) and avoidance of excess fluid intake to prevent, control, or eliminate edema.

Surgical Management

Coronary bypass surgery, PTCA, other innovative therapies as indicated (eg, mechanical assist devices, transplantation)

Pharmacologic Therapy

Alone or in combination: vasodilator therapy (angiotensin-converting enzyme [ACE] inhibitors), angiotensin II receptor blockers (ARBs), select beta-blockers, calcium channel blockers, diuretic therapy, cardiac glycosides (digitalis), and others

- Dobutamine, milrinone, anticoagulants, beta-blockers, as indicated
- Possibly antihypertensives or antianginal medications and anticoagulants

▌NURSING PROCESS: The Patient with Heart Failure

Assessment

Nursing assessment of the patient with heart failure is directed toward evaluating the therapeutic effectiveness of medical and nursing interventions and observing for signs and symptoms of pulmonary and systemic fluid overload. All untoward signs are recorded and reported.

- Note report of sleep disturbance due to shortness of breath, and number of pillows used for sleep.
- Note activities reported to cause shortness of breath.

- Respiratory: auscultate lungs at frequent intervals to determine presence or absence of crackles and wheezes. Note rate and depth of respirations.
- Cardiac: auscultate for S_3 heart sound, which may mean pump is beginning to fail; signs of fluid overload (orthopnea, PND, DOE).
- Assess sensorium and level of consciousness.
- Periphery: assess dependent parts of body for perfusion and edema and the liver for hepatojugular reflux and jugular vein distention
- Measure intake and output to detect oliguria or anuria; weigh patient daily.

Diagnosis

Nursing Diagnoses

- Activity intolerance (or risk for) related to imbalance between oxygen supply and demand secondary to decreased cardiac output
- Fatigue secondary to heart failure
- Excess fluid volume related to excess fluid or sodium intake or retention secondary to heart failure and its medical therapy
- Anxiety related to breathlessness and restlessness secondary to inadequate oxygenation
- Powerlessness related to inability to perform role responsibilities secondary to chronic illness and hospitalizations
- Noncompliance related to lack of knowledge
- Deficient knowledge of self-care program related to nonacceptance of necessary lifestyle changes

Collaborative Problems/Potential Complications

- Cardiogenic shock
- Thromboembolism
- Pericardial effusion and cardiac tamponade
- Dysrhythmias

Planning and Goals

Major goals of the patient may include promotion of activity while maintaining vital signs within identified range, reduced fatigue, relief of fluid overload symptoms, decreased anxiety or increased ability to manage anxiety, knowledge of self-care program, and ability to make decisions and influence outcomes.

Nursing Interventions

Promoting Activity Tolerance

- Monitor patient's response to activities. Instruct patient to avoid prolonged bed rest; patient should rest if symptoms are severe but otherwise should assume regular activity.
- Encourage patient to perform an activity more slowly than usual, for a shorter duration, or with assistance initially.
- Identify barriers that could limit patient's ability to perform an activity, and discuss methods of pacing an activity (eg, chop or peel vegetables while sitting at the kitchen table rather than standing at the kitchen counter).
- Take vital signs, especially pulse, before, during, and immediately after an activity to identify whether they are within the predetermined range; heart rate should return to baseline within 3 minutes. If patient tolerates the activity, develop short-term and long-term goals to increase gradually the intensity, duration, or frequency of activity.
- Refer to a cardiac rehabilitation program as needed, especially for patients with a recent myocardial infarction, recent open heart surgery, or increased anxiety.

Reducing Fatigue

- Collaborate with patient to develop a schedule that promotes pacing and prioritization of activities. Encourage patient to alternate activities with periods of rest and avoid having two significant energy-consuming activities occur on the same day or in immediate succession.
- Encourage family to stagger visits to allow for rest between visits or calls; identify a spokesperson to relay messages from and to other friends and family members.

- Identify patient's peak and low periods of energy, and plan energy-consuming activities accordingly.
- Explain that small, frequent meals tend to decrease the amount of energy needed for digestion while providing adequate nutrition.
- Help patient develop a positive outlook focused on strengths, abilities, and interests.

H

Managing Fluid Volume

- Administer diuretics early in the morning so that diuresis does not disturb nighttime rest.
- Monitor fluid status closely: auscultate lungs, compare daily body weights, monitor intake and output.
- Teach patient to adhere to a low-sodium diet by reading food labels and avoiding commercially prepared convenience foods.
- Assist patient to adhere to any fluid restriction by planning the fluid distribution throughout the day while maintaining dietary preferences.
- Monitor intravenous fluids closely; contact physician or pharmacist about the possibility of double-concentrating any medications.
- Position patient, or teach patient how to assume a position, to shift fluid away from the heart (increase number of pillows, elevate head of bed, place bed legs on 20- to 30-cm [8- to 10-inch] blocks), or patient may prefer to sit in a comfortable armchair to sleep.
- Assess for skin breakdown, and institute preventive measures (frequent changes of position, positioning to avoid pressure, elastic pressure stockings, and leg exercises).

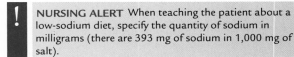

NURSING ALERT When teaching the patient about a low-sodium diet, specify the quantity of sodium in milligrams (there are 393 mg of sodium in 1,000 mg of salt).

Controlling Anxiety

- Decrease anxiety so that patient's cardiac work is also decreased.
- Administer oxygen during the acute stage to diminish the work of breathing and to increase comfort.
- When patient exhibits anxiety, promote physical comfort and psychological support; a family member's presence provides reassurance.
- Speak in a slow, calm, and confident manner; state specific, brief directions for an activity when necessary.
- When patient is comfortable, teach ways to control anxiety and avoid anxiety-provoking situations (relaxation techniques).
- Assist in identifying factors that contribute to anxiety (lack of sleep, lack of information, misinformation, or poor nutritional status).
- Provide accurate information.
- Screen for depression, which often accompanies or results from anxiety.

> **!** **NURSING ALERT** Cerebral hypoxia with superimposed carbon dioxide retention, if present in cardiac failure, may cause patient to react to sedative-hypnotic medications with confusion and increased anxiety. Administer sedative-hypnotic medications with caution because hepatic congestion may result in a decreased ability of the liver to metabolize the medication within a normal time frame to prevent toxicity. Avoid use of restraints in cases of confusion and anxiety reactions. The patient who insists on getting out of bed at night can be seated comfortably in an armchair.

Minimizing Powerlessness

- Assess for factors contributing to a perception of powerlessness, and intervene accordingly.
- Listen actively to patient often; encourage patient to express concerns and questions.

- If indicated, review hospital policies and standards that tend to promote powerlessness, and advocate for their elimination or change.
- Provide patient with decision-making opportunities with increasing frequency and significance; provide encouragement and praise while identifying patient's progress; assist patient to differentiate between factors that can be controlled and those that cannot.

Monitoring and Managing Potential Complications

- Monitor for hypokalemia caused by diuresis (potassium depletion). Signs are weak pulse, faint heart sounds, hypotension, muscle flabbiness, diminished deep tendon reflexes, and generalized weakness.
- To reduce the risk for hypokalemia, advise patient to increase dietary intake of potassium. Dried apricots, bananas, beets, figs, grapefruit (fresh and juice), orange or tomato juice, peaches, and prunes (dried plums), potatoes, raisins, spinach, squash, and watermelon are good sources of potassium.
- Assess electrolyte levels periodically to alert health team members to hypokalemia, hypomagnesemia, and hyponatremia.

Promoting Home and Community-Based Care

Teaching Patients Self-Care

- Provide patient education, and involve patient in implementing the therapeutic regimen to promote understanding and compliance.
- Support patient and family, and encourage them to ask questions so that information can be clarified and understanding enhanced.
- Adapt teaching plan according to cultural factors.
- Teach patients and family how the progression of the disease is influenced by compliance with the treatment plan.
- Convey that monitoring symptoms and daily weights, restricting sodium intake, avoiding excess fluids, preventing infection, avoiding noxious agents such as alcohol and

tobacco, and participating in regular exercise all aid in preventing the exacerbation of cardiac failure.

Continuing Care

- Reinforce and clarify information about diet and fluid restrictions, monitor symptoms and daily body weight, and reinforce follow-up health care expectations.
- Provide assistance in scheduling and keeping appointments.
- Encourage patient to increase self-care and responsibility for accomplishing the daily requirements of the therapeutic regimen.
- Refer patient for home care if indicated (elderly patients or patients who have long-standing heart disease and whose physical stamina is compromised). The home care nurse assesses the physical environment of the home and the patient's support system and suggests adaptations in the home to meet patient's activity limitations.

Evaluation

Expected Patient Outcomes

- Demonstrates tolerance for increased activity
- Experiences less fatigue and dyspnea
- Maintains fluid balance
- Experiences less anxiety
- Adheres to self-care regimen
- Makes decisions regarding care and treatment
- Avoids complications

For more information, see Chapter 30 in Smeltzer and Bare: *Brunner and Suddarth's Textbook of Medical-Surgical Nursing*, 11th edition. Philadelphia: Lippincott Williams & Wilkins, 2008.

Hemophilia

Hemophilia is a relatively rare disease. There are two hereditary bleeding disorders that are clinically indistinguishable but can be separated by laboratory tests: hemophilia A and hemophilia B. Hemophilia A is due to a defect of or deficiency of factor VIII clotting activity. Hemophilia B stems from a defect of or deficiency of factor IX. Factor VIII deficiency is about three times more common. Both types are inherited as X-linked traits. All ethnic groups are affected. Almost all affected people are male; their mothers and some sisters are carriers but do not have symptoms. The disease is usually recognized in early childhood, usually in toddlers. Mild hemophilia may not be diagnosed until trauma or surgery.

Clinical Manifestations

The frequency and severity of bleeding depend on the degree of factor deficiency and the intensity of trauma.

- Hemorrhage occurs into various body parts (large, spreading bruises and bleeding into muscles, joints, and soft tissues) after even minimal trauma.
- Pain in joints may occur before swelling and limitation of motion are apparent; pain occurs most often in knees, elbows, ankles, shoulders, wrists, and hips.
- Chronic pain or ankylosis (fixation) of the joint may occur with recurrent hemorrhage; many patients are crippled by joint damage before adulthood.
- Spontaneous hematuria and gastrointestinal bleeding can occur. Hematomas within the muscle can cause peripheral nerve compression with decreased sensation, weakness, and atrophy of the area.
- Some patients have a milder deficiency and bleed only after dental extractions or surgery; such hemorrhages can prove fatal if the cause is not recognized quickly. The most dangerous hemorrhage is within the head.

Assessment and Diagnostic Methods

Laboratory tests include clotting factor measurement and complete blood count.

Medical Management

- Factor VIII and IX concentrates are given when active
  bleeding occurs or as a prophylactic measure before dental
  extractions, lumbar puncture, or surgery.
- Aminocaproic acid (Amicar) may slow the dissolution of
  blood clots; DDAVP (desmopressin) induces transient
  increase in factor VIII.
- Aspirin and intramuscular injections are avoided.
- Good dental hygiene is a preventive measure.
- Use splints or other orthopedic devices in patients who
  have suffered joint or muscle hemorrhage.

NURSING PROCESS: The Patient with Hemophilia

Assessment

- Assess for evidence of internal bleeding, muscle
  hematomas, and hemorrhage into joint spaces.
- Monitor vital signs and hemodynamic pressure readings for
  hypovolemia.
- Assess all joints for swelling, mobility limitation, and pain.
  Perform range-of-motion exercises slowly to avoid more
  damage.
- Assess surgical sites frequently and carefully for bleeding.
- Determine how patient and family are coping with the
  condition and any limitations imposed on lifestyle and daily
  activities.

Diagnosis

Nursing Diagnoses

- Pain related to joint hemorrhage and subsequent ankylosis
- Ineffective health maintenance related to ongoing need for
  preventive health practices and coping with chronic illness
- Ineffective coping related to the chronicity of the condition
  and its effect on lifestyle

Collaborative Problems/Potential Complications

Bleeding

Planning and Goals

Patient goals may include relief or minimization of pain, compliance with measures to prevent bleeding, coping with chronicity and altered lifestyle, and absence of complications.

Nursing Interventions

Relieving or Minimizing Pain

- Give analgesics to alleviate pain.
- Encourage patient to move slowly and prevent stress on involved joints.
- Encourage warm baths to promote relaxation, improved mobility, and lessened pain.
- Avoid heat during bleeding episodes because it potentiates further bleeding.
- Use splints, canes, or crutches to shift body weight off painful joints.

Monitoring and Managing Complications

- Assess frequently for signs and symptoms of hypoxia to vital organs: restlessness, anxiety, confusion, pallor, cool and clammy skin, chest pain, and decreased urinary output.
- Assess for hypotension and tachycardia as a result of volume depletion.
- Monitor hemodynamic parameters; perform blood studies.
- Observe for bleeding from the skin, mucous membranes, and wounds and for internal bleeding.
- Apply cold compresses to bleeding sites when indicated.
- Administer parenteral medications with small-gauge needles to decrease trauma and bleeding.
- Administer blood, blood components, and medications as prescribed.
- Use safety precautions to prevent patient injury.

Promoting Home and Community-Based Care

Prevention

- Inform patient and family of risk of bleeding and necessary safety precautions.
- Teach family how to administer factor VIII or IX concentrate at home at the first sign of bleeding.
- Encourage patient and family to adapt the home environment to prevent physical trauma.
- Encourage electric razor for shaving and soft toothbrush for oral hygiene.
- Teach patient to avoid forceful nose blowing, coughing, and straining at stool; use stool softener as necessary.
- Teach patient to avoid aspirin and aspirin-containing drugs.
- Encourage noncontact sports such as swimming, hiking, and golf; discourage participation in contact sports.
- Encourage regular checkups and laboratory studies.

Coping with Chronicity and Lifestyle Changes

- Encourage patient to carry or wear medical identification.
- Assist patient and family in coping with the condition because it is chronic and places restrictions on lifestyle. It is an inherited disorder that can be passed to future generations.
- Encourage patient to be self-sufficient and to maintain independence.
- Encourage patient to work through feelings about condition to accept more responsibility for maintaining optimal health.
- If patient has the human immunodeficiency virus (HIV), support patient's and family's efforts to deal with anger. (The percentage of patients with hemophilia who are HIV positive is increasing.) Assist in finding support sources for those who are HIV positive.

Evaluation

Expected Outcomes

- Reports absence of or decrease in pain
- Complies with measures to prevent bleeding

- Demonstrates effective coping with chronicity and altered lifestyle
- Demonstrates no complications

For more information, see Chapter 33 in Smeltzer and Bare: *Brunner and Suddarth's Textbook of Medical-Surgical Nursing*, 11th edition. Philadelphia: Lippincott Williams & Wilkins, 2008.

H Hepatic Encephalopathy and Hepatic Coma

Hepatic encephalopathy, a complication of liver disease, occurs with profound liver failure and may result from the accumulation of ammonia and other toxic metabolites in the blood. Hepatic coma represents the most advanced stage of hepatic encephalopathy. Ammonia accumulates because the damaged liver cells fail to detoxify and convert the ammonia to urea. The increased ammonia concentration in the blood causes brain dysfunction and damage, resulting in hepatic encephalopathy and coma. Circumstances that increase serum ammonia levels precipitate or aggravate hepatic encephalopathy, such as digestion of dietary and blood proteins and ingestion of ammonium salts. Other factors that may cause hepatic encephalopathy include excessive diuresis, dehydration, infections, fever, surgery, and some medications. Portal system encephalopathy is the most common type of hepatic encephalopathy.

Clinical Manifestations

- Earliest symptoms of hepatic encephalopathy include minor mental changes and motor disturbances. Slight confusion and alterations in mood occur; the patient becomes unkempt, experiences disturbed sleep patterns, and tends to sleep during the day and to experience restlessness and insomnia at night.

- As coma progresses, patient may be difficult to awaken, and asterixis (flapping tremor of the hands) may occur. Simple tasks, such as handwriting, become difficult.
- In early stages, patient's reflexes are hyperactive; with worsening encephalopathy, reflexes disappear and extremities become flaccid.
- Occasionally fetor hepaticus, a characteristic breath odor like freshly mowed grass, acetone, or old wine, may be noticed.
- Gross disturbances of consciousness and complete disorientation occur as the disease progresses.
- With further progression, frank coma and seizures occur.

Assessment and Diagnostic Findings

- Electroencephalogram (EEG) shows slowing and increase in amplitude of brain waves.
- Serum ammonia measurements are evaluated.
- Assess symptoms in a susceptible patient: daily handwriting or drawing sample; constructional apraxia reveals progression.

Medical Management

- Administer lactulose (Cephulac) to reduce serum ammonia level. Observe for watery diarrheal stools, which indicate lactulose overdose.
- Reduce protein intake or eliminate if signs of impending encephalopathy or coma occur.
- Give enema as prescribed to reduce ammonia absorption from the gastrointestinal tract.
- Administer nonabsorbable antibiotics (neomycin) as an intestinal antiseptic.
- Monitor serum ammonia level daily; monitor electrolyte status, and correct if abnormal.
- Discontinue medications that may precipitate encephalopathy (eg, sedative medications, tranquilizers, analgesic agents).
- Administer benzodiazepine antagonists (flumazenil).

- Other treatments may include administration of intravenous glucose, vitamins, and oxygen.

Nursing Management

- Maintain a safe environment to prevent bleeding, injury, and infection.
- Assess neurologic status frequently. Keep daily record of handwriting and performance in arithmetic to monitor mental status.
- Monitor fluid intake and output and body weight daily; monitor vital signs at least every 4 hours.
- Monitor for peritoneal, pulmonary, or other infection, and report promptly.
- Instruct family to observe patient for subtle signs of recurrent encephalopathy. Explain that rehabilitation after recovery is likely to be prolonged.
- Instruct in maintenance of low-protein, high-calorie diet. Protein may then be added (10-g increments every 3 to 5 days). Reduce if relapse noted.
- Teach how to administer lactulose and monitor for side effects.
- Refer for home care nurse visits to assess patient's physical and mental status and compliance with prescribed therapeutic regimen.
- Emphasize importance of periodic follow-up.

For more information, see Chapter 39 in Smeltzer and Bare: *Brunner and Suddarth's Textbook of Medical-Surgical Nursing*, 11th edition. Philadelphia: Lippincott Williams & Wilkins, 2008.

Hepatic Failure, Fulminant

Fulminant hepatic failure is the clinical syndrome of sudden and severely impaired liver function in a previously healthy person. It is characterized by the development of first symptoms or jaundice within 8 weeks of the onset of disease. Three categories that have been cited are hyperacute, acute, and subacute. There is rapid clinical deterioration caused by massive hepatocellular injury and necrosis. Mortality is 50% to 85%. Viral hepatitis is the most common cause; other causes include toxic drugs, chemicals, metabolic disturbances, and structural changes.

Clinical Manifestations

- Jaundice and profound anorexia
- Often accompanied by coagulation defects, renal failure, electrolyte disturbances, infection, hypoglycemia, encephalopathy, and cerebral edema

Management

- Liver transplantation (treatment of choice)
- Blood or plasma exchanges, charcoal hemoperfusion, and corticosteroids (plasmapheresis)
- Liver support systems, such as hepatocytes within synthetic fiber columns, extracorporeal liver-assist devices, and bioartificial liver, until transplantation is possible

For more information, see Chapter 39 in Smeltzer and Bare: *Brunner and Suddarth's Textbook of Medical-Surgical Nursing*, 11th edition. Philadelphia: Lippincott Williams & Wilkins, 2008.

Hepatitis, Viral: Types A, B, C, D, E, and G

Hepatitis A

Hepatitis A is caused by an RNA virus of the Enterovirus family. Mode of transmission of this disease is the fecal-oral route, primarily through ingestion of foods or fluids infected by the virus. The virus is found in the stool of infected patients before the onset of symptoms and during the first few days of illness. The incubation period is estimated to be 2 to 7 weeks, with an average of 30 days. The course of illness may last 4 to 8 weeks. The virus is present only briefly in the serum; by the time jaundice appears, the patient is likely to be noninfectious. A person who is immune to hepatitis A may contract other forms of hepatitis. Recovery from hepatitis A is usual; it rarely progresses to acute liver necrosis and fulminant hepatitis. No carrier state exists, and no chronic hepatitis is associated with hepatitis A.

Clinical Manifestations

- Many patients are anicteric (without jaundice) and symptomless.
- When symptoms appear, they are of a mild, flulike, upper respiratory infection, with low-grade fever.
- Anorexia is an early symptom and is often severe.
- Later, jaundice and dark urine may be apparent.
- Indigestion is present in varying degrees.
- Liver and spleen may be moderately enlarged for a few days after onset.
- Adults are more likely to have symptoms than are children.
- Patient may have an aversion to cigarette smoke and strong odors; symptoms tend to clear when jaundice reaches its peak.

Assessment and Diagnostic Methods

- Stool analysis for hepatitis A antigen
- Serum hepatitis A virus antibodies; immunoglobulin

Prevention

- Scrupulous hand washing, safe water supply, proper control of sewage disposal

- Hepatitis vaccine is recommended for high-risk groups (be cautious of hypersensitivity).
- Administration of immune globulin to prevent hepatitis A if given within 2 weeks of exposure
- Hepatitis vaccine and immunoglobulin are recommended for those who travel to developing countries and settings with unsatisfactory hygiene or sanitation conditions.
- Immunoglobulin is recommended for household members and sexual contacts of people with hepatitis A.

Management

H

- Bed rest during the acute stage; encourage a nutritious diet.
- Give small, frequent feedings supplemented by intravenous glucose if necessary during period of anorexia.
- Promote gradual but progressive ambulation to hasten recovery. Patient is usually managed at home unless symptoms are severe.
- Assist patient and family to cope with the temporary disability and fatigue that are common problems in hepatitis.
- Teach patient and family the indications to seek additional health care if the symptoms persist or worsen.
- Instruct patient and family regarding diet, rest, follow-up blood work, avoidance of alcohol, and sanitation and hygiene measures (hand washing) to prevent spread of disease to other family members.
- Teach patient and family about reducing risk for contracting hepatitis A: good personal hygiene with careful hand washing; environmental sanitation with safe food and water supply and sewage disposal.

Hepatitis B

Hepatitis B virus (HBV) is a DNA virus transmitted primarily through blood. The virus has been found in saliva, semen, and vaginal secretions and can be transmitted through mucous membranes and breaks in the skin. Hepatitis B has a long incubation period. It replicates in the liver and remains in the serum for long periods, allowing transmission of the virus. Those at risk include all health care workers, patients in hemodialysis and oncology units, sexually active homosexual and bisexual men, and intravenous drug users. The incubation period is between 1 and 6 months. About 10% of patients progress to a carrier state or develop chronic hepatitis. Hepatitis B is the chief cause of cirrhosis and hepatocellular carcinoma worldwide.

Clinical Manifestations

- Symptoms may be insidious and variable; subclinical episodes frequently occur, fever and respiratory symptoms are rare; some patients have arthralgias and rashes.
- Loss of appetite, dyspepsia, abdominal pain, general aching, malaise, and weakness may occur.
- Jaundice may or may not be evident. With jaundice, there are light-colored stools and dark urine.
- Liver may be tender and enlarged; spleen is enlarged and palpable in a few patients. Posterior cervical lymph nodes may also be enlarged.

Assessment and Diagnostic Findings

Hepatitis B surface antigen appears in blood of up to 90% of patients. Additional antigens help to confirm diagnosis.

Gerontologic Considerations

Elderly patients who contract hepatitis B have a serious risk for severe liver cell necrosis or fulminant hepatic failure. The patient is seriously ill and the prognosis is poor.

Prevention

- Screening of blood donors
- Good personal hygiene

- Education
- Hepatitis B vaccine

Medical Management

- Alfa-interferon has shown promising results.
- Bed rest and restriction of activities until hepatic enlargement and elevation of serum bilirubin and liver enzymes have disappeared
- Maintain adequate nutrition; restrict proteins when the ability of the liver to metabolize protein byproducts is impaired.
- Administer antacids and antiemetics for dyspepsia and general malaise; avoid all medications if patient is vomiting.
- Convalescence may be prolonged and recovery may take 3 to 4 months; provide hospitalization and fluid therapy if vomiting persists.

Nursing Management

- Encourage gradual activity after complete clearing of jaundice.
- Consider psychological implications of the long disease course and isolation and separation from family and friends.
- Include family in planning patient's care and activities.
- Institute measures to control and prevent hepatitis B. Interrupt the chain of transmission; protect people at high risk with active immunization through use of hepatitis B vaccine; use passive immunization for unprotected people exposed to hepatitis B.
- Educate patient and family in home care and convalescence.
- Instruct patient and family to provide adequate rest and nutrition.
- Inform family and intimate friends about risks of contracting hepatitis B.
- Arrange for family and intimate friends to receive hepatitis B vaccine or hepatitis B immune globulin. Hepatitis B vaccine

is given in three doses, the second and third doses 1 and
6 months after the first dose.

- Caution patient to avoid drinking alcohol and eating raw
  shellfish.
- Inform family that follow-up home visits by home care
  nurse are indicated to assess progress and understanding,
  reinforce teaching, and answer questions.
- Teach those at risk the early signs of hepatitis B and ways to
  reduce risk by avoiding all modes of transmission.
- Encourage patient to use strategies to prevent exchange of
  body fluids, such as avoiding sexual intercourse or using
  condoms.

Hepatitis C

A significant portion of cases of viral hepatitis are neither A, B,
nor D; they are classified as hepatitis C. It is the primary form
of hepatitis associated with parenteral means (sharing contaminated needles, needlesticks or injuries to health care workers,
blood transfusions) or sexual contact. The incubation period is
variable and may range from 15 to 160 days. The clinical course
of hepatitis C is similar to that of hepatitis B; symptoms are
usually mild. A chronic carrier state occurs frequently. There is
an increased risk for cirrhosis and liver cancer after hepatitis C.
A combination of ribavirin (Rebetol) and interferon (Intron-A)
therapy is effective for treating patients with hepatitis C and in
treating relapses.

Hepatitis D

Hepatitis D (delta agent) occurs in some cases of hepatitis B.
Only patients with hepatitis B are at risk. The virus requires
hepatitis B surface antigen for its replication. It is common in
intravenous drug users, hemodialysis patients, and recipients
of multiple blood transfusions. Sexual contact is an important
mode of transmission of hepatitis B and D. Incubation varies
between 21 and 140 days. The symptoms are similar to those of
hepatitis B except that patients are more likely to have fulminant

hepatitis and progress to chronic active hepatitis and cirrhosis. Treatment is similar to that for other forms of hepatitis.

Hepatitis E

The hepatitis E virus is transmitted by the fecal-oral route, principally through contaminated water and poor sanitation. Incubation is variable and is estimated to range between 15 and 65 days. Onset and symptoms are similar to those of other types of viral hepatitis (resembles hepatitis A). Hepatitis E has a self-limiting course with abrupt onset. Jaundice is nearly always present; chronic forms do not develop. The major method of prevention is avoiding contact with the virus through hygiene (hand washing). The effectiveness of immune globulin in protecting against hepatitis E virus is uncertain.

Hepatitis G

Hepatitis G (the latest form) is a post-transfusion hepatitis with an incubation period of 14 to 145 days. Autoantibodies are absent. The risk factors are similar to those for hepatitis C.

For more information, see Chapter 39 in Smeltzer and Bare: *Brunner and Suddarth's Textbook of Medical-Surgical Nursing*, 11th edition. Philadelphia: Lippincott Williams & Wilkins, 2008.

Hiatal Hernia

In a hiatal (hiatus) hernia, the opening in the diaphragm through which the esophagus passes becomes enlarged, and part of the upper stomach tends to move up into the lower portion of the thorax. There are two types of hernias: sliding and para-esophageal. With a type I, or sliding, hiatal hernia, the upper stomach and the gastroesophageal junction are displaced upward and slide in and out of the thorax; this occurs in about 90% of patients with esophageal hiatal hernias. The less frequent paraesophageal hernias are classified by extent of herniation (type II, III, or IV) and occur when all or part of the stomach pushes through the diaphragm next to the gastroesophageal junction (GED). Hiatal hernia occurs more often in women than men.

Clinical Manifestations

Axial (Sliding) Hernia

- Heartburn, regurgitation, and dysphagia; at least half of cases are asymptomatic
- Often implicated in reflux

Paraesophageal Hernia

- Sense of fullness after eating or may be asymptomatic
- Reflux does not usually occur.
- Complications of hemorrhage, obstruction, and strangulation possible

Assessment and Diagnostic Methods

Diagnosis is confirmed by radiographic studies, barium swallow, and fluoroscopy.

Medical Management

- Frequent, small feedings that easily pass through the esophagus are given.
- Advise patient not to recline for 1 hour after eating (prevents reflux or hernia movement).
- Elevate head of bed on 4- to 8-inch blocks to prevent hernia from sliding upward.
- Surgery is indicated in about 15% of patients; paraesophageal hernias may require emergency surgery.
- Medical and surgical management of paraesophageal hernias is similar to that for gastroesophageal reflux: antacids, histamine blockers, gastric acid pump inhibitors,

or prokinetic agents (metoclopramide [Reglan], cisapride [Propulsid]).

NURSING PROCESS: The Patient with an Esophageal Condition and Reflux

Assessment

- Take a complete health history, including pain assessment and nutrition assessment.
- Determine if patient appears emaciated.
- Auscultate chest to determine presence of pulmonary complications.

Diagnosis

Nursing Diagnoses

- Imbalanced nutrition: Less than body requirements related to difficulty swallowing
- Risk for aspiration due to difficulty swallowing or tube feeding
- Acute pain related to difficulty swallowing, ingestion of abrasive agent, a tumor, or reflux
- Deficient knowledge about the esophageal disorder, diagnostic studies, treatments, and rehabilitation

Planning and Goals

Major goals may include adequate nutritional intake, avoidance of respiratory compromise from aspiration, relief of pain, and increased knowledge level.

Nursing Interventions

Encouraging Adequate Nutritional Intake

- Instruct patient to eat a low-fat, high-fiber diet.
- Encourage patient to eat slowly and chew all food thoroughly.

- Small, frequent feedings of nonirritating foods are recommended; sometimes drinking liquids with food helps passage.
- Prepare food in an appealing manner to help stimulate appetite; avoid irritants (tobacco, alcohol).
- Obtain a baseline weight, and record daily weights; assess nutrient intake.

Decreasing Risk of Aspiration

- If patient has difficulty swallowing or handling secretions, keep him or her in at least a semi-Fowler's position.
- Instruct patient in the use of oral suction to decrease risk of aspiration.

Relieving Pain

- Teach patient to eat small meals frequently (6 to 8 daily).
- Instruct patient to avoid caffeine, tobacco, carbonated beverages, very hot or very cold beverages, and spicy foods.
- Advise patient not to recline for 1 to 4 hours after eating to prevent reflux or movement of the hernia.
- Advise patient to avoid any activities that put strain on the thoracic region and increase pain.
- Elevate head of bed on 4- to 8-inch blocks; avoid tight clothes.
- Advise patient not to use over-the-counter antacids because of possible rebound acidity.
- Instruct in use of prescribed antacids or histamine antagonists.

Promoting Home and Community-Based Care

Teaching Patients Self-Care

- Reassure patient and discuss all procedures and their purposes.
- Give sufficient information for participation in care and diagnostic effort.
- Prepare patient for surgery if required.
- Help patient plan for needed physical and psychological adjustments and follow-up care if condition is chronic.

- Help in planning meals, using medications as prescribed, and resuming activity.
- Teach patient and family to use special equipment (enteral or parenteral feeding devices, suction).
- Educate about nutritional requirements and how to measure the adequacy of nutrition (particularly in elderly and debilitated patients). See Nursing Management under the Preoperative and Postoperative Patient for additional information.

Continuing Care

- Arrange for home health care nursing support and assessment when indicated.
- Teach patient to prepare blenderized or soft food if indicated.
- Assist patient to adjust medication schedule to daily activities when possible.
- Arrange for nutritionist, social worker, or hospice care when indicated.

For more information, see Chapter 35 in Smeltzer and Bare: *Brunner and Suddarth's Textbook of Medical-Surgical Nursing*, 11th edition. Philadelphia: Lippincott Williams & Wilkins, 2008.

Hodgkin's Disease

Hodgkin's disease is a rare cancer of unknown cause that is unicentric in origin and spreads along the lymphatic system. There is a familial pattern associated with Hodgkin's as well as an association with the Epstein-Barr virus (found in 40% to 50% of patients). It is more common in men and tends to peak in the early 20s and after 50 years of age. The Reed-Sternberg cell, a gigantic morphologically unique tumor cell that is thought to be of immature lymphoid origin, is the pathologic hallmark and essential diagnostic criterion for Hodgkin's disease. Most patients with Hodgkin's disease have the types currently designated "nodular sclerosis" or "mixed cellularity." The nodular sclerosis type tends to occur more often in young women and at an earlier stage but has a worse prognosis than the mixed cellularity subgroup, which occurs more commonly in men and causes more constitutional symptoms but has a better prognosis.

Clinical Manifestations

- Painless enlargement of the lymph nodes on one side of the neck. Individual nodes are firm and painless; common sites are the cervical, supraclavicular, and mediastinal nodes.
- Mediastinal lymph nodes may be visible on x-ray films and large enough to cause severe pressure symptoms (eg, dyspnea from pressure against the trachea; dysphagia from pressure against the esophagus).
- Symptoms may result from the tumor compressing other organs, causing cough and pulmonary effusion (from pulmonary infiltrates); jaundice (from hepatic involvement or bile duct obstruction); abdominal pain (from splenomegaly or retroperitoneal adenopathy); or bone pain (due to skeletal involvement).
- Pruritus is common and can be distressing; unclear etiology. Herpes zoster infection is common.
- Some patients (20%) experience brief but severe pain after drinking alcohol, usually at the site of the tumor.
- Mild anemia develops; the white blood cell count may be elevated or decreased; and anergy (an absence of or decreased response to skin sensitivity tests such as candidal infection, mumps) may be noted.
- Constitutional symptoms, for prognostic purposes referred to as B symptoms, include fever (without chills), drenching sweats (particularly at night), and unintentional loss of more than 10% of body weight (found in 40% of patients and more common in advanced disease).

Assessment and Diagnostic Methods

Diagnosis depends on identification of characteristic histologic features in an excised lymph node. After the diagnosis is confirmed, the total extent of tumor involvement is assessed, and its distribution is defined.

- Laboratory studies: complete blood count; platelet count, sedimentation rate, liver and renal function studies. RBC sedimentation rate and serum copper levels are used by some clinicians to assess disease activity.
- Excisional lymph node biopsy, bone marrow biopsy, characteristic presence of Reed-Sternberg cell; staging of node
- Chest x-ray and computed tomography (CT) of chest, abdomen, and pelvis; positron emission tomography (PET) to detect residual disease

H

Medical Management

Treatment is determined by the stage of the disease instead of the histologic type.

- Chemotherapy followed by radiation therapy is used in early-stage disease.
- Combination chemotherapy alone is now the standard treatment for more advanced disease.
- When Hodgkin's does recur, the use of high doses of chemotherapeutic medications, followed by autologous bone marrow or stem-cell transplantation, can be very effective.

Nursing Management

See Nursing Management under Cancer for additional information about nursing interventions for patients undergoing chemotherapy and radiation treatments.

- Help patient to cope with undesirable effects of radiation therapy, including esophagitis, anorexia, loss of taste, dry mouth, nausea and vomiting, diarrhea, skin reactions, and lethargy.
- Serve bland, soft foods at mild temperatures.
- Teach patient about proper dental hygiene.

- Administer antiemetics during peak times of nausea.
- Teach patient that skin reactions and the appearance of sunburned or tanned skin are common; rubbing the area and applying heat, cold, or lotion should be avoided.
- Encourage patient to rest and sleep to maintain a reasonable energy level; lethargy accompanies radiation.
- Help patient to prepare for alopecia by encouraging him or her to purchase a wig before hair loss.
- Encourage patient to report any sign of infection for immediate treatment.
- Instruct patient to use contraception during chemotherapy to prevent cytotoxic effects on the fetus.
- Encourage patient to keep all follow-up appointments.

For more information, see Chapter 33 in Smeltzer and Bare: *Brunner and Suddarth's Textbook of Medical-Surgical Nursing*, 11th edition. Philadelphia: Lippincott Williams & Wilkins, 2008.

Huntington's Disease

Huntington's disease is a chronic, hereditary disease of the nervous system that results in progressive involuntary choreiform (dance-like) movements and dementia. Researchers believe that glutamine abnormally collects in certain brain cell nuclei, causing cell death. Huntington's disease affects men and women of all races. It is transmitted as an autosomal dominant genetic disorder. Each child of a parent with Huntington's has a 50% risk of inheriting the illness. Onset usually occurs between 35 and 45 years of age.

Clinical Manifestations

- The most prominent clinical features are abnormal involuntary movements (chorea), intellectual decline, and emotional disturbance.

- Constant writhing, twisting, and uncontrollable movements of the entire body occur as the disease progresses.
- Facial movements produce tics and grimaces; speech becomes slurred, hesitant, often explosive, and then eventually unintelligible.
- Chewing and swallowing are difficult, and aspiration and choking are dangers.
- Gait becomes disorganized, and ambulation is eventually impossible; patient is eventually confined to a wheelchair.
- Bowel and bladder control is lost.
- Progressive intellectual impairment occurs with eventual dementia.
- Uncontrollable emotional changes occur but become less acute as the disease progresses. Patient may be nervous, irritable, or impatient. During the early stages of illness: uncontrollable fits of anger; profound, often suicidal depression; apathy; or euphoria.
- Hallucinations, delusions, and paranoid thinking may precede appearance of disjointed movements.
- Patient dies in 10 to 15 years from heart failure, pneumonia, or infection or as a result of a fall or choking.

Assessment and Diagnostic Findings

- Diagnosis is made on the basis of clinical presentation, positive family history, and exclusion of other causes.
- Imaging studies, such as computed tomography (CT) and magnetic resonance imaging (MRI), may show atrophy of the striatum.
- A genetic marker for Huntington's disease has been located. It offers no hope of cure or even specific determination of onset.

Medical Management

No treatment stops or reverses the process; palliative care is given.

- Medications such as phenothiazines (haloperidol), butyrophenones, and thioxanthenes, which block dopamine receptors, and reserpine and tetrabenazine. Anti-parkinsonism therapy (L-dopa) may improve chorea and temporarily decrease rigidity in some patients.
- Motor signs are continually assessed and evaluated. Akathisia (motor restlessness) in the overmedicated patient is dangerous and should be reported.
- Psychotherapy aimed at allaying anxiety and reducing stress may be beneficial; antidepressants are given for depression or suicidal ideation.
- Patient's needs and abilities are the focus of treatment.

Nursing Management

- Reinforce understanding that Huntington's disease takes emotional, physical, social, and financial tolls on every member of patient's family.
- Encourage genetic counseling, long-term psychological counseling, marriage counseling, and financial and legal support.
- Teach patient and family about medications, including signs indicating need for change in dosage or medication.
- Address strategies to manage symptoms (chorea, swallowing problems, ambulation problems, or altered bowel or bladder function).
- Arrange for consultation with a speech therapist, if needed.
- Emphasize the need for regular follow-up.
- Refer for home care nursing assistance, respite care, day care centers, and eventually skilled long-term care to assist patient and family to cope.
- Provide information about the Huntington's Disease Foundation of America, which gives information, referrals, education, and support for research.

For more information, see Chapter 65 in Smeltzer and Bare: *Brunner and Suddarth's Textbook of Medical-Surgical Nursing*, 11th edition. Philadelphia: Lippincott Williams & Wilkins, 2008.

Hyperglycemic Hyperosmolar Nonketotic Syndrome (HHNS)

Hyperglycemic hyperosmolar nonketotic syndrome (HHNS) is a serious condition in which hyperglycemia and hyperosmolarity predominate with alterations of the sensorium (sense of awareness). Ketosis is minimal or absent. The basic biochemical defect is lack of effective insulin (insulin resistance).

Pathophysiology

H

Persistent hyperglycemia causes osmotic diuresis, resulting in water and electrolyte losses. Although there is not enough insulin to prevent hyperglycemia, the small amount of insulin present is enough to prevent fat breakdown. This condition occurs most frequently in older people (50 to 70 years of age) who have had no previous history of diabetes or only mild type 2 diabetes. The acute development of the condition can be traced to some precipitating event, such as acute illness (pneumonia, myocardial infarction, stroke), ingestion of medications known to provoke insulin insufficiency (thiazide diuretics, propranolol), or therapeutic procedures (peritoneal dialysis or hemodialysis, hyperalimentation).

Clinical Manifestations

- History of days to weeks of polyuria and polydipsia
- Hypotension, tachycardia
- Profound dehydration (dry mucous membranes, poor skin turgor)
- Variable neurologic signs (alterations of sensorium, seizures, hemiparesis)

Assessment and Diagnostic Methods

- Blood work, including blood glucose, electrolytes, blood urea nitrogen (BUN), complete blood count, serum osmolality, and arterial blood gases
- Clinical picture of severe dehydration

Medical Management

The overall treatment of HHNS is similar to that of diabetic ketoacidosis (DKA): fluids, electrolytes, and insulin.

- Start fluid treatment with 0.9% or 0.45% normal saline, depending on sodium level and severity of volume depletion.
- Central venous or arterial pressure monitoring may be necessary to guide fluid replacement.
- Add potassium to replacement fluids when urinary output is adequate; guided by continuous electrocardiogram (ECG) monitoring and laboratory determinations of potassium.
- Insulin is usually given at a continuous low rate to treat hyperglycemia.
- Dextrose is added to replacement fluids when the glucose level decreases to 250 to 300 mg/dL.
- Other treatment modalities are determined by the underlying illness and results of continuing clinical and laboratory evaluation.
- Treatment is continued until metabolic abnormalities are corrected and neurologic symptoms clear (may take 3 to 5 days for neurologic symptoms to resolve).

Nursing Management

See Nursing Management under Diabetes Mellitus and Diabetic Ketoacidosis for additional information.

- Monitor fluid volume and electrolyte status for prevention of heart failure and cardiac dysrhythmias (because of increased age of typical patient).
- Reinforce that after recovery from HHNS, many patients can control diabetes with diet alone or with diet and oral hypoglycemic agents. Insulin may not be needed after the acute hyperglycemic complication is resolved.

For more information, see Chapter 41 in Smeltzer and Bare: *Brunner and Suddarth's Textbook of Medical-Surgical Nursing*, 11th edition. Philadelphia: Lippincott Williams & Wilkins, 2008.

Hypertension (and Hypertensive Crisis)

Hypertension is defined as a systolic blood pressure above 140 mm Hg or a diastolic pressure above 90 mm Hg, based on two or more measurements. Hypertension can be classified as follows:

- Normal: systolic <120 mmHg; diastolic <80 mmHg
- Prehypertension: systolic 120 to 139 mmHg; diastolic 80 to 89 mmHg
- Stage 1: systolic 140 to 159 mmHg; diastolic 90 to 99 mmHg
- Stage 2: systolic ≥160 mmHg; diastolic ≥100 mmHg

Hypertension is a major risk factor for atherosclerotic cardiovascular disease, heart failure, stroke, and kidney failure. Hypertension carries the risk for premature morbidity or mortality, which increases as systolic and diastolic pressures rise. Prolonged blood pressure elevation damages blood vessels in target organs (heart, kidneys, brain, and eyes).

Essential (Primary) Hypertension

In the adult population with hypertension, between 90% and 95% have essential (primary) hypertension, which has no identifiable medical cause; it appears to be a multifactorial, polygenic condition. For high blood pressure to occur, an increase in peripheral resistance and/or cardiac output must occur secondary to increased sympathetic stimulation, increased renal sodium reabsorption, increased renin-angiotensin-aldosterone system activity, decreased vasodilation of the arterioles, or resistance to insulin action.

On occasion, hypertension appears abruptly and severely and takes a "malignant" course that causes rapid deterioration, signaling an emergency state known as hypertensive crisis or hypertensive urgency (see Box H-1).

> ### BOX H–1   Emergency! Hypertensive Crisis
>
> Hypertensive crisis, or hypertensive emergency, exists when an elevated blood pressure level must be lowered immediately (not necessarily to less than 140/90 mm Hg) to halt or prevent target organ damage. Hypertensive urgency exists when blood pressure must be lowered within a few hours. Hypertensive crisis requires prompt treatment in an intensive care setting because of the risk for serious organ damage. The medication regimen (eg, nitroprusside, nicardipine hydrochloride) requires extremely close hemodynamic monitoring. Vital signs should be checked as often as every 5 minutes.

H

Emotional disturbances, obesity, excessive alcohol intake, and overstimulation with coffee, tobacco, and stimulatory drugs play a role. Hypertension is strongly familial. Hypertension affects more women than men, but African-American men are less able to tolerate the disease.

Secondary Hypertension

Secondary hypertension is characterized by elevations in blood pressure with a specific cause, such as arterial disease, renal disease, certain medications, tumors, and pregnancy. Hypertension can also be acute, a sign of an underlying condition that causes a change in peripheral resistance or cardiac output.

Clinical Manifestations

- Physical examination may reveal no abnormality other than high blood pressure.
- Changes in the retinas with hemorrhages (cotton-wool spots from small infarcts), exudates, narrowed arterioles, and papilledema may be seen in severe hypertension.
- Symptoms usually indicate vascular damage related to organ systems served by involved vessels.

- Coronary artery disease with angina or myocardial infarction is the most common sequela.
- Left ventricular hypertrophy may occur; left heart failure ensues.
- Pathologic changes may occur in the kidney (nocturia and increased blood urea nitrogen [BUN] and creatinine levels).
- Cerebrovascular involvement may occur (stroke or transient ischemic attack [ie, temporary hemiplegia, sudden falls, dizziness, weakness, or alterations in vision or speech]).

Assessment and Diagnostic Methods

H

- History and physical examination, including retinal examination; laboratory studies for organ damage, including urinalysis, blood chemistry (sodium, potassium, creatinine, fasting glucose, total and high-density lipoprotein); electrocardiogram (ECG); and echocardiography to assess left ventricular hypertrophy
- Special studies: intravenous pyelography, renal arteriography, split renal function studies, renin levels, 24-hour urine protein, creatinine clearance

Medical Management

The goal of any treatment program is to prevent death and complications by achieving and maintaining an arterial blood pressure below 140/90 mm Hg (130/80 mm Hg for people with diabetes mellitus or proteinuria >1 g/24 hours), whenever possible.

- Nonpharmacologic approaches include weight reduction; restriction of alcohol, sodium, tobacco; regular exercise and relaxation. A DASH (Dietary Approach to Stop Hypertension) diet high in fruit and vegetables and low in dairy products has been shown to lower elevated pressures.
- Select a drug class that has the greatest effectiveness, fewest side effects, and best chance of acceptance by patient. Two classes of drugs are available as first-line therapy: diuretics and beta-blockers.

- Promote compliance by avoiding complicated drug schedules.

NURSING PROCESS: The Patient with Hypertension

Assessment

- Assess blood pressure at frequent intervals; know baseline level. Note changes in pressure that would require a change in medication.
- Note the apical and peripheral pulse rate, rhythm, and character.
- Assess symptoms such as nosebleeds; anginal pain; shortness of breath; alterations in vision, speech, or balance (vertigo); headaches; or nocturia.
- Assess extent to which hypertension has affected patient personally, socially, or financially.

Diagnosis

Nursing Diagnoses

- Deficient knowledge regarding the relationship between the treatment regimen and control of the disease process
- Noncompliance related to side effects of prescribed therapy

Collaborative Problems/Potential Complications

- Retinal hemorrhage
- Heart failure
- Renal insufficiency and failure
- Cerebrovascular accident (CVA)
- Transient ischemic attack (TIA)
- Myocardial infarction
- Left ventricular hypertrophy

Planning and Goals

The major goals of the patient include understanding the disease process and its treatment, compliance with the self-care program, and absence of complications.

Nursing Interventions

Increasing Knowledge

- Emphasize the concept of controlling hypertension (with lifestyle changes and medications) rather than curing it.
- Arrange a consultation with a dietitian to help patient plan weight loss.
- Obtain patient education materials from the American Heart Association.
- Advise patient to limit alcohol intake and avoid use of tobacco.

H

Monitoring and Managing Potential Complications

- Assess all body systems when patient returns for follow-up care.
- Question patient about blurred vision, spots, or diminished visual acuity.
- Report any significant findings promptly to determine whether additional studies or changes in medications are required.

✿ Gerontologic Considerations

Isolated systolic hypertension is common in older adults as a result of age-related changes. Compliance with the therapeutic program is even more difficult for elderly people because medication therapy must be continuous, may be complicated, and may be expensive for a person on a fixed income.

- Promote monotherapy (treatment with a single agent) if appropriate to simplify the medication regimen and make it less expensive. The dosage of medication is often half that needed in younger patients.
- Make sure that patient understands the medication regimen, can read the instructions, can open the container, and is prepared to adjust to postural hypotensive effects of antihypertensive medications (change position slowly, use supportive devices).
- Include the family in the teaching program so that they understand the patient's needs, support adherence to the

therapeutic program, and know when to seek guidance from health professionals.

- Encourage return to the outpatient setting for follow-up care.
- Assess all body systems to detect evidence of vascular damage to vital organs, such as eyes (blurred vision, spots in front of eyes, diminished visual acuity), heart, nervous system, and kidneys.

Promoting Home and Community-Based Care

Teaching Patients Self-Care

- Support patient and promote adherence to therapy in a cost-effective manner; collaborate with patient to set goals.
- Reinforce the importance of taking medications as prescribed, scheduling regular follow-up appointments, maintaining dietary restrictions of sodium and fat, increasing fruits and vegetables, and controlling weight.
- Support patient in planning lifestyle changes, including an exercise program with regular physical activity.
- Encourage counseling, education, and weight control; cessation of smoking; and stress self-help groups for family and patient.

Promoting Compliance with Self-Care Program

- Encourage active participation of patient in the program, including self-monitoring of blood pressure and diet for increased compliance.
- Encourage patient to abstain from alcohol because alcohol may have a synergistic effect with medication.
- Discourage use of tobacco and nicotine products.
- Give patient written information regarding expected effects and side effects of medications.
- Teach patient and family how to measure blood pressure.

Continuing Care

- Reinforce importance of regular follow-up care.
- Obtain patient history and perform physical examination at each clinic visit.

- Assess for medication-related problems (orthostatic hypotension).

Evaluation

Expected Patient Outcomes

- Maintains adequate tissue perfusion
- Complies with self-care program
- Experiences no complications

H

For more information, see Chapter 32 in Smeltzer and Bare: *Brunner and Suddarth's Textbook of Medical-Surgical Nursing*, 11th edition. Philadelphia: Lippincott Williams & Wilkins, 2008.

Hyperthyroidism (Graves' Disease)

Hyperthyroidism is the second most common endocrine disorder, and Graves' disease is the most common type. It results from an excessive output of thyroid hormones due to abnormal stimulation of the thyroid gland by circulating immunoglobulins. Long-acting thyroid stimulator (LATS) is found in significant concentrations in the serum of many of these patients. The disorder affects women eight times more frequently than men and peaks between the second and fourth decades of life. It may appear after an emotional shock, stress, or infection, but the exact significance of these relationships is not understood. Other common causes include thyroiditis and excessive ingestion of thyroid hormone (eg, from the treatment of hypothyroidism).

Clinical Manifestations

Hyperthyroidism presents a characteristic group of signs and symptoms (thyrotoxicosis).

- Nervousness (emotionally hyperexcitable), irritability, apprehensiveness; inability to sit quietly; palpitations; rapid pulse on rest and exertion
- Poor tolerance of heat; excessive perspiration; skin that is flushed and likely to be warm, soft, and moist
- Dry skin and diffuse pruritus in the elderly
- Fine tremor of the hands
- Exophthalmos (bulging eyes) in some patients
- Increased appetite and dietary intake, progressive loss of weight, abnormal muscle fatigability, weakness, amenorrhea, and changes in bowel function (constipation or diarrhea)
- Pulse ranges between 90 and 160 beats/min with sinus tachycardia or dysrhythmias; systolic (but not diastolic) blood pressure elevation (increased pulse pressure)
- Atrial fibrillation; cardiac decompensation in the form of congestive heart failure, especially in the elderly
- Osteoporosis and fracture
- May include remissions and exacerbations, terminating with spontaneous recovery in a few months or years
- May progress relentlessly, causing emaciation, intense nervousness, delirium, disorientation, and eventually myocardial hypertrophy and heart failure

Assessment and Diagnostic Findings

- Thyroid gland is enlarged; it is soft and may pulsate; a thrill may be felt and a bruit heard over thyroid arteries.
- Laboratory tests show a decrease in serum TSH, an increase in serum thyroxine (T_4) level and an increase in ^{123}I or ^{125}I uptake in excess of 50%.

🌿 Gerontologic Considerations

Elderly patients commonly present with vague and nonspecific signs and symptoms. The major symptoms in the elderly patient may be depression and apathy, accompanied by significant weight loss and constipation in some. The patient may report cardiovascular symptoms and difficulty climbing stairs or rising from a chair because of muscle weakness; congestive failure may be noted. Elderly patients may experience a single manifestation, such as atrial fibrillation, anorexia, or weight loss. These general symptoms may mask underlying thyroid disease. Spontaneous remission of hyperthyroidism is rare in the elderly. Measurement of thyroid-stimulating hormone (TSH) uptake is indicated in elderly patients with unexplained physical or mental deterioration. Use of ^{123}I or ^{131}I is generally recommended for treatment of thyrotoxicosis rather than surgery unless an enlarged thyroid gland is pressing on the airway. Thyrotoxicosis must be controlled by antithyroid drugs before ^{131}I is used because radiation may precipitate thyroid storm, which has a high mortality rate in the elderly. Beta-blockers may be indicated. Use these agents with extreme caution and monitor closely for granulocytopenia. Modify dosages of other medications because of the altered rate of metabolism in hyperthyroidism.

Medical Management

Treatment is directed toward reducing thyroid hyperactivity for symptomatic relief and removing the cause of complications. Three forms of treatment are available:

- Irradiation involving the administration of ^{131}I or ^{123}I for destructive effects on the thyroid gland
- Pharmacotherapy with antithyroid medications
- Surgery with the removal of most of the thyroid gland

Radioactive Iodine (^{131}I)

- ^{131}I is given to destroy the overactive thyroid cells (most common treatment in the elderly).
- ^{131}I is contraindicated in pregnancy and nursing mothers because radioiodine crosses the placenta and is secreted in breast milk.

Pharmacotherapy

- The objective of pharmacotherapy is to inhibit hormone synthesis or release and reduce the amount of thyroid tissue.
- The most commonly used medications are propylthiouracil (Propacil, PTU) and methimazole (Tapazole) until patient is euthyroid.
- Maintenance dose is established, followed by gradual withdrawal of the medication over the next several months.
- Antithyroid drugs are contraindicated in late pregnancy because of a risk for goiter and cretinism in the fetus.
- Thyroid hormone may be administered to put the thyroid to rest.

Adjunctive Therapy

- Potassium iodide, Lugol's solution, and saturated solution of potassium iodide (SSKI) may be added.
- Beta-adrenergic agents may be used to control the sympathetic nervous system effects that occur in hyperthyroidism; for example, propranolol is used for nervousness, tachycardia, tremor, anxiety, and heat intolerance.

Surgical Intervention

- Surgical intervention (reserved for special circumstances) removes about five sixths of the thyroid tissue.
- Before surgery, patient is given propylthiouracil until signs of hyperthyroidism have disappeared.
- Iodine is prescribed to reduce thyroid size and vascularity and blood loss. Patient is monitored carefully for evidence of iodine toxicity (swelling buccal mucosa, excessive salivation, skin eruptions).
- Risk for relapse and complications necessitates long-term follow-up of patient undergoing treatment of hyperthyroidism.
- Surgery to treat hyperthyroidism is performed after thyroid function has returned to normal (4 to 6 weeks).

NURSING PROCESS: The Patient with Hyperthyroidism

Assessment

- Obtain a health history, including family history of hyperthyroidism, and note reports of irritability or increased emotional reaction and the impact of these changes on patient's interaction with family, friends, and coworkers.
- Assess stressors and patient's ability to cope with stress.
- Evaluate nutritional status and presence of symptoms; note excessive nervousness and changes in vision and appearance of eyes.
- Assess and monitor cardiac status periodically (heart rate, blood pressure, heart sounds, and peripheral pulses).
- Assess emotional state and psychological status.

Diagnosis

Nursing Diagnoses

- Imbalanced nutrition: Less than body requirements related to exaggerated metabolic rate, excessive appetite, and increased gastrointestinal activity
- Ineffective coping related to irritability, hyperexcitability, apprehension, and emotional instability
- Low self-esteem related to changes in appearance, excessive appetite, and weight loss
- Imbalanced body temperature

Collaborative Problems/Potential Complications

- Thyrotoxicosis or thyroid storm
- Hypothyroidism

Planning and Goals

Goals of the patient may be improved nutritional status, improved coping ability, improved self-esteem, normal body temperature, and absence of complications.

Nursing Interventions

Improving Nutritional Status

- Provide several small, well-balanced meals (up to six meals a day) to satisfy patient's increased appetite.
- Replace food and fluids lost through diarrhea and diaphoresis, and control diarrhea that results from increased peristalsis.
- Reduce diarrhea by avoiding highly seasoned foods and stimulants such as coffee, tea, cola, and alcohol; encourage high-calorie, high-protein foods.
- Provide quiet atmosphere during mealtime to aid digestion.
- Record weight and dietary intake daily.

Enhancing Coping Measures

- Reassure family and friends that symptoms are expected to disappear with treatment.
- Maintain a calm, unhurried approach, and minimize stressful experiences.
- Keep the environment quiet and uncluttered.
- Provide information regarding thyroidectomy and preparatory pharmacotherapy to alleviate anxiety.
- Assist patient to take medications as prescribed and encourage adherence to the therapeutic regimen.
- Repeat information often, and provide written instructions as indicated due to short attention span.

Improving Self-Esteem

- Convey to patient an understanding of concerns regarding problems with appearance, appetite, and weight, and assist in developing coping strategies.
- Provide eye protection if patient experiences eye changes secondary to hyperthyroidism; instruct regarding correct instillation of eyedrops or ointment to soothe the eyes and protect the exposed cornea.
- Arrange for patient to eat alone, if desired and if embarrassed by the large meals consumed due to increased metabolic rate. Avoid commenting on intake.

Maintaining Normal Body Temperature

- Provide a cool, comfortable environment and fresh bedding and gown as needed.
- Give cool baths and provide cool fluids; monitor body temperature.
- Explain to patient and family the importance of providing a cool environment.

Monitoring and Managing Potential Complications

- Monitor closely for signs and symptoms indicative of thyroid storm.
- Assess cardiac and respiratory function: vital signs, cardiac output, electrocardiogram (ECG) monitoring, arterial blood gases, pulse oximetry.
- Administer oxygen to prevent hypoxia.
- Give intravenous fluids to maintain blood glucose levels and replace lost fluids.
- Administer antithyroid medications to reduce thyroid hormone levels.
- Administer propranolol and digitalis to treat cardiac symptoms.
- Implement strategies to treat shock if needed.
- Monitor for hypothyroidism; encourage continued therapy.
- Antithyroid medications block utilization of iodine (thyroid hormone may be given in addition).

Promoting Home and Community-Based Care
Teaching Patients Self-Care

- Instruct how and when to take prescribed medications.
- Teach patient how the medication regimen fits in with the broader therapeutic plan. Explain the consequences of failing to take medications.
- Provide an individualized written plan of care for use at home.
- Teach patient and family about the desired effects and side effects of medications.
- Instruct patient and family about which adverse effects should be reported to the physician.

- Teach patient about what to expect from a thyroidectomy if this is to be performed.
- Teach patient to avoid situations that have the potential of stimulating thyroid storm.

Continuing Care

- Stress long-term follow-up care because of the possibility of hypothyroidism after thyroidectomy or treatment with antithyroid drugs or ^{131}I.
- Refer to home care for assessment of the home and family environment.
- Assess patient's and family's understanding of the importance of the therapeutic regimen and compliance with it; recommend follow-up monitoring.
- Assess for changes indicating return to normal thyroid function; assess for physical signs of hyperthyroidism and hypothyroidism.

Evaluation

Expected Patient Outcomes

- Shows improved nutritional status
- Demonstrates effective coping methods in dealing with family, friends, and coworkers
- Achieves increased self-esteem
- Maintains normal body temperature
- Displays absence of complications

For more information, see Chapter 42 in Smeltzer and Bare: *Brunner and Suddarth's Textbook of Medical-Surgical Nursing*, 11th edition. Philadelphia: Lippincott Williams & Wilkins, 2008.

Hypoglycemia (Insulin Reaction)

Hypoglycemia (abnormally low blood glucose level) occurs when the blood glucose falls below 50 to 60 mg/dL. It can be caused by too much insulin or oral hypoglycemic agents, too little food, or excessive physical activity. Hypoglycemia may occur at any time. It often occurs before meals, especially if meals are delayed or if snacks are omitted. Middle-of-the-night hypoglycemia may occur because of peaking evening NPH or Lente insulins, especially in patients who have not eaten a bedtime snack.

Clinical Manifestations

- The symptoms of hypoglycemia may be grouped into two categories: adrenergic symptoms and central nervous system symptoms.
- Hypoglycemic symptoms may occur suddenly and unexpectedly and vary from person to person.
- Patients who have blood glucose in the hyperglycemic range (200 mg/dL or greater) may feel hypoglycemic with adrenergic symptoms when blood glucose quickly drops to 120 mg/dL (6.6 mmol/L) or less.
- Patients with usual blood glucose levels in the low range of normal may not experience symptoms when blood glucose slowly falls under 50 mg/dL (2.7 mmol/L).
- A decreased hormonal (adrenergic) response to hypoglycemia may occur in patients who have had diabetes for many years. Patient must perform blood glucose checks frequently.
- As the glucose falls, the normal surge of adrenaline does not occur, and patient does not feel the usual adrenergic symptoms (sweating and shakiness).

Mild Hypoglycemia

The sympathetic nervous system is stimulated, producing sweating, tremor, tachycardia, palpitations, nervousness, and hunger.

Moderate Hypoglycemia

Moderate hypoglycemia produces impaired function of the central nervous system, including inability to concentrate, headache, lightheadedness, confusion, and memory lapses. Additional symptoms include numbness of the lips and tongue, slurred speech, impaired coordination, emotional changes, irrational or combative behavior, double vision, and drowsiness or any combination of these symptoms.

Severe Hypoglycemia

In severe hypoglycemia, central nervous system function is further impaired. The patient needs the assistance of another for treatment. Symptoms may include disoriented behavior, seizures, difficulty arousing from sleep, or loss of consciousness.

Assessment and Diagnostic Methods

Measurement of serum glucose levels

🌿 Gerontologic Considerations

Elderly people frequently live alone and may not recognize the symptoms of hypoglycemia. With decreasing renal function, it takes longer for oral hypoglycemic agents to be excreted by the kidneys. Teach patient to avoid skipping meals because of decreased appetite or financial limitations. Decreased visual acuity may lead to errors in insulin administration.

Medical Management

- The usual recommendation is 15 g of a fast-acting sugar orally: (1) three or four commercially prepared glucose tablets (glucagon tablets); (2) 4 to 6 ounces of fruit juice or regular soda; (3) 6 to 10 Life Savers or other hard candies; (4) 2 to 3 teaspoons of sugar or honey.
- Patient should avoid adding table sugar to juice, even "unsweetened" juice, which may cause a sharp increase in glucose, resulting in hyperglycemia hours later.

- Treatment is repeated if the symptoms persist more than 10 to 15 minutes; patient is retested in 15 minutes and retreated if blood glucose level is less than 70 to 75 mg/dL.
- Patient should eat a snack containing protein and starch (milk, or cheese and crackers) after the symptoms resolve or should eat a meal or snack within 30 to 60 minutes.
- Diabetic patients should carry a form of simple sugar with them at all times.
- Patient is discouraged from eating high-calorie, high-fat dessert foods to treat hypoglycemia, because high-fat snacks may slow absorption of the glucose.

H

Management of Hypoglycemia in the Unconscious Patient

- Glucagon, 1 mg subcutaneously or intramuscularly for patients who cannot swallow, or who refuse treatment; patient may take up to 20 minutes to regain consciousness. Give a simple sugar followed by snack when awake.
- From 25 to 50 mL of 50% dextrose in water is administered intravenously to patients who are unconscious or unable to swallow (in a hospital setting).

Nursing Management

- Teach patient to prevent hypoglycemia by following a consistent, regular pattern for eating, administering insulin, and exercising. Consume between-meal and bedtime snacks to counteract the maximum insulin effect.
- Reinforce that routine blood glucose tests are performed so that changing insulin requirements may be anticipated.
- Encourage patients taking insulin to wear an identification bracelet or tag indicating they have diabetes.
- Instruct patient to notify physician after severe hypoglycemia has occurred.
- Instruct patients and family about symptoms of hypoglycemia and use of glucagon.

- Teach family that hypoglycemia can cause irrational and unintentional behavior.
- Teach patient the importance of performing self-monitoring of blood glucose on a frequent and regular basis.
- Teach patients with type 2 diabetes who take oral hypoglycemic agents that symptoms of hypoglycemia may also develop.

For more information, see Chapter 41 in Smeltzer and Bare: *Brunner and Suddarth's Textbook of Medical-Surgical Nursing*, 11th edition. Philadelphia: Lippincott Williams & Wilkins, 2008

Hypoparathyroidism

The most common cause of hypoparathyroidism is inadequate secretion of parathyroid hormone after interruption of the blood supply or surgical removal of parathyroid gland tissue during thyroidectomy, parathyroidectomy, or radical neck dissection. Atrophy of the parathyroid glands of unknown etiology is a less common cause. Symptoms are due to deficiency of parathormone that results in an elevation of blood phosphate and decrease in blood calcium levels.

Clinical Manifestations

- Tetany is the chief symptom.
- Latent tetany: numbness, tingling, and cramps in the extremities; stiffness in the hands and feet
- Overt tetany: bronchospasm, laryngeal spasm, carpopedal spasm, dysphagia, photophobia, cardiac dysrhythmias, and seizures
- Other symptoms: anxiety, irritability, depression, and delirium. Electrocardiogram (ECG) changes and hypotension may also occur.

Assessment and Diagnostic Findings

- Latent tetany is suggested by a positive Trousseau's sign or a positive Chvostek's sign (tetany noted with serum calcium 5 to 6 mg/dL or 1.2 to 1/5 mmol/L).
- Diagnosis is difficult because of vague symptoms; laboratory studies show decreased serum calcium, increased serum phosphate; increased bone density and brain calcification on radiograph.

Medical Management

- Serum calcium level is raised to 9 to 10 mg/dL.
- When hypocalcemia and tetany occur after thyroidectomy, intravenous calcium gluconate is given immediately. Sedatives (pentobarbital) may be administered. Parenteral parathormone may be given, watching for an allergic reaction.
- Neuromuscular irritability is reduced by providing an environment that is free of noise, drafts, bright lights, or sudden movement.
- Emergency management with bronchodilating medications, tracheostomy, or mechanical ventilation for respiratory distress
- Chronic hypoparathyroidism is treated with a diet high in calcium and low in phosphorus. Patient should avoid milk, milk products, egg yolk, and spinach.
- Oral calcium tablets and vitamin D preparations and aluminum hydroxide or aluminum carbonate may be given.

Nursing Management

- Anticipate signs of tetany, convulsions, and respiratory difficulty.
- Keep calcium gluconate at bedside and observe for cardiac problems, such as dysrhythmias. If patient is receiving digitalis, then calcium gluconate must be administered slowly and cautiously.

H

- Provide continuous cardiac monitoring and careful assessment; calcium and digitalis increase systolic contraction and potentiate each other and the risk for fatal dysrhythmias.
- Provide oral tablets of calcium salts (calcium gluconate); give aluminum hydroxide gel after meals to bind phosphate.
- Provide vitamin D preparations to enhance calcium absorption from the gastrointestinal tract.
- Teach patient about medications and diet therapy and reason for high calcium and low phosphate intake; teach patient to contact physician if symptoms occur.
- Teach the importance of maintaining a diet high in calcium and low in phosphorus for patients with chronic hypoparathyroidism.
- Caution patient to restrict intake of milk, milk products, and egg yolk because they contain high levels of phosphorus and to eliminate spinach because it contains oxalate, which forms insoluble calcium substances.

For more information, see Chapter 42 in Smeltzer and Bare: *Brunner and Suddarth's Textbook of Medical-Surgical Nursing*, 11th edition. Philadelphia: Lippincott Williams & Wilkins, 2008.

Hypopituitarism

Hypopituitarism is pituitary insufficiency from destruction of the anterior lobe of the pituitary gland or hypofunction of the hypothalamus. Panhypopituitarism (Simmonds' disease) is total absence of all pituitary secretions and is rare. Postpartum pituitary necrosis (Sheehan's syndrome) is another uncommon cause of failure of the anterior pituitary. It is more likely to occur in women with severe blood loss, hypovolemia, and hypotension at the time of delivery. Hypopituitarism is also a complication of radiation therapy to the head and neck. Total destruction of the pituitary gland by trauma, tumor, or vascular lesion removes all stimuli that are normally received by the thyroid, gonads, and adrenal glands. The result is extreme weight loss, emaciation, atrophy of all endocrine glands and organs, hair loss, impotence, amenorrhea, hypometabolism, and hypoglycemia. Coma and death occur without replacement of missing hormones.

For more information, see Chapter 42 in Smeltzer and Bare: *Brunner and Suddarth's Textbook of Medical-Surgical Nursing*, 11th edition. Philadelphia: Lippincott Williams & Wilkins, 2008.

Hypothyroidism and Myxedema

Hypothyroidism is a condition of thyroid deficiency (suboptimal levels of thyroid hormone). Types of hypothyroidism include primary, which refers to dysfunction of the thyroid gland (more than 95% of cases); central, due to failure of the pituitary gland, hypothalamus, or both; secondary or pituitary, which is due entirely to a pituitary disorder; and hypothalamic or tertiary, due to a disorder of the hypothalamus resulting in inadequate secretion of thyroid-stimulating hormone (TSH) from decreased stimulation by thyrotropin-releasing hormone (TRH). Hypothyroidism occurs most often in older women. Its causes include autoimmune thyroiditis (Hashimoto's thyroiditis, most common type in adults); therapy for hyperthyroidism (radioiodine, surgery, or antithyroid drugs); radiation therapy for head and neck cancer; infiltrative diseases of the thyroid (amyloidosis and scleroderma); iodine deficiency; and iodine excess. When thyroid deficiency is present at birth, the condition is known as cretinism. The term "myxedema" refers to the accumulation of mucopolysaccharides in subcutaneous and other interstitial tissue and is used only to describe the extreme symptoms of severe hypothyroidism.

Clinical Manifestations

- Nonspecific early symptoms
- Extreme fatigue

- Hair loss, brittle nails, dry skin, and numbness and tingling of fingers
- Husky voice and hoarseness
- Menstrual disturbances; menorrhagia or amenorrhea; loss of libido
- Severe hypothyroidism: subnormal temperature and pulse rate; weight gain without corresponding increase in food intake; cachexia (with severe hypothyroidism)
- Sensation of cold in a warm environment
- Subdued emotional responses as the condition progresses; dulled mental processes and apathy
- Slowed speech; enlarged tongue, hands, and feet; constipation; possibly deafness
- Hypothyroidism (affects women five times more frequently than men); associated tendency toward atherosclerosis, with all consequences
- Advanced hypothyroidism: personality and cognitive changes, pleural effusion, pericardial effusion, and respiratory muscle weakness
- Myxedema: thickened skin, thinning hair or alopecia; expressionless and masklike facial features
- Advanced hypothyroidism with hypothermia: abnormal sensitivity to sedatives, opiates, and anesthetic agents (these drugs are given with extreme caution)

🌿 Gerontologic Considerations

The higher prevalence of hypothyroidism in the elderly population may be related to alterations in immune function with age. Depression, apathy, or decreased mobility or activity may be the major initial symptom. The effects of analgesics, sedatives, and anesthetic agents are prolonged in all patients with hypothyroidism, and these agents should be administered with caution. Thyroid hormone replacement must be started with low doses and gradually increased to prevent serious cardiovascular and neurologic side effects, such as angina. Regular testing of serum TSH is recommended for people over 60 years of age. Myxedema and myxedema coma generally occur in patients older than 50 years of age.

> **!** **NURSING ALERT** Patients with unrecognized hypothyroidism undergoing surgery are at increased risk for intraoperative hypotension, postoperative congestive heart failure, and altered mental status. Myocardial ischemia or infarction may occur in response to therapy in patients with severe, long-standing hypothyroidism or myxedema coma. Be alert for signs of angina, especially during the early phase of treatment, and discontinue administration of thyroid hormone immediately if symptoms occur.

Medical Management

The primary objective is to restore a normal metabolic state by replacing thyroid hormone. Additional treatment in severe hypothyroidism consists of maintaining vital functions, monitoring arterial blood gas (ABG) values, and administering fluids cautiously because of the danger of water intoxication.

Pharmacologic Therapy

- Synthetic levothyroxine (Synthroid or Levothroid) is the preferred preparation.
- External heat application is avoided because it increases oxygen requirements and may lead to vascular collapse.
- Concentrated glucose may be given if hypoglycemia is evident.
- If myxedema coma is present, thyroid hormone is given intravenously until consciousness is restored.

Interaction of Thyroid Hormones with Other Drugs

- Thyroid hormones increase blood glucose levels, which may necessitate adjustment in doses of insulin or oral hypoglycemic agents.
- The effects of thyroid hormone may be increased by phenytoin and tricyclic antidepressants.

- Thyroid hormone may increase the pharmacologic effect of digitalis, glycosides, anticoagulants, and indomethacin, requiring careful observation and assessment for side effects of these drugs.

> **!** **NURSING ALERT** Severe untreated hypothyroidism increases susceptibility to all hypnotic and sedative drugs.

NURSING PROCESS: The Patient with Hypothyroidism

Assessment

- Monitor and record vital signs for baseline.
- Monitor respiratory rate, depth, pattern, pulse oximetry, and ABG values.
- Assess all body systems; note any abnormal functions.
- Explore the impact of condition on patient and family and coping skills.

Diagnosis

Nursing Diagnoses

- Ineffective breathing pattern related to depressed ventilation
- Activity intolerance related to fatigue and depressed cognitive process
- Imbalanced body temperature
- Constipation related to depressed gastrointestinal function
- Deficient knowledge about the therapeutic regimen for lifelong thyroid replacement therapy
- Impaired thought processes related to depressed metabolism and altered cardiovascular and respiratory status

Planning and Goals

The major goals of the patient may include tolerance of moderate activity, normal body temperature and effective breathing pattern, prevention of constipation, understanding of therapeutic regimen, and effective thought processes.

Nursing Interventions

Improving Respiratory Status

- Encourage deep breathing and coughing.
- Administer medications with caution (hypnotics and sedatives).
- Maintain patent airway through suction and ventilatory support if indicated.

Increased Participation in Activities

- Support patient by assisting with care and hygiene while encouraging him or her to participate in activities within tolerance to prevent complications of immobility (major role of nurse).
- Space activities to promote rest and exercise as tolerated.
- Monitor vital signs and cognitive level closely during diagnostic workup and initiation of treatment to detect: (1) deterioration in physical and mental status, (2) symptoms indicating that an increased metabolic rate exceeds the ability of the cardiovascular and pulmonary systems to respond, and (3) continued limitations and complications of myxedema.

Maintaining Normal Body Temperature and Promoting Comfort

- Provide extra clothing and blankets for chilling and extreme intolerance to cold.
- Avoid heating pads and electric blankets; patient could be burned because of delayed responses and decreased mental status.
- Monitor body temperature, and report decreases from baseline.
- Protect from exposure to cold and drafts.

H

Promoting Return of Bowel Function

- Encourage increased fluid intake within limits of fluid restriction.
- Provide foods high in fiber.
- Instruct patient about foods with high water content.
- Monitor bowel function.
- Encourage increased mobility within exercise tolerance.
- Advise patient to use laxatives and enemas sparingly.

Providing Emotional Support

- Assist patient and family in dealing with emotional reactions to changes in appearance and body image.
- Inform patient that symptoms will subside when hypothyroidism is treated.
- Provide assistance and counseling to deal with emotional concerns and reactions.

Improving Thought Processes

- Orient patient to time, place, date, and events.
- Provide stimulation through conversation and nonthreatening activities.
- Explain to patient and family that change in cognitive and mental functioning is a result of disease process.
- Monitor cognitive and mental processes and responses of these to medication and other therapy.

Monitoring and Preventing Complications

- Monitor increasing severity of signs and symptoms of hypothyroidism.
- Assist in ventilatory support if needed.
- Administer medications (thyroxine) with caution.
- Turn and reposition patient at intervals.
- Avoid use of hypnotic, sedative, and analgesic agents in myxedema.
- Document and report subtle signs and symptoms that indicate inadequate thyroxine hormone.

Promoting Home and Community-Based Care

Teaching Patients Self-Care

- Provide follow-up, teaching, and health care before hospital discharge.
- Provide dietary instructions to promote weight loss after medication therapy has been initiated and to promote return of normal bowel pattern.
- Instruct family about treatment goals, medication schedules, and signs of overdose or underdose or side effects to be reported.

Continuing Care

- Give encouragement and assistance in daily administration of medications; encourage development of schedule and administration checklist.
- Reinforce knowledge that continued thyroid hormone replacement is necessary, with periodic follow-up testing.
- If indicated, arrange a weekly visit from the home care nurse to assess patient's physical and cognitive status and ability to cope with recent changes.

For more information, see Chapter 42 in Smeltzer and Bare: *Brunner and Suddarth's Textbook of Medical-Surgical Nursing*, 11th edition. Philadelphia: Lippincott Williams & Wilkins, 2008.

Idiopathic Thrombocytopenia Purpura

Idiopathic thrombocytopenia purpura (ITP) is a disease affecting all ages but is more common in children and young women. Although the precise cause remains unknown, viral infection sometimes precedes the disease in children. Other conditions (eg, systemic lupus erythematosus, pregnancy) or medications (eg, sulfa drugs) can also produce ITP. Antiplatelet autoantibodies are produced, which attack platelets; platelet lifespan is markedly shortened. The body attempts to compensate for this destruction by increasing platelet production within the marrow. There are two forms: acute (primarily in children) and chronic.

Clinical Manifestations

- Many patients have no symptoms.
- Petechiae and easy bruising (dry purpura)
- Heavy menses and mucosal bleeding (wet purpura, high risk of intracranial bleeding)
- Platelet count generally below 20,000 mm^3
- Acute form self-limiting, possibly with spontaneous remissions

Assessment and Diagnostic Findings

Usually the diagnosis is based on the decreased platelet count and survival time and increased bleeding time and ruling out other causes of thrombocytopenia. Key diagnostic procedures include platelet count, complete blood count, and bone marrow aspiration, which shows an increase in megakaryocytes (platelet precursors). Many patients are infected with *Helicobacter pylori*.

To date, effectiveness of *H. pylori* treatment in relation to management of ITP is unknown.

Medical Management

Primary goal of treatment is a safe platelet count. Splenectomy is sometimes performed (thrombocytopenia may return months or years later).

Pharmacologic Therapy

Immunosuppressive medications, such as corticosteroids, are the treatment of choice. The bone mineral density of patients receiving chronic corticosteroid therapy needs to be monitored. These patients may benefit from calcium and vitamin D supplementation or bisphosphonate therapy to prevent significant bone disease.

- Intravenous gamma globulin (very expensive) and vincristine are also effective.
- A new approach involves using anti-D (WinRho) for patients who are Rh(D) positive.
- Epsilon aminocaproic acid (EACA; Amicar) may be useful for patients with significant mucosal bleeding who are refractory to other treatment modalities.
- Platelet infusions are avoided except to stop catastrophic bleeding.

Nursing Management

- Obtain history of medication use, including over-the-counter medications, herbs, and nutritional supplements; recent viral illness; or complaints of headache or visual disturbances (intracranial bleed). Be alert for sulfa-containing medications and medications that alter platelet function (eg, aspirin or other NSAIDs). Physical assessment should include a thorough search for signs of bleeding, neurologic assessment, and vital sign measurement.

- To minimize bleeding, instruct patient to avoid all medications that interfere with platelet function (eg, quinine, sulfa-containing medication, aspirin, NSAIDs). Avoid administering medications by injection or rectal route.
- Monitor for complications, including osteoporosis, proximal muscle wasting, cataract formation, and dental caries.
- Teach patient to recognize exacerbations of disease (petechiae, ecchymoses); how to contact health care personnel; and the names of medications that induce ITP.
- Provide information about medications (tapering schedule, if relevant), frequency of platelet count monitoring, and medications to avoid.
- Instruct patient to avoid constipation, the Valsalva maneuver, and tooth flossing.
- Encourage patient to use electric razor for shaving and soft-bristled toothbrushes instead of stiff-bristled brushes.
- Advise patient to refrain from vigorous sexual intercourse when platelet count is less than $10,000/mm^3$.

For more information, see Chapter 33 in Smeltzer and Bare: *Brunner and Suddarth's Textbook of Medical-Surgical Nursing*, 11th edition. Philadelphia: Lippincott Williams & Wilkins, 2008.

Impetigo

Impetigo is a superficial infection of the skin caused by staphylococci, streptococci, or multiple bacteria. Exposed areas of the body, face, hands, neck, and extremities are most frequently involved. Impetigo is contagious and may spread to other parts of the skin or to other members of the family who touch the patient or who use towels or combs that are soiled with the exudate of the lesion. Impetigo is particularly common among children living in poor hygienic conditions. Chronic health problems, poor hygiene, and malnutrition may predispose adults to impetigo.

Clinical Manifestations

- Lesions begin as small, red macules that become discrete, thin-walled vesicles that rupture and become covered with a honey-yellow crust.
- These crusts, when removed, reveal smooth, red, moist surfaces on which new crusts develop.
- If the scalp is involved, the hair is matted, distinguishing the condition from ringworm.
- Bullous impetigo, a deep-seated infection of the skin caused by *Staphylococcus aureus*, is characterized by the formation of bullae from original vesicles. The bullae rupture, leaving a raw, red area.

Medical Management
Pharmacologic Therapy

Systemic antibiotic therapy is the usual treatment for impetigo. It reduces contagious spread and prevents the possible aftermath of glomerulonephritis.

- Agents for nonbullous impetigo: benzathine penicillin, or oral penicillin or erythromycin
- Agents for bullous impetigo: penicillinase-resistant penicillin or erythromycin
- Topical antibacterial therapy is the usual treatment for disease that is limited to a small area. The topical preparation is applied to lesions several times daily for 1 week. Lesions are soaked or washed with soap solution to remove central site of bacterial growth and to give the topical antibiotic an opportunity to reach the infected site.

Nursing Management

- Use antiseptic solutions (chlorhexidine [Hibiclens]) to cleanse the skin and reduce bacterial content and prevent spread.
- Wear gloves when giving care to patients with impetigo.

- Instruct patient and family to bathe at least once daily with bactericidal soap.
- Encourage cleanliness and good hygiene practices to prevent spread of lesion from one skin area to another and from one person to another.
- Instruct patient and family not to share bath towels and washcloths and to avoid physical contact between the infected person and other people until lesions heal.

For more information, see Chapter 56 in Smeltzer and Bare: *Brunner and Suddarth's Textbook of Medical-Surgical Nursing*, 11th edition. Philadelphia: Lippincott Williams & Wilkins, 2008.

Increased Intracranial Pressure

Increased intracranial pressure (ICP) is the result of the amount of brain tissue, blood, and cerebrospinal fluid (CSF) within the skull at any one time. The volume and pressure of these three components are usually in a state of equilibrium. Because there is limited space for expansion within the skull, an increase in any of these components causes a change in the volume of the others by displacing or shifting CSF, increasing the absorption of CSF, or decreasing cerebral blood volume. The normal ICP is 10 to 20 mm Hg. Although elevated ICP is most commonly associated with head injury, an elevated pressure may be seen secondary to brain tumors, subarachnoid hemorrhage, and toxic and viral encephalopathies. Increased ICP from any cause decreases cerebral perfusion, stimulates swelling, and produces distortion and shifts of brain tissue. Life-threatening herniation may result.

Clinical Manifestations

When ICP increases to the point where the brain's ability to adjust has reached its limits, neural function is impaired. Increased ICP is manifested by changes in level of consciousness and abnormal respiratory and vasomotor responses.

- Level of responsiveness and consciousness is the most important indicator of the patient's condition.
- Lethargy is the earliest sign of increasing ICP. Slowing of speech and delay in response to verbal suggestions are early indicators.
- Sudden change in condition, such as restlessness (without apparent cause), confusion, or increasing drowsiness, has neurologic significance.
- Decreased cerebral perfusion pressure (CPP) can result in a Cushing's response and Cushing's triad (bradycardia, bradypnea, and hypertension); widening pulse pressure is an ominous sign.
- As pressure increases, patient becomes stuporous and may react only to loud auditory or painful stimuli. This indicates serious impairment of brain circulation, and immediate surgical intervention may be required. With further deterioration, coma and abnormal motor responses in the form of decortication, decerebration, or flaccidity may occur.
- When coma is profound, pupils are dilated and fixed, respirations are impaired, and death is usually inevitable.

Assessment and Diagnostic Methods

- Cerebral angiography, computed tomography (CT), magnetic resonance imaging (MRI), positron emission tomography (PET), transcranial Doppler studies, or electrophysiologic monitoring may be done. Lumbar puncture is avoided to prevent risking herniation.
- ICP monitoring provides useful information (ventriculostomy, subarachnoid bolt/screw, epidural monitor, fiberoptic monitor).

Medical Management

Increased ICP is a true emergency and must be treated promptly. Immediate management involves invasive monitoring of ICP, decreasing cerebral edema, lowering the volume of CSF, and decreasing blood volume while maintaining cerebral perfusion.

Pharmacologic Therapy

- Osmotic diuretics and corticosteroids are administered, fluid is restricted, CSF is drained, patient is hyperventilated, fever is controlled (using antipyretics, hypothermia blanket, with chlorpromazine [Thorazine] to control shivering), and cellular metabolic demands are reduced (with barbiturates, paralyzing agents).
- If patient does not respond to conventional treatment, cellular metabolic demands may be reduced by administering high doses of barbiturates or administering pharmacologic paralyzing agents, such as pancuronium (Pavulon).
- Patient requires care in a critical care unit.

NURSING PROCESS:
The Unconscious Patient

Assessment

- Obtain patient history with subjective data, including events leading to present illness.
- Complete a neurologic examination as patient's condition allows. Evaluate mental status, LOC, cranial nerve function, cerebellar function (balance and coordination), reflexes, and motor and sensitivity function.
- Use the Glasgow Coma Scale to assess verbal response, motor response, and eye opening behaviors.
- Note subtle changes, such as restlessness, headache, forced breathing, mental cloudiness, and purposeless movements, which may be early indications of rising ICP.
- Assess headache (usually constant, increasing in intensity, and aggravated by movement or straining).
- Note recurrent or projectile vomiting, which indicates increased pressure.
- Monitor ICP closely as an essential part of management.
- Inspect pupils for change: observe size, configuration, reaction to light, and gaze (conjugate [paired and working

together] or disconjugate). Also assess ability of eyes to abduct or adduct. Inspect retina and optic nerve for hemorrhage and papilledema.

> **NURSING ALERT** Changes in vital signs may be a late sign of increased ICP. As ICP increases, pulse rate and respiratory rate decrease, and blood pressure and temperature rise. Observe for widening pulse pressure, bradycardia, and respiratory irregularity: Cheyne-Stokes breathing and ataxic breathing (Cushing's triad). Widened pulse pressure is a serious development. Immediate surgical intervention is indicated if the major circulation begins to decrease as a result of brain compression.

Diagnosis

Nursing Diagnoses

- Ineffective airway clearance related to accumulation of secretions secondary to depressed level of responsiveness
- Ineffective cerebral tissue perfusion related to effects of increased ICP
- Ineffective breathing patterns related to neurologic dysfunction (brain stem compression, structural displacement)
- Deficient fluid volume related to fluid restriction
- Risk for infection related to ICP monitoring system (fiberoptic or intraventricular catheter)

Collaborative Problems/Potential Complications

- Brain stem herniation
- Diabetes insipidus
- Syndrome of inappropriate antidiuretic hormone (SIADH) secretion

Planning and Goals

The major goals of the patient may include adequate cerebral tissue perfusion through reduction of ICP, normal respiration, patent airway, restored fluid balance, normal urine and bowel elimination, absence of infection, and absence of complications.

Nursing Interventions

Maintaining a Patent Airway

- Maintain patency of the airway; oxygenate patient before and after suctioning.
- Auscultate lung fields for adventitious sounds every 8 hours.
- Elevate head of bed to help clear secretions and improve venous drainage of the brain.
- Discourage coughing and straining.

Attaining Normal Respiratory Pattern

- Monitor constantly for respiratory irregularities.
- Collaborate with respiratory therapist in monitoring arterial carbon dioxide pressure ($PaCO_2$), which is usually maintained between 30 and 35 mm Hg when hyperventilation therapy is used.
- Maintain continuous neurologic observation record with repeated assessments.

Optimizing Cerebral Tissue Perfusion

- Monitor for bradycardia, bradypnea, and rising blood pressure (Cushing's reflex or response).
- Avoid raising jugular venous pressure and ICP by keeping patient's head in a neutral (midline) position and maintaining slight elevation of the head to aid in venous drainage.
- Avoid extreme rotation and flexion of the neck, because compression or distortion of the jugular veins increases ICP.
- Avoid extreme hip flexion: this position causes an increase in intra-abdominal and intrathoracic pressures, which produce a rise in ICP.
- Instruct patient to exhale when moving or turning in bed to avoid the Valsalva maneuver.
- Provide stool softeners and a high-fiber diet if patient can eat; note any abdominal distention.
- Avoid isometric muscle contractions.

- Avoid suctioning longer than 15 seconds; hyperventilate on ventilator with 100% oxygen before suctioning.
- Maintain a calm atmosphere and reduce environmental stimuli; avoid emotional stress.
- Avoid enemas and cathartics.
- Pace interventions to prevent transient increases in ICP. During nursing care, ICP should not rise above 25 mm Hg and should return to baseline within 5 minutes.

Maintaining Negative Fluid Balance

- Assess skin turgor, mucous membranes, and serum and urine osmolality for signs of dehydration.
- Monitor vital signs to assess fluid volume status.
- Give oral hygiene for mouth dryness.
- Insert indwelling catheter to assess renal and fluid status.
- Monitor urine output every hour in the acute phase.
- Administer intravenous fluids by pump at a slow to moderate rate; monitor patients receiving mannitol for congestive failure.
- Administer corticosteroids and dehydrating agents as ordered.
- Test stools for blood if patient is on high doses of corticosteroids (gastrointestinal bleeding is a complication).

Preventing Infection

- Strictly adhere to the facility's written protocols for managing ICP monitoring systems.
- Keep dressings over ventricular catheters dry, because wet dressings are conducive to bacterial growth.
- Use aseptic technique at all times when managing the ventricular drainage system and changing drainage bag.
- Check carefully for any loose connections that cause leaking and contamination of the ventricular system and contamination of CSF as well as inaccurate ICP readings.
- Check character of CSF drainage for signs of infection (cloudiness or blood). Report changes.
- Monitor for signs and symptoms of meningitis: fever, chills, nuchal (neck) rigidity, and increasing or persistent headache.

I

Monitoring and Managing Potential Complications

- ICP elevation: monitor ICP closely for continuous elevation or significant increase over baseline; assess vital signs at time of ICP increase. Assess for and immediately report manifestations of increasing ICP.
- Impending brain herniation: monitor for increase in blood pressure, decrease in pulse, and change in pupillary response.
- Patients not on paralyzing agents may change from decerebrate to decorticate posturing to a flaccid or rag-doll appearance; this requires rapid intervention using mannitol or drainage of CSF. Monitor urine output closely.
- Diabetes insipidus requires fluid and electrolyte replacement and administration of vasopressin; monitor serum electrolytes for replacement.
- SIADH requires fluid restriction and serum electrolyte monitoring.

Evaluation

Expected Patient Outcomes

- Remains free of excessive airway secretions; airway is patent
- Attains normal respirations
- Demonstrates improved cerebral tissue perfusion
- Attains improved fluid balance
- Has no sign of infection
- Remains free of complications

For more information, see Chapter 61 in Smeltzer and Bare: *Brunner and Suddarth's Textbook of Medical-Surgical Nursing*, 11th edition. Philadelphia: Lippincott Williams & Wilkins, 2008.

Influenza

Influenza is an acute viral disease that causes worldwide epidemics every 2 to 3 years with a highly variable degree of severity.

The virus is easily spread from host to host through droplet exposure. Previous infection with influenza does not guarantee protection from future exposure. Mortality is probably attributable to accompanying pneumonia (viral or superimposed bacterial pneumonia) and other chronic cardiopulmonary sequelae. Transmission is most likely to occur in the first 3 days of illness.

Management

Goals of medical and nursing management include relieving symptoms, treating complications, and preventing transmission. See Nursing and Medical Management under Pharyngitis and Pneumonia for additional information.

Prevention

Annual influenza vaccinations are recommended for those at high risk for complications of influenza. These include people over age 50; residents of extended care facilities; people with chronic pulmonary or cardiovascular diseases, diabetes, immunosuppression, or renal dysfunction; children 6 to 23 months old; children who require long-term aspirin therapy, which puts them at increased risk of developing Reye's syndrome; health care personnel; and pregnant women.

For more information, see Chapters 23 and 70 in Smeltzer and Bare: *Brunner and Suddarth's Textbook of Medical-Surgical Nursing*, 11th edition. Philadelphia: Lippincott Williams & Wilkins, 2008.

K

Kaposi's Sarcoma

Kaposi's sarcoma (KS) is the most common cancer related to the human immunodeficiency virus (HIV) and involves the endothelial layer of blood and lymphatic vessels. It is subdivided into three categories: classic KS, African (endemic) KS, and KS (acquired) associated with immunosuppressant therapy.

Classic KS occurs predominantly in men between the ages of 40 and 70 years who are of Eastern European ancestry. This type of KS is chronic, relatively benign, and rarely fatal. The endemic form, found most often in young men and also in children in equatorial Africa, may infiltrate and progress to lymphadenopathic forms. Immunosuppressive therapy–associated KS occurs when patients are treated with immunosuppressive agents. The greater the immunosuppression, the higher the incidence of KS. Although the histopathologic features of all forms of KS are virtually identical, the clinical manifestations differ with AIDS-related KS, which exhibits a more variable and aggressive course, ranging from localized cutaneous lesions to disseminated disease involving multiple organ systems. Internal organ involvement leads to organ failure, hemorrhage, infection, and death.

Clinical Manifestations

- Cutaneous lesions can occur anywhere on the body and are brownish pink to deep purple. They characteristically present as lower-extremity skin lesions.
- AIDS-related KS has a more variable and aggressive course.
- AIDS-related KS lesions may be flat or raised and surrounded by ecchymosis and edema; they develop rapidly and cause extensive disfigurement.
- The location and size of the lesions can lead to venous stasis, lymphedema, and pain. Common sites of visceral

involvement include the lymph nodes, gastrointestinal tract, and lungs.

- KS associated with immunosuppressive therapy, as in transplant recipients, is characterized by local skin lesions and disseminated visceral and mucocutaneous disease.

Assessment and Diagnostic Findings

- Diagnosis is confirmed by biopsy of suspected lesions.
- Prognosis depends on extent of tumor, presence of constitutional symptoms, and the CD4+ count.
- Pathologic findings indicate that death occurs from tumor progression, but more often from other complications of HIV infection or AIDS.

Medical Management

The treatment goal is reduction of symptoms by decreasing the size of the skin lesions, reducing discomfort associated with edema and ulcerations, and controlling symptoms associated with mucosal or visceral involvement. Localized treatment includes surgical excision of the lesions or application of liquid nitrogen to lesions and injection of intraoral lesions with dilute vinblastine. Radiation therapy is effective as a palliative measure to relieve localized pain from KS lesions in the mouth, conjunctiva, face, and soles of the feet.

Pharmacologic Therapy

- Patients with cutaneous KS treated with alpha-interferon have experienced tumor regression and improved immune system function.
- Pain management may include nonsteroidal anti-inflammatory drugs (NSAIDs) and opioids.

Nursing Management

- Provide thorough and meticulous skin care, involving regular turning, cleansing, and application of medicated ointments and dressings.

K

- Provide analgesic agents at regular intervals around the clock.
- Teach patient relaxation and guided imagery, which may be helpful in reducing pain and anxiety.
- Teach patient to self-administer alpha-interferon at home or arrange for patient to receive it in an outpatient setting.
- Support patient in coping with disfigurement of the condition; stress that lesions are temporary, when applicable (after immunotherapy is discontinued).
- Provide supportive care and treatment as ordered to minimize pain and edema, address complications, and promote healing.

For more information, see Chapter 52 in Smeltzer and Bare: *Brunner and Suddarth's Textbook of Medical-Surgical Nursing*, 11th edition. Philadelphia: Lippincott Williams & Wilkins, 2008.

K

Leukemia

The common feature of the leukemias is an unregulated proliferation or accumulation of white blood cells (WBCs) in the bone marrow, replacing normal marrow elements. There is also proliferation in the liver and spleen and invasion of nonhematologic organs, such as the meninges, lymph nodes, gums, and skin. The leukemias are often classified as either lymphocytic or myelocytic and according to the stem cell line involved. Leukemia is also classified as acute (abrupt onset) or chronic (evolves over months to years). Its cause is unknown. There is some evidence that genetic influence and viral pathogenesis may be involved. Bone marrow damage from radiation exposure or chemicals and alkylating agents can also cause leukemia.

Clinical Manifestations

Cardinal signs and symptoms include weakness and fatigue, bleeding tendencies, petechiae and ecchymoses, pain, headache, vomiting, fever, and infection.

Assessment and Diagnostic Findings

Blood and bone marrow studies confirm proliferation of WBCs (leukocytes) in the bone marrow.

🌱 Gerontologic Considerations

Aging is accompanied by a gradual decline of physiologic processes, among which is a reduction in the immune function, resulting in increased susceptibility to infections.

Older patients often delay reporting symptoms because of lack of knowledge, financial resources, or support systems. The complications of leukemia can be devastating to the already decreased reserves of the elderly patient. Comprehensive nursing care is crucial in assisting the older patient to tolerate the side effects and treatment of the disease and to cope with the psychological and financial aspects.

NURSING MANAGEMENT: The Patient with Leukemia

Assessment

- Identify range of signs and symptoms reported by patient in nursing history and physical examination.
- Assess results of blood studies, and report alterations of WBCs, hematocrit, platelets, electrolytes, absolute neutrophil count (ANC), hepatic function tests and creatinine findings, and culture results.

Diagnosis

Nursing Diagnoses

- Impaired gas exchange
- Risk for infection and bleeding
- Impaired mucous membranes from changes in epithelial lining of the gastrointestinal tract from chemotherapy or antimicrobial medications
- Acute pain and discomfort related to mucositis, leukocytic infiltration of systemic tissues, fever, and infection
- Imbalanced nutrition: less than body requirements related to hypermetabolic state, anorexia, mucositis, pain, and nausea
- Diarrhea from altered gastrointestinal flora, mucosal denudation
- Fluid imbalance from potential for bleeding and renal dysfunction
- Risk for excess fluid volume related to renal dysfunction, hypoproteinemia, need for multiple IV medications and blood products

L

- Hyperthermia related to tumor lysis and infection
- Fatigue and activity intolerance related to anemia and infection
- Impaired skin integrity and alopecia related to toxic effects of chemotherapy
- Grieving related to anticipatory loss and altered role functioning
- Disturbed body image related to change in appearance, function, and roles
- Self-care deficits related to fatigue and malaise
- Risk for spiritual distress
- Deficient knowledge of disease process, treatment, complication management, and self-care measures
- Anxiety due to uncertain future

Collaborative Problems/Potential Complications

- Infection
- Bleeding
- Renal dysfunction
- Tumor lysis syndrome
- Nutritional depletion
- Mucositis

Planning and Goals

The major goals of the patient may include self-care, activity tolerance, attainment or maintenance of comfort, attainment or maintenance of adequate nutrition, promotion of positive body image, understanding of the disease process and its treatment, ability to cope with the diagnosis and prognosis, and absence of complications.

Nursing Interventions

Preventing or Managing Bleeding

- Assess for thrombocytopenia, granulocytopenia, and anemia.
- Report any increase in petechiae, melena, hematuria, or nosebleeds.

- Avoid trauma and injections; use small-gauge needles when analgesics are administered parenterally, and apply pressure after injections to avoid bleeding.
- Use acetaminophen instead of aspirin for analgesia.
- Give prescribed hormonal therapy to prevent menses.
- Manage hemorrhage with bed rest and transfuse red blood cells and platelets as ordered.

Preventing Infection

- Infection is a major cause of death in leukemia patients.
- Assess temperature elevation, flushed appearance, chills, tachycardia, and appearance of white patches in the mouth.
- Observe for redness, swelling, heat, or pain in eyes, ears, throat, skin, joints, abdomen, and rectal and perineal areas.
- Assess for cough and changes in character or color of sputum.
- Give frequent oral hygiene.
- Wear sterile gloves to start infusions.
- Provide daily IV site care; observe for signs of infection.
- Ensure normal elimination; avoid rectal thermometers, enemas, and rectal trauma; avoid vaginal tampons.
- Avoid catheterization unless essential. Practice scrupulous asepsis if catheterization is necessary.

> **!**   **NURSING ALERT**   The usual manifestations of infection are altered in patients with leukemia. Corticosteroid therapy may blunt the normal febrile and inflammatory responses to infection.

Managing Mucositis

- Assess the oral mucosa thoroughly; identify and describe lesions; note color and moisture (remove dentures first).
- Assist patient with oral hygiene with soft-bristled toothbrush.
- Avoid drying agents, such as lemon-glycerin swabs and commercial mouthwashes (use saline or saline and baking soda).

- Emphasize the importance of oral rinse medications to prevent yeast infections.
- Instruct patient to cleanse the perirectal area after each bowel movement; monitor frequency of stools, and stop stool softener with loose stool.

Easing Pain and Providing Comfort

- Prevent undue pain in the abdomen, lymph node areas, bones, and joints with careful positioning of patient.
- Avoid sudden movements, and promote comfort with soft supports such as pillows; back and shoulder massage may provide comfort.
- Administer acetaminophen rather than aspirin for analgesia.
- Sponge patient with cool water for fever; avoid cold water or ice packs.
- Provide oral hygiene (for stomatitis), and assist the patient with use of patient-controlled analgesia (PCA) for pain.
- Use creative strategies to permit uninterrupted sleep (a few hours). Assist the patient when awake to balance rest and activity to prevent deconditioning.
- Listen actively to patients enduring pain.

Attaining and Maintaining Adequate Nutrition

- Encourage adequate nutrition by careful timing of chemotherapeutic drug administration and prophylactic use of antiemetics.
- Give frequent oral hygiene (before and after meals) to prevent oral lesions and promote appetite; with oral anesthetics, caution patient to prevent self-injury and to chew carefully.
- Maintain nutrition with palatable, small, frequent feedings of soft nonirritating foods and fluids that are high in protein and vitamins.
- Maintain calorie counts and formal nutritional assessment; monitor daily body weights.
- Encourage intake of low-microbial diet. Administer parenteral nutrition (PN) as ordered.

Maintaining Fluid and Electrolyte Balance

- Measure intake and output accurately; weigh the patient daily.
- Assess for signs of fluid overload or dehydration.
- Monitor laboratory tests (electrolytes, blood urea nitrogen [BUN], creatinine), and replace blood, fluids, and electrolyte components as ordered and indicated.

Decreasing Fatigue and Deconditioning

- Assist in choosing activity priorities; help patient balance activity and rest; suggest a stationary bicycle and sitting up in chair.
- Assist patient in using a high-efficiency particulate air (HEPA) filter mask to ambulate outside room.
- Assess for dyspnea, tachycardia, and other evidence of inadequate oxygen supply to vital organs.
- Arrange for physical therapy when indicated.

Improving Self-Care

- Encourage the patient to do as much as possible.
- Listen empathetically to the patient.
- Assist patient to resume more self-care during recovery from treatment.

Managing Anxiety and Grief

- Provide emotional support, and discuss the impact of uncertain future.
- Assess patient's understanding of illness, treatment, and potential complications.
- Assist patient to identify the source of grief, and encourage patient to allow time to adjust to the major life changes rendered by the illness.
- Arrange to have communication with nurses across care settings to reassure patient that he or she has not been abandoned.

Promoting Positive Body Image

- Prepare patient for the occurrence of alopecia, and help patient to express and resolve feelings.
- Help patient to adjust to body image problems by encouraging involvement and support of family or support system.

Encouraging Spiritual Well-Being

- Assess the patient's spiritual and religious practices, and offer relevant services.
- Assist the patient to maintain realistic hope over the course of the illness (initially for a cure, in later stages for a quiet, dignified death).

Promoting Home and Community-Based Care

Teaching Patients Self-Care

- Ensure that patients and their families have a clear understanding of disease and complications (risk for infection and bleeding).
- Teach family members about home care while patient is still in the hospital, particularly vascular access device management if applicable.

Continuing Care

- Maintain communication between the patient and nurses across care settings.
- Provide specific instructions regarding when and how to seek care from the physician.

Terminal Care

- Respect the patient's choices about treatment, including measures to prolong life, when there is no longer any response to therapy. Provide for advance directives and living wills to give the patient control during terminal phase.
- Support families and coordinate home care services to alleviate anxiety about managing the patient's care in the home.

L

- Provide respite for the caregivers and patient with hospice volunteers.
- Give the patient and caregivers assistance to cope with changes in their roles and responsibilities (that is, anticipatory grieving).
- Provide information on hospital-based hospice programs for patients to receive palliative care in the hospital when care at home is no longer possible.

Evaluation

Expected Patient Outcomes

- Demonstrates absence of infection
- Demonstrates absence of bleeding
- Exhibits intact oral mucous membranes
- Attains optimal level of nutrition
- Reports satisfaction with pain and discomfort levels
- Experiences less fatigue and increases activity
- Maintains fluid and electrolyte balance
- Participates in self-care
- Copes with anxiety and grief
- Experiences absence of complications

For more information, see Chapter 33 in Smeltzer and Bare: *Brunner and Suddarth's Textbook of Medical-Surgical Nursing*, 11th edition. Philadelphia: Lippincott Williams & Wilkins, 2008.

Leukemia, Lymphocytic, Acute

Acute lymphocytic leukemia (ALL) results from an uncontrolled proliferation of immature cells (lymphoblasts) from the lymphoid stem cell. It is most common in young children; boys are affected more frequently than girls, with a peak incidence at 4 years of age. After age 15, ALL is uncommon. Therapy for this childhood leukemia has improved to the extent that about 80% of children survive at least 5 years.

Clinical Manifestations

- Immature lymphocytes proliferate in marrow and crowd development of normal myeloid cells.
- Normal hematopoiesis is inhibited, and leukopenia, anemia, and thrombocytopenia develop.
- Pain results from enlarged liver or spleen or is felt in bone; headache and vomiting are due to leukemic cell infiltration into other organs (more common with ALL than with other forms of leukemia).
- Erythrocyte and platelet counts are low.
- Leukocyte counts are low or high but always include immature cells.

Medical Management

The major form of treatment is chemotherapy with vinca alkaloids and glucocorticoids.

- Combinations of vincristine, prednisone, daunorubicin, and asparaginase are used for initial induction therapy.
- Combinations of medications are used for maintenance (maintenance doses of medications for up to 3 years).
- Irradiation of the cerebrospinal region and intrathecal injection of chemotherapeutic drugs help prevent central nervous system recurrence.

Nursing Management

See Nursing Management under Leukemia for additional information.

For more information, see Chapter 33 in Smeltzer and Bare: *Brunner and Suddarth's Textbook of Medical-Surgical Nursing*, 11th edition. Philadelphia: Lippincott Williams & Wilkins, 2008.

Leukemia, Lymphocytic, Chronic

Chronic lymphocytic leukemia (CLL) is a common cancer of older adulthood (two thirds of patients are older than 60 years of age). It is derived from a malignant clone of B lymphocytes. These cells escape apoptosis (programmed cell death), leading to excessive accumulation. There are more mature leukemia cells than immature cells, so it tends to be a mild disorder compared with the acute form. The disease is classified into three or four stages (two classification systems are in use). In the early stage, an elevated lymphocyte count is seen; it can exceed 100,000. The disease is usually diagnosed during physical examination or treatment for another disease.

Clinical Manifestations

- Many cases are asymptomatic.
- CLL patients can develop "B symptoms": fevers, sweats (especially night), and unintentional weight loss. Infections are common.
- Anergy (decreased or absent reaction to skin sensitivity tests) reveals the defect in cellular immunity.
- Lymphadenopathy (enlargement of lymph nodes), which is sometimes severe and painful, and hepatomegaly and splenomegaly may be noted.
- Erythrocyte and platelet counts may be normal or decreased.
- Lymphocytosis is always present.
- In the later stages, anemia and thrombocytopenia may develop.

Medical Management

- In its early stages, CLL may require no treatment. For severe symptoms, chemotherapy with steroids and chlorambucil (Leukeran) is a choice. Other agents may include cyclo-phosphamide, vincristine, and doxorubicin, as well as monoclonal antibodies.

- Patients who do not respond to ordinary therapy may achieve remission with fludarabine monophosphate therapy.
- Intravenous immunoglobulin may prevent recurrent bacterial infections in selected patients.

Nursing Management

See Nursing Management under Leukemia for additional information.

For more information, see Chapter 33 in Smeltzer and Bare: *Brunner and Suddarth's Textbook of Medical-Surgical Nursing*, 11th edition. Philadelphia: Lippincott Williams & Wilkins, 2008.

Leukemia, Myeloid, Acute

L

- Acute myeloid leukemia (AML) results from a defect in the hematopoietic stem cell that differentiates into all myeloid cells: monocytes, granulocytes (basophils, neutrophils, eosinophils), erythrocytes, and platelets. AML can be further classified into seven different subgroups, based on cytogenetics, histology, and morphology (appearance) of the blasts. All age groups are affected; incidence rises with age and peaks at 60 years of age. It is the most common nonlymphocytic leukemia. Death usually occurs secondary to infection or hemorrhage.

Clinical Manifestations

- Most signs and symptoms evolve from insufficient production of normal blood cells: fever and infection result from neutropenia, weakness and fatigue are due to anemia, bleeding tendencies are a result of thrombocytopenia. Major hemorrhage occurs with a platelet count of less than 10,000/mm^3. The most common sites of bleeding are gastrointestinal, pulmonary, and intracranial.

- Proliferation of leukemic cells within organs leads to a variety of additional symptoms: pain from enlarged liver or spleen, hyperplasia of the gums, lymphadenopathy, headache or vomiting secondary to meningeal leukemia, and bone pain from expansion of marrow.
- AML has its onset without warning; symptoms develop over 1 to 6 weeks or over months.
- Peripheral blood shows decreased erythrocyte and platelet counts.
- The leukocyte count is low, normal, or high; the percentage of normal cells is usually vastly decreased.

Assessment and Diagnostic Methods

- Bone marrow specimen (excess of immature blast cells)
- Complete blood count (decreased platelet count and erythrocyte count)

Medical Management

The objective is to achieve complete remission, typically with chemotherapy (induction therapy), which in some instances results in remissions lasting a year or longer.

Chemotherapy

- Daunorubicin (Cerubidine), cytarabine (Cytosar-U)
- Mercaptopurine (Purinethol), mitoxantrone, or idarubicin
- Consolidation therapy (postremission therapy with chemotherapy agents)

Supportive Care

- Administration of blood products
- Prompt treatment of infections

- Granulocyte colony-stimulating factor (G-CSF [filgrastim]) or granulocyte-macrophage colony-stimulating factor (GM-CSF [sargramostim]) to decrease neutropenia

Bone Marrow Transplantation

Bone marrow transplantation is used when a tissue match of a close relative can be obtained. The transplantation procedure follows destruction of the leukemic marrow by chemotherapy.

Nursing Management

See Nursing Management under Leukemia for additional information.

For more information, see Chapter 33 in Smeltzer and Bare: *Brunner and Suddarth's Textbook of Medical-Surgical Nursing*, 11th edition. Philadelphia: Lippincott Williams & Wilkins, 2008.

L

Leukemia, Myelogenous, Chronic

Chronic myelogenous leukemia (CML) arises from a mutation in the myeloid stem cells. A wide spectrum of cell types exists within the blood, from blast forms through mature neutrophils. More normal cells are present than in the acute form, however, and the disease is milder. A cytogenetic abnormality termed the Philadelphia chromosome is found in 90% to 95% of patients. CML is uncommon before 20 years of age, but the incidence rises with age (median age of onset is 40 to 50 years). CML has three stages: chronic, transformation, and accelerated or blast crisis. Marrow expands into cavities of the long bones, and cells are formed in the liver and spleen, with resultant painful enlargement problems. Infection and bleeding are rare until the disease transforms to the acute phase.

Clinical Manifestations

The clinical picture of CML is similar to that of acute myeloid leukemia, but signs and symptoms are less severe. Many patients are without symptoms for years.

- Onset is insidious; patients demonstrate malaise, anorexia, weight loss.
- Leukocytosis is always present, sometimes at extraordinary levels. Patient may be short of breath or slightly confused from leukostasis.
- Splenomegaly with tenderness and hepatomegaly are common.
- In the transforming phase, bone pain, fever, weight loss, anemia, and thrombocytopenia are noted.

Medical Management

Pharmacologic Therapy

- Drug therapies of choice are busulfan (Myleran) and hydroxyurea, or chlorambucil (Leukeran) alone or with steroids. An anthracycline chemotherapeutic agent (eg, daunomycin) may be used.
- Bone marrow transplantation increases survival significantly and is best if done in the chronic phase.
- Other drug choices are alpha-interferon, fludarabine (Fludara), and cytosine, or oral chemotherapy (hydroxyurea or busulfan) in the chronic phase.
- An oral formulation of a tyrosine kinase inhibitor, STI-571 (marketed as Gleevec, or imatinib mesylate)
- Leukapheresis may be needed if the white blood cell count exceeds 300,000/mm.
- In the transformation phase, treatment is the same chemotherapy regimen that is used in ALL.
- Bone marrow transplant and peripheral blood stem cell transplantation are additional treatment strategies.

Nursing Management

Nursing management is similar to that for chronic lymphocytic leukemia. See Nursing Management under Leukemia for additional information.

For more information, see Chapter 33 in Smeltzer and Bare: *Brunner and Suddarth's Textbook of Medical-Surgical Nursing*, 11th edition. Philadelphia: Lippincott Williams & Wilkins, 2008.

Lung Abscess

A lung abscess is a localized necrotic lesion of the lung parenchyma containing purulent materials; the lesion collapses and forms a cavity. Most lung abscesses occur because of aspiration of nasopharyngeal or oral anaerobes into the lung. Abscesses may also occur secondary to mechanical or functional obstruction of the bronchi. At-risk patients include those with impaired cough reflexes, loss of glottal closures, or swallowing difficulties, which may cause aspiration of foreign material. Other at-risk patients include those with central nervous system disorders (seizure, stroke, altered mental status, drug or alcohol addiction) or esophageal disease, those with compromised immune function, and those fed by nasogastric tube. The site of lung abscess is related to gravity and is determined by the patient's position. For patients in a recumbent position, the posterior segment of the upper right lobe is the most common site. The organisms most frequently associated with lung abscess are *Klebsiella* species and *Staphylococcus aureus*.

Clinical Manifestations

- The clinical features vary from a mild productive cough to acute illness.
- Fever is accompanied by a productive cough of moderate to copious amounts of foul-smelling sputum, often bloody.

- Pleurisy, or dull chest pain, dyspnea, weakness, anorexia, and weight loss are common.
- Chest dullness on percussion and decreased or absent breath sounds are found, with an intermittent pleural friction rub and possibly crackles on auscultation.

Assessment and Diagnostic Methods

Chest radiograph, sputum culture, and fiberoptic bronchoscopy are performed. A computed tomography (CT) scan of the chest may be required.

Medical Management

Prevention

To reduce the risk for lung abscess, give appropriate antibiotic therapy before dental procedures and maintain adequate dental and oral hygiene. Give appropriate antimicrobial therapy for pneumonia.

Treatment

Findings of the history, physical examination, chest radiograph, and sputum culture indicate type of organism and treatment.

- Coughing, postural drainage (chest physiotherapy), and possibly percutaneous catheter placement or, infrequently, bronchoscopy for abscess drainage are used.
- The patient is advised to eat a high-protein, high-calorie diet.
- Surgical intervention is rare. Pulmonary resection (lobectomy) is performed when there is massive hemoptysis or no response to medical management.

Pharmacologic Therapy

- Intravenous antimicrobial therapy: clindamycin (Cleocin) is the medication of choice. Meropenem (Merrem) or piperacillin/tazobactam (Zosyn) is also prescribed. Large intravenous doses are required because the antibiotic must penetrate necrotic tissue and abscess fluid.

- Antibiotics are administered orally instead of intravenously after signs of improvement (normal temperature, lowered white blood cell count, and improvement on chest x-ray [reduction in size of cavity]). Antibiotic therapy may last 4 to 8 weeks.

Nursing Management

- Administer antibiotic and intravenous therapy as prescribed, and monitor for any adverse effects.
- Initiate chest physiotherapy as prescribed to drain abscess.
- Teach patient deep-breathing and coughing exercises.
- Encourage diet high in protein and calories.
- Provide emotional support; abscess may take a long time to resolve.
- Teach patient or caregiver how to change dressings to prevent skin excoriation and offensive odor.
- Perform deep-breathing and coughing exercises every 2 hours during the day.
- Teach postural drainage and percussion techniques to caregiver.
- Provide counseling for attaining and maintaining an optimal state of nutrition.
- Emphasize importance of completing antibiotic regimen, rest, and appropriate activity levels to prevent relapse.
- Arrange home health nursing and visits by an intravenous therapy nurse to administer intravenous antibiotic therapy.

For more information, see Chapter 23 in Smeltzer and Bare: *Brunner and Suddarth's Textbook of Medical-Surgical Nursing*, 11th edition. Philadelphia: Lippincott Williams & Wilkins, 2008.

Lymphedema and Elephantiasis

Lymphedema is classified as primary (congenital malformations) or secondary (acquired obstruction). Tissues in the extremities swell because of an increased quantity of lymph that results from an obstruction of the lymphatic vessels. It is especially marked when the extremity is in a dependent position. The most common type is congenital lymphedema (lymphedema praecox), caused by hypoplasia of the lymphatic system of the lower extremity. It is usually seen in women and appears first between the ages of 15 and 25 years. The obstruction may be in both the lymph nodes and the lymphatic vessels. At times, it is seen in the arm after a radical mastectomy and in the leg in association with varicose veins or a chronic thrombophlebitis (from lymphangitis). Lymphatic obstruction caused by a parasite (filaria) is seen frequently in the tropics. When chronic swelling is present, there may be frequent bouts of infection (high fever and chills) and increased residual edema after inflammation resolves. These lead to chronic fibrosis, thickening of the subcutaneous tissues, and hypertrophy of the skin. The condition in which chronic swelling of the extremity recedes only slightly with elevation is referred to as elephantiasis.

L

Medical Management

- Strict bed rest with leg elevation to help mobilize fluids
- Active and passive exercise to assist in moving lymphatic fluid into the bloodstream; also manual lymphatic drainage (a massage technique)
- External compression devices
- Custom-fitted elastic stockings, when patient is ambulatory

Pharmacologic Therapy

- Diuretic therapy, initially with furosemide (Lasix) to prevent fluid overload, and other diuretic therapy palliatively for lymphedema
- Antibiotic therapy if lymphangitis or cellulitis is present

Surgical Management

Excision of affected tissue and fascia with skin grafting, or relocation of lymphatic vessels if edema is severe and uncontrolled by medical therapy, if infection is present, or if mobility is severely compromised

Nursing Management

- Teach patient to perform self-care by inspecting the skin for evidence of infection, elevating the extremities, and performing passive and active exercises.
- If the patient undergoes surgery, provide standard postsurgical care of skin grafts and flaps, elevate the affected extremity, and observe for complications constantly (eg, flap necrosis, hematoma, or abscess under the flap, cellulitis).
- Instruct the patient receiving antibiotics to take the medication exactly as prescribed.

For more information, see Chapter 31 in Smeltzer and Bare: *Brunner and Suddarth's Textbook of Medical-Surgical Nursing*, 11th edition. Philadelphia: Lippincott Williams & Wilkins, 2008.

Mastoiditis and Mastoid Surgery

Mastoiditis is an inflammation of the mastoid resulting from an infection of the middle ear (otitis media). Since the discovery of antibiotics, acute mastoiditis has been rare. Chronic otitis media may cause chronic mastoiditis. Chronic mastoiditis can lead to the formation of cholesteatoma (ingrowth of the skin of the external layer of the eardrum into the middle ear). If mastoiditis is untreated, osteomyelitis may occur.

Clinical Manifestations

- Pain and tenderness behind the ear (postauricular)
- Discharge from the middle ear (otorrhea)
- Mastoid area that becomes erythematous and edematous
- Otoscopic evaluation of the tympanic membrane reveals cholesteatoma

Medical Management

General symptoms are usually successfully treated with antibiotics; occasionally, myringotomy is required.

Surgical Management

If recurrent or persistent tenderness, fever, headache, and discharge from the ear are evident, mastoidectomy may be necessary to remove the cholesteatoma and gain access to diseased structures.

▌ NURSING MANAGEMENT: The Patient Undergoing Mastoid Surgery

Assessment

- During the health history, collect data about the ear problem, including infection, otalgia, otorrhea, hearing loss and vertigo, duration and intensity, causation, prior treatments, health problems, current medications, family history, and drug allergies.
- During the physical assessment, observe for erythema, edema, otorrhea, lesions, and odor and color of discharge.
- Review results of audiogram.

Diagnosis

Nursing Diagnoses

- Acute pain related to mastoid surgery
- Risk for infection related to mastoidectomy, placement of grafts, prostheses, or electrodes; surgical trauma to surrounding tissues and structures
- Anxiety related to surgical procedure, potential loss of hearing, potential taste disturbance, and potential loss of facial movement
- Disturbed auditory sensory perception related to ear disorder, surgery, or packing and to potential damage to facial nerve (cranial nerve VII) and chorda tympani nerve
- Risk for trauma related to balance difficulties or vertigo
- Impaired skin integrity related to surgery
- Deficient knowledge about mastoid disease, surgical procedure, and postoperative care and expectations

Planning and Goals

Major goals for mastoidectomy include reduced anxiety; comfort; prevention of infection; stable or improved hearing and communication; absence of injury or vertigo; absence of, or adjustment to, sensory perceptual alterations; return of skin

M

integrity; and increased knowledge regarding disease, surgical procedure, and postoperative care.

Nursing Interventions

Reducing Anxiety

Reinforce information the otologic surgeon has discussed: anesthesia, the location of the incision (postauricular), and expected surgical results (hearing, balance, taste, and facial movement). Encourage patient to discuss any anxiety or concerns.

Relieving Pain

- Administer prescribed analgesic agent for the first 24 hours postoperatively and then only as needed.
- Instruct patient in use of and side effects of medication.
- If a tympanoplasty is also performed, inform patient that he or she may have packing or a wick in the external auditory canal and may experience sharp shooting pains in the ear for 2 to 3 weeks postoperatively.

Preventing Infection

- Explain prescribed prophylactic antibiotic regimen.
- Instruct patient to keep water from entering the ear for 6 weeks and to keep postauricular incision dry for 2 days.
- Observe for and report signs of infection (fever, purulent drainage).
- Inform patient that some serous drainage is normal postoperatively.

Improving Hearing and Communication

- Initiate measures to improve hearing and communication: reduce environmental noise, face patient when speaking, speak clearly and distinctly without shouting. Provide good lighting if patient must speech-read and use nonverbal clues.
- Instruct family that patient will have temporarily reduced hearing from surgery as a result of edema, packing, and fluid in middle ear; instruct family in ways to improve communication with patient.

Increasing Knowledge

- Inform patient about the surgery and operating room environment.
- Discuss postoperative expectations to decrease anxiety about the unknown.
- Provide postoperative instructions for mastoid surgery as appropriate for particular otologic surgeon's preferences.

Improving Sensory Perception

- Reinforce to patient that a taste disturbance and dry mouth may be experienced on the operated side for several months until the nerve regenerates.
- Instruct patient to report immediately any evidence of facial nerve (cranial nerve VII) weakness, such as drooping of the mouth on the operated side.
- Stress the importance of safety measures at home to prevent falls and injury.

M

Promoting Home and Community-Based Care

- Provide instructions about prescribed medications: analgesics, antivertiginous agents, and antihistamines for balance disturbance.
- Inform patient about the expected effects and potential side effects of the medications.
- Instruct patient about any activity restrictions.
- Teach patient to monitor for possible complications, such as infection, facial nerve weakness, or taste disturbances, including signs and symptoms to report immediately.
- Refer patients, particularly elderly patients, for home care nursing.
- Caution caregiver and patient that patient may experience some vertigo and will therefore require help with ambulation to avoid falling.
- Instruct patient to report promptly any symptoms of complications to the surgeon.
- Stress the importance of scheduling and keeping follow-up appointments.

Evaluation

Expected Patient Outcomes

- Demonstrates reduced anxiety about surgical procedure
- Remains free of discomfort or pain
- Demonstrates no signs or symptoms of infection
- Exhibits signs that hearing has stabilized or improved
- Remains free of injury and trauma secondary to vertigo
- Experiences adjustment to or remains free of altered sensory perception
- Demonstrates no skin breakdown
- Demonstrates understanding (as confirmed by conversation) about the reasons for and methods of care and treatment

---

For more information, see Chapter 59 in Smeltzer and Bare: *Brunner and Suddarth's Textbook of Medical-Surgical Nursing*, 11th edition. Philadelphia: Lippincott Williams & Wilkins, 2008.

M

Ménière's Disease

Ménière's disease is an abnormal inner ear fluid balance (too much circulatory fluid) caused by malabsorption in the endolymphatic sac or blockage in the duct. Endolymphatic hydrops, a dilation in the endolymphatic space, develops. Either increased pressure in the system or rupture of the inner ear membranes occurs, producing symptoms. Although it has been reported in children, Ménière's disease is more common in adults, with the average age of onset in the fourth decade of life. There is no cure. There are two possible subsets of the disease: cochlear and vestibular.

Clinical Manifestations

Ménière's disease presents with four major symptoms: (1) episodic incapacitating vertigo (lasting minutes to hours, with nausea and vomiting), (2) tinnitus or a roaring sound, (3) fluctuating progressive sensorineural hearing loss, and (4) a feeling of pressure or fullness in the ear. At the onset, only one or two symptoms are manifested. Attacks occur with increasing frequency until eventually all of the symptoms develop.

Cochlear Disease

Cochlear disease is recognized as a fluctuating progressive sensorineural hearing loss associated with tinnitus and aural pressure without vertigo.

Vestibular Disease

Vestibular disease is characterized by the episodic vertigo associated with the aural pressure and no cochlear symptoms. Diaphoresis and a persistent feeling of disequilibrium may last for days. Usually only one ear is involved, but both ears are affected in about 20% of patients.

Assessment and Diagnostic Methods

- Disease is not diagnosed until the four major symptoms are present; careful history of vertigo and nausea and vomiting contributes to diagnosis.
- There is no absolute diagnostic test for this disease.
- Audiovestibular diagnostic procedures, including Weber's test, are used with finding of sensorineural hearing loss in the affected ear.
- Electronystagmogram may be normal or may show reduced vestibular response.
- Other laboratory and radiographic tests are performed to rule out other causes for symptoms.

Medical Management

Goals of treatment may include recommendations for changes in lifestyle and habits or surgical treatment. The treatment is designed to eliminate vertigo or to stop the progression of or stabilize the disease.

- Treatment approaches are rehabilitative, dietary, medical, and surgical.

M

- Psychological evaluation may be indicated if patient is anxious, uncertain, fearful, or depressed.

Pharmacologic Therapy

- Tranquilizers and antihistamines such as meclizine (Antivert) to control vertigo and to suppress the vestibular system; antiemetics for nausea and vomiting
- Diuretics to lower pressure in the endolymphatic system
- Vasodilators are often used in conjunction with other therapies.
- Middle and inner ear perfusion or systemic injections of ototoxic medications: streptomycin, gentamicin to eliminate vertigo; procedure is highly successful in decreasing vertigo but is accompanied by a significant risk for hearing loss

Dietary Management

- Low sodium (2,000 mg/day)
- Avoidance of alcohol, nicotine, and caffeine

Surgical Management

- Endolymphatic sac decompression or shunt
- Middle and inner ear perfusion with placement of intraotologic catheters for drainage and infusion of medication (see Pharmacologic Therapy)
- Labyrinthectomy (destruction of inner ear)
- Vestibular nerve section (eighth cranial nerve)

NURSING MANAGEMENT: The Patient with Vertigo

Assessment

- Obtain a history of symptoms, causative factors, and alleviating factors.

- Determine extent of disability related to activities of daily living as well as emotional response to symptoms.
- Elicit medications being taken, including over-the-counter drugs.

Diagnosis

Nursing Diagnoses

- Risk for injury related to altered mobility because of gait disturbance and vertigo
- Impaired adjustment related to disability requiring change in lifestyle because of unpredictability of vertigo
- Risk for fluid volume imbalance and deficit related to increased fluid output, altered intake, and medications
- Anxiety related to threat of, or change in, health status and disabling effects of vertigo
- Ineffective coping related to personal vulnerability and unmet expectations stemming from vertigo
- Feeding, bathing/hygiene, dressing/grooming, and toileting self-care deficits related to labyrinth dysfunction and episodes of vertigo

M

Planning and Goals

Patient goals include avoidance of injuries associated with imbalance or falls; adjustments to lifestyle to decrease disability and exert maximum control and independence; normal fluid and electrolyte balance; decreased anxiety; self-care ability; and absence of complications.

Nursing Interventions

Preventing Injury

- Assess for vertigo.
- Assist patient in identifying aura that suggests an impending attack.
- Encourage patient to sit down when dizzy.

- Recommend that patient keep eyes open and stare straight ahead when lying down and experiencing vertigo; place pillows on side of head to restrict movement.
- Reinforce vestibular and balance therapy as prescribed.
- Administer and teach about antivertiginous medication and vestibular sedation; instruct in side effects.

Adjusting to Disability

- Encourage patient to identify personal strengths and roles that can be fulfilled.
- Provide information about vertigo and what to expect.
- Include family and significant others in rehabilitative process.
- Encourage patient in making decisions and assuming more responsibility for care.

Maintaining Fluid Volume

- Assess intake and output; monitor laboratory values.
- Assess indicators of dehydration.
- Encourage oral fluids as tolerated; avoid caffeine (a vestibular stimulant).
- Teach about antiemetics and antidiarrheal medications.

Relieving Anxiety

- Assess level of anxiety; help identify successful coping skills.
- Encourage patient to discuss anxieties and explore concerns about vertigo attacks.
- Teach stress management; provide comfort measures.

Monitoring and Managing Complications

- Assist patient in preparing for diagnostic tests.
- Prepare patient for surgery if indicated.
- Observe for potential complications.
- Assist unsteady patient as required; expect vertigo and nausea after labyrinthectomy.
- Arrange for psychosocial and family support as necessary.
- Provide patient and family with hearing aid information.

Promoting Home and Community-Based Care
Teaching Patients Self-Care

- Teach patient to administer antiemetic and other prescribed medications to relieve nausea and vomiting.
- Encourage patient to care for bodily needs when free of vertigo.
- Review diet with patient and caregivers; offer fluids as necessary.

For more information, see Chapter 59 in Smeltzer and Bare: *Brunner and Suddarth's Textbook of Medical-Surgical Nursing*, 11th edition. Philadelphia: Lippincott Williams & Wilkins, 2008.

Meningitis

Meningitis is an inflammation of the meninges (membranes surrounding the brain and spinal cord). Types of meningitis include aseptic, septic, and tuberculous. The aseptic form may be viral or secondary to lymphoma, leukemia, or brain abscess. The septic form is caused by bacteria such as *Neisseria meningitidis*.

Pathophysiology

The causative organism enters the bloodstream, crosses the blood-brain barrier, and triggers an inflammatory reaction in the meninges. Independent of the causative agent, inflammation of the subarachnoid and pia mater occurs. Increased intracranial pressure (ICP) results. Meningeal infections generally originate in one of two ways: either through the bloodstream from other infections (cellulitis) or by direct extension (after a traumatic injury to the facial bones). In a few cases, the cause is iatrogenic or secondary to invasive procedures (lumbar puncture) or devices (ICP monitoring devices) or to opportunistic infections, such as acquired immunodeficiency syndrome (AIDS) or Lyme disease.

Bacterial meningitis is the most significant form. The common bacterial pathogens are *N. meningitidis* (meningococcal meningitis), *Streptococcus pneumoniae* (in adults), and *Haemophilus influenzae* (in children and young adults). These three organisms account for about 75% of the cases. Mode of transmission is direct contact, including droplets and discharges from the nose and throat of carriers or infected people. Bacterial meningitis starts as an infection of the oropharynx and is followed by septicemia, which extends to the meninges of the brain and upper region of the spinal cord.

Clinical Manifestations of Bacterial Meningitis

Severe headache and fever are frequently initial symptoms; these symptoms result from infection and increased ICP. Additional manifestations include changes in level of consciousness and disorientation and memory impairment early in the illness. Lethargy, unresponsiveness, and coma may develop as the illness progresses. Signs of meningeal irritation include the following:

- Nuchal rigidity (stiff neck) is an early sign.
- Positive Kernig's sign: when lying with thigh flexed on abdomen, patient cannot completely extend leg
- Positive Brudzinski's sign: flexing patient's neck produces flexion of the knees and hips; passive flexion of lower extremity of one side produces similar movement for opposite extremity
- Photophobia (extreme sensitivity to light) is common.
- Seizures (secondary to focal areas of cortical irritability) and increased ICP: signs of increasing ICP include focal motor deficits, widened pulse pressure and bradycardia, respiratory irregularity, headache, vomiting, and depressed levels of consciousness
- Rash (*N. meningitidis*): ranges from petechial rash with purpuric lesions to large areas of ecchymosis

Clinical Manifestations of Meningococcal Meningitis

Ten percent of patients present with a fulminating infection, with signs of overwhelming septicemia.

- Abrupt onset of high fever
- Extensive purpuric lesions (over face and extremities)
- Shock and signs of disseminated intravascular coagulopathy (DIC)
- Death is possible within a few hours of onset of infection.
- In AIDS patients there are few if any symptoms because of the blunted inflammatory response.

Assessment and Diagnostic Findings

Infecting organisms are usually identified through culture and Gram staining of cerebrospinal fluid and blood (polysaccharide antigens support a diagnosis of bacterial meningitis).

Prevention

People who have close contact with patients should be considered candidates for antimicrobial prophylaxis (rifampin). Close contacts of patients should be observed and examined immediately if fever or other signs and symptoms of meningitis develop.

Meningococcal vaccination may be beneficial, particularly for college students and some travelers visiting countries that are experiencing epidemic meningococcal disease. Vaccination should be considered as an adjunct to antibiotic chemoprophylaxis for anyone living with a patient who has meningococcal disease. Polysaccharide vaccine (Haemophilus B polysaccharide vaccine) against invasive *Haemophilus influenzae* type B infection is used routinely in children to prevent meningitis.

Medical Management
Pharmacologic Therapy

- Antimicrobial therapy: penicillin (or piperacillin or ampicillin), or one of the cephalosporins. The treatment for cryptococcal meningitis is intravenous administration of amphotericin B; may be used with or without 5-flucytosine.
- Vancomycin hydrochloride, alone or in combination with rifampin, may be used if resistant strains of bacteria are identified.

- Dexamethasone may be beneficial as adjunct therapy for acute bacterial meningitis and pneumococcal meningitis.
- Fluid volume expanders are used to treat dehydration and shock.
- Diazepam (Valium) or phenytoin (Dilantin) is used to control seizures.
- An osmotic diuretic, such as mannitol, is used to treat cerebral edema.

Nursing Management

Prognosis depends largely on the supportive care provided. Related nursing interventions include the following:

- Monitor vital signs constantly. Determine oxygenation from arterial blood gas values and pulse oximetry.
- Insert cuffed endotracheal tube (or tracheostomy), and place patient on mechanical ventilation as prescribed.
- Give oxygen to maintain arterial partial pressure of oxygen.
- Monitor central venous pressure (CVP) for incipient shock, which precedes cardiac or respiratory failure.
- Note generalized vasoconstriction, circumoral cyanosis, and cold extremities.
- Reduce high fever to decrease load on heart and brain from oxygen demands.
- Rapid intravenous fluid replacement may be prescribed, but take care not to overhydrate patient because of risk of cerebral edema.
- If syndrome of inappropriate antidiuretic hormone (SIADH) secretion is suspected, monitor closely for body weight, serum electrolytes, and urine volume, specific gravity, and osmolality.
- Assess clinical status continuously; evaluate skin and oral hygiene; promote comfort; and protect patient during seizures and while comatose.
- Implement infection control precautions and respiratory isolation until 24 hours after start of antibiotic therapy.

- Inform family about patient's condition and permit family to see patient at appropriate intervals.

For more information, see Chapter 64 in Smeltzer and Bare: *Brunner and Suddarth's Textbook of Medical-Surgical Nursing*, 11th edition. Philadelphia: Lippincott Williams & Wilkins, 2008.

Mitral Regurgitation (Insufficiency)

Mitral regurgitation results when the margins of the mitral valve are unable to close during systole. There is a problem with one or more of the leaflets, the annulus, or the papillary muscles, preventing closure of the leaflets. At each beat, the left ventricle forces some blood back into the left atrium, causing the agent to dilate and hypertrophy. This backward flow of blood from the ventricle eventually causes the lungs to become congested, which adds strain to the right ventricle, resulting in cardiac failure.

M

Clinical Manifestations

Chronic mitral regurgitation is often asymptomatic; but acute regurgitation (after MI) usually presents as severe heart failure.

- Usual symptoms include dyspnea, shortness of breath on exertion, fatigue, weakness, palpitations of the heart, and cough due to chronic passive pulmonary congestion.
- Irregular pulse as a result of either extrasystole or atrial fibrillation may persist indefinitely.

Assessment and Diagnostic Methods

A high-pitched, blowing systolic murmur is heard at the apex. The pulse may be regular and of good volume, or it may be irregular due to dysrhythmia. Doppler echocardiography is used to diagnose and monitor the progression of mitral regurgitation. Transesophageal echocardiography provides good images of the mitral valve.

Medical Management

Management is the same as for heart failure. Surgical intervention consists of mitral valve replacement or valvuloplasty.

For more information, see Chapter 29 in Smeltzer and Bare: *Brunner and Suddarth's Textbook of Medical-Surgical Nursing*, 11th edition. Philadelphia: Lippincott Williams & Wilkins, 2008.

Mitral Stenosis

M

Mitral stenosis is the progressive thickening and contracture of the mitral valve leaflets and chordae tendineae that causes narrowing of the orifice and progressive obstruction to blood flow from the left atrium into the left ventricle. Normally, the mitral valve opening is as wide as three fingers. In cases of marked stenosis, the opening narrows to the width of a pencil. The left atrium dilates and hypertrophies because it has great difficulty moving blood into the ventricle and because of the increased blood volume the atria must now hold. Because there is no valve to protect the pulmonary veins from the backward flow of blood from the atrium, the pulmonary circulation becomes congested. The resulting high pulmonary pressure can eventually lead to right ventricular failure.

Clinical Manifestations

- The first symptom is often dyspnea on exertion (due to pulmonary venous hypertension).
- Progressive fatigue (result of low cardiac output), hemoptysis and cough, and repeated respiratory infections may be noted.

- Weak and often irregular pulse (because of atrial fibrillation) may also be noted.

Assessment and Diagnostic Methods

- Electrocardiography (ECG): atrial dysrhythmia
- Echocardiography to reveal stenosis
- Cardiac catheterization with angiography to reveal severity of stenosis

Medical Management

See Medical Management and Nursing Management under Cardiac Failure for additional information. Additional management measures include:

- Prophylactic antibiotic therapy to prevent recurrence of infections; anticoagulant therapy to reduce risk of thrombi
- Treatment of anemia if required
- Cardiotonics and diuretics for treatment of congestive heart failure
- Strenuous excercise restrictions
- Surgical intervention (valvuloplasty, commissurotomy, or replacement of the mitral valve)
- Percutaneous transluminal valvuloplasty for palliation of symptoms

M

For more information, see Chapter 29 in Smeltzer and Bare: *Brunner and Suddarth's Textbook of Medical-Surgical Nursing*, 11th edition. Philadelphia: Lippincott Williams & Wilkins, 2008.

Mitral Valve Prolapse

Mitral valve prolapse is a dysfunction of the mitral valve leaflets that prevents the mitral valve from closing completely during systole. Blood then regurgitates from the left ventricle back into the left atrium. It occurs more frequently in women.

Clinical Manifestations

The syndrome may produce no symptoms or may progress rapidly and result in sudden death.

- Patients may experience symptoms of fatigue, shortness of breath (not correlated with activity), lightheadedness, dizziness, syncope, palpitations, chest pain, and anxiety.
- Fatigue may be present regardless of the person's activity level and amount of rest or sleep.
- During the physical examination, a mitral (systolic) click is identified. Presence of a click indicates early valvular incompetence.
- The mitral click may deteriorate into a murmur over time as the valve leaflets become more dysfunctional.
- As the murmur progresses, there may be signs and symptoms of heart failure (not common).

Medical Management

Medical management is directed at controlling symptoms.

- Antidysrhythmic agents are prescribed.
- In advanced stages, mitral valve replacement may be necessary.
- Dietary restrictions; avoidance of alcohol and coffeine.

Nursing Management

- Teach patient about antidysrhythmic or antianginal medications, if prescribed.
- Explain that alcohol, ephedrine, and epinephrine, which may be in over-the-counter preparations, may stimulate dysrhythmias. Teach patient to read product labels to avoid these agents.
- Educate patient about the need for prophylactic antibiotic therapy before undergoing invasive procedures (eg, dental work, genitourinary procedures, or gastrointestinal procedures). Patient should consult physician if in doubt about need for antibiotics before a procedure.

- Teach patient about the diagnosis and the possibility that the disorder is hereditary.

For more information, see Chapter 29 in Smeltzer and Bare: *Brunner and Suddarth's Textbook of Medical-Surgical Nursing*, 11th edition. Philadelphia: Lippincott Williams & Wilkins, 2008.

Multiple Myeloma

Multiple myeloma is a malignant disease of plasma cells (B lymphocytes) that infiltrates bone, lymph nodes, liver, spleen, and kidneys. It is not classified as a lymphoma. The malignant cell is the plasma cell, and the neoplastic proliferation takes place mainly in the bone marrow. Median survival is 3 to 5 years, with death resulting from infection or renal failure.

Clinical Manifestations

- Normochromic, normocytic anemia, back pain, and sometimes leukopenia or thrombocytopenia due to bone marrow infiltration by malignant plasma cells
- Constant bone pain that may be incapacitating
- Hypercalcemia and bone fractures are common, especially in the vertebrae or ribs

Assessment and Diagnostic Methods

- Aspiration or biopsy of the bone marrow
- Bence Jones proteins (fragments of abnormal globulins) excreted in urine

Gerontologic Considerations

The incidence of multiple myeloma increases with age. The disease rarely occurs before age 40. Closely investigate any back pain, which is a common presenting complaint.

Medical Management

- Melphalan (Alkeran), cyclophosphamide, and steroids to decrease tumor mass and relieve bone pain
- Radiation to relieve bone pain
- Vertebroplasty and bisphosphonate therapy
- Good hydration to prevent renal damage resulting from Bence Jones proteins in the renal tubules, hypercalcemia, and hyperuricemia
- Narcotic analgesics, thalidomide, and bortezomib for refractory disease and severe pain

Nursing Management

- Assess patient for signs and symptoms of renal insufficiency.
- Administer medications as recommended for pain relief.
- Teach patient to recognize and report signs and symptoms of hypercalcemia.
- Keep patient as active as possible to prevent pathologic fractures, but patient should avoid heavy lifting (10 pounds or more).
- Observe for bacterial infections (pneumonia).
- Avoid fasting regimens for diagnostic tests because dehydration can precipitate acute renal failure.
- Instruct patient in appropriate infection prevention measures.

For more information, see Chapter 33 in Smeltzer and Bare: *Brunner and Suddarth's Textbook of Medical-Surgical Nursing*, 11th edition. Philadelphia: Lippincott Williams & Wilkins, 2008.

Multiple Sclerosis

Multiple sclerosis (MS) is a chronic, degenerative, progressive disease of the central nervous system characterized by small patches of demyelination in the brain and spinal cord.

Demyelination (destruction of myelin) results in impaired transmission of nerve impulses.

Pathophysiology

The cause of MS is not known, but a defective immune response probably plays a major role. In MS, sensitized T cells inhabit the CNS and facilitate the infiltration of other agents that damage the immune system. The immune system attack leads to inflammation that destroys myelin and oligodendroglial cells that produce myelin in the CNS. Plaques of sclerotic tissue appear on demyelinated axons, further interrupting the transmission of impulses. Demyelination interrupts the flow of nerve impulses.

MS is more common in people living in northern temperate zones. It is one of the most disabling neurologic diseases of young adults (20 to 40 years), and it affects more women than men.

Disease Course

M

MS has various courses:

- Relapsing-remitting course, with complete recovery between relapses
- Chronic primary progressive course from the onset, with a progressive decline in function and the potential development of quadriparesis, cognitive dysfunction, visual loss and brain-stem syndromes
- Benign course with a normal life span; symptoms are so mild that patients do not seek treatment

Clinical Manifestations

- Signs and symptoms are varied and multiple and reflect the location of the lesion (plaque) or combination of lesions.
- Primary symptoms: pain, fatigue, weakness, numbness, difficulty in coordination, and loss of balance
- Visual disturbances: blurring of vision, double vision, patchy blindness (scotoma), or total blindness

- Spastic weakness of the extremities and loss of abdominal reflexes; ataxia and tremor
- Sensory dysfunction
- Cognitive and psychosocial problems; depression, emotional lability, and euphoria
- Bladder, bowel, and sexual problems possible

Secondary Manifestations Related to Complications

- Urinary tract infections, constipation
- Pressure ulcers, contracture deformities, dependent pedal edema
- Pneumonia
- Reactive depressions and decreased bone mass
- Emotional, social, marital, economic, and vocational problems

M

Exacerbations and Remissions

- Relapses may be associated with periods of emotional and physical stress.
- There is evidence that remyelination occurs in some patients.

Assessment and Diagnostic Findings

- Magnetic resonance imaging (MRI) (primary diagnostic tool) to visualize small plaques, evaluate course and effect of treatment
- Electrophoresis study of the cerebrospinal fluid (CSF); abnormal immunoglobulin G antibody (oligoclonal bonding) appears in the CSF in up to 95% of patients
- Neuropsychological testing as indicated to assess cognitive impairment
- Sexual history to identify changes in sexual function
- Evoked potential studies and urodynamic studies

Medical Management

Because no cure exists for MS, the goals of treatment are to delay the progression of the disease, manage chronic symptoms, and treat acute exacerbations. An individualized treatment program is indicated to relieve symptoms (spasticity, fatigue, bladder dysfunction, and ataxia) and provide support. Management strategies target the various motor and sensory symptoms and effects of immobility that can occur. Radiation therapy may be used to induce immunosuppression.

Pharmacologic Therapy

- "ABC" drugs: interferon-beta-1a (Avonex) and beta-1b (Betaseron) and glatiramer acetate (Copaxone) for relapsing-remitting MS
- Mitoxantrone (Novantrone) is an antineoplastic agent recently approved to treat secondary progressive MS.
- Immunotherapeutic medications to modulate the immune response and reduce the rate at which the disease progresses and the frequency and severity of exacerbations (azathioprine, interferon, cyclophosphamide)
- Corticosteroids (eg, intravenous methylprednisolone) and adrenocorticotropic hormone (ACTH) as anti-inflammatory agents and to improve nerve conduction
- Amantadine (Symmetrel), pemoline (Cylert), or fluoxetine (Prozac) to treat fatigue
- Medications used to treat ataxia include beta-adrenergic blockers (Inderal), antiseizure agents (Neurontin), and benzodiazepines (Klonopin, Valium).
- Baclofen: treatment of choice for spasticity

Management of Related Bowel and Bladder Problems

Anticholinergics, alpha-adrenergic blockers, or antispasmodic agents may be used to treat problems related to elimination, and patients may be taught to perform intermittent self-catheterization as well. Additional measures include assessment of urinary tract infections; ascorbic acid to acidify urine; antibiotics when appropriate.

NURSING PROCESS: The Patient with Multiple Sclerosis

Assessment

- Assess actual and potential problems associated with the disease: neurologic problems, secondary complications, and impact of disease on patient and family.
- Assess patient's function, particularly ambulation, when patient is well rested and when fatigued; look for weakness, spasticity, visual impairment, and incontinence.
- Assess lifestyle and sexual history for specific areas of concern.

Diagnosis

Nursing Diagnoses

- Impaired physical mobility related to weakness, muscle paresis, spasticity
- Risk for injury related to sensory and visual impairment
- Impaired urinary and bowel elimination related to nervous system dysfunction
- Disturbed thought processes (loss of memory, dementia, euphoria) related to cerebral dysfunction
- Ineffective individual coping related to uncertainty of diagnosis
- Impaired home maintenance management related to physical, psychological, and social limits imposed by MS
- Impaired speech and swallowing related to cranial nerve involvement
- Potential for sexual dysfunction related to spinal cord involvement or psychological reactions to condition

Planning and Goals

The major goals of the patient may include physical mobility, avoidance of injury, bladder and bowel continence, improved cognitive function, coping skills, improved self-care, adaptation to sexual dysfunction, and adequate speech and swallowing.

Nursing Interventions

Promoting Physical Mobility

- Encourage progressive resistance exercises to strengthen weak muscles.
- Encourage patient to work up to a point just short of fatigue. Relaxation and coordination exercises promote muscle efficiency.
- Advise patient to take frequent short rest periods, preferably lying down, to prevent extreme fatigue.
- Encourage walking exercises to improve gait.
- Apply warm packs to spastic muscles; avoid hot baths due to sensory loss.
- Encourage daily exercises for muscle stretching to minimize joint contractures.
- Encourage swimming, stationary bicycling, and progressive weight bearing to relieve spasticity in legs.
- Avoid hurrying patient in any activity, because hurrying increases spasticity.
- Prevent complications of immobility by assessment and maintenance of skin integrity and through coughing and deep-breathing exercises.

M

Preventing Injury

- Teach patient to walk with feet wide apart to increase walking stability if motor dysfunction causes incoordination.
- Teach patient to watch the feet while walking if there is a loss of position sense.
- Provide a wheelchair or motorized scooter if gait remains insufficient after gait training (walker, cane, braces, crutches, parallel bars, and physical therapy).
- Assess skin for pressure ulcers if patient is confined to wheelchair.

Enhancing Bladder and Bowel Control

- Keep bedpan or urinal readily available because the need to void must be heeded immediately.
- Set up a voiding schedule, with gradual lengthening of time intervals.
- Instruct patient to drink a measured amount of fluid every 2 hours and to attempt to void 30 minutes after drinking.
- Encourage patient to take prescribed medications for bladder spasticity.
- Teach intermittent self-catheterization, if necessary.
- Provide adequate fluids, dietary fiber, and a bowel-training program for bowel problems, including constipation, fecal impaction, and incontinence.

Improving Sensory and Cognitive Function

- Provide an eye patch or eyeglass occluder to block visual impulses of one eye when diplopia (double vision) occurs.
- Advise patient about free talking-book services.
- Refer patient and family to a speech-language pathologist when mechanisms of speech are involved.
- Provide compassion and emotional support to patient and family to adapt to new self-image and to cope with life disruption.
- Keep a structured environment; use lists and other memory aids to help patient maintain a daily routine.

Strengthening Coping Mechanisms

- Alleviate stress, and make referrals for counseling and support to minimize adverse effects of dealing with chronic illness.
- Provide information on the illness to patient and family.
- Help patient define problems and develop alternatives for management.

Improving Self-Care Abilities

- Suggest modifications that allow independence in self-care activities at home (raised toilet seat, bathing aids, telephone

modifications, long-handled comb, tongs, modified clothing).
- Avoid physical and emotional stress when possible.
- Maintain moderate environmental temperature; heat increases fatigue and muscle weakness and extreme cold may increase spasticity.

Managing Speech and Swallowing Difficulties

- Arrange for evaluation by a speech therapist. Reinforce this instruction and encourage patient and family to adhere to the plan.
- Reduce the risk for aspiration by careful feeding, proper positioning for eating, having suction apparatus available.

Promoting Sexual Function

Suggest a sexual counselor to assist patient and partner with sexual dysfunction (eg, erectile and ejaculatory disorders in men; orgasmic dysfunction and adductor spasms of the thigh muscles in women; bladder and bowel incontinence; urinary tract infections).

M

Promoting Home and Community-Based Care

Teaching Patients Self-Care

- Teach patient and family about use of assistive devices, self-catheterization, and administration of medications.
- Assist patient and family to deal with new disabilities and changes as disease progresses.

Continuing Care

- Refer for home health care nursing assistance as indicated.
- Encourage patient to contact the local chapter of the National Multiple Sclerosis Society for services, publications, and contact with other MS patients.
- Teach and reinforce new self-care techniques.
- Assess changes in patient's health status and coping strategies.
- Reinforce the importance of follow-up care.

Evaluation

Expected Patient Outcomes

- Reports improved physical mobility
- Remains free of injury
- Attains or maintains improved bladder and bowel control
- Participates in gait training and rehabilitation programs
- Compensates for altered thought processes
- Demonstrates improved coping strategies
- Adheres to plan for home maintenance management
- Participates in strategies to improve speech and swallowing
- Adapts to changes in sexual function

For more information, see Chapter 64 in Smeltzer and Bare: *Brunner and Suddarth's Textbook of Medical-Surgical Nursing*, 11th edition. Philadelphia: Lippincott Williams & Wilkins, 2008.

M | Muscular Dystrophies

Muscular dystrophies are a group of chronic muscle disorders characterized by a progressive weakening and wasting of the skeletal or voluntary muscles. Most are inherited. The pathologic features include degeneration and loss of muscle fibers, variation in muscle fiber size, phagocytosis and regeneration, and replacement of muscle tissue by connective tissue. Types of symptoms are affected by patterns of inheritance, muscles involved, age of onset, and rate of progression.

Clinical Manifestations

Muscle wasting and weakness; cardiomyopathy is a common complication in all forms of muscular dystrophy.

Assessment and Diagnostic Findings

- Abnormal elevation in serum creatinine phosphokinase (CPK)
- Myopathic electromyography (EMG) pattern
- Myopathic findings on muscle biopsy

Medical Management

Treatment focuses on supportive care and prevention of complications. Supportive management is intended to keep patients active and functioning as normally as possible and to minimize functional deterioration. A therapeutic exercise program is individualized to prevent muscle tightness, contractures, and disuse atrophy. Night splints and stretching exercises are employed to delay joint contractures (especially ankles, knees, and hips). Braces may be used to compensate for muscle weakness. The patient may be fitted with an orthotic jacket to improve sitting stability, reduce trunk deformity, and support cardiovascular status. Spinal fusion may be performed to maintain spinal stability. All upper respiratory infections and fractures from falls are treated vigorously to minimize immobilization and to prevent joint contractures.

Advise genetic counseling because of the genetic nature of this disease. Also advise patient to consult with appropriate caregivers for dental and speech problems and gastrointestinal tract problems that result in gastric dilation, rectal prolapse, and fecal impaction.

M

Nursing Management

The goals are to maintain function at optimal levels and enhance the quality of life.

- Attend to patient's physical requirements and emotional and developmental needs.
- Actively involve patient and family in decision making, including end-of-life decisions.
- During hospitalization for treatment of complications, assess knowledge and expertise of patient and family responsible for giving care in the home. Assist patient and family to maintain coping strategies used at home while in the hospital.
- Provide patient and family with information about the disorder, its anticipated course, and care and management strategies that will optimize patient's growth and development and physical and psychological status.

- Communicate recommendations to all members of the health care team so that they work toward common goals.
- Encourage patient to use self-help devices to achieve greater independence; assist adolescents to make transition to adulthood. Encourage education and job tracking as appropriate.
- Encourage range-of-motion exercises to prevent disabling contractures.
- When teaching family to monitor patient for respiratory problems, give information regarding appropriate respiratory support, such as negative-pressure devices and positive-pressure ventilators.
- Assist family in adjusting home environment to maximize functional independence; patient may require manual or electric wheelchair, gait aids, seating systems, bathroom equipment, lifts, ramps, and additional activity of daily living aids.
- Assess for signs of depression, prolonged anger, bargaining, or denial and help patient to cope and adapt to chronic disease. Arrange for referral to a psychiatric nurse clinician or other mental health professional if indicated to assist patient to cope and adapt to the disease.
- Provide a hopeful, supportive, and nurturing environment.

For more information, see Chapter 65 in Smeltzer and Bare: *Brunner and Suddarth's Textbook of Medical-Surgical Nursing*, 11th edition. Philadelphia: Lippincott Williams & Wilkins, 2008.

Musculoskeletal Trauma (Contusions, Strains, Sprains and Joint Dislocations)

Injury to one part of the musculoskeletal system usually results in injury or dysfunction of adjacent structures and of structures enclosed or supported by them. If the bone is broken, the muscles cannot function, and blood vessels and nerves in the vicinity of the fracture may be injured. If motor nerves do not send impulses to the muscles, as in paralysis, the bones cannot move. If the joint surfaces do not articulate normally, neither the bones nor the muscles can function properly.

Contusions, Strains, and Sprains

A contusion is a soft tissue injury produced by blunt force (eg, a blow, kick, or fall). Many small blood vessels rupture and bleed into soft tissues (ecchymosis, or bruising). A hematoma develops when the bleeding is sufficient to cause an appreciable collection of blood. Most contusions resolve in 1 to 2 weeks.

A strain is a "muscle pull" from overuse, overstretching, or excessive stress. Strains are microscopic, incomplete muscle tears with some bleeding into the tissue.

A sprain is an injury to the ligaments surrounding a joint, caused by a wrenching or twisting motion. A torn ligament loses its stabilizing ability. Blood vessels rupture and edema occurs.

M

Joint Dislocations

A dislocation of a joint is a condition in which the articular surfaces of the bones forming the joint are no longer in anatomic contact. The bones are literally "out of joint." Dislocations may be congenital, present at birth (most often the hip); spontaneous or pathologic, due to disease of the articular or the periarticular structures; or traumatic, resulting from injury in which the joint is disrupted by force. A subluxation is a partial dislocation of the articulating surfaces. Traumatic dislocations are orthopedic emergencies because the associated joint structures, blood supply, and nerves are distorted and severely stressed. If the dislocation is not treated promptly, avascular necrosis (tissue death due to anoxia and diminished blood supply) and nerve palsy may occur.

Clinical Manifestations

- Contusion: local symptoms (pain, swelling, and discoloration)
- Strain: soreness or sudden pain with local tenderness on muscle use and isometric contraction
- Sprain: tenderness of the joint, painful movement; increased disability and pain the first 2 to 3 hours after injury because of associated swelling and bleeding
- Dislocation or subluxation: pain, change in contour of joint, change in length of extremity, loss of normal mobility, and change in the axis of the dislocated bones

Assessment and Diagnostic Methods

X-ray examination to evaluate for bone injury (eg, avulsion fracture, in which a bone fragment is pulled away by a ligament or tendon), which may be associated with a sprain

M

Medical Management

Treatment of injury of the musculoskeletal system involves providing support for the injured part until healing is complete. Treatment of contusions, strains, and sprains consists of rest, applying ice, applying a compression bandage, and elevating the affected part (RICE: rest, ice, compression, elevation).

- Ice or some form of moist or dry cold is applied intermittently for 20 to 30 minutes during the first 24 to 48 hours after injury to produce vasoconstriction, which decreases bleeding, edema, and discomfort. Avoid excessive cold because it could cause skin and tissue damage.
- An elastic compression bandage controls bleeding, reduces edema, and provides support for the injured tissues.
- Elevation controls the swelling. If the sprain is severe (torn muscle fibers and disrupted ligaments), surgical repair or

cast immobilization may be necessary so that the joint will not lose its stability.

- After the acute inflammatory stage (eg, 24 to 48 hours after injury), heat may be applied intermittently (for 15 to 30 minutes, four times a day) to relieve muscle spasm and to promote vasodilation, absorption, and repair.
- Depending on the severity of injury, progressive passive and active exercises may begin in 2 to 5 days.
- Severe sprains may require 1 to 3 weeks of immobilization before protected exercises are initiated.
- Strains and sprains take weeks or months to heal. Splinting may be used to prevent reinjury.
- With a dislocation, the affected joint needs to be immobilized while the patient is transported to the hospital.
- The dislocation is promptly reduced (ie, displaced parts brought into normal position) to preserve joint function. Analgesia, muscle relaxants, and possibly anesthesia are used to facilitate closed reduction.
- The joint is immobilized by bandages, splints, casts, or traction and is maintained in a stable position.
- Several days to weeks after reduction, gentle, progressive, active, and passive movement three or four times a day is begun to preserve range of motion and restore strength.
- The joint is supported between exercise sessions.

Nursing Management

- Administer analgesic agents and provide measures to promote comfort.
- Evaluate neurovascular status frequently (eg, circulation, motion, sensation).
- Protect the joint during healing.
- Teach patient about pain management, medications (analgesics, antibiotics), cast care, wound care, possible complications (eg, altered neurovascular status, infection, skin breakdown), and self-care.

- Teach patient proper use of ambulatory devices, the healing process, and activity limitations to promote healing.
- Teach patient how to manage the immobilizing devices and how to protect the joint from reinjury.

For more information, see Chapter 69 in Smeltzer and Bare: *Brunner and Suddarth's Textbook of Medical-Surgical Nursing*, 11th edition. Philadelphia: Lippincott Williams & Wilkins, 2008.

Myasthenia Gravis

Myasthenia gravis (MG) is an autoimmune disorder affecting the myoneural junction. Antibodies (most often autoantibodies) are directed at the neurotransmitter (acetylcholine) receptor on the motor end plate, disrupting the transmission to the voluntary muscles of the body. Excessive weakness and fatigability occur. It affects women between the ages of 20 and 40 years and men older than 40 years.

M

Clinical Manifestations

MG is purely a motor disorder, with no effect on sensation or coordination. Symptoms include extreme muscular weakness and easy fatigability, which worsen after effort and are relieved by rest. Symptoms vary according to the muscles affected:

- Early symptoms: diplopia and ptosis
- Sleepy, masklike expression because facial muscles are affected
- Dysphonia (voice impairment), with nasal sound or difficulty in articulation
- Problems with chewing and swallowing, which can present danger of choking and aspiration
- Weakness of arm and hand muscles, less commonly leg muscles
- Progressive weakness of diaphragm and intercostal muscles, which may produce respiratory distress (an acute emergency)

Assessment and Diagnostic Findings

- Presumptive diagnosis is based on history and physical examination. A patient presenting with ocular, bulbar symptoms or fluctuating weakness will need a diagnostic workup for MG.
- Injection of edrophonium (Tensilon) is used to confirm the diagnosis (have atropine available for side effects). Improvement in muscle strength represents a positive test and usually confirms the diagnosis.
- MRI may demonstrate an enlarged thymus gland.
- Tests include serum analysis for acetylcholine receptor and electromyography (EMG) to measure electrical potential of muscle cells.

Complications
Myasthenic Crisis

This sudden onset of muscle weakness is usually the result of undermedication or no cholinergic medication at all. Myasthenic crisis may result from progression of the disease, emotional upset, systemic infections, medications, surgery, or trauma. The crisis is manifested by the sudden onset of acute respiratory distress and inability to swallow or speak.

Cholinergic Crisis

Caused by overmedication with cholinergic or anticholinesterase drugs, cholinergic crisis produces muscle weakness and the respiratory depression of myasthenic crisis as well as gastrointestinal symptoms (nausea, vomiting, diarrhea), sweating, increased salivation, and bradycardia.

Medical Management

Management is directed at improving function through the administration of anticholinesterase medications and by reducing and removing circulating antibodies. Patients with MG are usually managed on an outpatient basis unless hospitalization is required for managing symptoms or complications.

M

Anticholinesterase Medications

Pyridostigmine bromide (Mestinon) or neostigmine bromide (Prostigmin) is administered to increase the response of the muscles to nerve impulses and improve strength; effect can be expected within 1 hour after administration.

Immunosuppressive Therapy

Immunosuppressive therapy aims to reduce the production of antireceptor antibody or remove it directly by plasma exchange. Corticosteroids are given to suppress the immune response, decreasing the amount of blocking antibody. Plasma exchange (plasmapheresis) produces a temporary reduction in the titer of circulating antibodies. Thymectomy (surgical removal of the thymus) produces substantial remission, especially in patients with tumor or hyperplasia of the thymus gland.

M | NURSING PROCESS: The Patient with Myasthenia Gravis

Assessment

- Assess health history, focusing on muscle weakness (respiratory and esophageal muscles), eye and vision changes, and patient's and family's knowledge about the disease and the drug treatment program.
- Assess patient's functional capability and support system to determine discharge needs for services.
- Ongoing assessment for respiratory failure is essential.

Diagnosis

Nursing Diagnoses

- Ineffective breathing pattern related to respiratory muscle weakness
- Impaired physical mobility related to neuromuscular impairment and resulting muscle weakness

- Impaired verbal communication related to weakened speech muscles
- Disturbed sensory perception related to impaired vision
- Risk for aspiration related to weakness of bulbar muscles

Collaborative Problems/Potential Complications

- Myasthenic crisis
- Cholinergic crisis

Planning and Goals

The major goals of the patient may include improved respiratory function, increased physical mobility, improved ability to communicate, avoidance of aspiration, and absence of complications (myasthenic and cholinergic crisis).

Nursing Interventions

Improving Respiratory Function

- Assess respiratory status frequently (respiratory rate, depth, and breath sounds) and monitor the results of pulmonary function tests to detect pulmonary problems before changes in arterial blood gas levels appear.
- Provide chest physical therapy, including postural drainage, to mobilize secretions, and suction to remove secretions. (Postural drainage should not be performed for 30 minutes after tube feeding.) Administer oxygen if needed.
- Acknowledge patient's fears and give assurance. If impending respiratory failure is noted, initiate appropriate action.
- Avoid sedatives and tranquilizers because they aggravate hypoxia and hypercapnia and can cause respiratory and cardiac depression.

Increasing Physical Mobility

- Teach patient about anticholinesterase drugs: action, timing, dosage, symptoms of overdose, and toxic effects.
- Emphasize importance of taking medications on time to improve strength and endurance.

- Encourage patient to keep a diary of symptoms.
- Teach patient to avoid factors that may increase weakness and precipitate myasthenic crisis: emotional upset, infections (respiratory), vigorous physical activity, exposure to heat and cold.
- Advise patient to wear an identification bracelet.
- Educate patient regarding self-help devices; provide as desired.

Improving Communication

Teach patients with weakened speech muscles techniques for improving communication (eg, blink eyes, wiggle fingers or toes).

Providing Eye Care

- Help patient cope with impaired vision (eg, taping eyes open for short intervals, instilling artificial tears to prevent corneal damage).
- Suggest patient use a patch over one eye for double vision and wear sunglasses to diminish the effects of bright light that increase eye problems.

Preventing Aspiration

- Assess for drooling, regurgitation through the nose, and choking while attempting to swallow.
- Provide standby suction.
- Encourage rest before meals; place patient in an upright position to facilitate swallowing.
- Provide soft foods that are easily swallowed.
- Schedule meals to coincide with the peak effects of anticholinesterase.
- Assist with gastrostomy feedings if necessary.

Monitoring and Managing Potential Complications: Myasthenic and Cholinergic Crises

Respiratory distress combined with varying signs of dysphagia (difficulty swallowing), dysarthria (difficulty speaking), eyelid ptosis, diplopia, and prominent muscle weakness are symptoms of a crisis of either type.

- Provide immediate ventilatory assistance.
- Suction as needed.
- Monitor arterial blood gases, serum electrolytes, intake and output, and daily weights.
- Assist with endotracheal intubation and mechanical ventilation; place patient in intensive care unit for constant monitoring.
- Assist with administration of intravenous edrophonium to differentiate type of crisis; this agent improves myasthenic crisis but temporarily worsens cholinergic crisis. Neostigmine methylsulfate is given with myasthenic crisis.
- Assist with nasogastric tube feedings if patient is unable to swallow.
- Avoid sedatives and tranquilizing drugs because they aggravate hypoxia and hypercapnia and can cause respiratory and cardiac depression.

Promoting Home and Community-Based Care

Teaching Patients Self-Care

M

- Instruct patient to consult with physician before taking any new medications. Many medications aggravate myasthenia gravis (antibiotics, cardiovascular medications, antiseizure and psychotropic medications, morphine, quinine and related agents, beta-blockers, and nonprescription medications).
- Teach patient the importance of taking medications as prescribed.
- Inform patient and family about crisis intervention, ways to deal with daily needs, and ways to cope with the disease.
- Teach family emergency measures that may be needed; provide opportunity to practice these.

> **!** **NURSING ALERT** A nursing priority is to give the prescribed anticholinesterase drug according to an exact time schedule to control symptoms; any delay in drug administration may result in inability to swallow.

Continuing Care

Inform patient of community and support groups provided by the Myasthenia Gravis Foundation.

Evaluation

Expected Patient Outcomes

- Achieves adequate respiratory function
- Adapts to impaired mobility
- Uses communication methods
- Reports ability to see objects and people in environment
- Experiences no aspiration
- Recovers from myasthenic and cholinergic crisis

For more information, see Chapter 64 in Smeltzer and Bare: *Brunner and Suddarth's Textbook of Medical-Surgical Nursing*, 11th edition. Philadelphia: Lippincott Williams & Wilkins, 2008.

M Myocardial Infarction

Myocardial infarction (MI) refers to the process by which myocardial tissue is destroyed in regions of the heart that are deprived of an adequate blood supply because of reduced coronary artery blood flow. The cause is usually a critical narrowing of a coronary artery due to atherosclerosis or complete occlusion of an artery due to embolus or thrombus. Decreased coronary blood flow may also result from vasospasm of a coronary artery, decreased oxygen supply (eg, shock and hemorrhage), or increased demand for oxygen (eg, tachycardia, thyrotoxicosis, or ingestion of cocaine). In each case, there is a profound imbalance between myocardial oxygen supply and demand. An MI may be defined by the location of the injury to the heart muscle or by the point in time in the process of infarction (acute, evolving, old).

Clinical Manifestations

- Chest pain that occurs suddenly and continues despite rest and medication is the primary presenting symptom. ECG may be abnormal or normal.

- In many cases, the signs and symptoms cannot be distinguished from those of unstable angina.
- Pain may radiate to the jaw, neck, shoulders, and arm (usually left).
- Pain may be accompanied by cool skin, pallor, clammy diaphoresis, tachycardia, and tachypnea if stimulation of the sympathetic nervous system occurs.
- Patients with diabetes mellitus may not experience severe pain because the neuropathy that accompanies diabetes can interfere with neuroreceptors, dulling the pain.

Assessment and Diagnostic Methods

- Patient history (description of presenting symptom; history of previous illnesses and family health history, particularly of heart disease). Previous history should also include information about patient's risk factors for heart disease.
- ECG within 10 minutes of pain onset or arrival at the emergency department; echocardiography to evaluate ventricular function
- Serial serum enzymes and isoenzymes (creatine kinase and isoenzymes), myoglobin, and troponin; other laboratory tests known as cardiac biomarkers

🌿 Gerontologic Considerations

The gerontologic considerations for MI are the same as those for angina. The mortality rate is higher in elderly (older than age 65) patients with an acute MI. Age, other illnesses, and preexisting conditions may prevent the patient from receiving otherwise indicated treatment for acute MI.

Medical Management

The goals of medical management are to minimize myocardial damage, preserve myocardial function, and prevent complications such as lethal dysrhythmias and cardiogenic shock.

- Oxygen administration is initiated at the onset of chest pain.

M

- Reperfusion via emergency use of thrombolytic medications or percutaneous coronary intervention (PCI)
- Coronary artery bypass or minimally invasive direct coronary artery bypass (MIDCAB)

Pharmacologic Therapy

- Nitrates (nitroglycerin) to increase oxygen supply
- Anticoagulants (aspirin, heparin)
- Analgesics (morphine sulfate)
- Angiotensin-converting enzyme (ACE) inhibitors
- Beta-blocker initially, and a prescription to continue its use after hospital discharge
- Thrombolytics (streptokinase, tissue-type plasminogen activator [t-PA]), alteplase [Activase], reteplase [r-PA, TNKase], anistreplase [Eminase]): most effective if administered as early as possible after the onset of chest pain, before transmural tissue necrosis occurs

M

NURSING PROCESS: The Patient with Myocardial Infarction

Assessment

Obtain baseline data on current status of patient for comparison with ongoing status. Include history of chest pain or discomfort, dyspnea, palpitations, faintness, or sweating. Perform a complete physical assessment, which is crucial for detecting complications and any change in status. The examination should include the following:

- Assess level of consciousness.
- Evaluate chest pain (most important clinical finding).
- Assess heart rate and rhythm; dysrhythmias may indicate not enough oxygen to the myocardium.
- Assess heart sounds; S_3 can be an early sign of impending left ventricular failure.

- Measure blood pressure to determine response to pain and treatment; note pulse pressure, which may be narrowed after an MI, suggesting ineffective ventricular contraction.
- Assess peripheral pulses: rate, rhythm, and volume.
- Evaluate skin color and temperature.
- Auscultate lung fields at frequent intervals for signs of ventricular failure (crackles in lung bases).
- Assess bowel motility; mesenteric artery thrombosis is a potentially fatal complication.
- Observe urinary output and check for edema; an early sign of cardiogenic shock is hypotension with oliguria.
- Examine IV lines and sites frequently.

Diagnosis

Nursing Diagnoses

- Acute pain
- Ineffective cardiac tissue perfusion related to reduced coronary blood flow from coronary thrombus and atherosclerotic plaque
- Risk for imbalanced fluid volume resulting in impaired gas exchange
- Risk for ineffective peripheral tissue perfusion related to decreased cardiac output from left ventricular dysfunction
- Death anxiety
- Deficient knowledge about post-MI self-care

Collaborative Problems/Potential Complications

- Dysrhythmias and cardiac arrest
- Acute pulmonary edema
- Heart failure
- Thromboembolism
- Myocardial rupture
- Pericardial effusion and cardiac tamponade

Planning and Goals

The major goals of the patient include relief of symptoms of ischemia (chest pain, ST segment changes), absence of respiratory

M

difficulties, adequate tissue perfusion, reduced anxiety, adherence to self-care program, and prevention or early recognition of complications.

Nursing Interventions

Relieving Chest Pain

- Administer vasodilator (eg, nitroglycerin), anticoagulant (heparin) medications, and aspirin as prescribed to preserve heart muscle.
- Provide thrombolytic therapy if patient clinically qualifies.
- Administer analgesic agents (morphine sulfate).
- Administer oxygen in tandem with analgesia to ensure maximum relief of pain (inhalation of oxygen reduces pain associated with low levels of circulating oxygen).
- Assess vital signs as long as patient is experiencing pain.
- Assist patient to rest with back elevated or in cardiac chair to decrease chest discomfort and dyspnea.

> ! **NURSING ALERT** Resolution of pain is the primary clinical indicator that myocardial oxygen demand and supply are in equilibrium.

Improving Respiratory Function

- Assess respiratory function to detect early signs of complications.
- Pay attention to fluid volume status to prevent overloading the heart and lungs.
- Encourage patient to breathe deeply and change position often to prevent pooling of fluid in lung bases.

Promoting Adequate Tissue Perfusion

- Keep patient on bed or chair rest to reduce cardiac workload.
- Check skin temperature and peripheral pulses frequently to determine adequate tissue perfusion.
- Administer oxygen to enrich supply of circulating oxygen.

Reducing Anxiety

- Develop a trusting and caring relationship with patient.
- Provide frequent and private opportunities to share concerns and fears.
- Provide an atmosphere of acceptance to help patient know that his or her feelings are realistic and normal.

Monitoring and Managing Complications

Monitor closely for cardinal signs and symptoms that signal onset of complications.

Promoting Home and Community-Based Care

Teaching Patients Self-Care

- Educate about the disease process.
- Work with patient to develop a plan to meet specific needs to enhance compliance.

Preparing for Cardiac Rehabilitation

Goals of rehabilitation for the patient with MI are to extend and improve quality of life. The immediate objectives are to limit the effects and progression of atherosclerosis, return patient to work and pre-illness lifestyle, enhance patient's psychosocial and vocational status, and prevent another cardiac event.

- Encourage physical activity and physical conditioning.
- Educate patient and family.
- Provide counseling and behavioral interventions when necessary.

Evaluation

Expected Patient Outcomes

- Experiences relief of pain
- Shows no signs of respiratory difficulties
- Maintains adequate tissue perfusion
- Expresses less anxiety

M

- Complies with self-care program
- Experiences absence of complications

For more information, see Chapter 28 in Smeltzer and Bare: *Brunner and Suddarth's Textbook of Medical-Surgical Nursing,* 11th edition. Philadelphia: Lippincott Williams & Wilkins, 2008.

Myocarditis

Acute myocarditis is an inflammatory process involving the myocardium. When the muscle fibers of the heart are damaged, life is threatened. Myocarditis usually results from an infectious process (eg, viral, bacterial, mycotic, parasitic, protozoal, or spirochetal). It may be produced in systemic infections, such as rheumatic fever, in patients receiving immunosuppressive therapy, or in patients with infective endocarditis. Myocarditis can cause heart dilation, mural thrombi (on the heart wall), infiltration of circulating blood cells around coronary vessels and between muscle fibers, and degeneration of muscle fibers.

Clinical Manifestations

- Clinical features depend on the type of infection, degree of myocardial damage, and capacity of the myocardium to recover.
- Symptoms may be moderate, mild, or absent.
- Patient may report fatigue and dyspnea, palpitations, and occasional discomfort in the chest and upper abdomen.
- Patient may develop severe congestive heart failure or sustain sudden cardiac death.
- Pericardial friction rub may be heard if myocarditis is associated with pericarditis.
- Pulsus alternans may be present.
- Fever and tachycardia are common, and symptoms of congestive heart failure may develop.

Assessment and Diagnostic Findings

Cardiac enlargement, faint heart sounds, gallop rhythm, and systolic murmur may be found on clinical examination. Diagnosis is confirmed by endomyocardial biopsy.

Medical Management

Appropriate immunizations and early treatment are recommended to decrease the incidence of myocarditis. If myocarditis develops, management involves treating the underlying cause and the following measures:

- Bed rest to decrease cardiac workload and prevent complications
- Continuous cardiac monitoring if dysrhythmia occurs
- Medications to slow the heart rate and augment myocardial contractility (digitalis) when there is evidence of congestive heart failure

Nursing Management

M

- Because patients with myocarditis are sensitive to digitalis, monitor for digitalis toxicity (dysrhythmia, anorexia, nausea, vomiting, bradycardia, headache, malaise).
- Apply, and instruct patient and family in use of, elastic stockings and passive and active exercises to prevent thrombosis.
- Instruct patient to increase physical activity slowly and to report any symptoms that occur with increased activity, including rapid heart rate.
- Instruct patient to avoid competitive sports and alcohol.
- If patient develops heart failure, the management is essentially the same as for all causes of heart failure.

For more information, see Chapter 29 in Smeltzer and Bare: *Brunner and Suddarth's Textbook of Medical-Surgical Nursing*, 11th edition. Philadelphia: Lippincott Williams & Wilkins, 2008.

N

Nephrotic Syndrome

Nephrotic syndrome is a primary glomerular disease characterized by proteinuria, hypoalbuminemia, edema, and hyperlipidemia. It is seen in any condition that seriously damages the
glomerular capillary membrane, causing increased glomerular
permeability with loss of protein in the urine. Generally a disorder of childhood, it does occur in adults, including the elderly.
Causes include chronic glomerulonephritis and diabetes mellitus, among other conditions.

Clinical Manifestations

- Major manifestation is edema (usually periorbital, in
  dependent areas [sacrum, ankles, and hands], and ascites).
- Malaise, headache, irritability, and fatigue

Assessment and Diagnostic Findings

- Protein electrophoresis and immunoelectrophoresis to
  determine type of proteinuria exceeding 3 to 3.5 g/day
- Serum markers (Anti-C1q)
- Microscopic hematuria, urinary casts
- Needle biopsy of the kidney for histologic examination to
  confirm diagnosis

Medical Management

Objective of management is to preserve renal function and prevent complications.

- Bed rest for a few days to promote diuresis and reduce
  edema

- Dietary restrictions of protein and cholesterol to lower lipidemia
- Low sodium, low saturated fat, liberal potassium

Pharmacologic Therapy

- Diuretics for severe edema, in combination with angiotensin-converting enzyme (ACE) inhibitors
- Adrenocorticosteroids to reduce proteinuria
- Antineoplastic agents (Cytoxan) or immunosuppressive agents (Imuran, Leukeran, or cyclosporine)

Nursing Management

- In the early stages, nursing management is similar to that of acute glomerulonephritis.
- As the disease worsens, management is similar to that of chronic renal failure.
- Monitor intake and output; note signs of low plasma volume and impaired circulation with prerenal acute renal failure.
- Instruct patient receiving steroids or cyclosporine regarding medication and signs and symptoms that must be reported to physician.
- Instruct patient in selecting a therapeutic diet.

N

For more information, see Chapter 44 in Smeltzer and Bare: *Brunner and Suddarth's Textbook of Medical-Surgical Nursing,* 11th edition. Philadelphia: Lippincott Williams & Wilkins, 2008.

O

Obesity, Morbid

Morbid obesity is the term applied to people whose body weight is greater than 100 pounds over ideal body weight, those who weigh more than twice their ideal body weight, or those whose body mass index (BMI) exceeds 30 kg/m^2 (BMI is the patient's weight in pounds divided by the patient's height in inches squared, multiplied by 704.5). Patients with morbid obesity are at higher risk for health problems such as cardiovascular disease, hypertension, stroke, sleep apnea, arthritis, asthmatic bronchitis, and diabetes. They frequently suffer from low self-esteem, impaired body image, and depression.

Medical Management

A weight loss diet in conjunction with behavioral modification and exercise is usually unsuccessful. Depression can be treated using bupropion hydrochloride (Wellbutrin). Some physicians recommend acupuncture and hypnosis before recommending surgery.

Pharmacologic Management

- Sibutramine HCl (Meridia) decreases appetite by inhibiting the reuptake of serotonin and norepinephrine. Check drug precautions.
- Orlistat (Xenical) reduces caloric intake by inhibiting digestion of triglycerides. Review side effects; multivitamin is usually recommended.

Surgical Management

- Bariatric surgery (surgery for morbid obesity) includes gastric restriction procedures such as gastric bypass and vertical banded gastroplasty (performed laparoscopically or by open surgical technique).
- Body contouring after weight loss involves lipoplasty to remove fat deposits or a panniculectomy to remove excess abdominal skinfolds.

NURSING PROCESS: The Patient Having Surgery for Morbid Obesity

Assessment

Assess for risk of complications associated with surgery to treat morbid obesity: peritonitis, stomal obstruction, stomal ulcers, atelectasis and pneumonia, thromboembolism, and metabolic imbalances resulting from prolonged vomiting and diarrhea.

Diagnosis

Nursing Diagnoses

- Risk for infection and bleeding
- Pain and discomfort related to incision
- Imbalanced nutrition: Less than body requirements related to hypermetabolic state, anorexia, mucositis, pain, and nausea
- Disturbed body image related to change in appearance
- Deficient knowledge about treatment, complication management, and self-care measures

Collaborative Problems/Potential Complications

- Infection
- Bleeding

Planning and Goals

Major goals may include self-care, attainment and maintenance of ideal weight, adequate nutrition, positive body image, understanding of the postoperative process and its treatment, and absence of complications.

Nursing Interventions

- Provide six small feedings consisting of a total of 600 to 800 calories per day (after bowel sounds have returned and oral intake is resumed).
- Encourage fluid intake to prevent dehydration.

Promoting Home and Community-Based Care

Teaching Patients Self-Care

- Advise patient that usually he or she will be discharged in 4 to 5 days with detailed dietary instructions.
- Explain that deviations from dietary instructions, such as eating too much or too fast or eating high-calorie liquid and soft foods, will likely result in vomiting and painful esophageal distention.
- Instruct patient to report signs and symptoms of infection and/or excessive thirst or concentrated urine (sign of dehydration).
- Discuss essential psychosocial modifications: changes in eating behaviors and coping with changes in body image.
- Encourage patient to schedule and keep monthly outpatient visits.
- Instruct patient to monitor for long-term side effects, including increased risk for gallstones, nutritional deficiencies, and potential to regain weight.

Evaluation

Expected Patient Outcomes

Experiences absence of complications

For more information, see Chapters 18 and 37 in Smeltzer and Bare: *Brunner and Suddarth's Textbook of Medical-Surgical Nursing*, 11th edition. Philadelphia: Lippincott Williams & Wilkins, 2008.

Osteoarthritis (Degenerative Joint Disease)

Osteoarthritis (OA), also known as degenerative joint disease or osteoarthrosis, is the most common joint disorder. It is characterized by a progressive loss of joint cartilage. Besides age, risk factors for OA include female gender, genetic predisposition, obesity, mechanical joint stress, joint trauma, congenital and developmental disorders of the hip, previous bone and joint disorders, inflammatory joint diseases, and endocrine and metabolic diseases. OA has been classified as primary (idiopathic) and secondary (related to risk factors). Obesity, in addition to being a risk factor for osteoarthritis, increases the pain and discomfort of the disease. OA peaks between the fifth and sixth decades of life.

Clinical Manifestations

- Pain, stiffness, and functional impairment are primary clinical manifestations.
- Stiffness is most common in the morning after awakening. It usually lasts less than 30 minutes and decreases with movement.
- Functional impairment is due to pain on movement and limited joint motion when structural changes develop.
- OA occurs most often in weight-bearing joints (hips, knees, cervical and lumbar spine); finger joints are also involved.
- Bony nodes may be present (painless unless inflamed).

Assessment and Diagnostic Findings

- X-ray study shows narrowing of joint space and osteophytes (spurs) at the joint margins and on the subchondral bone. These two findings together are sensitive and specific.
- Serum studies are not useful in the diagnosis of this disorder.
- There is a weak correlation between joint pain and synovitis.

Medical Management

Management focuses on slowing and treating symptoms because there is no treatment available that stops the degenerative joint disease process.

Prevention

- Weight reduction
- Prevention of injuries
- Perinatal screening for congenital hip disease
- Ergonomic modifications

Pharmacologic Therapy

- Acetaminophen; nonsteroidal anti-inflammatory drugs (NSAIDs) if joint symptoms persist
- The newer COX-2 inhibitors (for patients with increased risk for GI bleeding)
- Topical analgesics such as capsaicin and methylsalicylate
- Newer therapeutic approaches: glucosamine and chondroitin; viscosupplementation (intra-articular injection of hyaluronic acid); intra-articular injections of corticosteroids for acute joint inflammation (short-term only)

Conservative Measures

- Heat, weight reduction, joint rest, and avoidance of joint overuse
- Orthotic devices to support inflamed joints (splints, braces)
- Isometric and postural exercises, and aerobic exercise
- Occupational and physical therapy

Surgical Management

Use when pain is intractable and function is lost.

- Tidal irrigation, osteotomy.

- Joint arthroplasty (replacement) is used in patients with end-stage disease.

Nursing Management

The nursing care of the patient with OA is generally the same as the basic care plan for the patient with rheumatic disease (see Arthritis, Rheumatoid). Managing pain and optimizing functional ability are major goals of nursing intervention, and helping patients understand their disease process and symptom pattern is critical to a plan of care.

- Assist patients with management of obesity (weight loss and an increase in aerobic activity) and other health problems or diseases, if applicable.
- Refer patient for physical therapy or to an exercise program.
- Provide and encourage use of canes or other assistive devices for ambulation as indicated.

For more information, see Chapter 54 in Smeltzer and Bare: *Brunner and Suddarth's Textbook of Medical-Surgical Nursing*, 11th edition. Philadelphia: Lippincott Williams & Wilkins, 2008.

Osteomalacia

Osteomalacia is a metabolic bone disease characterized by inadequate mineralization of bone. The primary defect is a deficiency in activated vitamin D (calcitriol), which causes an imbalance of calcium and phosphate and faulty bone calcification/mineralization of calcium. Osteomalacia results from failed calcium absorption (malabsorption) or excessive loss of calcium (celiac disease, biliary tract obstruction, chronic pancreatitis, bowel resection) and loss of vitamin D (liver and kidney disease). Additional risk factors include dietary deficiencies, malabsorption, gastrectomy, chronic renal failure, prolonged anticonvulsant therapy, and insufficient vitamin D (eg, from inadequate dietary intake or inadequate sunlight exposure).

Clinical Manifestations

- Bone pain and tenderness
- Muscle weakness from calcium deficiency
- Waddling or limping gait; legs bowed in more advanced disease
- Pathologic fractures
- Softened vertebrae become compressed, shortening patient's trunk and deforming thorax (kyphosis).
- Weakness and unsteadiness, presenting risk of falls and fractures

Assessment and Diagnostic Findings

- Radiograph, bone biopsy shows increased osteoid (demineralized bone matrix)
- Laboratory studies show low serum calcium and phosphorus levels, moderately elevated alkaline phosphatase level, decreased urine calcium and creatinine excretion.

🌿 Gerontologic Considerations

Promote adequate intake of calcium and vitamin D and a nutritious diet in disadvantaged elderly patients. Encourage patient to spend time in the sun. Reduce incidence of fractures with prevention, identification, and management of osteomalacia. When osteomalacia is combined with osteoporosis, the incidence of fracture increases.

Medical Management

- Underlying cause is corrected when possible (eg, diet modifications, vitamin D and calcium supplements, sunlight).
- Long-term monitoring is undertaken to ensure stabilization or reversal.
- Orthopedic deformities may be treated with braces or surgery (osteotomy).

- Physical, psychological, and pharmacologic measures are used to reduce pain and discomfort.

NURSING PROCESS: The Patient with Osteomalacia

Assessment

- Assess for generalized bone pain in the low back and extremities, with associated tenderness.
- Assess for fracture.
- Obtain information about coexisting diseases (malabsorption syndrome) and dietary habits.
- Note skeletal deformities on physical examination and any muscle weakness.

Nursing Diagnoses

- Acute pain related to bone tenderness and possible fracture
- Disturbed body image related to bowing legs, waddling gait, spinal deformities
- Deficient knowledge about disease process and treatment regimen

Planning and Goals

Major goals may include knowledge of the disease process and treatment regimen, relief of pain, and improved self-concept.

Nursing Interventions

Relieving Pain

- Assist patient in reducing discomfort by physical and psychological measures and medications.
- Change positions often to decrease discomfort from immobility.
- Administer prescribed analgesic agents as needed.

Improving Body Image

- Establish a trusting relationship, and encourage patient to discuss any changes in body image and methods of coping.
- Encourage patient to recognize and use existing strengths.
- Include patient in plan of care to promote self-control and improve feelings of self-worth.

Teaching Patients Self-Care

- Educate patient about the cause of osteomalacia and approaches to controlling it.
- Instruct patient about dietary sources of calcium and vitamin D and safe use of vitamin supplements.
- Inform patient that high doses of vitamin D are toxic and increase risk of hypercalcemia.
- Note importance of monitoring serum calcium levels.
- Encourage outdoor activities to expose skin to sunshine.

For more information, see Chapter 68 in Smeltzer and Bare: *Brunner and Suddarth's Textbook of Medical-Surgical Nursing*, 11th edition. Philadelphia: Lippincott Williams & Wilkins, 2008.

Osteomyelitis

Osteomyelitis is an infection of the bone. It may occur by extension of soft tissue infections, direct bone contamination (eg, bone surgery, gunshot wound), or hematogenous (bloodborne) spread from other foci of infection. *Staphylococcus aureus* causes 70% to 80% of bone infections. Other pathogenic organisms frequently found include *Proteus* and *Pseudomonas* species and *Escherichia coli*. Penicillin-resistant nosocomial gram-negative and anaerobic infections are increasing. Patients at risk include poorly nourished, elderly, and obese patients; those with impaired immune systems and chronic illness (eg, diabetes); and those on long-term corticosteroid therapy. The condition may be prevented by prompt treatment and management of focal and soft tissue infections.

Clinical Manifestations

Hematogenous Infection

- Onset is sudden, occurring with clinical manifestations of sepsis (eg, chills, high fever, rapid pulse, and general malaise).
- Extremity becomes painful, swollen, warm, and tender.
- Patient may describe a constant pulsating pain that intensifies with movement (due to the pressure of collecting pus).
- When osteomyelitis is caused by adjacent infection or direct contamination, there are no symptoms of sepsis.
- With chronic osteomyelitis, there is a continually draining sinus or recurrent periods of pain, inflammation, swelling, and drainage.

Assessment and Diagnostic Findings

- Early x-ray films show only soft tissue swelling.
- Bone scans and magnetic resonance imaging (MRI) may be performed.
- Blood studies and blood cultures are taken (elevated sedimentation rate and leukocytes).
- Chronic osteomyelitis: x-ray shows large, irregular cavities, a raised periosteum, sequestra, or dense bone formations

Medical Management

Initial goal is to control and arrest the infective process.

- Affected area is immobilized; warm saline soaks are provided for 20 minutes several times a day.
- Blood and wound cultures are performed to identify organisms and select the antibiotic.
- Intravenous antibiotic therapy is given around-the-clock.
- Antibiotic medication is administered orally (on empty stomach) when infection appears to be controlled; the medication regimen is continued for up to 3 months.

- Surgical débridement of bone is performed with irrigation; adjunctive antibiotic therapy is maintained.

NURSING PROCESS: The Patient with Osteomyelitis

Assessment

- Assess for risk factors (eg, older age, diabetes, long-term steroid therapy) and for previous injury, infection, or orthopedic surgery.
- Observe for guarded movement of infected area and generalized weakness due to systemic infection.
- Observe for swelling and warmth of affected area, purulent drainage, and elevated temperature.
- Note that patients with chronic osteomyelitis may have minimal temperature elevations, occurring in the afternoon or evening.

Nursing Diagnoses

- Acute pain related to inflammation and swelling
- Impaired physical mobility associated with pain, immobilization devices, and weight-bearing limitations
- Risk for extension of infection: bone abscess formation
- Deficient knowledge about treatment regimen

Planning and Goals

Major goals may include relief of pain, improved mobility within therapeutic limitations, control and eradication of infection, and knowledge of treatment regimen.

Nursing Interventions

Relieving Pain

- Restrict activity and immobilize affected part with splint to decrease pain and muscle spasm.

- Place joints above and below the affected part gently through range of motion.
- Handle affected part with great care to avoid pain.
- Elevate affected part to reduce swelling and discomfort.
- Administer prescribed analgesic agents and use other techniques to reduce pain.
- Monitor neurovascular status of affected extremity.

Improving Physical Mobility

- Teach the rationale for activity restrictions (bone is weakened by the infective process).
- Encourage activities of daily living within physical limitations.

Controlling Infectious Process

- Monitor response to antibiotic therapy. Observe intravenous sites for evidence of phlebitis or infiltration. Monitor for signs of superinfection with long-term, intensive antibiotic therapy (eg, oral or vaginal candidiasis; loose or foul-smelling stools).
- If surgery was necessary, ensure adequate circulation (wound suction, elevation of area, avoidance of pressure on grafted area); maintain immobility as needed; comply with weight-bearing restrictions. Change dressings using aseptic technique to promote healing and prevent cross-contamination.
- Monitor general health and nutrition of patient.
- Provide a balanced diet high in protein and vitamin C to ensure positive nitrogen balance and promote healing; encourage adequate hydration.

Promoting Home and Community-Based Care

Teaching Patients Self-Care

- Advise patient and family to adhere strictly to the therapeutic regimen of antibiotics and prevention of falls or other injury that could result in fracture.
- Teach patient how to maintain and manage the intravenous access site and intravenous administration equipment.

- Provide in-depth medication education (eg, drug name, dosage, frequency, administration rate), including need for laboratory monitoring.
- Instruct patient to observe for and report odor, increased inflammation, elevated temperature, drainage, adverse reactions, and signs of superinfection.
- Teach patient and family how to perform aseptic dressing changes and warm compress techniques.

Continuing Care

- Complete home assessment to determine patient's and family's ability to continue therapeutic regimen.
- Refer for a home care nurse if indicated.
- Monitor patient for response to treatment, signs and symptoms of superinfection, and adverse drug reactions.
- Stress importance of follow-up health care appointments.

Evaluation

Expected Patient Outcomes

- Experiences pain relief
- Increases mobility
- Shows absence of infection
- Complies with therapeutic plan

For more information, see Chapter 68 in Smeltzer and Bare: *Brunner and Suddarth's Textbook of Medical-Surgical Nursing*, 11th edition. Philadelphia: Lippincott Williams & Wilkins, 2008.

Osteoporosis

Osteoporosis is a disorder in which there is a reduction of bone density and a change in bone structure. The rate of bone resorption is greater than the rate of bone formation. The bones become progressively porous, brittle, and fragile, and they fracture easily. Multiple compression fractures of the vertebrae result in skeletal deformity (kyphosis). This kyphosis is sometimes associated with loss of height. Patients at risk include postmenopausal women and small-framed, non-obese white women of European ancestry.

Risk factors include inadequate nutrition, inadequate vitamin D and calcium, and lifestyle choices (eg, smoking, caffeine, and alcohol consumption); genetics; and lack of physical activity. Age-related bone loss begins soon after peak bone mass is achieved (about 35 years of age). Withdrawal of estrogens at menopause or oophorectomy causes decreased calcitonin and accelerated bone resorption, which continues during menopausal years. Endogenous and exogenous catabolic agents may contribute to osteoporosis: excessive corticosteroids, Cushing's syndrome, hyperthyroidism, and hyperparathyroidism. Further causes include coexisting medical conditions, such as malabsorption syndromes, lactose intolerance, renal failure, liver failure, and endocrine disorders. Contributing medications may include isoniazid, heparin, tetracycline, aluminum-containing antacids, furosemide, anticonvulsants, and thyroid supplements. Immobility contributes to the development of osteoporosis.

Assessment and Diagnostic Findings

- Osteoporosis is identified on routine x-ray films when there has been 25% to 40% demineralization.
- Laboratory studies, including serum calcium and serum phosphate, and radiographs are used to exclude other diagnoses.
- Dual-energy x-ray absorptiometry (DEXA; DXA) provides information about spine and hip bone mass and bone mineral density (BMD).
- Quantitative ultrasound (QUS) studies of the heel are used for diagnosis and to predict risk for fracture.

🌿 Gerontologic Considerations

Elderly people fall frequently as a result of environmental hazards, neuromuscular disorders, diminished senses, and cardiovascular responses to medications. Environmental hazards, such as scatter rugs, pets underfoot, and clutter, that may cause the elderly patient to fall need to be identified and eliminated. The patient and family must be included in establishing continuing care and preventive regimens. The home should be well lit and should include safety features such as grab-bars in the bathroom and sturdy railings on the stairs. The patient should wear properly fitting, nonskid shoes and hip protectors, if appropriate.

Medical Management

- Adequate, balanced diet rich in calcium and vitamin D
- Increased calcium intake in adolescents and elderly, or prescribe a calcium supplement with meals or beverages high in vitamin C
- Regular weight-bearing exercise to promote bone formation (20 to 30 minutes aerobic exercise 3 days/week)
- Other medications: the bisphosphonates alendronate (Fosamax), risedronate (Actonel), and ibandronate, selective receptor modulators (SERMs), raloxifene (Evista), calcitonin

> **!** **NURSING ALERT** Female patients who use hormone replacement therapy (HRT) to retard bone loss should have regular breast examinations and Pap tests.

NURSING PROCESS: Vertebral Fracture

Assessment

- To identify risk for and recognition of problems associated with osteoporosis, interview patient regarding family history, previous fractures, intake of calcium, alcohol, caffeine, and cigarettes, exercise patterns, onset of menopause, and use of steroids.
- On physical examination, observe for fracture, kyphosis of thoracic spine, or shortened stature.

Nursing Diagnoses

- Deficient knowledge of osteoporotic process and treatment regimen
- Acute pain related to fracture and muscle spasm
- Risk for constipation related to immobility or development of ileus
- Risk for injury: fracture related to osteoporotic bone

Planning and Goals

Major goals may include knowledge about osteoporosis and the treatment regimen, relief of pain, improved bowel elimination, and absence of additional fracture.

Nursing Interventions

Explaining Osteoporosis and Treatment Regimen

- Focus patient teaching on factors influencing the development of osteoporosis, interventions to slow or arrest the process, and measures to relieve symptoms.
- Inform patient about importance of adequate dietary or supplemental calcium, regular weight-bearing exercise, and modification of lifestyle (eg, reduced use of caffeine, smoking and alcohol cessation).
- Emphasize importance of weight-bearing exercise and physical activity to develop dense bones.
- Inform patient about foods high in calcium, such as skim or whole milk, Swiss cheese, canned salmon with bones.
- Encourage patient to take calcium supplements with meals and adequate fluids.
- Instruct patient who is taking nasal calcitonin to alternate the nostril used to administer the medication.
- Inform patient that at menopause, a calcium-preserving regimen may be prescribed. If alendronate is prescribed, it should be taken on an empty stomach.
- Inform patient taking HRT that estrogen has been associated with increased incidence of breast and endometrial cancer;

therefore, patient should perform breast self-examination monthly and should have regular pelvic examinations.
• Encourage elderly patients to continue to take sufficient calcium and vitamin D, to expose skin to sunshine, and to exercise to minimize the osteoporotic process.

Relieving Pain

• Teach relief of back pain through bed rest and use of a firm, nonsagging mattress, knee flexion, intermittent local heat, and back rubs.
• Instruct patient to move the trunk as a unit and avoid twisting; encourage good posture and good body mechanics.
• Encourage patient to apply lumbosacral corset for immobilization and temporary support when out of bed.

Improving Bowel Elimination

• Encourage patient to eat a high-fiber diet, increase fluids, and use prescribed stool softeners.
• Monitor patient's intake, bowel sounds, and bowel activity; ileus may develop if the vertebral collapse involves T10 to L2 vertebrae.

Preventing Injury

• Promote physical activity to strengthen muscles, prevent disuse atrophy, and retard progressive bone demineralization.
• Encourage patient to perform isometric exercises to strengthen trunk muscles.
• Encourage walking, good body mechanics, and good posture.
• Instruct patient to avoid sudden bending, jarring, and strenuous lifting.
• Encourage outdoor activity in the sunshine to enhance body's ability to produce vitamin D.

Evaluation

Expected Patient Outcomes

- Acquires knowledge about osteoporosis and treatment regimen
- Achieves pain relief
- Demonstrates normal bowel elimination
- Experiences no new fractures

For more information, see Chapter 68 in Smeltzer and Bare: *Brunner and Suddarth's Textbook of Medical-Surgical Nursing*, 11th edition. Philadelphia: Lippincott Williams & Wilkins, 2008.

Otitis Media, Acute

Acute otitis media is an acute infection of the middle ear, usually lasting less than 6 weeks. The primary cause is the entrance of pathogenic bacteria into the normally sterile middle ear when there is eustachian tube dysfunction due to obstruction caused by upper respiratory infections, inflammation of surrounding structures (sinusitis), or allergic reactions (allergic rhinitis). Causative organisms are *Streptococcus pneumoniae*, *Haemophilus influenzae*, and *Moraxella catarrhalis*. Modes of entry of the bacteria are the eustachian tube from contaminated secretions in the nasopharynx, and the middle ear from a tympanic membrane perforation. The disorder is most common in children.

Clinical Manifestations

- Symptoms vary with the severity of the infection and may be either mild and transient or severe; usually unilateral in adults.
- Pain in and about the ear (otalgia) may be intense and relieved only after spontaneous perforation of the eardrum or after myringotomy.
- Fever; drainage from the ear

- Tympanic membrane is erythematous and often bulging or perforated.
- Conductive hearing loss due to exudate in the middle ear
- Even if the condition becomes subacute (3 weeks to 3 months) with purulent discharge, permanent hearing loss is rare.

Complications

- Perforation of the tympanic membrane may persist and develop into chronic otitis media.
- Secondary complications involve the mastoid (mastoiditis), meningitis, or brain abscess (rare).

Management

- With early and appropriate broad-spectrum antibiotic therapy, otitis media may clear with no serious sequelae. If drainage occurs, an antibiotic otic preparation may be prescribed.
- Patient must take antibiotic as prescribed and must complete all the prescribed medication.
- Outcome depends on efficiency of antibiotic therapy, virulence of bacteria, and physical status of patient.

Myringotomy (Tympanotomy)

If mild cases of otitis media are treated effectively, a myringotomy may not be necessary. If it is, an incision is made into the tympanic membrane to relieve pressure and to drain serous or purulent fluid from the middle ear. This painless procedure usually takes less than 15 minutes. If episodes of acute otitis media recur and there is no contraindication, a ventilating, or pressure-equalizing, tube may be inserted.

For more information, see Chapter 59 in Smeltzer and Bare: *Brunner and Suddarth's Textbook of Medical-Surgical Nursing*, 11th edition. Philadelphia: Lippincott Williams & Wilkins, 2008.

Otitis Media, Chronic

Chronic otitis media results from repeated episodes of acute otitis media, causing irreversible tissue pathology and persistent perforation of the eardrum. Chronic infections of the middle ear cause damage to the tympanic membrane, can destroy the ossicles, and can involve the mastoid.

Clinical Manifestations

- Symptoms may be minimal, with varying degrees of hearing loss and a persistent or intermittent foul-smelling otorrhea (discharge).
- Pain may be present if acute mastoiditis occurs; when mastoiditis is present, postauricular area is tender; erythema and edema may be present.
- Cholesteatoma (sac filled with degenerated skin and sebaceous material) may be present as a white mass behind the tympanic membrane visible through an otoscope. If untreated, the cholesteatoma continues to grow and destroys structures of the temporal bone, possibly causing damage to the facial nerve and horizontal canal and destruction of other surrounding structures. Auditory tests often show a conductive or mixed hearing loss.

Medical Management

- Careful suctioning and cleansing of the ear are done under microscopic guidance.
- Antibiotic drops are instilled or antibiotic powder is applied to treat purulent discharge.
- Tympanoplasty procedures (myringoplasty and more extensive types) may be performed to prevent recurrent infection, reestablish middle ear function, close the perforation, and improve hearing.
- Mastoidectomy may be done to remove cholesteatoma.
- Ossiculoplasty may be done to reconstruct the middle ear bones to restore hearing.

Nursing Management

See Nursing Management under Mastoiditis for additional information.

For more information, see Chapter 59 in Smeltzer and Bare: *Brunner and Suddarth's Textbook of Medical-Surgical Nursing*, 11th edition. Philadelphia: Lippincott Williams & Wilkins, 2008.

O

Pancreatitis, Acute

Pancreatitis (inflammation of the pancreas) is a serious disorder that can range in severity from a relatively mild, self-limiting disorder to a rapidly fatal disease that does not respond to any treatment.

Acute pancreatitis is commonly described as an autodigestion of this organ by the exocrine enzymes it produces, principally trypsin. Common causes of acute episodes are biliary tract disease and long-term alcohol use; 5% of patients with gallstones develop pancreatitis. Less common forms include bacterial or viral infection, with pancreatitis as a complication. Many disease processes and conditions have been associated with an increased incidence of pancreatitis: surgery on or near the pancreas, medications, hypercalcemia, and hyperlipidemia. Up to 20% of cases are idiopathic, and there is a small incidence of hereditary pancreatitis.

Mortality is high because of shock, anoxia, hypotension, or fluid and electrolyte imbalances. Complete recovery may occur, or the condition may become chronic.

Clinical Manifestations

Severe abdominal pain is the major symptom.

- Pain in the mid-epigastrium may be accompanied by abdominal distention, a poorly defined palpable abdominal mass, and decreased peristalsis.
- Frequently acute in onset (24 to 48 hours after a heavy meal or alcohol ingestion); may be more severe after meals and unrelieved by antacids
- Patient appears acutely ill.
- Abdominal guarding; rigid or boardlike abdomen

- Soft abdomen in the absence of peritonitis
- Ecchymosis in the flank or around the umbilicus, which may indicate severe hemorrhagic pancreatitis
- Nausea and vomiting, fever, jaundice, mental confusion, agitation
- Hypotension related to hypovolemia and shock
- Acute renal failure common
- May develop tachycardia, cyanosis, and cold, clammy skin
- Respiratory distress and hypoxia
- Dyspnea
- Tachypnea
- Abnormal blood gas values
- Diffuse pulmonary infiltrates
- Myocardial depression, hypocalcemia, hyperglycemia, and disseminated intravascular coagulation (DIC)

Assessment and Diagnostic Findings

Diagnosis is based on history of abdominal pain, known risk factors, and selected diagnostic findings (increased urine amylase level and white blood cell count; hypocalcemia; transient hyperglycemia; glucosuria and increased serum bilirubin levels in some patients). X-rays of abdomen and chest, ultrasound, and CT scan may be performed.

Serum amylase and serum lipase levels are most indicative (rise to more than three times normal within 24 hours; amylase returns to normal within 48 to 72 hours; lipase remains elevated 5 to 7 days). Peritoneal fluid is evaluated for increase in pancreatic enzymes.

🖋 Gerontologic Considerations

The mortality from acute pancreatitis increases with advancing age. Patterns of complications change with age (eg, the incidence of multiple organ failure increases with age). Close observation of major organ function (lungs and kidneys) is indicated, and aggressive treatment is necessary to reduce mortality in the elderly.

Medical Management: Acute Phase

During the acute phase, management is symptomatic and directed toward preventing or treating complications.

- Oral intake is withheld to inhibit pancreatic stimulation and secretion of pancreatic enzymes.
- Parenteral nutrition (PN) is administered to the debilitated patient.
- Nasogastric suction is used to relieve nausea and vomiting, decrease painful abdominal distention and paralytic ileus, and remove hydrochloric acid so that it does not stimulate the pancreas.
- Histamine$_2$ antagonists (cimetidine, ranitidine) or, sometimes, proton pump inhibitors are given to decrease hydrochloric acid secretion.
- Adequate pain medication, such as morphine, is administered.
- Correction of fluid, blood loss, and low albumin levels is necessary.
- Antibiotics are administered if infection is present.
- Insulin is necessary if significant hyperglycemia occurs.
- Aggressive respiratory care is provided for pulmonary infiltrates, effusion, and atelectasis.
- Biliary drainage (drains and stents) results in decreased pain and increased weight gain.
- Surgical intervention may be performed for diagnosis, drainage, resection, or débridement.

P

Medical Management: Postacute Phase

- Antacids are given when the acute episode begins to resolve.
- Oral feedings low in fat and protein are initiated gradually.
- Caffeine and alcohol are eliminated.
- Medications (eg, thiazide diuretics, glucocorticoids, or oral contraceptives) are discontinued.

NURSING PROCESS: The Patient with Pancreatitis

Assessment

- Assess presence and character of pain, its relationship to eating and to alcohol consumption; note effect of patient's efforts to obtain pain relief.
- Assess nutritional and fluid status and history of gallbladder attacks and alcohol use.
- Elicit history of gastrointestinal problems: fatty stools, diarrhea, nausea, and vomiting.
- Assess respiratory status, including rate, pattern, and breath sounds.
- Assess abdomen for pain, tenderness, guarding, and bowel sounds; note boardlike or soft abdomen.

Diagnosis

Nursing Diagnoses

- Acute pain and discomfort related to edema, distention of the pancreas, and peritoneal irritation
- Imbalanced nutrition: Less than body requirements related to inadequate dietary intake, impaired absorption, reduced food intake, and increased metabolic demands
- Ineffective breathing pattern related to severe pain, pulmonary infiltrates, pleural effusion, and atelectasis
- Impaired skin integrity resulting from poor nutritional status, bed rest, surgical wound

Collaborative Problems/Potential Complications

- Fluid and electrolyte disturbances
- Necrosis of the pancreas
- Shock and multiple organ dysfunction syndrome

Planning and Goals

The major goals of the patient include relief of pain and discomfort, improved fluid and nutritional status, improved respiratory function, and absence of complications.

Nursing Interventions

Relieving Pain and Discomfort

- Administer morphine as ordered. This is the drug of choice.
- Withhold oral fluids to decrease formation and secretion of secretin.
- Use nasogastric suctioning to remove gastric secretions and relieve abdominal distention; avoid tension on tube and use water-soluble lubricant around nares; give frequent oral hygiene.
- Maintain patient on bed rest to decrease metabolic rate and reduce secretion of pancreatic enzymes; report increased pain (may be pancreatic hemorrhage or inadequate analgesic dosage).
- Provide explanations about treatment; patient may have clouded sensorium from pain, fluid imbalances, and hypoxemia.

Improving Nutritional Status

- Monitor laboratory test results, daily weights, and anthropometric measures.
- Assess nutritional status and increased metabolic requirements (note increased body temperature, restlessness, increased physical activity) and fluid lost through diarrhea.
- Provide mouth care; patient should receive nothing by mouth during an attack.
- Administer fluids, electrolytes, and parenteral nutrition (PN) as prescribed.
- Monitor serum glucose level every 4 to 6 hours, and give insulin as prescribed.
- Introduce oral feedings gradually as symptoms subside.
- Avoid heavy meals, alcoholic beverages, excessive use of coffee, and spicy foods.

Improving Respiratory Function

- Maintain patient in semi-Fowler's position to decrease pressure on diaphragm.

P

- Change position frequently to prevent atelectasis and pooling of respiratory secretions.
- Administer anticholinergic medications to decrease gastric and pancreatic secretions; dry respiratory tract secretions.
- Assess respiratory status frequently (pulse oximetry, arterial blood gas values) and teach patient techniques of coughing and deep breathing.

Providing Wound Care

- Assess the wound, drainage sites, and skin carefully for signs of infection, inflammation, and breakdown.
- Carry out wound care as prescribed, and take precautions to protect intact skin from contact with drainage; consult with an enterostomal therapist as needed to identify appropriate skin care devices and protocols.
- Turn patient every 2 hours; use of specialty beds may be indicated to prevent skin breakdown. Surgical wound may be irrigated and repacked every 2 to 3 days.

Monitoring and Managing Complications

Fluid and Electrolyte Disturbances

- Assess fluid and electrolyte status by noting skin turgor and moistness of mucous membranes.
- Weigh daily; measure all fluid intake and output.
- Assess for factors that may affect fluid and electrolyte status: fever, fluid loss through diarrhea, vomiting, nasogastric suctioning, or wound drainage.
- Observe for ascites, and measure abdominal girth.
- Administer intravenous fluids, electrolytes, blood, and albumin to maintain volume and prevent or treat shock.
- Assist patient to turn and change positions every 2 hours.
- Report decreased blood pressure, reduced urine output, and low serum calcium and magnesium.

Pancreatic Necrosis

- Transfer patient to intensive care unit for close monitoring.
- Administer fluids, medications, and blood products.
- Assist with supportive management, such as mechanical ventilation.

Shock and Multiple Organ Dysfunction Syndrome

- Monitor patient closely for early signs of neurologic, cardiovascular, renal, and respiratory dysfunction.
- Prepare for rapid changes in patient status, treatment, and therapies; respond quickly.
- Inform family of status and progress of patient; allow time with patient.

Promoting Home and Community-Based Care
Teaching Patients Self-Care

- Provide patient and family with facts and explanations of the acute phase of illness; provide necessary repetition and reinforcement. Offer printed teaching materials.
- Reinforce the need for a low-fat diet, avoidance of heavy meals, and avoidance of alcohol.
- Provide additional explanations on dietary modifications if biliary tract disease is the cause.

Continuing Care

- Assess the home situation and reinforce teaching.
- Refer for home care (often indicated).
- Provide information about resources and support groups, particularly if alcohol is the cause of acute pancreatitis.
- Permit patient and family to air questions and concerns, and provide education and emotional support.

Evaluation

Expected Patient Outcomes

- Reports relief of pain and discomfort
- Achieves nutritional and fluid and electrolyte balance
- Experiences improved respiratory function
- Exhibits intact skin
- Remains free of complications

P

For more information, see Chapter 40 in Smeltzer and Bare: *Brunner and Suddarth's Textbook of Medical-Surgical Nursing*, 11th edition. Philadelphia: Lippincott Williams & Wilkins, 2008.

Pancreatitis, Chronic

Chronic pancreatitis is an inflammatory disorder characterized by progressive anatomic and functional destruction of the pancreas. Cells are replaced by fibrous tissue with repeated attacks of pancreatitis. The end result is mechanical obstruction of the pancreatic and common bile ducts and duodenum. In addition, the secreting cells of the pancreas become inflamed and destruction ensues. Alcohol consumption in Western societies and malnutrition worldwide are the major causes. Among alcoholics, the incidence of pancreatitis is 50 times the rate in the nondrinking population.

Pathophysiology

Chronic consumption of alcohol produces hypersecretion of protein in pancreatic secretions. The result is protein plugs and calculi within the pancreatic ducts. Alcohol has a direct toxic effect on the cells of the pancreas. Damage is more severe in patients with diets low in protein and very high or very low in fat.

P

Clinical Manifestations

- Recurring attacks of severe upper abdominal and back pain, accompanied by vomiting; narcotics may not provide relief
- There may be continuous severe pain or dull, nagging, constant pain.
- Risk of addiction to opiates is high because of the severe pain.
- Weight loss is a major problem.
- Altered digestion (malabsorption) of foods (proteins and fats) results in frequent, frothy, and foul-smelling stools with a high fat content (steatorrhea).
- As disease progresses, calcification of the gland may occur and calcium stones may form within the ducts.

Assessment and Diagnostic Methods

- Endoscopic retrograde cholangiopancreatography (ERCP) is the most useful study.
- A glucose tolerance test evaluates pancreatic islet cell function.

Medical Management

Treatment is directed toward preventing and managing acute attacks.

- Pain and discomfort are relieved with analgesics.
- Patient should avoid alcohol and foods that produce abdominal pain and discomfort. No other treatment will relieve pain if patient continues to consume alcohol.
- Diabetes mellitus resulting from dysfunction of pancreatic islet cells is treated with diet, insulin, or oral hypoglycemic agents. Patient and family are taught the hazard of severe hypoglycemia related to alcohol use.
- Pancreatic enzyme replacement therapy is instituted for malabsorption and steatorrhea.
- Surgery is done to relieve abdominal pain and discomfort, restore drainage of pancreatic secretions, and reduce frequency of attacks (pancreaticojejunostomy).
- Morbidity and mortality after surgical procedures are high because of patient's poor physical condition before surgery and concomitant occurrence of cirrhosis.

Nursing Management

See Nursing Management under Pancreatitis, Acute, for treatment guidelines.

For more information, see Chapter 40 in Smeltzer and Bare: *Brunner and Suddarth's Textbook of Medical-Surgical Nursing*, 11th edition. Philadelphia: Lippincott Williams & Wilkins, 2008.

Parkinson's Disease

Parkinson's disease is a slowly progressive degenerative neurologic disorder affecting the brain centers that are responsible for control and regulation of movement. The degenerative or idiopathic form of Parkinson's disease is the most common; there is also a secondary form with a known or suspected cause. The cause of the disease is mostly unknown. The disease usually first appears in the fifth decade of life and is the fourth most common neurodegenerative disease.

Pathophysiology

Stores of the neurotransmitter dopamine are lost in the substantia nigra and the corpus striatum because of a degenerative process. The loss of dopamine stores in this area of the brain results in more excitatory neurotransmitters than inhibitory neurotransmitters, leading to an imbalance that affects voluntary movement. Other neurotransmitter pathways (responsible for cell metabolism, growth, nutrition, and so forth) may be involved as well. Cellular degeneration causes impairment of the extrapyramidal tracts that control semiautomatic functions and coordinated movements. Regional cerebral blood flow is reduced, and there is a high prevalence of dementia. Biochemical and pathologic data suggest that patients with Parkinson's disease and dementia may have coexistent Alzheimer's disease.

Clinical Manifestations

The three cardinal signs of Parkinson's disease are tremor, rigidity, and bradykinesia (abnormally slow movements).

- Impaired movement: bradykinesia includes difficulty in initiating, maintaining, and performing motor activities; muscle stiffness or rigidity
- Resting tremors: a slow, unilateral turning of the forearm and hand and a pill-rolling motion of the thumb against the

fingers; tremor at rest and increasing with concentration and anxiety
- Muscle weakness
- Hypokinesia (abnormally diminished movement), gait disturbances, flexed posture, and postural instability (loss of postural reflexes, and the freezing phenomenon)

Other Characteristics

Patients tend to develop micrographia (shrinking, slow hand-writing) as dexterity declines. Additional characteristics include:

- Dysphonia (soft, slurred, low-pitched, and less audible speech)
- Masklike facial expression
- Loss of postural reflexes: patient stands with head bent forward and walks with propulsive gait (shuffling gait); difficulty pivoting and loss of balance, resulting in risk for falls
- Depression and psychiatric manifestations (personality changes, psychosis, dementia, and confusion)
- Sleep disorders, uncontrolled sweating, orthostatic hypotension, gastric and urinary retention, and constipation

P

Assessment and Diagnostic Methods

- Patient's history and presence of two of the three cardinal manifestations: tremor, muscle rigidity, and bradykinesia
- Positron emission tomography (PET) scanning
- Neurologic examination and response to pharmacologic management

Medical Management

Goal of treatment is to control symptoms and maintain functional independence; no approach prevents disease progression.

Pharmacologic Therapy

- Levodopa therapy (converts to dopamine): most effective agent to relieve symptoms; usually given in combination with carbidopa (Sinemet), which prevents levodopa breakdown
- Budipine is a non-dopaminergic, antiparkinson medication that significantly reduces akinesia, rigidity, and tremor.
- Antihistamine drugs to allay tremors
- Dopamine agonists (eg, pergolide [Permax], bromocriptine mesylate [Parlodel]), ropinirole, and pramipexole are used to postpone the initiation of carbidopa and levodopa therapy.
- Anticholinergic therapy to control the tremor and rigidity
- Amantadine hydrochloride (Symmetrel), an antiviral agent, to reduce rigidity, tremor, and bradykinesia
- Monoamine oxidase inhibitors (MAOIs) to inhibit dopamine breakdown
- Antidepressant drugs
- Trials of catechol-O-methyltransferase (COMT) inhibitors

Surgical Management

- Surgery to destroy a part of the thalamus (stereotactic thalamotomy and pallidotomy) to interrupt nerve pathways and alleviate tremor or rigidity
- Transplantation of neural cells from fetal tissue of human or animal source to reestablish normal dopamine release
- Deep brain stimulation with pacemaker-like brain implants shows promise but is waiting for FDA approval.

▌NURSING PROCESS: The Patient with Parkinson's Disease

Assessment

The nurse notes how disease affects the patient's activities of daily living and functional abilities and also observes for changes in physical and behavioral function (how patient moves about, walks, thinks, speaks, and drinks) and for the patient's responses to medication throughout the day. The following questions may facilitate observations:

- Do you have leg or arm stiffness?
- Have you experienced any irregular jerking of your arms or legs?
- Does your mouth water excessively?
- Have you (or others) noticed yourself grimacing or making faces or chewing movements?
- What specific activities do you have difficulty doing?
- Have you ever been "frozen" or rooted to the spot and unable to move?

Nursing Diagnoses

- Impaired physical mobility related to muscle rigidity and motor weakness
- Self-care deficits (eating, drinking, dressing, hygiene, and toileting) related to tremor and motor disturbance
- Constipation related to medication and reduced activity
- Imbalanced nutrition: Less than body requirements related to tremor, slowness in eating, difficulty in chewing and swallowing
- Impaired verbal communication related to decreased speech volume, slowness of speech, inability to move facial muscles
- Ineffective coping related to depression and dysfunction due to disease progression
    Other possible nursing diagnoses include:
- Sleep pattern disturbances
- Deficient knowledge
- Compromised family coping
- Disturbed thought processes
- Risk for injury

Planning and Goals

Patient goals may include improved functional mobility, independence in activities of daily living, adequate bowel elimination, acceptable nutritional status, effective communication, and positive coping mechanisms.

Nursing Interventions

Improving Mobility

- Help patient plan progressive program of daily exercise to increase muscle strength, improve coordination and dexterity, reduce muscular rigidity, and prevent contractures.
- Encourage exercises for joint mobility (eg, stationary bike, walking).
- Instruct in stretching and range-of-motion exercises to increase joint flexibility.
- Encourage postural exercises to counter the tendency of the head and neck to be drawn forward and down. Teach patient to walk erect, watch the horizon, use a wide-based gait, swing arms with walking, walk heel-toe, and practice marching to music. Also encourage breathing exercises while walking and frequent rest periods to prevent fatigue or frustration.
- Advise patient that warm baths and massage help relax muscles.

Enhancing Self-Care and Using Assistive Devices

- Encourage, teach, and support patient during activities of daily living.
- Modify environment to compensate for functional disabilities.
- Enlist assistance of an occupational therapist as indicated.
- Obtain special devices/equipment as needed to assist patient (plate stabilizer, nonspill cup, eating utensils with built-up handles).

Improving Bowel Function

- Establish a regular bowel routine.
- Increase fluid intake; eat foods with moderate fiber content.
- Provide raised toilet seat for easier toilet use.

Improving Swallowing and Nutrition

- Promote swallowing and prevent aspiration by having patient sit in upright position during meals.
- Provide semisolid diet with thick liquids that are easier to swallow.
- Remind patient to hold head upright and to make a conscious effort to swallow to control buildup of saliva.
- Provide supplementary feeding and, as disease progresses, tube feedings.
- Consult a dietitian regarding patient's nutritional needs.
- Monitor patient's weight on a weekly basis.

Improving Communication

- Remind patient to face the listener, speak slowly and deliberately, and exaggerate pronunciation of words.
- Instruct patient to speak in short sentences and take a few breaths before speaking.
- Enlist a speech therapist to assist the patient.

Supporting Coping Abilities

- Encourage faithful adherence to exercise and walking program; point out activities that are being maintained through active participation.
- Provide continuous encouragement and reassurance.
- Assist and encourage patient to set achievable goals.
- Encourage patient to carry out daily tasks to retain independence.

Promoting Home and Community-Based Care

Teaching Patients Self-Care

Explain the importance of remaining as functionally independent for as long as possible. The education plan should include a clear explanation of the disease and its management to offset disabling anxieties and fears. The patient and family also need to know about the effects and side effects of medications and the importance of reporting side effects to the physician.

Continuing Care

- Acknowledge the stress the family is under living with a disabled member.
- Include caregiver in planning and counsel caregiver to learn stress reduction techniques.
- Provide family with information about treatment and care to prevent complications.
- Encourage caregiver to obtain periodic relief from responsibilities, to have a yearly health assessment, and to participate in health promotion activities.
- Give family members permission to express feelings of frustration, anger, and guilt.

Evaluation

Expected Patient Outcomes

- Strives toward improved mobility
- Progresses toward self-care
- Maintains bowel function
- Attains improved nutritional status
- Achieves a method of communication

For more information, see Chapter 65 in Smeltzer and Bare: *Brunner and Suddarth's Textbook of Medical-Surgical Nursing*, 11th edition. Philadelphia: Lippincott Williams & Wilkins, 2008.

Pelvic Infection (Pelvic Inflammatory Disease)

Pelvic infection is an inflammatory condition of the pelvic cavity that may involve the uterus, fallopian tubes, ovaries, pelvic peritoneum, or pelvic vascular system. Infection may be acute, subacute, recurrent, or chronic and may be localized or widespread. It is usually bacterial but may be caused by a virus, fungus, or parasite.

Pathophysiology

Pathogenic organisms usually enter the body through the vagina, pass through the cervical canal into the uterus, and may proceed to one or both fallopian tubes and ovaries, and into the pelvis. Infection most commonly occurs through sexual transmission but also may be caused by invasive procedures such as endometrial biopsy, surgical abortion, hysteroscopy, or insertion of an intrauterine device (IUD). The most common organisms involved are gonorrhea, chlamydia, and mycoplasma. The infection is usually bilateral. Risk factors include early age at first intercourse, multiple sex partners, frequent intercourse, risky sexual behaviors (intercourse without condoms, history of sexually transmitted diseases).

Clinical Manifestations

Symptoms may be acute and severe or low-grade and subtle.

- Vaginal discharge, lower abdominal pelvic pain, and tenderness after menses; pain increases during voiding or defecating
- Systemic symptoms include fever, general malaise, anorexia, nausea, headache, and possibly vomiting.
- Intense tenderness is noted on palpation of the uterus or movement of cervix (cervical motion tenderness) during pelvic examination.

Complications

- Pelvic or generalized peritonitis, abscess formation, strictures, and obstruction of fallopian tubes
- Adhesions that eventually may require removal of the uterus, tubes, and ovaries

- Bacteremia with septic shock and thrombophlebitis with possible embolization

Medical Management

Broad-spectrum antibiotic therapy is instituted, with mild to moderate infections being treated on an outpatient basis. If the patient is acutely ill, hospitalization may be required. Once hospitalized, the patient is placed on a regimen of bed rest, intravenous fluids, and intravenous antibiotic therapy. Nasogastric intubation and suction are used if ileus is present; vital signs are monitored. Treatment of sexual partners is necessary to prevent reinfection.

Nursing Management

Nursing measures include nutritional support of the patient and administration of antibiotic therapy as prescribed. Vital signs are assessed, as are characteristics of the disorder and the amount of vaginal discharge.

Comfort measures include applying heat safely to the abdomen and administering analgesic agents for pain relief. Another nursing intervention is prevention of transmission of infection to others by impeccable hand washing and use of barrier precautions and hospital guidelines for disposing of biohazardous articles (eg, pads).

Hospitalized patients must maintain bed rest. While in bed, they remain in semi-Fowler's position to facilitate dependent drainage. Before discharge, patients are taught self-care measures:

- Inform patient that IUDs may increase the risk for infection and that antibiotics may be prescribed.
- Instruct patient to use proper perineal care, wiping from front to back.
- Instruct patient to avoid douching, which can reduce natural flora.

- Teach patient to consult with health care provider if unusual vaginal discharge or odor is noted.
- Educate patient to maintain optimal health with proper nutrition, exercise, weight control, and safer sex practices (eg, using condoms, avoiding multiple sexual partners).
- Advise patient to have a gynecologic examination at least once a year.
- Evaluate any pelvic pain or abnormal discharge, particularly after sexual exposure, childbirth, or pelvic surgery.
- Instruct patient that her partner should wear a condom before and during intercourse if there is any chance of transmitting infection.
- Provide information about signs and symptoms of ectopic pregnancy (pain, abnormal bleeding, faintness, dizziness, and shoulder pain).

For more information, see Chapter 47 in Smeltzer and Bare: *Brunner and Suddarth's Textbook of Medical-Surgical Nursing*, 11th edition. Philadelphia: Lippincott Williams & Wilkins, 2008.

Pemphigus

P

Pemphigus is a group of serious diseases of the skin characterized by the appearance of bullae (blisters) on apparently normal skin and mucous membranes (mouth, vagina). Evidence indicates that pemphigus is an autoimmune disease involving immunoglobulin G (IgG).

Pathophysiology

A blister forms from the antigen-antibody reaction. The level of serum antibody is predictive of disease severity. The condition may be associated with ingestion of penicillin and captopril and with myasthenia gravis. Genetic factors may also play a role, with the highest incidence in those of Jewish or Mediterranean descent. It occurs with equal frequency in men and women in middle and late adulthood.

Clinical Manifestations

- Most cases present with oral lesions appearing as irregularly shaped erosions that are painful, bleed easily, and heal slowly.
- Skin bullae enlarge, rupture, and leave large, painful eroded areas with crusting and oozing.
- A characteristic offensive odor emanates from the bullae.
- Blistering or sloughing of uninvolved skin occurs when minimal pressure is applied (Nikolsky's sign).
- Eroded skin heals slowly, and eventually huge areas of the body are involved. Fluid and electrolyte imbalance and hypoalbuminemia may result from loss of fluid and protein.
- Bacterial superinfection is common.

Assessment and Diagnostic Findings

Diagnosis is confirmed by histologic examination of a biopsy specimen and immunofluorescent examination of the serum, which show circulating pemphigus antibodies.

Medical Management

Goals of therapy are to bring the disease under control as rapidly as possible, prevent loss of serum and development of secondary infection, and promote re-epithelialization of the skin.

- Primary treatment: systemic, high-dose oral corticosteroids. Essential to therapeutic management are daily evaluations of body weight, blood pressure, blood glucose levels, and fluid balance.
- Adjunct therapy: immunosuppressive agents (eg, azathioprine [Imuran], cyclophosphamide [Cytoxan]), gold
- Plasmapheresis is usually reserved for life-threatening cases.

▮ NURSING PROCESS: The Patient with Pemphigus

Assessment

Disease activity is monitored by examining the skin for the appearance of new blisters as well as signs and symptoms of infection.

Diagnosis

Nursing Diagnoses

- Acute pain of oral cavity and skin related to blistering and erosions
- Impaired skin integrity related to ruptured bullae and denuded areas of skin
- Anxiety and ineffective coping related to appearance of skin and no hope of a cure
- Deficient knowledge about medications and side effects

Collaborative Problems/Potential Complications

- Infection and sepsis related to loss of protective barrier of skin and mucous membranes
- Fluid volume deficit and electrolyte imbalance related to loss of tissue fluids

Planning and Goals

The major goals may include relief of discomfort from lesions, skin healing, reduced anxiety, improved coping ability, and absence of complications.

Nursing Interventions

Relieving Oral Discomfort

- Provide meticulous oral hygiene for cleanliness and regeneration of epithelium.
- Provide frequent prescribed mouthwashes to rinse mouth of debris. Avoid commercial mouthwashes.

- Keep lips moist with lanolin, petrolatum, or lip balm.
- Humidify environmental air.

Enhancing Skin Integrity

- Provide cool, wet dressings or baths (protective and soothing).
- Premedicate with analgesic agents before skin care is initiated.
- Dry skin carefully and dust with nonirritating powder.
- Avoid use of tape, which may produce more blisters.
- Keep patient warm to avoid hypothermia.
    See Nursing Management under Burn Injury for additional information.

Reducing Anxiety

- Demonstrate a warm and caring attitude; allow patient to express anxieties, discomfort, and feelings of hopelessness.
- Educate patient and family regarding the disease.
- Refer to psychological counseling as needed.

Monitoring and Managing Potential Complications

- Keep skin clean to eliminate debris and dead skin and to prevent infection.
- Inspect oral cavity for secondary infections and *Candida albicans* infection from high-dose steroid therapy; report if noted.
- Investigate all "trivial" complaints or minimal changes, because corticosteroids mask typical symptoms of infection.
- Monitor for temperature fluctuations and chills; monitor secretions and excretions for changes suggestive of infection.
- Administer antimicrobial agents as prescribed, and note response to treatment.
- Employ effective hand drying techniques; use protective isolation measures and standard precautions.
- Avoid environmental contamination (have housekeeping department dust with a damp cloth and wash floor with a wet mop).

Achieving Fluid and Electrolyte Balance

- Administer saline infusion for sodium chloride depletion.
- Administer blood component therapy to maintain blood volume and hemoglobin and plasma protein concentrations if necessary.
- Encourage adequate oral intake.
- Monitor serum albumin, hemoglobin, hematocrit, and protein levels.
- Provide cool, nonirritating fluids (grape or apple juice) for hydration; provide small, frequent feedings of high-protein, high-calorie foods and snacks.
- Provide parenteral nutrition if patient cannot eat.

Promoting Home and Community-Based Care

Encourage continuing therapy, because disease is characterized by recurrent relapses. Monitor for side effects of cortisone regularly. Encourage patient to report for health-care follow-up regularly.

Evaluation

Expected Patient Outcomes

- Achieves relief from pain of oral lesions
- Achieves skin healing
- Experiences decreased anxiety and increased ability to cope
- Experiences no infection
- Experiences no complications

P

For more information, see Chapter 56 in Smeltzer and Bare: *Brunner and Suddarth's Textbook of Medical-Surgical Nursing*, 11th edition. Philadelphia: Lippincott Williams & Wilkins, 2008.

Peptic Ulcer

A peptic ulcer is an excavation formed in the mucosal wall of the stomach, pylorus, duodenum, or esophagus. It is frequently referred to as a gastric, duodenal, or esophageal ulcer, depending on its location. It is caused by the erosion of a circumscribed area of mucous membrane. Peptic ulcers are more likely to be in the duodenum than in the stomach. They tend to occur singly, but there may be several present at one time. Chronic ulcers usually occur in the lesser curvature of the stomach, near the pylorus. Peptic ulcer has been associated with bacterial infection, such as *Helicobacter pylori* (present in 70% of patients with gastric ulcers and 95% of patients with duodenal ulcers, not associated with esophageal ulcers). The greatest frequency is noted in people between the ages of 40 and 60 years. After menopause, the incidence among women is almost equal to that in men. Predisposing factors include family history of peptic ulcer, blood type O, chronic use of nonsteroidal anti-inflammatory drugs (NSAIDs), alcohol ingestion, excessive smoking, and, possibly, high stress. Esophageal ulcers result from the backward flow of hydrochloric acid from the stomach into the esophagus.

Zollinger-Ellison syndrome (gastrinoma) is suspected when a patient presents with severe peptic ulcer or ulcer that is resistant to standard medical therapy. This syndrome involves extreme gastric hyperacidity (hypersecretion of gastric juice), duodenal ulcer, and gastrinomas (islet cell tumors, which are gastrin-secreting, benign or malignant tumors of the pancreas). About 90% of tumors are found in the gastric triangle. About one third of gastrinomas are malignant. Diarrhea and steatorrhea (unabsorbed fat in the stool) may be evident. These patients may have coexistent parathyroid adenomas or hyperplasia and exhibit signs of hypercalcemia. The most frequent complaint is epigastric pain. The presence of *H. pylori* is not a risk factor.

Stress ulcer (not to be confused with Cushing's or Curling's ulcers) is a term given to acute mucosal ulceration of the duodenal or gastric area that occurs after physiologically stressful events, such as burns, shock, severe sepsis (particularly in ventilator-dependent posttraumatic or postsurgical patients), and multiple organ trauma. Fiberoptic endoscopy within 24 hours of injury shows shallow erosions of the stomach wall; by 72 hours, multiple gastric erosions are observed, and as the stressful condition continues, the ulcers spread. When the patient recovers, the lesions are reversed; this pattern is typical of stress ulceration.

Clinical Manifestations

- Symptoms of duodenal ulcer (most common peptic ulcer) may last days, weeks, or months and may subside only to reappear without cause. Many patients have asymptomatic ulcers.
- Dull, gnawing pain and a burning sensation in the mid-epigastrium or in the back are characteristic.
- Pain is relieved by eating or taking alkali; once the stomach has emptied or the alkali wears off, the pain returns.
- Sharply localized tenderness is elicited by gentle pressure on the epigastrium or slightly right of the midline; some relief is obtained with local pressure to the epigastrium.
- Other symptoms include pyrosis (heartburn) and a burning sensation in the esophagus and stomach, which moves up to the mouth, occasionally with sour eructation (burping).
- Vomiting is rare in uncomplicated duodenal ulcer; it may or may not be preceded by nausea and usually follows a bout of severe pain and bloating; it is relieved by ejection of the acid gastric contents.
- Constipation or diarrhea may result from diet and medications.
- Bleeding (15% of patients with gastric ulcers) and tarry stools may occur; a small portion of patients who bleed from an acute ulcer have no previous digestive complaints but develop symptoms later.

P

Assessment and Diagnostic Methods

- Physical examination (epigastric tenderness, abdominal distention)
- Endoscopy (preferred, but upper gastrointestinal barium study may be done)
- Diagnostic tests include analysis of stool specimens for occult blood, gastric secretory studies, and biopsy and histology with culture to detect *H. pylori* (a breath test may also detect *H. pylori*).

Medical Management

Lifestyle Changes

The goals of treatment are to eradicate *H. pylori* and manage gastric acidity.

- Stress reduction and rest are priority interventions. The patient needs to identify situations that are stressful or exhausting (eg, rushed lifestyle and irregular schedules) and implement changes, such as establishing regular rest periods during the day in the acute phase of the disease. Biofeedback, hypnosis, or behavioral modification may also be useful.
- Smoking cessation is strongly encouraged because smoking raises duodenal acidity and significantly inhibits ulcer repair. Support groups may be helpful.
- Dietary modification may be helpful. Patients should eat whatever agrees with them; small, frequent meals are not necessary if antacids or histamine blockers are part of therapy. Oversecretion and hypermotility of the gastrointestinal tract can be minimized by avoiding extremes of temperature and overstimulation by meat extracts. Alcohol and caffeinated beverages such as coffee (including decaffeinated coffee, which stimulates acid secretion) should be avoided. Diets rich in milk and cream should be avoided also because they are potent acid stimulators. The patient is encouraged to eat three regular meals a day.

Pharmacologic Therapy

- Antibiotics combined with proton pump inhibitors and bismuth salts to suppress *H. pylori*
- H_2-receptor antagonists to decrease stomach acid secretion; maintenance doses of H_2-receptor antagonists are usually recommended for 1 year. Proton pump inhibitors (in high doses in patients with Zollinger-Ellison syndrome) may also be prescribed.

- Cytoprotective agents (protect mucosal cells from acid or NSAIDs)
- Antacids in combination with cimetidine (Tagamet) or ranitidine (Zantac) for treatment of stress ulcer and for prophylactic use
- Anticholinergics (inhibit acid secretion)
- Patient should adhere to the prescribed medication program to ensure complete healing of the ulcer.

Surgical Management

- With the advent of H_2-receptor antagonists, surgical intervention is less common.
- If recommended, surgery is usually for intractable ulcers (particularly with Zollinger-Ellison syndrome), life-threatening hemorrhage, perforation, or obstruction. Surgical procedures include vagotomy, vagotomy with pyloroplasty, or Billroth I or II.

NURSING PROCESS: The Patient with Peptic Ulcer

P

Assessment

- Assess pain and methods used to relieve it; take a thorough history, including a 72-hour food intake history.
- If patient has vomited, determine whether emesis is bright red or coffee ground in appearance. This helps identify source of the blood.
- Assess for blood in the stools with an occult blood test.
- Ask patient about usual food habits, alcohol, smoking, medication use (NSAIDs), and level of tension or nervousness.
- Ask how patient expresses anger (especially at work and with family), and determine whether patient is experiencing occupational stress or family problems.
- Obtain a family history of ulcer disease.

- Assess vital signs for indicators of anemia (tachycardia, hypotension).
- Palpate abdomen for localized tenderness.
- Assess for malnutrition and weight loss.

Diagnosis

Nursing Diagnoses

- Acute pain related to the effect of gastric acid secretion on damaged tissue
- Imbalanced nutrition: Less than body requirements related to changes in diet
- Anxiety related to coping with an acute disease
- Deficient knowledge about preventing symptoms and managing the condition

Collaborative Problems/Potential Complications

- Hemorrhage: upper gastrointestinal
- Perforation
- Penetration
- Pyloric obstruction (gastric outlet obstruction)

Planning and Goals

The major goals of the patient may include relief of pain, reduced anxiety, maintenance of nutritional requirements, knowledge about management and prevention of ulcer recurrence, and absence of complications.

Nursing Interventions

Relieving Pain and Improving Nutrition

- Administer prescribed medications.
- Avoid aspirin, which is an anticoagulant, and foods and beverages that contain acid-enhancing caffeine (colas, tea, coffee, chocolate).
- Encourage patient to eat regularly spaced meals in a relaxed atmosphere; obtain regular weights and encourage dietary modifications.

- Encourage relaxation techniques, and assist patient to cope with stress and pain and to stop smoking.

Reducing Anxiety

- Assess what patient wants to know about the disease, and evaluate level of anxiety; encourage patient to express fears openly and without criticism.
- Explain diagnostic tests; administer medications on schedule.
- Reassure patient that nurses are always available to help with problems.
- Interact in a relaxing manner, help in identifying stressors, and explain effective coping techniques and relaxation methods.
- Encourage family to participate in care, and give emotional support.

Monitoring and Managing Complications

If hemorrhage is a concern:

- Assess for faintness or dizziness and nausea, before or with bleeding; test stool for occult or gross blood; monitor vital signs frequently (tachycardia, hypotension, and tachypnea).
- Monitor intake and output; insert and maintain an intravenous line for infusing fluid and blood.
- Monitor laboratory values (hemoglobin and hematocrit).
- Insert and maintain a nasogastric tube and monitor drainage; provide lavage as ordered.
- Treat hypovolemic shock as indicated (see Nursing Management under Shock for additional information).

If perforation and penetration are concerns:

- Note and report symptoms of penetration (back and epigastric pain not relieved by medications that were effective in the past).
- Note and report symptoms of perforation (sudden abdominal pain, referred pain to shoulders, vomiting and collapse, extremely tender and rigid abdomen, hypotension and tachycardia, or other signs of shock).

See Preoperative and Postoperative Nursing Management for additional information.

Promoting Home and Community-Based Care

Teaching Patients Self-Care

- Assist the patient in understanding the condition and factors that help or aggravate it.
- Teach patient about prescribed medications, including name, dosage, frequency, and possible side effects. Also identify medications such as aspirin that patient should avoid.
- Instruct patient about particular foods that will upset the gastric mucosa, such as coffee, tea, colas, and alcohol, which have acid-producing potential.
- Encourage patient to eat regular meals in a relaxed setting and to avoid overeating.
- Explain that smoking may interfere with ulcer healing; refer patient to programs to assist with smoking cessation.
- Help patient to reduce and manage stress by identifying sources of stress in family and work environments, by resting during the day if possible, and by using psychological counseling if desired.
- Alert patient to signs and symptoms of complications that should be reported, including hemorrhage (cool skin, confusion, increased heart rate, labored breathing, blood in stool); perforation (severe abdominal pain, rigid and tender abdomen, vomiting, elevated temperature, increased heart rate); pyloric obstruction/gastric outlet obstruction (nausea, vomiting, distended abdomen, abdominal pain). To identify obstruction, insert and monitor nasogastric tube; more than 400 mL residual suggests obstruction.

Continuing Care

- Teach patient that follow-up supervision is necessary for about 1 year.
- Tell patient that the ulcer could recur; advise patient to seek medical assistance if symptoms recur.

- Inform patient and family that surgery is no guarantee of cure. Discuss possible postoperative sequelae, such as intolerance to dairy products and sweet foods.

Evaluation

Expected Patient Outcomes

- Remains free of pain between meals
- Experiences less anxiety by avoiding stress
- Complies with therapeutic regimen
- Experiences no complications

For more information, see Chapter 37 in Smeltzer and Bare: *Brunner and Suddarth's Textbook of Medical-Surgical Nursing*, 11th edition. Philadelphia: Lippincott Williams & Wilkins, 2008.

Pericarditis (Cardiac Tamponade)

Pericarditis refers to an inflammation of the pericardium, the membranous sac enveloping the heart. It may be primary or may develop in the course of a variety of medical and surgical disorders. Some causes are unknown; others include infection (usually viral, rarely bacterial or fungal), connective tissue disorders, hypersensitivity states, diseases of adjacent structures, neoplastic disease, radiation therapy, trauma, renal disorders, and tuberculosis.

Pericarditis may be acute or chronic and may be classified by the layers of the pericardium becoming attached to each other (adhesive) or by what accumulates in the pericardial sac: serum (serous), pus (purulent), calcium deposits (calcific), clotting proteins (fibrinous), or blood (sanguinous). Frequent or prolonged episodes of pericarditis may lead to thickening and decreased elasticity that restrict the heart's ability to fill properly with blood (constrictive pericarditis). The pericardium may also become calcified, which restricts ventricular contraction. Pericarditis can lead to an accumulation of fluid in the pericardial sac (pericardial effusion) and increased pressure on the heart, leading to cardiac tamponade.

Clinical Manifestations of Pericarditis

- Characteristic symptom is pain. Pain, which is felt over the precordium or beneath the clavicle and in the neck and left scapular region, is aggravated by breathing, turning in bed, and twisting the body; it is relieved by sitting up (or leaning forward).
- Dyspnea may occur as a result of pericardial compression of the heart's movements.
- Other signs may include fever, high white blood cell count, and friction rub, or extremely ill appearance.

Clinical Manifestations of Cardiac Tamponade

- Falling blood pressure, rising venous pressure (distended neck veins), and distant (muffled) heart sounds with pulsus paradoxus
- Anxious, confused, and restless state
- Dyspnea, tachypnea, and precordial pain
- Elevated central venous pressure (CVP)

Assessment and Diagnostic Methods

Diagnosis is based on signs and symptoms, echocardiogram, and electrocardiogram (ECG). CT and MRI are useful diagnostic tools as well.

Medical Management

Objectives of management are to determine the cause, to administer therapy for the specific cause (when known), and to watch for cardiac tamponade (compression of the heart from fluid in the pericardial sac).

Bed rest is instituted when cardiac output is impaired until fever, chest pain, and friction rub have disappeared. Then a gradual increase in activity is permitted as the patient's condition improves.

Pharmacologic Therapy: Pericarditis

- Narcotic analgesic agents for pain relief during the acute phase
- Analgesic agents and nonsteroidal anti-inflammatory drugs (NSAIDs) to relieve pain and hasten reabsorption of fluid in rheumatic pericarditis. Colchicine may also be used as an alternative medication.
- Corticosteroids to control symptoms, hasten resolution of the inflammatory process, and prevent recurring pericardial effusion
- Penicillin for pericarditis of rheumatic fever
- Isoniazid, ethambutol, rifampin, and streptomycin for pericarditis of tuberculosis
- Amphotericin B for fungal pericarditis

P

Surgical Management: Cardiac Tamponade

- Thoracotomy for penetrating cardiac injuries
- Pericardiocentesis for pericardial fluid removal
- Surgical removal of the tough encasing pericardium (pericardiectomy) if indicated

! **NURSING ALERT** Nursing assessment skills are key to anticipating and identifying the triad of symptoms of cardiac tamponade: falling arterial pressure, rising venous pressure, and distant heart sounds. Search diligently for a pericardial friction rub.

NURSING PROCESS: The Patient with Pericarditis

Assessment

- Assess pain by observation and evaluation while having patient vary positions to determine precipitating or intensifying factors. (Is pain influenced by respiratory movements?)
- Monitor temperature frequently, because pericarditis causes an abrupt onset of fever in a previously afebrile patient.
- Assess pericardial friction rub (a pericardial friction rub is continuous, distinguishing it from a pleural friction rub). Ask patient to hold breath to help in differentiation: audible on auscultation, synchronous with heartbeat, best heard at the left sternal edge in the fourth intercostal space where the pericardium comes into contact with the left chest wall, scratchy or leathery sound, louder at the end of expiration and may be best heard with patient in sitting position.

Diagnosis

Nursing Diagnoses

- Acute pain related to inflammation of the pericardium

Collaborative Problems/Potential Complications

- Pericardial effusion
- Cardiac tamponade

Planning and Goals

The major goals of the patient may include relief of pain and absence of complications.

Nursing Interventions

Relieving Pain

- Advise bed rest or chair rest in a sitting-upright and leaning-forward position.

- Instruct patient to resume activities of daily living as chest pain and friction rub abate.
- Administer medications; monitor and record responses.
- Instruct patient to resume bed rest if chest pain and friction rub recur.

Monitoring and Managing Potential Complications

- Observe for pericardial effusion, which can lead to cardiac tamponade: arterial pressure falls; systolic pressure falls while diastolic pressure remains stable; pulse pressure narrows; heart sounds progress from being distant to imperceptible.
- Observe for neck vein distention and other signs of rising central venous pressure.
- Notify physician immediately upon observing any of the above symptoms, and prepare for pericardiocentesis. Reassure patient and continue to assess and record signs and symptoms until physician arrives.

Evaluation

Expected Patient Outcomes

- Is free of pain
- Experiences no complications
- Returns to normal activities of daily living

For more information, see Chapters 29 and 30 in Smeltzer and Bare: *Brunner and Suddarth's Textbook of Medical-Surgical Nursing*, 11th edition. Philadelphia: Lippincott Williams & Wilkins, 2008.

Perioperative Nursing Management

Preoperative Concerns

Surgery, whether elective or emergency, is a stressful, complex event. Surgery may be performed for a variety of reasons. It may be diagnostic (eg, biopsy specimen, exploratory laparotomy). It may be curative (eg, excision of tumor mass). It may be reparative (eg, repair of wounds). It may be reconstructive or cosmetic (eg, a facelift). It may be palliative (eg, pain relief). Surgery may also be classified according to the degree of urgency involved (emergency, urgent, required, elective, and optional).

Whatever its classification, current surgery involves many more ambulatory procedures than ever before and administrative processes that are new to nursing and other health-care staff. However, perioperative nursing concerns still focus on the patient and his or her well-being. Inpatient or outpatient, all surgical procedures require a comprehensive preoperative nursing assessment and interventions to prepare the patient and family before surgery.

Nursing Management

Informed Consent

- Reinforce information provided by surgeon.
- Notify physician if patient needs additional information to make his or her decision.
- Ascertain that the consent form has been signed before administering psychoactive premedication. Informed consent is required for invasive procedures, such as incision, biopsy, cystoscopy, or paracentesis; procedures requiring sedation and/or anesthesia; nonsurgical procedures that pose more than slight risk to the patient (arteriography); and procedures involving radiation.
- Arrange for a responsible family member or legal guardian to be available to give consent when the patient is a minor or is unconscious or incompetent (an emancipated minor [married or independently earning own living] may sign his or her own surgical consent form).
- Place the signed consent form in a prominent place on the patient's chart.

Assessment: Inpatient Surgery

- Obtain a health history and perform a physical examination to establish vital signs and a database for future comparisons.
- Determine the existence of allergies, previous allergic reactions, any sensitivities to medications, and past adverse reactions to these agents; report a history of bronchial asthma to the anesthesiologist.
- During the physical examination, note significant physical findings such as physical abuse, pressure ulcers, edema, or abnormal breath sounds that further describe the patient's overall condition.
- Obtain and document medication history; include dosage and frequency of prescribed and over-the-counter (OTC) preparations, particularly adrenal corticosteroids, diuretics, phenothiazines, antidepressants, tranquilizers, insulin, and antibiotics.
- Assess patient's usual level of functioning and typical daily activities to assist in patient's care and recovery or rehabilitation plans.
- Determine nutritional needs based on patient's height and weight, body mass index (BMI), triceps skinfold thickness, upper arm circumference, serum protein levels, or nitrogen balance. Nutrition deficiencies should be corrected before surgery.
- Assess mouth for dental caries, dentures, and partial plates. Decayed teeth or dental prostheses may become dislodged during intubation for anesthetic delivery and occlude the airway.
- Assess cardiovascular status to meet oxygen and circulatory demands.
- Determine the value and reliability of patient's support systems; determine role of patient's family or friends.
- Elicit patient concerns that can have a bearing on the surgical experience.
- Identify the ethnic group to which the patient relates and the customs and beliefs the patient holds about illness and health care providers.

P

- Monitor obese patients for abdominal distention; phlebitis; and cardiovascular, endocrine, hepatic, and biliary diseases, which occur more readily in obese patients.
- Be alert for a history of drug or alcohol abuse when obtaining the patient's history; remain patient, ask frank questions, and maintain a nonjudgmental attitude.
- Investigate the mildest symptoms or slightest temperature elevation in patients with disorders affecting the immune system (eg, acquired immunodeficiency syndrome [AIDS], leukemia); use strict asepsis.

Assessment: Ambulatory Surgery

- Obtain the health history of the ambulatory or same-day surgical patient by telephone interview or at preadmission testing. Ask about recent and past health history, allergies, medications, preoperative preparation, and psychosocial and demographic factors.
- Complete the physical assessment the day of surgery.

🌱 Gerontologic Considerations

Monitor the older person undergoing surgery for subtle clues that indicate underlying problems because elderly patients have less physiologic reserve (cardiac, renal, and hepatic function and gastrointestinal activity) than younger patients. Also monitor elderly patients for dehydration, hypovolemia, and electrolyte imbalances, which can be a significant problem in the elderly population.

Nursing Diagnoses

- Anxiety related to the surgical experience (anesthesia, pain) and the outcome of surgery
- Risk for ineffective therapeutic management regimen related to deficient knowledge of preoperative procedures and protocols and postoperative expectations
- Fear related to perceived threat of the surgical procedure and separation from support system
- Deficient knowledge related to the surgical process

Planning and Goals

The surgical patient's major goals may include relief of preoperative anxiety, adequate nutrition and fluids, optimal respiratory and cardiovascular status, optimal hepatic and renal function, mobility and active body movement, spiritual comfort, and knowledge of preoperative preparations and postoperative expectations.

Nursing Interventions

Reducing Anxiety and Fear: Providing Psychosocial Support

- Be a good listener, be empathetic, and provide information that helps alleviate concerns.
- During preliminary contacts, give the patient opportunities to ask questions and to become acquainted with those who might be providing care during and after surgery.
- Acknowledge patient concerns or worries about impending surgery by listening and communicating therapeutically.
- Explore any fears with patient, and arrange for the assistance of other health professionals if required.
- Teach patient cognitive strategies that may be useful for relieving tension, overcoming anxiety, and achieving relaxation, including imagery, distraction, or optimistic affirmations.

Managing Nutrition and Fluids

- Provide nutritional support as ordered to correct any nutrient deficiency before surgery to provide enough protein for tissue repair.
- Instruct patient that oral intake of food or water should be withheld 8 to 10 hours before the operation (most common), unless physician allows clear fluids up to 3 to 4 hours before surgery.
- Inform patient that a light meal may be permitted on the preceding evening when surgery is scheduled in the

morning, or provide a soft breakfast, if prescribed, when surgery is scheduled to take place after noon and does not involve any part of the gastrointestinal tract.

- In dehydrated patients, and especially in older patients, encourage fluids by mouth, as ordered, before surgery, and administer fluids intravenously as ordered.
- Monitor the patient with a history of chronic alcoholism for malnutrition and other systemic problems that increase the surgical risk as well as for alcohol withdrawal (delirium tremens up to 72 hours after alcohol withdrawal).

Promoting Optimal Respiratory and Cardiovascular Status

- Urge patient to stop smoking 2 months before surgery (or at least 24 hours before).
- Teach patient breathing exercises and how to use an incentive spirometer if indicated.
- Assess patient with underlying respiratory disease (eg, asthma, chronic obstructive pulmonary disease [COPD]) carefully for current threats to pulmonary status; assess patient's use of medications that may affect postoperative recovery.
- In the patient with cardiovascular disease, avoid sudden changes of position, prolonged immobilization, hypotension or hypoxia, and overloading of the circulatory system with fluids or blood.

Supporting Hepatic and Renal Function

- If patient has a disorder of the liver, carefully assess various liver function tests and acid-base status.
- Frequently monitor blood glucose levels of the patient with diabetes before, during, and after surgery.
- Report the use of steroid medications for any purpose by the patient during the preceding year to the anesthesiologist and surgeon.
- Monitor patient for signs of adrenal insufficiency.

- Assess patients with uncontrolled thyroid disorders for a history of thyrotoxicosis (with hyperthyroid disorders) or respiratory failure (with hypothyroid disorders).

Promoting Mobility and Active Body Movement

- Explain the rationale for frequent position changes after surgery (to improve circulation, prevent venous stasis, and promote optimal respiratory function) and show patient how to turn from side to side and assume the lateral position without causing pain or disrupting intravenous lines, drainage tubes, or other apparatus.
- Discuss any special position patient will need to maintain after surgery (eg, adduction or elevation of an extremity) and the importance of maintaining as much mobility as possible despite restrictions.
- Instruct patient in exercises of the extremities, including extension and flexion of the knee and hip joints (similar to bicycle riding while lying on the side); foot rotation (tracing the largest possible circle with the great toe); and range of motion of the elbow and shoulder.
- Use proper body mechanics, and instruct patient to do the same. Maintain patient's body in proper alignment when patient is placed in any position.

P

Respecting Spiritual and Cultural Beliefs

- Help patient obtain spiritual help if he or she requests it; respect and support the beliefs of each patient.
- Ask if the patient's spiritual adviser knows about the impending surgery.
- When assessing pain, remember that some cultural groups are unaccustomed to expressing feelings openly. Individuals from some cultural groups may not make direct eye contact with others; this lack of eye contact is not avoidance or a lack of interest but a sign of respect.
- Listen carefully to patient, especially when obtaining the history. Correct use of communication and interviewing

skills can help the nurse acquire invaluable information and insight. Remain unhurried, understanding, and caring.

Providing Preoperative Patient Education

- Teach each patient as an individual, with consideration for any unique concerns or learning needs.
- Begin teaching as soon as possible, starting in the physician's office and continuing during the preadmission visit, when diagnostic tests are being performed, through arrival in the operating room.
- Space instruction over a period of time to allow patient to assimilate information and ask questions.
- Combine teaching sessions with various preparation procedures to allow for an easy flow of information. Include descriptions of the procedures and explanations of the sensations the patient will experience.
- During the preadmission visit, arrange for the patient to meet and ask questions of the perianesthesia nurse, view audiovisuals, and review written materials. Provide a telephone number for patient to call if questions arise closer to the date of surgery.
- Reinforce information about the possible need for a ventilator and the presence of drainage tubes or other types of equipment to help the patient adjust during the postoperative period.
- Inform the patient when family and friends will be able to visit after surgery and that a spiritual advisor will be available if desired.

Teaching the Ambulatory Surgical Patient

- For the same-day or ambulatory surgical patient, teach about discharge and follow-up home care. Education can be provided by a videotape, over the telephone, or during a group meeting, night classes, preadmission testing, or the preoperative interview.
- Answer questions and describe what to expect.

- Tell the patient when and where to report, what to bring (insurance card, list of medications and allergies), what to leave at home (jewelry, watch, medications, contact lenses), and what to wear (loose-fitting, comfortable clothes; flat shoes).
- During the last preoperative phone call, remind the patient not to eat or drink as directed; brushing teeth is permitted, but no fluids should be swallowed.

Teaching Deep-Breathing and Coughing Exercises

- Teach the patient how to promote optimal lung expansion and consequent blood oxygenation after anesthesia by assuming a sitting position, taking deep and slow breaths (maximal sustained inspiration), and exhaling slowly.
- Demonstrate how patient can splint the incision line to minimize pressure and control pain (if there will be a thoracic or abdominal incision).
- Inform patient that medications are available to relieve pain, and that they should be taken regularly for pain relief to enable effective deep-breathing and coughing exercises.

Explaining Pain Management

- Instruct patient to take medications as frequently as prescribed during the initial postoperative period for pain relief.
- Discuss the use of oral analgesic agents with patient before surgery, and assess patient's interest and willingness to participate in pain relief methods.
- Instruct patient in the use of a pain rating scale to promote postoperative pain management.

Preparing the Bowel for Surgery

- If ordered preoperatively, administer or instruct the patient to take the antibiotic and a cleansing enema or laxative the evening before surgery and repeat it the morning of surgery.

- Have the patient use the toilet or bedside commode rather than the bedpan for evacuation of the enema, unless the patient's condition presents some contraindication.

Preparing Patient for Surgery

- Instruct patient to use detergent-germicide for several days at home (if the surgery is not an emergency).
- If hair is to be removed, remove it immediately before the operation using electric clippers.
- Dress patient in a hospital gown that is left untied and open in the back.
- Cover patient's hair completely with a disposable paper cap; if patient has long hair, it may be braided; hairpins are removed.
- Inspect patient's mouth and remove dentures or plates.
- Remove jewelry, including wedding rings (if patient objects, securely fasten the ring with tape).
- Give all articles of value, including dentures and prosthetic devices, to family members, or if needed label articles clearly with patient's name and store in a safe place according to agency policy.
- Assist patients (except those with urologic disorders) to void immediately before going to the operating room.
- Administer preanesthetic medication as ordered, and keep the patient in bed with the side rails raised. Observe patient for any untoward reaction to the medications. Keep the immediate surroundings quiet to promote relaxation.

Transporting Patient to Operating Room

- Send the completed chart with patient to operating room; attach surgical consent form and all laboratory reports and nurses' records, noting any unusual last-minute observations that may have a bearing on the anesthesia or surgery at the front of the chart in a prominent place.
- Take the patient to the preoperative holding area, and keep the area quiet, avoiding unpleasant sounds or conversation.

NURSING ALERT Someone should be with the preoperative patient at all times to ensure safety and provide reassurance (verbally as well as nonverbally by facial expression, manner, or the warm grasp of a hand).

Attending to Special Needs of Older Patients

- Assess the older patient for dehydration, constipation, and malnutrition; report if present.
- Maintain a safe environment for the older patient with sensory limitations such as impaired vision or hearing and reduced tactile sensitivity.
- Initiate protective measures for the older patient with arthritis, which may affect mobility and comfort. Use adequate padding for tender areas. Move patient slowly and protect bony prominences from prolonged pressure. Provide gentle massage to promote circulation.
- Take added precautions when moving an elderly patient because decreased perspiration leads to dry, itchy, fragile skin that is easily abraded.
- Apply a lightweight cotton blanket as a cover when the elderly patient is moved to and from the operating room, because decreased subcutaneous fat makes older people more susceptible to temperature changes.
- Provide the elderly patient with an opportunity to express fears; this enables patient to gain some peace of mind and a sense of being understood.

Attending to the Family's Needs

- Assist the family to the surgical waiting room, where the surgeon may meet the family after surgery.
- Reassure the family they should not judge the seriousness of an operation by the length of time the patient is in the operating room.
- Inform those waiting to see the patient after surgery that the patient may have certain equipment or devices in place (ie, intravenous lines, indwelling urinary catheter, nasogastric

P

tube, suction bottles, oxygen lines, monitoring equipment, and blood transfusion lines).
- When the patient returns to the room, provide explanations regarding the frequent postoperative observations.

Evaluation

Expected Patient Outcomes

- Reports decreased fear and anxiety
- Voices understanding of surgical intervention

Postoperative Nursing Management

The postoperative period extends from the time the patient leaves the operating room until the last follow-up visit with the surgeon (as short as 1 week or as long as several months). During the postoperative period, nursing care is directed at reestablishing the patient's physiologic equilibrium, alleviating pain, preventing complications, and teaching the patient self-care. Careful assessment and immediate intervention assist the patient in returning to optimal function quickly, safely, and as comfortably as possible. Ongoing care in the community through home care, telephone follow-up, and clinic or office visits promotes an uncomplicated recovery.

Postanesthesia care in some hospitals and ambulatory surgical centers is divided into three phases. Phase I, the immediate recovery phase, requires intensive nursing care. In phase II, the patient is prepared for self-care or care in the hospital or an extended care setting. In phase III, the patient is prepared for discharge.

Nursing Management in the PACU

Patients still under anesthesia or recovering from it are placed in the postanesthesia care unit (PACU), formerly called the postanesthesia recovery room, which is located adjacent to the operating rooms. Patients may be in the PACU for as long as 4 to 6 hours or for as little as 1 to 2 hours. In some cases, the patient is discharged home directly from this unit. Documentation of information and events germane to PACU care includes the following:

- Medical diagnosis and type of surgery performed
- Patient's age and general condition, airway patency, vital signs
- Anesthetic and other medications used (eg, opioids and other analgesics, muscle relaxant, antibiotics)
- Any problems that occurred in the operating room that might influence postoperative care (eg, extensive hemorrhage, shock, cardiac arrest)
- Fluid administered, estimated blood loss and replacement
- Any tubing, drains, catheters, or other supportive aids
- Specific information about which the surgeon, anesthesiologist, or anesthetist wishes to be notified
- Pathology encountered (if malignancy, whether the patient or family has been informed)

The nursing management objectives for the patient in the PACU are to provide care until the patient has recovered from the effects of anesthesia (ie, until return of motor and sensory functions), is oriented, has stable vital signs, and shows no evidence of hemorrhage.

Role of PACU Nurse

The PACU nurse obtains frequent assessments of the patient's oxygen saturation, pulse volume and regularity, depth and nature of respirations, skin color, level of consciousness, and ability to respond to commands. In some cases, end-tidal carbon dioxide ($ETCO_2$) levels are monitored as well. The nurse also performs a baseline assessment followed by checking the surgical site for drainage or hemorrhage and connecting all drainage tubes and monitoring lines. After the initial assessment, the nurse monitors vital signs and assesses the patient's general physical status at least every 15 minutes, including assessment of cardiovascular function with the above assessments. The nurse maintains airway patency and supplemental oxygen; maintains cardiovascular stability with prevention, prompt recognition, and treatment of hemorrhage, hypertension, dysrhythmias, hypotension and shock; relieves pain and anxiety; and controls nausea and vomiting. The nurse also notes any pertinent information from the patient's history that may be significant (eg, hard of hearing, blind, history of seizures, diabetes, allergies to certain medications or other substances).

Usually the following measures are used to determine the patient's readiness for discharge from the PACU:

- Uncompromised pulmonary function
- Pulse oximetry readings of adequate oxygen saturation
- Stable vital signs
- Orientation to place, events, and time
- Urine output not less than 30 mL/h
- Nausea and vomiting under control
- Minimal pain

Patients being discharged directly to home are given teaching, written instructions, and information about follow-up care. Usually, the nurse makes sure they are transported home safely by a responsible person.

Nursing Management in Same-Day Surgery

- Inform the patient and caregiver (ie, family member or friend) about expected outcomes and immediate postoperative changes anticipated in the patient's capacity for self-care.
- Provide written instructions about wound care, activity and dietary recommendations, medication, and follow-up visits to the same-day surgery unit or the surgeon. Provide caregiver with verbal and written instructions about what to observe the patient for and about the actions to take if complications occur.
- Give prescriptions to patient, provide the nurse's or surgeon's telephone number, and encourage patient and

caregiver to call if questions arise. Follow-up telephone calls from the nurse or surgeon may be used to assess patient's progress and to answer any questions.

- Instruct patient to limit activity for 24 to 48 hours (avoid driving a vehicle, drinking alcoholic beverages, or performing tasks that require energy or skill); to consume fluids as desired; and to consume smaller than normal amounts of food.
- Caution patient not to make important decisions at this time because the medications, anesthesia, and surgery may affect thinking ability.
- Refer patient for home care as indicated (elderly or frail patients, those who live alone, and patients with other health care problems that may interfere with self-care or resumption of usual activities).

Postoperative Nursing Management in Home Care

- The home care nurse assesses the patient's physical status (eg, respiratory and cardiovascular status, adequacy of pain management, surgical incision) and the patient's and family's ability to adhere to the recommendations given at the time of discharge. Previous teaching is reinforced as needed.
- The home care nurse may change surgical dressings or catheters or teach the patient or family how to do so, monitor the patency of a drainage system, administer medications or teach the patient and family to do so, and assess for surgical complications.
- The home care nurse determines if any additional services are needed and assists the patient and family to arrange for them (needed supplies, resources or support groups the patient may want to contact).
- The home care nurse reinforces previous teaching and reminds the patient to keep follow-up appointments. The patient and family are instructed about signs and symptoms to report to the surgeon.

Postoperative Nursing Management in the Clinical Unit

- Prepare the patient's unit by assembling the necessary equipment and supplies: intravenous pole, drainage receptacle holder, emesis basin, tissues, disposable pads (Chux), blankets, and postoperative charting forms.

- Receive report from the PACU nurse containing baseline data, including demographic data, medical diagnosis, procedure performed, comorbid conditions, unexpected intraoperative events, estimated blood loss, type and amount of fluids received, medications administered for pain, whether patient has voided, information patient and family have received about patient's condition, and specific information about which the surgeon, anesthesiologist or anesthetist wishes to be notified.

- Review the postoperative orders, admit patient to unit, perform an initial assessment, and attend to patient's immediate needs.

- During the first hours after surgery, interventions focus on helping the patient recover from the effects of anesthesia, performing frequent assessments, monitoring for complications, managing pain, and implementing measures to promote self-care, successful management of the therapeutic regimen, discharge to home, and full recovery.

- In the initial hours after admission to the clinical unit, adequate ventilation, hemodynamic stability, incisional pain, surgical site integrity, nausea and vomiting, neurologic status, and spontaneous voiding are primary concerns.

P

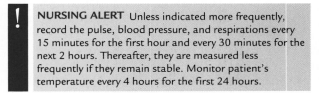

NURSING ALERT Unless indicated more frequently, record the pulse, blood pressure, and respirations every 15 minutes for the first hour and every 30 minutes for the next 2 hours. Thereafter, they are measured less frequently if they remain stable. Monitor patient's temperature every 4 hours for the first 24 hours.

Nursing Interventions

Maintaining Patent Airway

- Check the orders for and apply supplemental oxygen. Assess respiratory rate and depth, ease of respirations, oxygen saturation, and breath sounds.
- Monitor patient for airway obstruction in which the tongue falls backward and patient has choking, noisy, and irregular respirations and, within minutes, a blue, dusky color (cyanosis) of the skin. Maintain hard rubber or plastic airway in patient's mouth or nose until gag reflex resumes.
- Encourage patient to turn frequently and take deep breaths and cough at least every 2 hours.
- Carefully assist patient to splint an abdominal or thoracic incision site to help patient overcome the fear that the exertion of coughing might open the incision.
- Administer pain medications to permit more effective coughing; suction patient as needed.
- Assist and encourage patient to use incentive spirometer hourly while awake (10 breaths per hour).

> **NURSING ALERT** Coughing is contraindicated in patients who have head injuries or who have undergone intracranial surgery, eye surgery, or plastic surgery.

Maintaining Cardiovascular Stability

- Monitor cardiovascular stability by assessing patient's mental status; vital signs; cardiac rhythm; skin temperature, color, and moisture; and urine output.
- Assess patency of all intravenous lines.
- On patient's arrival in the clinical unit, observe the surgical site for bleeding, type and integrity of dressing, and drains (eg, Penrose, Hemovac, and Jackson-Pratt).
- Assess output from wound drainage systems and amount of bloody drainage on the surgical dressing frequently. Mark

and time spots of drainage on dressings; report excess
drainage or fresh blood to surgeon immediately.

- Reinforce dressing with sterile gauze bandages and record
the time. Do not change initial dressing; surgeon will
usually wish to be present.

> **!** **NURSING ALERT** A systolic blood pressure of less than
> 90 mm Hg is usually considered reportable at once.
> However, the patient's preoperative or baseline blood
> pressure is used to make informed postoperative
> comparisons. A previously stable blood pressure that
> shows a downward trend of 5 mm Hg at each 15-minute
> reading should also be reported.

Assessing and Managing Pain

- Assess pain level using a verbal or visual analog scale, and
assess the characteristics of the pain.
- Discuss options in pain relief measures with patient to
determine the best medication. Assess effectiveness of
medication periodically beginning 30 minutes after
administration (sooner if given intravenously).
- Administer medication at prescribed intervals, or if ordered
as needed, before pain becomes severe or unbearable. Risk
of addiction is negligible with use of opioids for short-term
pain control.
- Provide other pain relief measures (changing patient's
position, using distraction, applying cool washcloths to the
face, and rubbing the back with a soothing lotion) to relieve
general discomfort temporarily.

Maintaining Normal Body Temperature

- Monitor body system function and vital signs with
temperature every 4 hours for the first 24 hours and every
shift thereafter.

- Report signs of hypothermia to physician. This is a particular risk in elderly patients and those with long surgeries.
- Maintain the room at a comfortable temperature, and provide blankets to prevent chilling.
- Monitor patient for cardiac dysrhythmias.
- Take efforts to identify malignant hyperthermia and to treat it early.

Assessing Mental Status

- Assess mental status (level of consciousness, speech, and orientation) and compare to preoperative baseline; change may be related to anxiety, pain, medications, oxygen deficit, or hemorrhage.
- Assess for possible causes of discomfort, such as tight, drainage-soaked bandages or distended bladder.
- Address sources of discomfort, and report signs of complications to surgeon for immediate treatment.
- Assess neurovascular status (have patient move the hand or foot distal to the surgical site through a full range of motion, ensuring that all surfaces have intact sensation and assessing peripheral pulses).

P

Assessing and Managing Gastrointestinal Function and Promoting Nutrition

- If in place, maintain nasogastric tube and monitor patency and drainage.
- Provide symptomatic therapy, including antiemetic medications for nausea and vomiting.
- Administer phenothiazine medications as prescribed for severe, persistent hiccups.
- Assist patient to return to normal dietary intake gradually at a pace set by patient (liquids first, then soft foods, such as gelatin, junket, custard, milk, and creamed soups, are added gradually, then solid food).

- Remember that paralytic ileus and intestinal obstruction are potential postoperative complications that occur more frequently in patients undergoing intestinal or abdominal surgery. See specific gastrointestinal disorders for discussion of treatment.
- Arrange for patient to consult with the dietitian to plan appealing, high-protein meals that provide sufficient fiber, calories, and vitamins. Nutritional supplements, such as Ensure or Sustacal, may be recommended.
- Instruct patient to take multivitamins, iron, and vitamin C supplements if prescribed postoperatively.

> **!**   **NURSING ALERT** At the slightest indication of nausea, turn patient completely on one side to promote mouth drainage and prevent aspiration of vomitus, which can cause asphyxiation and death.

Assessing and Managing Voluntary Voiding

- Assess for bladder distention and urge to void on patient's arrival in the unit and frequently thereafter (patient should void within 8 hours of surgery).
- Obtain order for catheterization before the end of the 8 hour time limit if patient has an urge to void and cannot, or if the bladder is distended and no urge is felt or patient cannot void.
- Initiate methods to encourage the patient to void (eg, letting water run, applying heat to perineum).
- Warm the bedpan to reduce discomfort and automatic tightening of muscles and urethral sphincter.
- Assist patient who complains of not being able to use the bedpan to use a commode or stand or sit to void (males), unless contraindicated.
- Take safeguards to prevent the patient from falling or fainting due to loss of coordination from medications or orthostatic hypotension.
- Note the amount of urine voided (report less than 30 cc/h) and palpate the suprapubic area for distention or

tenderness, or use a portable ultrasound device to assess residual volume.

- Continue intermittent catheterization every 4 to 6 hours until patient can void spontaneously and postvoid residual is less than 100 mL.

Encouraging Activity

- Encourage most surgical patients to ambulate as soon as possible.
- Remind patient of the importance of early mobility in preventing complications (helps overcome fears).
- Anticipate and avoid orthostatic hypotension (postural hypotension: 20-mm Hg fall in systolic blood pressure or 10-mm Hg fall in diastolic blood pressure, weakness, dizziness, and fainting).
- Assess patient's feelings of dizziness and his or her blood pressure first in the supine position, after patient sits up, again after patient stands, and 2 to 3 minutes later.
- Assist patient to change position gradually. If patient becomes dizzy, return to supine position and delay getting out of bed for several hours.
- When patient gets out of bed, remain at patient's side to give physical support and encouragement.
- Take care not to tire patient.
- Initiate and encourage patient to perform bed exercises to improve circulation (range of motion to arms, hands and fingers, feet, and legs; leg flexion and leg lifting; abdominal and gluteal contraction).
- Encourage frequent position changes early in the postoperative period to stimulate circulation. Avoid positions that compromise venous return (raising the knee gatch or placing a pillow under the knees, sitting for long periods, and dangling the legs with pressure at the back of the knees).
- Apply antiembolism stockings, and assist patient in early ambulation. Check postoperative activity orders before getting patient out of bed. Then have patient sit on the edge

P

of bed for a few minutes initially; advance to ambulation as tolerated.

Promoting Fluid Balance

- Monitor patient closely to detect and correct conditions such as fluid volume deficit, altered tissue perfusion, and decreased cardiac output.
- Assess patency of intravenous lines, ensuring that appropriate fluids are administered at prescribed rate (up to 24 hours or until patient is tolerating oral fluids).
- Record intake and output, including emesis and output from wound drainage systems, separately and add them to determine fluid balance (with indwelling urinary catheter, monitor outputs hourly and report rates of less than 30 mL/h; if the patient is voiding, report an output of less than 240 mL per shift).
- Monitor electrolyte levels and hemoglobin and hematocrit levels.

Promoting Self-Care

- Have patient perform as much routine hygiene care as possible on first postoperative day (setting up patient to bathe with a bedside wash basin, or, if possible, assisting patient to bathroom to sit at a chair at the sink).
- Assist patient to build up to ambulating a functional distance (length of house or apartment), get in and out of bed unassisted, and be independent with toileting, to prepare for discharge to home.
- Ask patient to perform as much as possible and then to call for assistance. Collaborate with patient for progressive activity, and assess vital signs before, during, and after a scheduled activity.
- Provide physical support to maintain patient's safety, and provide a positive attitude about patient's ability to perform the activity, promoting confidence.
- While changing the dressing, teach patient how to care for incision and change dressings at home. Observe for

indicators that patient is ready to learn, such as looking at the incision, expressing interest, or assisting in the dressing change.

Maintaining a Safe Environment

- Keep side rails up and bed in the low position.
- Assess level of consciousness and orientation.
- Determine whether patient needs his or her eyeglasses or hearing aid and provide them as soon as possible.
- Place all objects patient may need within reach, including, of course, the call bell.
- Implement any immediate postoperative orders concerning special positioning, equipment, or intervention.
- Ask patient to seek assistance with any activity.
- Use restraints only if needed (disoriented patient), and assess neurovascular status frequently.

Providing Emotional Support
to Patient and Family

- Help patient and family work through their anxieties by providing reassurance and information and by spending time listening to and addressing their concerns.
- Describe hospital routines and what to expect in the hours and days until discharge.
- Explain the purpose of nursing assessments and interventions.
- Inform patients when they can take fluids or eat, when they will be getting out of bed, when tubes and drains will be removed, and so forth, to help them gain a sense of control and participation in recovery.
- Acknowledge family's concerns, and accept and encourage their participation in patient's care.
- Manipulate the environment to enhance rest and relaxation: provide privacy, reduce noise, adjust lighting, provide enough seating for family members, and perform any other supportive measures.

P

Monitoring and Preventing Postoperative Complications

Preventing Deep Vein Thrombosis

- Monitor for symptoms of deep vein thrombosis (DVT), which may include a pain or a cramp in the calf elicited on ankle dorsiflexion (Homans' sign); pain and tenderness may be followed by a painful swelling of the entire leg and may be accompanied by a slight fever and sometimes chills and perspiration.
- Administer prophylactic treatment for postoperative patients at risk (low-dose subcutaneous heparin, and then warfarin, external pneumatic compression, and thigh-high elastic pressure stockings).
- Avoid using blanket rolls, pillow rolls, or any form of elevation that can constrict vessels under the knees. Even prolonged "dangling" (having the patient sit on the edge of the bed with legs hanging over the side) can be dangerous and is not recommended in susceptible patients.
- Encourage adequate hydration (offer juices and water throughout the day).

P

Monitoring and Treating Hypotension and Shock

- Monitor closely for signs of shock (a fall in venous pressure, a rise in peripheral resistance, and tachycardia, or a fall in blood pressure). If the amount of blood loss exceeds 500 mL (especially if the loss is rapid), replacement is usually indicated.
- Monitor for the classic signs of shock: pallor; cool, moist skin; rapid breathing; cyanosis of the lips, gums, and tongue; a rapid, weak, thready pulse; decreasing pulse pressure; low blood pressure; and concentrated urine.
- Prevent hypovolemic shock by timely administration of intravenous fluids, blood, and medications that elevate blood pressure.

- Control pain by making patient as comfortable as possible and by using opioids judiciously. Avoid exposure, and maintain normothermia to prevent vasodilation.
- Administer volume replacement as ordered (lactated Ringer's solution or blood component therapy).
- Administer oxygen by nasal cannula, face mask, or mechanical ventilation.
- Administer cardiotonics, vasodilators, or steroids to improve cardiac function and reduce peripheral vascular resistance. Keep the patient warm; however, avoid overheating to prevent vessel dilation.
- Place patient flat in bed with legs elevated.
- Monitor respiratory and pulse rate, blood pressure, oxygen concentration, urinary output, level of consciousness, central venous pressure, pulmonary artery pressure, pulmonary capillary wedge pressure, and cardiac output to provide information about respiratory and cardiovascular status.
- Monitor vital signs continuously until condition has stabilized.

Detecting and Minimizing Hemorrhage

- Note signs of extreme blood loss (apprehensiveness, restlessness, and thirst; cold, moist, pale skin; increased pulse rate; decreasing temperature; and rapid and deep respirations, often of the gasping type spoken of as "air hunger").
- If the hemorrhage progresses untreated, cardiac output decreases, arterial and venous blood pressure and hemoglobin level fall rapidly, the lips and the conjunctivae become pallid, spots appear before the eyes, a ringing is heard in the ears, and the patient grows weaker but remains conscious until near death.
- Administer blood or blood product transfusion, and determine the cause of hemorrhage.
- Inspect surgical site and incision for bleeding. If bleeding is evident, apply a sterile gauze pad and a pressure dressing, and elevate the site of the bleeding to the level of the heart,

P

if possible; place patient in the shock position (lying flat on back with legs elevated at a 20-degree angle while knees are kept straight). If indicated, prepare patient for return to surgery.

- Give special considerations to patients who decline blood transfusions, such as Jehovah's Witnesses, and to those who identify specific requests on their advance directives or living will.

> **!** **NURSING ALERT** Giving too large a quantity of intravenous fluid or administering it too rapidly may raise the blood pressure enough to start the bleeding again.

Managing Wound Complications

- Hematoma: Monitor for bleeding beneath the skin at the surgical site, which may result in clot formation (hematoma) within the wound. (If clot is large, the wound may bulge, and healing is delayed unless the clot is removed.) Prepare patient for removal of several sutures by the physician, evacuation of the clot, and light wound packing with gauze. Healing occurs usually by granulation, or a secondary closure may be performed.

- Infection (wound sepsis): Monitor for (or instruct patient and family to monitor for) wound infection, which may not present until postoperative day 5. Risk factors for wound sepsis include wound contamination, foreign body, faulty suturing, devitalized tissue, hematoma, debilitation, dehydration, malnutrition, anemia, advanced age, extreme obesity, shock, length of preoperative hospitalization, duration of surgery, and associated disorders (eg, diabetes mellitus, immunosuppression). Signs and symptoms of infection include elevated pulse and temperature; increased white blood cell count; wound swelling, warmth, tenderness, or discharge and incisional pain. Local signs may be absent if the infection is deep.
- If wound infection results from beta-hemolytic streptococci or *Clostridium* species, take care not to spread infection to

others; provide intensive nursing care and care for open incision and drain if present. If needed, prepare patient for incision and drainage if the infection is deep. Administer antimicrobial therapy, and initiate wound care regimen.

- Wound dehiscence and evisceration: Monitor for wound dehiscence (disruption of surgical incision or wound) and evisceration (protrusion of wound contents), which are serious complications, especially when they involve abdominal incisions or wounds. The earliest sign may be a gush of bloody (serosanguineous) peritoneal fluid from the wound; coils of intestine may push out of the abdomen, pain and vomiting may be noted, and frequently the patient will say that "something gave way." Monitor patients with risk factors particularly closely (patients with infection, marked distention, strenuous cough, increasing age, poor nutritional status, and the presence of pulmonary or cardiovascular disease in patients who undergo abdominal surgery). If wound disruption occurs, place patient in low Fowler's position and instruct him or her to lie quietly to minimize protrusion of body tissues. Cover the protruding tissue or coils of intestine with sterile dressings moistened with sterile saline, and notify the surgeon at once. Apply an abdominal binder as a prophylactic measure against an abdominal incision evisceration.

P

Promoting Home and Community-Based Care

Although certain needs are germane to individual patients and the specific procedures they have undergone, patient education needs for postoperative care include the following:

- Provide detailed discharge instructions to assist patient in becoming proficient in self-care needs after surgery.
- Arrange for care by community-based services, such as a home care nurse, if necessary (older patients, patients who live alone, or patients without family support).
- Arrange for necessary services early in the acute care hospitalization.

- Wound care, drain management, catheter care, infusion therapy, and physical or occupational therapy are some of the needs addressed by community health care providers.
- Instruct patient to continue to perform bed exercises, wear pressure stockings when in bed, and rest as needed. Spray silicone over the adhesive used to hold dressings in place; the silicone waterproofs the dressing so that the patient can bathe or swim, and it isolates the area from contamination.

🌿 Gerontologic Considerations

Elderly patients continue to be at increased risk for postoperative complications. Age-related physiologic changes in respiratory, cardiovascular, and renal function and the increased incidence of comorbid conditions demand skilled assessment to detect early signs of deterioration. Anesthetics and opioids can cause confusion in the older adult, and altered pharmacokinetics results in delayed excretion and prolonged respiratory depressive effects. Careful monitoring of electrolyte, hemoglobin, and hematocrit levels and urine output is essential because the older adult is less able to correct and compensate for fluid and electrolyte imbalances. Elderly patients may need frequent reminders and demonstrations to participate in care effectively.

P

- Maintain physical activity while patient is confused. Physical deterioration can worsen delirium and place patient at increased risk for other complications.
- Avoid restraints, because they can also worsen confusion. If possible, family or staff member is asked to sit with patient instead.
- Administer haloperidol (Haldol) or lorazepam (Ativan) as ordered during episodes of acute confusion; discontinue these medications as soon as possible to avoid side effects.
- Assist the older postoperative patient in early and progressive ambulation to prevent the development of problems such as pneumonia, altered bowel function, DVT, weakness, and functional decline; avoid sitting positions that promote venous stasis in the lower extremities.

- Provide assistance to keep patient from bumping into objects and falling. A physical therapy referral may be indicated to promote safe, regular exercise for the older adult.
- Provide easy access to call bell and commode; prompt voiding to prevent urinary incontinence.
- Provide extensive discharge planning to coordinate both professional and family care providers; the nurse, social worker, or nurse case manager may institute the plan for continuing care.

Evaluation

Expected Patient Outcomes

- Experiences decreased pain
- Maintains optimal respiratory function
- Does not develop DVT
- Exercises and ambulates as prescribed
- Wound heals without complication
- Resumes oral intake and normal bowel function
- Acquires knowledge and skills necessary to manage therapeutic regimen
- Experiences no complications and has normal vital signs

P

For more information, see Chapters 18 through 20 in Smeltzer and Bare: *Brunner and Suddarth's Textbook of Medical-Surgical Nursing*, 11th edition. Philadelphia: Lippincott Williams & Wilkins, 2008.

Peripheral Arterial Occlusive Disease

Arterial insufficiency of the extremities is found more often in men and predominantly in the legs. The age of onset and the severity are influenced by the type and number of atherosclerotic risk factors present. Obstructive lesions are predominantly confined to segments of the arterial system extending from the aorta, below the renal arteries, to the popliteal artery.

Clinical Manifestations

Intermittent Claudication

- Claudication, the hallmark of peripheral arterial occlusive disease, is insidious and described as aching, cramping, fatigue, or weakness. Patient may report increased pain with ambulation.
- Rest pain is persistent, aching, or boring and is usually present in distal extremities with severe disease.
- Elevation or horizontal placement of the extremity aggravates the pain; lowering the extremity to a dependent position reduces pain.

Other Manifestations

- Coldness or numbness in the extremities accompanies intermittent claudication.
- Extremities may be cool and exhibit pallor on elevation or a ruddy, cyanotic color when in a dependent position.
- Skin and nail changes, ulcerations, gangrene, and muscle atrophy are present.
- Bruits may be auscultated and peripheral pulses may be diminished or absent.
- Inequality of pulses between extremities or absence of a normally palpable pulse is a reliable sign of occlusion.
- Nails may be thickened and opaque, and the skin shiny, atrophic, and dry, with sparse hair growth.
- Upper extremity occlusions are less symptomatic or asymptomatic, although arm fatigue and pain with exercise may be experienced.
- Patient may report vertigo, ataxia, syncope, and bilateral visual changes.

Assessment and Diagnostic Methods

- History of symptoms and physical examination (peripheral pulses)
- Imaging studies (eg, continuous wave [CW] Doppler device ultrasonic flow studies, ankle-brachial indices, angiography, digital subtraction angiography [DSA])
- Treadmill testing for claudication, duplex ultrasound

Medical Management

Key treatment measures include pharmacotherapy and surgery. Antiplatelet aggregating agents such as cilostazol (Pletal), aspirin, ticlopidine (Ticlid), and clopidogrel (Plavix) are tried and may be followed by vascular bypass grafting or endarterectomy, which is the treatment of choice when the limb is at risk for amputation. Another procedure that may be helpful is percutaneous transluminal angioplasty (PTA) for stenosis or occlusion of the vessel (short focal lesion in upper extremity artery). Exercise programs combined with weight reduction and smoking cessation often improve activity limitations.

Nursing Management

Promoting Circulation

Before surgery, patient education is a major nursing activity. The nurse instructs the patient to:

- Maintain meticulous cleanliness of the feet; wash feet daily, dry carefully, and do not rub with a towel.
- Keep feet warm; protect feet from injury.
- Wear comfortable shoes.
- Prevent constriction of blood vessels: do not cross legs and avoid any activity that cuts off blood supply to legs and feet.
- Exercise to stimulate circulation and tissue repair.
- Report redness, blistering, swelling, pain, any peeling or itching.
- Avoid tobacco in any form, because it aggravates peripheral vascular circulation.

P

Maintaining Circulation Postoperatively

The primary objective in postoperative management of patients who have had vascular procedures is to maintain adequate circulation through the arterial repair.

- Check pulses of affected extremity, and compare with other every hour for the first 24 hours.
- Notify surgeon immediately if a peripheral pulse disappears; this may indicate thrombotic occlusion of the graft.
- Monitor color and temperature of extremity, capillary refill, and sensory and motor functions for 24 hours with Doppler pulse evaluation of vessels distal to bypass graft and ankle/arm indices every 2 hours, and report changes.
- Monitor ankle-brachial index (ABI) every 8 hours for the first 24 hours.

Monitoring and Managing Potential Complications

- Monitor urine output (more than 30 mL/h), central venous pressure, mental status, and pulse rate and volume to permit early recognition and treatment of fluid imbalances.
- Instruct patient to avoid leg crossing and prolonged extremity dependence.
- Teach patient to perform leg elevation and to exercise limbs while in bed to reduce edema.
- Monitor for compartment syndrome (severe limb edema, pain, and decreased sensation).

Promoting Home and Community-Based Care

- Assess patient's ability to manage independently or availability of family and friends to assist.
- Determine patient's motivation to make lifestyle changes needed with chronic disease.
- Assess patient's knowledge and ability to assess for postoperative complications, such as infection, occlusion of graft, and decreased blood flow.

- Determine if patient wants to stop smoking and encourage all efforts to do so.

For more information, see Chapter 31 in Smeltzer and Bare: *Brunner and Suddarth's Textbook of Medical-Surgical Nursing*, 11th edition. Philadelphia: Lippincott Williams & Wilkins, 2008.

Peritonitis

Peritonitis, inflammation of the peritoneum, is usually the result of bacterial infection, with the organisms coming from disease of the gastrointestinal tract, or, in women, the internal reproductive organs. It can also result from external sources, such as injury or trauma or an inflammation from an extraperitoneal organ, such as the kidney.

Pathophysiology

Peritonitis is caused by leakage of contents from abdominal organs into the abdominal cavity, usually as a result of inflammation, infection, ischemia, trauma, or tumor perforation. The most common bacteria implicated are *Escherichia coli*, and *Klebsiella*, *Proteus*, and *Pseudomonas* species. Other common causes are appendicitis, perforated ulcer, diverticulitis, and bowel perforation. Peritonitis may also be associated with abdominal surgical procedures and peritoneal dialysis. Sepsis is the major cause of death from peritonitis (shock, from sepsis or hypovolemia). Intestinal obstruction from bowel adhesions may develop.

Clinical Manifestations

Clinical features depend on the location and extent of inflammation.

- Diffuse pain becomes constant, localized, and more intense near site of the process.
- Pain is aggravated by movement.

- Affected area of the abdomen becomes extremely tender and distended, and muscles become rigid.
- Rebound tenderness and ileus may be present.
- Temperature and pulse increase; leukocyte count is elevated.
- Nausea and vomiting occur and peristalsis is diminished.

Assessment and Diagnostic Methods

- Leukocytes (elevated), complete blood count, hemoglobin, hematocrit, and serum electrolytes (altered potassium, sodium and chloride)
- Abdominal x-rays, computed tomography (CT) scan, and peritoneal aspiration with culture and sensitivity studies

Medical Management

- Fluid, colloid, and electrolyte replacement with an isotonic solution is the major focus of medical management.
- Analgesics are administered for pain; antiemetics are administered for nausea and vomiting.
- Intestinal intubation and suction are used to relieve abdominal distention.
- Oxygen therapy by nasal cannula or mask is instituted to improve ventilatory function.
- Occasionally, airway intubation and ventilatory assistance are required.
- Massive antibiotic therapy may be instituted (sepsis is the major cause of death).
- Surgical objectives include removal of infected material; surgery is directed toward excision (appendix), resection (intestine), repair (perforation), or drainage (abscess).

Nursing Management

Pain Assessment

- Assess nature of pain, location in the abdomen, and shifts of pain and location.
- Assess vital signs, gastrointestinal function, fluid and electrolyte balance.

- Monitor central venous and pulmonary artery pressures frequently.
- Administer analgesic medication and position for comfort (eg, on side with knees flexed to decrease tension on abdominal organs).
- Record intake and output and central venous pressure.
- Administer and monitor intravenous fluids closely.
- Observe and record character of any surgical drainage.
- Observe for decrease in temperature and pulse rate, softening of the abdomen, return of peristaltic sounds, and passage of flatus and bowel movements, which indicate peritonitis is subsiding.
- Increase food and oral fluids gradually, and decrease parenteral fluid intake when peritonitis subsides.
- Observe and record character of drainage from post-operative wound drains if inserted; take care to avoid dislodging drains.
- Postoperatively, prepare patient and family for discharge; teach care of incision and drains if still in place at discharge.

For more information, see Chapter 38 in Smeltzer and Bare: *Brunner and Suddarth's Textbook of Medical-Surgical Nursing*, 11th edition. Philadelphia: Lippincott Williams & Wilkins, 2008.

P

Pharyngitis, Acute

Acute pharyngitis is an infection or inflammation in the throat, usually (70%) caused by a viral organism. The inflammatory response results in sore throat with pain, fever, vasodilation, edema, and tissue damage (redness and swelling in the tonsillar pillars, uvula, and soft palate). Uncomplicated viral infections usually subside within 3 to 10 days after onset. When caused by bacteria, the most common organism is group A streptococcus ("strep throat"). Pharyngitis caused by streptococcus is a more severe illness because of dangerous complications, including sinusitis, otitis media, mastoiditis, cervical adenitis, and peritonsillar abscess. Rarely, infection may lead to bacteremia, rheumatic fever, meningitis, pneumonia, and nephritis.

Clinical Manifestations

- Fiery red pharyngeal membrane and tonsils
- Lymphoid follicles swollen and freckled with white-purple exudate
- Cervical lymph nodes enlarged and tender
- Fever, malaise, and sore throat
- Hoarseness

Assessment and Diagnostic Methods

- Rapid screening test for streptococcal antigens, optical immunoassay (OIA), streptolysin titers, and throat cultures
- Nasal swabbings and blood cultures

Medical Management

Viral pharyngitis is treated with supportive measures, whereas antibiotic agents are used to treat pharyngitis caused by bacteria: penicillin for group A streptococci and cephalosporins for patients with penicillin allergies or erythromycin resistance. Antibiotics are administered for at least 10 days. In addition, liquid or soft diet is recommended during the acute stage. In some instances, intravenous fluids are administered if the patient cannot swallow. If the patient can swallow, he or she is encouraged to drink 2,000 to 3,000 mL of fluid daily.

Analgesic medications are given at 3- to 6-hour intervals, and antitussive medications (codeine, dextromethorphan [Robitussin DM] or hydrocodone [Hycodan]) are given to control persistent and painful cough.

Nursing Management

- Encourage bed rest during febrile stage of illness.
- Implement secretion precautions to prevent spread of infection.
- Examine skin once or twice daily for possible rash because acute pharyngitis may precede some other communicable disease.

- Secure nasal swabbings and throat and blood specimens for culture as needed.
- Administer warm saline gargles or irrigations (105°F–110°F [40.5°–43.3°C]) to ease pain. Also instruct patient regarding purpose and technique for warm gargles (as warm as patient can tolerate) to promote maximum effectiveness.
- Apply an ice collar for symptomatic relief.
- Administer analgesic drugs or antitussive medications.
- Perform mouth care to prevent fissures of lips and inflammation in the mouth.
- Permit gradual resumption of activity.
- Advise patient of importance of taking the full course of antibiotic therapy.
- Inform patient and family of symptoms to watch for that may indicate development of complications, including nephritis and rheumatic fever.

For more information, see Chapter 22 in Smeltzer and Bare: *Brunner and Suddarth's Textbook of Medical-Surgical Nursing*, 11th edition. Philadelphia: Lippincott Williams & Wilkins, 2008.

Pharyngitis, Chronic

Chronic pharyngitis is common in adults who work or live in dusty surroundings, use their voice to excess, suffer from chronic cough, and habitually use alcohol and tobacco. Three types are recognized: hypertrophic, a general thickening and congestion of the pharyngeal mucous membranes; atrophic, a late stage of type 1; and chronic granular, marked by numerous swollen lymph follicles of the pharyngeal wall.

Clinical Manifestations

- Constant sense of irritation or fullness in the throat
- Mucus that collects in the throat and is expelled by coughing
- Difficulty in swallowing

Medical Management

Treatment is based on symptom relief, avoidance of exposure to irritants, and correction of any upper respiratory, pulmonary, or cardiac condition that might be responsible for chronic cough. Nasal sprays (ephedrine sulfate or phenylephrine hydrochloride) are used to relieve nasal congestion. Aspirin (adults only) or acetaminophen may be recommended to control inflammation and relieve discomfort.

Nursing Management

- Advise patient to avoid contact with others until fever has subsided completely to prevent infection from spreading.
- Instruct patient to avoid alcohol, tobacco, secondhand smoke, exposure to cold, and environmental and occupational pollutants. Suggest wearing a disposable mask for protection.
- Encourage patient to drink plenty of fluids, and encourage gargling with warm salt water to relieve throat discomfort. Using lozenges may help to keep the throat moist.

For more information, see Chapter 22 in Smeltzer and Bare: *Brunner and Suddarth's Textbook of Medical-Surgical Nursing*, 11th edition. Philadelphia: Lippincott Williams & Wilkins, 2008.

Pheochromocytoma

A pheochromocytoma is a tumor (usually benign) that originates from the chromaffin cells of the adrenal medulla. In 90% of patients, the tumor arises in the medulla; in the remaining patients, it occurs in the extra-adrenal chromaffin tissue located in or near the aorta, ovaries, spleen, or other organs. It occurs at any age, but peak incidence is between 40 and 50 years of age; it affects men and women equally and has familial tendencies. Although uncommon, it is one cause of hypertension that is usually cured by surgery, but without detection and treatment it is usually fatal.

Clinical Manifestations

Classic symptoms are known as the five H's: hypertension, headache, hyperhidrosis (excessive sweating), hypermetabolism, and hyperglycemia.

- Blood pressure as high as 250/150 mm Hg
- Hypertension and other cardiovascular disturbances
- Intermittent or persistent hypertension (half of cases difficult to distinguish)
- May precipitate life-threatening complications: cardiac dysrhythmias, dissecting aneurysm, stroke, and acute renal failure
- Postural hypotension in most (70%) untreated cases
- Tremor
- Flushing
- Anxiety

Symptoms of Paroxysmal Form of Pheochromocytoma

- Acute, unpredictable attacks, lasting seconds or several hours, during which patient is extremely anxious, tremulous, and weak
- Headache, vertigo, blurring of vision, tinnitus, air hunger, and dyspnea
- Polyuria, nausea, vomiting, diarrhea, abdominal pain, and feeling of impending doom
- Palpitations and tachycardia
- Life-threatening blood pressure elevation (more than 250/150 mmHg)

Assessment and Diagnostic Methods

- Urine and plasma catecholamine levels. Catecholamines in 24-hour urine (metanephrine [MN] and vanillylmandelic acid [VMA]) and plasma (norepinephrine and epinephrine) offer the most direct and conclusive test.

- Imaging studies (eg, computed tomography [CT] and magnetic resonance imaging [MRI] scans, ultrasound, 131I-metaiodobenzylguanidine [MIBG] scintigraph) to determine location of tumor

Medical Management

- Preliminary preparation includes control of blood pressure and blood volume, carried out over 10 days to 2 weeks (eg, cautious use of alpha-adrenergic blocking agents or beta-adrenergic blockers and smooth muscle relaxants).
- Bed rest is recommended.
- Treatment is surgical removal of the tumor, usually with adrenalectomy (hypertension usually subsides with treatment).
- Patient is hydrated before, during, and after surgery.
- Postoperative corticosteroid replacement is required after bilateral adrenalectomy.
- Patient is monitored for several days in the intensive care unit, with attention given to electrocardiogram (ECG) changes, arterial pressures, fluid and electrolyte balance, and blood glucose levels.
- Blood pressure is monitored; hypertension can persist or recur if blood vessels have been damaged or if not all pheochromocytoma tissue has been removed.
- Postoperative urine and plasma levels of catecholamines are measured; when levels return to normal, patient may be discharged.

Nursing Management

- Advise bed rest, with head of bed elevated to promote orthostatic decrease in blood pressure.
- Monitor ECG changes, arterial pressures, fluid and electrolyte balance and blood glucose levels.

- Administer alpha-adrenergic blocking agents (phentolamine [Regitine]) or smooth muscle relaxants (sodium nitroprusside [Nipride]) to lower blood pressure.
- Encourage patient to schedule follow-up appointments to observe for return of normal blood pressure and serum and urine levels of catecholamines.
- Give verbal and written instructions on collecting 24-hour urine specimen.
- Give instructions regarding long-term steroid therapy, including the risk of skipping doses or stopping medication abruptly.
- Assess compliance to the medication schedule.
- Teach patient and family how to measure blood pressure and when to notify physician about changes in blood pressure.
- Refer for home care nurse if indicated.
- Reinforce prior teaching about management and monitoring.
- Assist in dealing with problems that may result from long-term steroid use.
- Give encouragement and support, because patient may be fearful of repeated attacks.

For more information, see Chapter 42 in Smeltzer and Bare: *Brunner and Suddarth's Textbook of Medical-Surgical Nursing*, 11th edition. Philadelphia: Lippincott Williams & Wilkins, 2008.

P

Pituitary Tumors

Pituitary tumors are of three principal types, representing an overgrowth of eosinophilic cells, basophilic cells (hyperadrenalism), or chromophobic cells (cells with no affinity for either eosinophilic or basophilic stains). They are usually benign.

Clinical Manifestations

Eosinophilic Tumors Developing Early in Life

- Gigantism: patient may be more than 7 feet tall and large in all proportions
- Patient is weak and lethargic, hardly able to stand.

Eosinophilic Tumors Developing in Adulthood

- Acromegaly (excessive skeletal growth of the feet, hands, superciliary ridges, molar eminences, nose, and chin)
- Enlargement of every tissue and organ of the body
- Severe headaches and visual disturbances because the tumors exert pressure on the optic nerves
- Loss of color discrimination, diplopia (double vision), or blindness of a portion of the field of vision
- Decalcification of the skeleton, muscular weakness, and endocrine disturbances, similar to those occurring in hyperthyroidism

Basophilic Tumors

Cushing's syndrome: masculinization and amenorrhea in females; truncal obesity, hypertension, osteoporosis, and polycythemia in males and females

Chromophobic Tumors (90% of Pituitary Tumors)

Symptoms of hypopituitarism:

- Obesity and somnolence
- Fine, scanty hair; dry, soft skin; pasty complexion; small bones
- Headaches, loss of libido, and visual defects progressing to blindness
- Polyuria, polyphagia, lowering of the basal metabolic rate, and subnormal body temperature

Assessment and Diagnostic Methods

- History and physical examination (visual field assessment)
- Computed tomography (CT) and magnetic resonance imaging (MRI)
- Serum levels of pituitary hormone

Medical Management of Pituitary Tumors and Acromegaly

- Surgical removal through a transsphenoidal approach is the treatment of choice.
- Stereotactic radiotherapy is used to deliver external-beam radiation therapy to the tumor with minimal effect on normal tissue.
- Traditional radiation therapy and the use of bromocriptine (dopamine agonist) and octreotide (somatostatin analogue) inhibit production or release of growth hormone.
- Hypophysectomy is used to remove primary tumors surgically.

For more information, see Chapter 42 in Smeltzer and Bare: *Brunner and Suddarth's Textbook of Medical-Surgical Nursing*, 11th edition. Philadelphia: Lippincott Williams & Wilkins, 2008.

P

Pleural Effusion

Pleural effusion, a collection of fluid in the pleural space, is usually secondary to other diseases (eg, pneumonia, pulmonary infections, nephrotic syndrome, connective tissue disease, neoplastic tumors, congestive heart failure). The effusion can be relatively clear fluid, which may be a transudate due to altered formation or reabsorption of pleural fluid or an exudate resulting from inflammation by bacterial products or tumors, or it can be blood or pus. Pleural fluid accumulates due to an imbalance in hydrostatic or oncotic pressures (transudate) or as a result of inflammation by bacterial products or tumors (exudate).

Clinical Manifestations

Some symptoms are caused by the underlying disease. Pneumonia causes fever, chills, and pleuritic chest pain. Malignant effusion may result in dyspnea and coughing. The size of effusion and the time course of development determine the severity of symptoms.

- Large effusion: shortness of breath to acute respiratory distress
- Small to moderate effusion: dyspnea may not be present
- Dullness or flatness to percussion over areas of fluid, minimal or absence of breath sounds, and tracheal deviation away from the affected side

Assessment and Diagnostic Methods

- Chest x-rays (lateral decubitus)
- Chest CT scan
- Ultrasound
- Thoracentesis
- Pleural biopsy
- Pleural fluid analysis (culture, chemistry, cytology)

Medical Management

Objectives of treatment are to discover the underlying cause, to prevent reaccumulation of fluid, and to relieve discomfort, dyspnea, and respiratory compromise. Specific treatment is directed at the underlying cause.

- Thoracentesis is performed to remove fluid, collect specimen for analysis, and relieve dyspnea.
- Chest tube and water-seal drainage may be necessary for drainage and lung re-expansion.

- Chemical pleurodesis: adhesion formation is promoted when drugs are instilled into the pleural space to obliterate the space and prevent further accumulation of fluid.
- Other treatment modalities include surgical pleurectomy (insertion of a small catheter attached to a drainage bottle).
- Educate patient and family about management of catheter and drainage system with outpatient therapy.

Nursing Management

- Implement medical regimen: prepare and position patient for thoracentesis and offer support throughout the procedure.
- Assist patient in pain relief. Assist patient to assume positions that are least painful. Administer pain medication as prescribed and needed to continue frequent turning and ambulation.
- Monitor chest tube drainage and water-seal system; record amount of drainage at prescribed intervals.
- Administer nursing care related to the underlying cause of the pleural effusion.

See Nursing Management under the disorder describing the underlying condition.

P

For more information, see Chapter 23 in Smeltzer and Bare: *Brunner and Suddarth's Textbook of Medical-Surgical Nursing*, 11th edition. Philadelphia: Lippincott Williams & Wilkins, 2008.

Pleurisy

Pleurisy refers to inflammation of both the visceral and parietal pleurae. When inflamed, pleural membranes rub together. The result is severe, sharp, knifelike pain with breathing that is intensified on inspiration. Pleurisy may develop with pneumonia or upper respiratory tract infection, tuberculosis, or a collagen disease; after chest trauma, pulmonary infarction, or embolism; in primary and metastatic cancer; and after thoracotomy.

Clinical Manifestations

- Pain usually occurs on one side and worsens with deep breaths, coughing, or sneezing.
- Pain is decreased when the breath is held. Pain is localized or radiates to the shoulder or abdomen.
- As pleural fluid develops, pain lessens. A friction rub can be auscultated but disappears as fluid accumulates.

Assessment and Diagnostic Methods

- Auscultation for pleural friction rub
- Chest x-rays
- Sputum culture
- Thoracentesis, pleural fluid examination, pleural biopsy (less common)

Medical Management

Objectives of management are to discover the underlying condition causing the pleurisy and to relieve the pain.

- Patient is monitored for signs and symptoms of pleural effusion: shortness of breath, pain, and decreased excursion of the chest.
- Prescribed analgesics, such as nonsteroidal anti-inflammatory drugs (NSAIDs), are given to relieve pain and allow effective coughing.
- Applications of heat or cold are provided for symptomatic relief.
- A procaine intercostal nerve block is done for severe pain.

Nursing Management

- Enhance comfort by turning patient frequently on affected side to splint chest wall.

- Teach patient to use hands to splint rib cage while coughing.
- Position patient to decrease pain.

See Nursing Management under Pneumonia for additional information.

For more information, see Chapter 23 in Smeltzer and Bare: *Brunner and Suddarth's Textbook of Medical-Surgical Nursing*, 11th edition. Philadelphia: Lippincott Williams & Wilkins, 2008.

Pneumonia

Pneumonia is an inflammation of the lung parenchyma commonly caused by microbial agents. Classically, pneumonia has been categorized as being bacterial or typical, atypical, anaerobic/cavitary, or opportunistic. Another classification scheme categorizes pneumonias as community-acquired (CAP), hospital-acquired (HAP or nosocomial), pneumonia in the immunocompromised host, and aspiration pneumonia. Those at risk for pneumonia often have chronic underlying disorders, severe acute illness, a suppressed immune system from disease or medications, immobility, and other factors that interfere with normal lung protective mechanisms.

Pathophysiology

An inflammatory reaction may occur in the alveoli, producing an exudate that partially occludes the bronchi or alveoli; bronchospasm may also occur if the patient has reactive airway disease that interferes with gas exchange. (Bronchopneumonia, the most common form, is distributed in a patchy fashion extending from the bronchi to surrounding lung parenchyma. Lobar pneumonia is the term used if a substantial part of one or more lobes is involved.) The elderly are also at high risk. Pneumonias are caused by a variety of microbial agents in the various settings. Common organisms include *Pseudomonas aeruginosa* and *Klebsiella* species, *Staphylococcus aureus*, *Haemophilus influenzae*, *Staphylococcus pneumoniae*, and enteric gram-negative bacilli, fungi, and viruses (most common in children).

Clinical Manifestations

Clinical features vary depending on the causative organism and the patient's disease.

- Sudden chills, rapidly rising fever (38.5°C to 40.5°C), and profuse perspiration
- Pleuritic chest pain aggravated by respiration and coughing
- Severely ill patient has marked tachypnea (25 to 45 breaths/min) and dyspnea; orthopnea when not propped up
- Pulse rapid and bounding; may increase 10 beats/min per degree of temperature elevation (Celsius)
- A relative bradycardia for the amount of fever suggests viral infection or *Mycoplasma* or *Legionella* species infection.
- Sputum purulent, rusty, blood-tinged, viscous, or green depending on etiologic agent
- Other signs: fever, headache and myalgia, crackles, and signs of lobar consolidation; initial upper respiratory tract symptoms (nasal congestion, sore throat)
- Severe pneumonia: flushed cheeks; lips and nail beds demonstrating central cyanosis

Assessment and Diagnostic Methods

- Primarily history, physical examination
- Chest x-rays, blood and sputum cultures, Gram stain

🌿 Gerontologic Considerations

In older patients and in those with chronic obstructive pulmonary disease (COPD), symptoms may develop insidiously. Classic symptoms of cough, chest pain, sputum production, and fever are often absent. Pneumonia may also occur spontaneously or as a complication of a chronic disease. Onset of pneumonia may be signaled by general deterioration, confusion, tachycardia, tachypnea, anorexia, and abdominal symptoms.

Pulmonary infections are difficult to treat and are associated with a higher mortality in elderly patients than in younger patients. The presence of some signs may be misleading; chest radiography may be performed to assist in differentiating the diagnosis.

Supportive treatment includes increased fluid intake (with caution regarding fluid overload); oxygen therapy; assistance with deep breathing, coughing, sputum production, and position changes; and early ambulation. Assess the elderly patient for alterations in mental status, prostration, and heart failure. Vaccination against pneumococcal and influenza viral infections is recommended for people older than 65 years, nursing home residents, debilitated patients, and those with diabetes and cardiovascular disease.

Medical Management

- Antibiotics are prescribed based on Gram stain results and antibiotic guidelines (resistance patterns, risk factors, etiology must be considered). Combination therapy may also be used.
- Supportive treatment includes hydration, antipyretics, antihistamines, or nasal decongestants.
- Bed rest is recommended until infection shows signs of clearing.
- Oxygen therapy is given for hypoxemia.
- Respiratory support includes endotracheal intubation, high inspiratory oxygen concentrations, and mechanical ventilation.
- Treatment of atelectasis, pleural effusion, shock, respiratory failure, or superinfection is instituted, if needed.
- For groups at high risk for community-acquired pneumonia, pneumococcal vaccination is advised.

P

NURSING PROCESS: The Patient with Pneumonia

Assessment

- Assess for fever, chills, night sweats, pleuritic-type pain, fatigue, tachypnea, use of accessory muscles, bradycardia or relative bradycardia, coughing, and purulent sputum, and auscultate breath sounds for consolidation.

- Note changes in temperature; pulse; amount, odor, and color of secretions; and breath sounds.
- Frequency and severity of cough
- Degree of tachypnea or shortness of breath
- Changes in chest x-ray findings
- Assess for complications, including continuing or recurring fever, failure to resolve, atelectasis, pleural effusion, cardiac complications, and superinfection.
- Assess the elderly patient for altered mental status, dehydration (excessive fatigue), and congestive heart failure.

Diagnosis

Nursing Diagnoses

- Ineffective airway clearance related to copious tracheobronchial secretions
- Risk for deficient fluid volume related to fever and dyspnea
- Activity intolerance related to impaired respiratory function
- Imbalanced nutrition: Less than body requirements
- Deficient knowledge about treatment regimen and preventive health measures

Collaborative Problems/Potential Complications

- Hypotension and shock
- Respiratory failure
- Atelectasis
- Pleural effusion
- Confusion
- Superinfection

Planning and Goals

The major goals of the patient may include improved airway patency, rest to conserve energy, proper fluid volume, adequate nutrition, an understanding of the treatment protocol and preventive measures, and absence of complications.

Nursing Interventions

Improving Airway Patency

- Encourage hydration: fluid intake (2 to 3 L/day) to loosen secretions.
- Provide humidified air using high-humidity face mask.
- Encourage patient to cough effectively, and provide correct positioning, chest physiotherapy, and incentive spirometry.
- Provide nasotracheal suctioning if necessary.
- Provide appropriate method of oxygen therapy.
- Monitor effectiveness of oxygen therapy.

Promoting Activity Tolerance

- Counsel patient to rest and to avoid overexertion, which may exacerbate symptoms.
- Assist patient into a comfortable position that maximizes breathing (eg, semi-Fowler's).
- Change position frequently (particularly in elderly patients).

Promoting Fluid Intake and Maintaining Nutrition

- Encourage fluids (2 L/day minimum with electrolytes and calories).
- Administer intravenous fluids and nutrients, if necessary.

Informing Patient

- Instruct on cause of pneumonia and management of symptoms.
- Explain treatments in simple manner and using appropriate language.
- Repeat instructions and explanations as needed.

Monitoring and Preventing Potential Complications

- Assess for signs and symptoms of shock, multisystem organ failure, and respiratory failure (eg, evaluate vital signs, pulse oximetry, and hemodynamic monitoring parameters).
- Administer intravenous fluids and medications and respiratory support as ordered.
- Initiate preventive measures for atelectasis.
- Assess for atelectasis and pleural effusion.

- Assist with thoracentesis, and monitor patient for pneumothorax after procedure.
- Monitor for superinfection (rise in temperature, increased cough), and assist in therapy.
- Assess for confusion or cognitive changes; assess underlying factors.

Promoting Home and Community-Based Care

Teaching Patients Self-Care

- Instruct patient to continue taking full course of antibiotics as prescribed.
- Advise patient to increase activities gradually after fever subsides.
- Advise patient that fatigue and weakness may linger.
- Encourage breathing exercises to promote lung expansion and clearing.
- Encourage follow-up chest x-rays.
- Encourage patient to stop smoking.
- Instruct patient to avoid fatigue, sudden changes in temperature, and excessive alcohol intake, which lower resistance to pneumonia.
- Review principles of adequate nutrition and rest.
- Recommend influenza vaccine and Pneumovax to all patients at risk (elderly; cardiac and pulmonary disease patients).
- Refer patient for home care to facilitate adherence to therapeutic regimen, as indicated.

For more information, see Chapter 23 in Smeltzer and Bare: *Brunner and Suddarth's Textbook of Medical-Surgical Nursing*, 11th edition. Philadelphia: Lippincott Williams & Wilkins, 2008.

Pneumothorax and Hemothorax

Pneumothorax occurs when the parietal or visceral pleura is breached and the pleural space is exposed to positive atmospheric pressure. Air enters the pleural space, and a lung or a portion of it collapses. Types of pneumothorax include simple, traumatic, and tension pneumothorax. A simple pneumothorax may occur in an apparently healthy person or may be associated with interstitial lung disease or emphysema. A traumatic pneumothorax can occur with blunt chest trauma, penetrating trauma to the chest, abdominal or diaphragmatic tears, or invasive thoracic procedures. An open traumatic pneumothorax includes a mediastinal swing that produces serious circulatory problems. Hemothorax is the collection of blood in the chest cavity because of torn intercostal vessels or laceration of the lungs injured through trauma. Often both blood and air are found in the chest cavity (hemopneumothorax).

Clinical Manifestations

Signs and symptoms associated with pneumothorax depend on its size and cause:

- Pleuritic pain of sudden onset
- Minimal respiratory distress with small pneumothorax; acute respiratory distress if large
- Anxiety, dyspnea, air hunger, use of accessory muscles, and central cyanosis (with severe hypoxemia), accompanied by tachypnea, tympanic sound on percussion of the chest wall, decreased or absent breath sounds, and tactile fremitus of affected side

P

Medical Management

The goal is evacuation of air or blood from the pleural space while maintaining fluid balance.

- A large-diameter chest tube is inserted, usually in the fourth or fifth intercostal space, for hemothorax.
- A small chest tube is inserted near the second intercostal space for a pneumothorax.
- Autotransfusion is begun if excessive bleeding from chest tube occurs.

- Traumatic open pneumothorax is plugged (petroleum gauze); patient is asked to inhale and strain against a closed glottis to eject air from the thorax until the chest tube is inserted, with water-seal drainage.

Tension Pneumothorax

A tension pneumothorax occurs when air is drawn into the pleural space and is trapped with each breath. Tension builds up in the pleural space, causing lung collapse. Mediastinal shift (shift of the heart and great vessels and trachea toward the unaffected side of the chest) is a life-threatening medical emergency. Both respiratory and circulatory functions are compromised.

Clinical Manifestations

- Air hunger, anxiety, and agitation
- Increasing hypoxemia, cyanosis
- Hypotension, tachycardia, and profuse diuresis
- Tracheal shift away from the affected side

Medical Management

- Pulse oximetry is used to monitor blood oxygen levels in cases of hypoxia.
- Conversion to simple pneumothorax is accomplished by insertion of a large-bore needle into the pleural space to relieve pressure.
- Chest tube is inserted with suction to remove remaining air and fluid.
- Surgery may be necessary to close the leak.

> **!** **NURSING ALERT** Pneumothorax requires emergency treatment.

Open Pneumothorax

Open pneumothorax is an opening in the chest wall large enough to allow air to pass freely in and out of the thoracic cavity with respiration (sucking wounds). The lung is collapsed; the heart and great vessels are shifted toward the uninjured side with each inspiration and in the opposite direction with expiration (mediastinal flutter).

 NURSING ALERT To stop the flow of air through the opening in the chest wall, use anything large enough to fill the hole (towel, handkerchief, heel of hand). Have patient inhale and strain against a closed glottis (if conscious). When possible, plug the opening by sealing with petrolatum-impregnated gauze. Apply pressure dressing.

Medical Management

A thoracatomy is performed or a chest tube is connected to water-seal drainage for exit of air and fluid, and antibiotics are administered to combat infection from contamination. Autotransfusion is performed if bleeding is excessive.

Nursing Management

P

- Promote early detection through assessment and identification of high-risk population; report symptoms.
- Assist in chest tube insertion; maintain chest drainage or water-seal.
- Monitor respiratory status and reexpansion of lung, with interventions (pulmonary support) performed in collaboration with other health care professionals (eg, physician, respiratory therapist, physical therapist).
- Provide information and emotional support to patient and family.

For more information, see Chapter 23 in Smeltzer and Bare: *Brunner and Suddarth's Textbook of Medical-Surgical Nursing*, 11th edition. Philadelphia: Lippincott Williams & Wilkins, 2008.

Polycythemia

Polycythemia is an increased volume of red blood cells. The hematocrit is elevated by more than 55% in men or more than 50% in women. Polycythemia is classified as either primary or secondary.

Secondary Polycythemia

Secondary polycythemia is caused by excessive production of erythropoietin. This may occur in response to a hypoxic stimulus, as in chronic obstructive pulmonary disease or cyanotic heart disease, or in certain hemoglobinopathies in which the hemoglobin has an abnormally high affinity for oxygen, or it can occur from a neoplasm, such as renal cell carcinoma. Management of secondary polycythemia involves treatment of the primary problem. If the cause cannot be corrected, phlebotomy may be necessary to reduce hypervolemia and hyperviscosity.

Polycythemia Vera (Primary)

Polycythemia vera, or primary polycythemia, is a proliferative disorder in which the myeloid stem cells do not respond to normal control mechanisms. The bone marrow is hypercellular, and in the peripheral blood, the red cell count (predominant with hematocrit more than 50%), white cell count, and platelets are often elevated. Diagnosis is made by complete blood count (elevated red and white cells and platelets). The erythropoietin level may not be as low as would be expected with an elevated hematocrit.

Clinical Manifestations

Patients typically have a ruddy complexion and splenomegaly. The symptoms are due to the increased blood volume (headache, tinnitus, paresthesias, dizziness, fatigue, and blurred vision) or to increased blood viscosity (angina, claudication, dyspnea, and thrombophlebitis). Bleeding is a complication, and pruritus is another common and bothersome complication. Erythromyalgia (a burning sensation in the fingers and toes) may be reported.

Medical Management

The objective of management is to reduce the high red blood cell mass.

- Phlebotomy is performed repeatedly to keep the hemoglobin within normal range; iron supplements are avoided.
- Radioactive phosphorus or chemotherapeutic agents are used to suppress marrow function (may increase risk for leukemia).
- Allopurinol is used to prevent gouty attacks when the uric acid level is elevated.
- Antihistamines may be administered to control pruritus (not very effective).
- Interferon alfa-2b to manage itching related to the disease
- Anegrelide (Agrylin) may be used to inhibit platelet aggregation and control the thrombocytosis related to polycythemia.

Nursing Management

- Teach patient to recognize signs and symptoms of thrombosis.
- Advise patient to avoid aspirin and medications containing aspirin (if patient has a history of bleeding).
- Advise patient to minimize alcohol intake and avoid iron and vitamins containing iron.
- Suggest a cool or tepid bath for pruritus, along with cocoa butter–based lotions and bath products to relieve itching.

For more information, see Chapter 33 in Smeltzer and Bare: *Brunner and Suddarth's Textbook of Medical-Surgical Nursing*, 11th edition. Philadelphia: Lippincott Williams & Wilkins, 2008.

Prostatitis

Prostatitis is an inflammation of the prostate gland caused by infectious agents (bacteria, fungi, mycoplasma) or various other problems (eg, urethral stricture, prostatic hyperplasia). Microorganisms are usually carried to the prostate from the urethra. Prostatitis may be classified as bacterial or abacterial, depending on the presence or absence of microorganisms in the prostatic fluid. *Escherichia coli* is the most commonly isolated organism.

Clinical Manifestations

Signs and symptoms include perineal discomfort, burning, urgency, frequency, and pain with or after ejaculation. An additional manifestation is prostatodynia (pain in the prostate) manifested by painful voiding or by perineal pain without evidence of inflammation or bacterial growth in prostatic fluid.

Symptoms of Acute Bacterial Prostatitis

Although some patients do not develop symptoms, others complain of sudden fever and chills; perineal, rectal, or low back pain; and urinary symptoms of frequency, urgency, nocturia, and dysuria.

Symptoms of Chronic Prostatitis

In addition to the above symptoms, occasional urethral discharge may be noted. Prostatitis may cause relapsing urinary tract infection (UTI).

Assessment and Diagnostic Methods

- History, culture of prostatic fluid or tissue
- Histologic examination of tissue (occasionally)
- Segmental urine culture and urinalysis
- Expressed prostatic fluid examination

Medical Management

The goal of management is to avoid complications, which include abscess formation and septicemia. Broad-spectrum antimicrobial agents are administered for 10 to 14 days and the patient is encouraged to remain on bed rest to alleviate symptoms rapidly. Analgesics, antispasmodics, bladder sedatives, sitz baths (for 10 to 20 minutes), and stool softeners promote comfort.

Management of Chronic Bacterial Prostatitis

A priority is treatment of relapsing UTI (if noted). Pharmacologic therapy includes antimicrobials (trimethoprim-sulfamethoxazole, tetracycline, minocycline, doxycycline), and continuous suppressive treatment with low-dose antimicrobial drugs may be indicated. Additional medications include alpha-adrenergic blockers to relax the prostate and bladder. Comfort measures are the same as for acute bacterial prostatitis.

Management of Nonbacterial Prostatitis

Measures to obtain symptomatic relief include sitz baths and analgesics.

P

Nursing Management

- Administer antibiotics as prescribed.
- Recommend comfort measures: analgesics, sitz baths for 10 to 20 minutes several times daily.
- Instruct patient to complete prescribed course of antibiotics.
- Encourage fluids to satisfy thirst but do not "force" them, because effective drug levels must be maintained in urine.
- Instruct patient to avoid foods and drinks that have diuretic action or increase prostatic secretions, including alcohol, coffee, tea, chocolate, cola, and spices.
- Instruct patient to avoid sexual arousal and intercourse during periods of acute inflammation.

- Teach patient that ejaculation by sexual intercourse or masturbation may be beneficial for chronic prostatitis by reducing retention of prostatic fluids.
- Advise patient to avoid sitting for long periods to minimize discomfort.
- Emphasize that medical follow-up is necessary for at least 6 months to 1 year.

> **!** **NURSING ALERT** Be alert for collaborative problems and potential complications, such as urinary retention from prostate swelling, epididymitis, bacteremia, and pyelonephritis.

For more information, see Chapter 49 in Smeltzer and Bare: *Brunner and Suddarth's Textbook of Medical-Surgical Nursing*, 11th edition. Philadelphia: Lippincott Williams & Wilkins, 2008.

Pruritus

Pruritus (itching) is one of the most common dermatologic complaints. Scratching the itchy area causes the inflamed cells and nerve endings to release histamine, which produces more pruritus and, in turn, a vicious itch-scratch cycle. Scratching can result in altered skin integrity with excoriation, redness, raised areas (wheals), infection, or changes in pigmentation. Although pruritus usually is due to primary skin disease, it may also reflect systemic disease, such as diabetes mellitus; renal, hepatic, thyroid, or blood disorders; or cancer. Pruritus may be caused by certain oral medications (aspirin, antibiotics, hormones, opioids), contact with irritating agents (soaps, chemicals), or prickly heat (miliaria). It may also be a side effect of radiation therapy, a reaction to chemotherapy, or a symptom of infection. It may occur in elderly patients as a result of dry skin. It may also be caused by psychological factors (emotional stress).

Clinical Manifestations

- Itching and scratching, often more severe at night (itch-scratch-itch cycle)
- Excoriations, redness, raised areas on the skin (wheals), as a result of scratching
- Infections or changes in pigmentation
- Debilitating itching, in severe cases

Medical Management

The cause of pruritus needs to be identified and treated. The patient is advised to avoid washing with soap and hot water. Cold compresses, ice cubes, or cool agents that contain soothing menthol and camphor may be applied.

- Bath oils (Lubriderm or Alpha Keri) are prescribed, except for elderly patients or those with impaired balance, who should not add oil to the bath because of the danger of slipping.
- Topical steroids are prescribed to decrease itching.
- Oral antihistamines (diphenhydramine [Benadryl]) are sometimes used.
- Tricyclic antidepressants (doxepin [Sinequan]) may be prescribed when pruritus is of neuropsychogenic origin.

P

Nursing Management

- Reinforce reasons for the prescribed therapeutic regimen.
- Remind patient to use tepid (not hot) water and to shake off excess water and blot between intertriginous areas (body folds) with a towel.
- Advise patient to avoid rubbing vigorously with towel, which overstimulates skin, causing more itching.
- Instruct patient to avoid scratching and to trim nails short to prevent skin damage and infection.
- Advise patient to avoid situations that cause vasodilation (warm environment, ingestion of alcohol or hot foods and liquids).

- Lubricate skin with an emollient that traps moisture (specifically after bathing).
- Keep room cool and humidified.
- Advise patient to wear soft cotton clothing next to skin and avoid activities that result in perspiration.
- When the underlying cause of pruritus is unknown and further testing is required, explain each test and the expected outcome.

For more information, see Chapter 56 in Smeltzer and Bare: *Brunner and Suddarth's Textbook of Medical-Surgical Nursing*, 11th edition. Philadelphia: Lippincott Williams & Wilkins, 2008.

Psoriasis

Psoriasis is a chronic, noninfectious, inflammatory disease of the skin in which the production of epidermal cells occurs at a rate that is about six to nine times faster than normal. Onset may occur at any age but is most common between the ages of 15 and 35 years. Main sites of the body affected are the scalp, areas over the elbows and knees, lower part of the back, and genitalia. Bilateral symmetry often exists. Psoriasis may be associated with asymmetric rheumatoid factor–negative arthritis of multiple joints. An exfoliative psoriatic state may develop in which the disease progresses to involve the total body surface (erythrodermic psoriatic state).

Pathophysiology

The basal skin cells divide too quickly, and the newly formed cells become evident as profuse scales or plaques of epidermal tissue. Psoriatic cells may travel from the basal cell layer of the epidermis to the stratum corneum (skin surface) and be cast off in 3 to 4 days, in sharp contrast to the normal 26 to 28 days. Because of the rapid cell passage, the normal events of cell maturation and growth cannot take place and the normal protective layers of the skin cannot form. There appears to be an interplay between genetics, the immune system, and environmental factors. The primary defect is unknown. Periods of emotional stress and anxiety aggravate the condition, and trauma, infections, and seasonal and hormonal changes are trigger factors.

Clinical Manifestations

Symptoms range from a cosmetic annoyance to a physically disabling and disfiguring affliction.

- Lesions appear as red, raised patches of skin covered with silvery scales.
- If scales are scraped away, the dark-red base of lesion is exposed, with multiple bleeding points.
- Patches are dry and may or may not itch.
- The condition may involve nail pitting, discoloration, crumbling beneath the free edges, and separation of the nail plate.
- If psoriasis occurs on the palms and soles, pustular lesions may develop.
- In erythrodermic psoriasis, the patient is acutely ill, with fever, chills, and an electrolyte imbalance.

P

Psychological Considerations

- Psoriasis may cause despair and frustration; observers may stare, comment, ask embarrassing questions, or even avoid the person.
- The condition can eventually exhaust resources, interfere with work, and make life miserable in general.
- Teenagers are especially vulnerable to its psychological effects.
- Psoriasis can cause family disruption because of time-consuming treatments, messy salves, and constant shedding of scales.

Assessment and Diagnostic Methods

- Classic plaque-type lesions (change histologically progressing from early to chronic plaques)
- Signs of nail and scalp involvement and positive family history

Medical Management

Goals of management are to slow the rapid turnover of epidermis and to promote resolution of the psoriatic lesions. There is no known cure. The therapeutic approach should be understandable, cosmetically acceptable, and not too disruptive of lifestyle.

First, any precipitating or aggravating factors are addressed. An assessment is made of lifestyle, because psoriasis is significantly affected by stress. The most important principle of psoriasis treatment is gentle removal of scales (bath oils, coal tar preparations, and a soft brush used to scrub the psoriatic plaques). After bathing, the application of emollient creams containing alpha-hydroxy acids (Lac-Hydrin, Penederm) or salicylic acid will continue to soften thick scales. Four types of therapy are standard: topical, intralesional, oral, and injectable.

P

Topical Therapy

- Topical treatment is used to slow the overactive epidermis without affecting other tissues.
- Topical corticosteroid therapy acts to reduce inflammation.
- Medications include tar preparations and anthralin (irritating), alpha-hydroxy or salicylic acid, and corticosteroids. Calcipotriene (Dovonex; not recommended for use by elderly patients because of their more fragile skin, or in pregnant or lactating women); and tazarotene (Tazorac) as well as vitamin D are additional nonsteroidal agents. Occlusive (plastic) dressing may improve effectiveness. Medications may be in the form of lotions, ointments, pastes, creams, and shampoos.

NURSING ALERT Assess the flammability of any plastic substances used; caution patient not to smoke or go near open flame.

Intralesional Therapy

Intralesional injections of triamcinolone acetonide (Aristocort, Kenalog-10, Trymex)

NURSING ALERT Ensure that normal skin is not injected with the medication.

Systemic Therapy: Oral and Injectable

- Systemic cytotoxic preparations (methotrexate) may be used in treating unresponsive psoriasis. Other systemic medications in use include hydroxyurea (Hydrea) and cyclosporine A (CyA).
- Laboratory studies are monitored to ensure that hepatic, hematopoietic, and renal systems are functioning adequately.
- Patient should avoid drinking alcohol while taking methotrexate (increases possibility of liver damage).
- Oral retinoids (synthetic derivatives of vitamin A and vitamin A acid), etretinate may be prescribed.

Photochemotherapy

- Psoralens and ultraviolet A (PUVA) therapy may be used for severely debilitating psoriasis.
- Photochemotherapy is associated with long-term risks of skin cancer, cataracts, and premature aging of the skin.
- Ultraviolet B (UVB) light therapy may be used to treat generalized plaque and may be combined with topical coal

P

tar (Goeckerman's therapy). Excimer laser therapy may be another treatment.

NURSING PROCESS: The Patient with Psoriasis

Assessment

Assessment focuses on how the patient is coping with the skin condition, the appearance of "normal" skin, and the appearance of skin lesions.

- Note major skin manifestations (red, scaling papules that coalesce to form oval, well-defined plaques).
- Examine areas especially affected: elbows, knees, scalp, gluteal cleft, fingers, and toenails (for small pits).

Diagnosis

Nursing Diagnoses

- Deficient knowledge of disease and its treatment
- Impaired skin integrity related to lesions and inflammatory response
- Disturbed body image related to embarrassment over appearance and self-perception of uncleanliness

Collaborative Problems/Potential Complications

- Psoriatic arthritis
- Infection

Planning and Goals

Major goals include increased understanding of psoriasis and the treatment regimen, smoother skin with control of lesions, self-acceptance, and absence of complications.

Nursing Interventions

Promoting Understanding

- Explain with sensitivity that there is no cure and that lifetime management is necessary; the disease process can usually be controlled.
- Review pathophysiology of psoriasis and factors that provoke it: any irritation or injury to the skin (cut, abrasion, sunburn), any current illness, emotional stress, unfavorable environment (cold), and drug (caution patient about nonprescription medication).
- Review and explain treatment regimen to ensure compliance; provide patient education materials in addition to face-to-face discussions.

Increasing Skin Integrity

- Advise patient not to pick or scratch areas.
- Encourage patient to prevent the skin from drying out; dry skin causes psoriasis to worsen.
- Inform patient that water should not be too hot and skin should be dried by patting with a towel.
- Teach patient to use bath oil or emollient cleansing agent for sore and scaling skin.

P

Improving Self-Concept and Body Image

Introduce coping strategies and suggestions for reducing or coping with stressful situations to facilitate a more positive outlook and acceptance of the disease.

Monitoring and Managing Complications

- Psoriatic arthritis: note joint discomfort and evaluate further
- Assist patient to rest joint, apply heat, and take salicylates.
- Educate patient about care and treatment and need for compliance.

Promoting Home and Community-Based Care

Teaching Patients Self-Care

- Advise patient that the topical agent anthralin leaves a brownish-purple stain that subsides when treatment stops. Lesions should be covered to prevent staining clothing, furniture, and bed linens.
- Advise patient that topical corticosteroid preparations on face and around eyes predispose to cataract development. Follow strict guidelines to avoid overuse.
- Provide helpful tips on application of tar preparations.
- Teach patient to avoid exposure to sun when undergoing PUVA treatments.
- Remind patient to schedule ophthalmic examinations on a regular basis.
- Instruct patient to prevent nausea by taking methoxsalen with food.
- Instruct patient to use lubricants and bath oils to remove scales and dryness.
- Advise female patients of childbearing age that PUVA therapy is teratogenic (can cause fetal defects). They may want to consider using contraceptives during therapy.
- Encourage patient to join a support group and to contact the National Psoriasis Foundation for information.

P

Evaluation

Expected Patient Outcomes

- Demonstrates knowledge and understanding of disease and its treatment
- Demonstrates self-acceptance
- Achieves smoother skin and control of lesions
- Experiences relief of itching and discomfort
- Experiences no complications

For more information, see Chapter 56 in Smeltzer and Bare: *Brunner and Suddarth's Textbook of Medical-Surgical Nursing*, 11th edition. Philadelphia: Lippincott Williams & Wilkins, 2008.

Pulmonary Edema, Acute

Pulmonary edema is the abnormal accumulation of fluid in the lung tissue or alveoli. The major factor is usually blood backing up into the pulmonary circulation, resulting in high pressures. Fluid leaks through the capillary walls, permeating the airways and giving rise to severe dyspnea. This is a severe, life-threatening condition, usually resulting from abnormal cardiac function. Noncardiac pulmonary edema has a wide variety of causes, including sudden increase in intravascular pressure in the lung, such as after pneumonectomy, and rapid inflation of the lungs after aspiration of a pneumothorax or evacuation of a pleural effusion, toxic inhalants, drug overdose, and neurogenic pulmonary edema. The most common cause of pulmonary edema is cardiac disease related to atherosclerosis, hypertension, and valvular and myopathic disorders. If appropriate measures are taken promptly, attacks can be aborted, and patients can survive.

Clinical Manifestations

- A typical attack occurs at night after lying down for a few hours and is usually preceded by increasing restlessness, anxiety, and inability to sleep.
- The patient experiences sudden onset of breathlessness and a sense of suffocation; the hands become cold and moist, nailbeds become cyanotic, and skin turns gray.
- Pulse is weak and rapid; neck veins are distended.
- Incessant coughing produces increasing quantities of frothy, blood-tinged sputum.
- As pulmonary edema progresses, anxiety develops into near panic; the patient becomes confused, then stuporous.
- Breathing is noisy and moist; the patient can suffocate with blood-tinged, frothy fluid (can drown in own fluid).

Assessment and Diagnostic Methods

- Clinical manifestations resulting from pulmonary congestion (lung crackles with left-sided failure; with or without right-sided failure)

- Chest x-ray to confirm diagnosis
- Hemodynamic testing: pulmonary artery capillary pressure and wedge pressure, and cardiac output by pulmonary artery catheter
- Pulse oxymetry to assess arterial blood gas levels

Medical Management

Goals of medical management are to improve ventricular function and increase respiratory exchange using a combination of oxygen and medication therapies.

Oxygenation

- Oxygen in concentrations adequate to relieve hypoxia and dyspnea
- Oxygen by intermittent or continuous positive pressure, if signs of hypoxemia persist
- Endotracheal intubation and mechanical ventilation, if respiratory failure occurs
- Positive end-expiratory pressure (PEEP)
- Monitoring of pulse oximetry and arterial blood gases (ABGs)

Pharmacologic Therapy

- Morphine given intravenously in small doses to reduce anxiety and dyspnea; contraindicated in cerebral vascular accident, chronic pulmonary disease, or cardiogenic shock; have naloxone hydrochloride (Narcan) available for excessive respiratory depression
- Diuretics: furosemide (Lasix) or hydrochlorothiazide (HydroDIURIL) to produce a rapid diuretic effect
- Digitalis: to improve cardiac contractility; administer with extreme caution to patients with acute myocardial infarction
- Vasodilators and various intravenous medications: for example, milrinone to dilate the arteries, or nesiritide (Natrecor) to improve stroke volume

Nursing Management

- Assist with intubation and administering oxygen.
- Position patient upright (in bed if necessary) or with legs and feet down to promote circulation. Preferably position patient with legs dangling over the side of bed.
- Provide psychological support by reassuring patient. Use touch to convey a sense of concrete reality. Maximize time at the bedside.
- Give frequent, simple, concise information about what is being done to treat the condition and what the responses to treatment mean.
- Identify any anxiety-inducing factors (eg, a pet left alone at home, the presence of an unwelcome family member) and take steps to reduce cause of anxiety if possible.
- Monitor effects of medications. Observe patient for excessive respiratory depression, hypotension, and vomiting. Keep a morphine antagonist available (eg, naloxone hydrochloride [Narcan]). Insert and maintain an indwelling catheter if ordered or provide bedside commode.
- Recognize early stages of complications when presenting signs and symptoms are those of pulmonary congestion. Auscultate lung fields of patients with cardiac disease.
- Promote mobility and circulation. Place patient in an upright position with feet and legs dependent.
- Eliminate overexertion and emotional stress to reduce left ventricular load.

For more information, see Chapters 23 and 30 in Smeltzer and Bare: *Brunner and Suddarth's Textbook of Medical-Surgical Nursing*, 11th edition. Philadelphia: Lippincott Williams & Wilkins, 2008.

Pulmonary Embolism

Pulmonary embolism refers to the obstruction of the base or one or more branches of the pulmonary arteries by a thrombus (or thrombi) that originates somewhere in the venous system or in the right side of the heart. Gas exchange is impaired in the lung mass supplied by the obstructed vessel. Massive pulmonary embolism is life-threatening and can cause death within the first 1 to 2 hours after the embolic event. It is a common disorder associated with trauma, surgery (orthopedic, major abdominal, pelvic, gynecologic), pregnancy, oral contraceptive use, congestive heart failure, age older than 50 years, hypercoagulable states, and prolonged immobility. Most thrombi originate in the deep veins of the legs.

Clinical Manifestations

Symptoms depend on the size of the thrombus and the area of the pulmonary artery occlusion.

- Dyspnea is the most common symptom. Tachypnea is the most frequent sign.
- Chest pain is common, usually sudden in onset and pleuritic in nature; it can be substernal and may mimic angina pectoris.
- Fever, tachycardia, apprehension, cough, diaphoresis, hemoptysis, syncope, shock, and sudden death may occur.
- Multiple small emboli in the terminal pulmonary arterioles simulate symptoms of bronchopneumonia or heart failure.

Assessment and Diagnostic Methods

- Ventilation-perfusion scan, pulmonary angiography, chest x-ray
- Electrocardiogram (ECG) to assess PR interval and T-wave changes, peripheral vascular studies, impedance plethysmography, and arterial blood gas (ABG) analysis (for hypoxemia)

Prevention

- Ambulation or leg exercises in patients on bed rest
- Anticoagulant therapy before abdominothoracic surgery and every 8 to 12 hours until discharge from hospital
- Application of sequential compression devices

Medical Management

Immediate objective is to stabilize the cardiorespiratory system.

- Nasal oxygen is administered immediately to relieve hypoxemia, respiratory distress, and cyanosis.
- An infusion is started to establish an intravenous route for drugs or fluids.
- In some circumstances pulmonary angiography, spiral CT, perfusion lung scans, hemodynamic measurements, and ABGs are performed.
- An indwelling urethral catheter is inserted to monitor urinary output, if embolism is massive and patient is hypotensive.
- Hypotension is treated by infusion of dobutamine or dopamine.
- ECG is monitored continuously for dysrhythmias and right ventricular failure.
- Digitalis glycosides, intravenous diuretics, and anti-arrhythmic agents are administered when appropriate.
- Blood is drawn for serum electrolyte, complete blood count, and hematocrit analyses.
- Patient is placed on a volume-controlled ventilator if clinical assessment and ABGs indicate.
- Small doses of intravenous morphine are given to relieve anxiety, alleviate chest discomfort, help patient tolerate endotracheal tube, and ease adaptation to mechanical ventilator.

Anticoagulation Therapy

- The partial thromboplastin time (PTT) is maintained at 1.5 to 2.0 times normal, or an INR of 2.0 to 2.5.
- Heparin is administered for 5 to 7 days.
- Warfarin (Coumadin) is begun within 24 hours following the start of heparin therapy and continued for 3 to 6 months.

Thrombolytic Therapy

- Thrombolytic therapy may include urokinase alteplase, anistreplase, reteplase, and streptokinase (tissue plasminogen activator). It is reserved for pulmonary embolism affecting a significant area and causing hemodynamic instability.

- Bleeding is a significant side effect; nonessential invasive procedures are avoided.

Surgical Management

- Embolectomy by means of thoracotomy with cardiopulmonary bypass technique
- Transvenous catheter embolectomy with or without insertion of an inferior vena caval filter (eg, Greenfield)

NURSING PROCESS: The Patient with Pulmonary Embolism

Assessment

- Examine for a positive Homans' sign, which indicates impending thrombosis of the leg veins.
- Identify patients at high risk for pulmonary embolism; suspect pulmonary embolism in conditions predisposing to slowing of venous return.
- Assess frequently for signs of hypoxia; monitor pulse oximetry values.
- Be alert for potential complications of cardiogenic shock or right ventricular failure.

Diagnosis

Nursing Diagnoses

- Impaired gas exchange related to pulmonary vessel obstruction
- Risk for altered tissue perfusion related to thrombus formation
- Pain related to vascular obstruction and decreased tissue perfusion

- Anxiety related to uncertain outcome and lack of knowledge about condition and treatment
- Risk for infection related to surgical wound
- Risk for injury: hemorrhage related to decreased clotting

Planning and Goals

The major goals include adequate oxygenation, absence of additional thrombus, effective pharmacologic therapy, minimal chest pain and anxiety, positive postoperative status, and effective home and community care.

Nursing Interventions

Providing General Care

- Ensure understanding of need for continuous oxygen therapy.
- Provide nebulizers, incentive spirometry, or percussion and postural drainage.
- Encourage deep-breathing exercises.

Preventing Thrombus Formation

- Encourage early ambulation and active and passive leg exercises.
- Instruct patient to move legs in a "pumping" exercise.
- Advise patient to avoid prolonged sitting, immobility, and constrictive clothing.
- Do not permit dangling of legs and feet in a dependent position.
- Instruct patient to place feet on floor or chair and to avoid crossing legs.
- Do not leave intravenous catheters in veins for prolonged periods.

Monitoring Anticoagulant and Thrombolytic Therapy

- Advise bed rest, monitor vital signs every 2 hours, limit invasive procedures.

P

- Measure PT or activated PTT every 3 to 4 hours after thrombolytic infusion is started to confirm activation of fibrinolytic systems.
- Perform only essential ABG studies on upper extremities, with manual compression of puncture site for at least 30 minutes.

Minimizing Chest Pain, Pleuritic

- Place patient in semi-Fowler's position; turn and reposition frequently.
- Administer analgesics as prescribed for severe pain.

Alleviating Anxiety

- Encourage patient to express feelings and concerns.
- Answer questions concisely and accurately.
- Explain therapy, and describe how to recognize untoward effects early.

Managing Oxygen Therapy

Assess for hypoxia (pulse oximetry), deep breathing, incentive spirometry, nebulizer therapy, percussion, and postnasal drainage.

Providing Postoperative Nursing Care

- Measure pulmonary arterial pressure and urinary output.
- Assess insertion site of arterial catheter for hematoma formation and infection.
- Maintain blood pressure to ensure perfusion of vital organs.
- Encourage isometric exercises, antiembolism stockings, and walking when permitted out of bed; elevate foot of bed when patient is resting.
- Discourage sitting; hip flexion compresses large veins in the legs.

Promoting Home and Community-Based Care
Teaching Patients Self-Care

- Before discharge and at follow-up clinic or home visits, teach patient how to prevent recurrence and which signs and symptoms should alert patient to seek medical attention.

- Teach patient to look for bruising and bleeding when taking anticoagulants and to avoid bumping into objects. Advise patient to use a toothbrush with soft bristles to prevent gingival bleeding.
- Instruct patient not to take aspirin (an anticoagulant) or antihistamine drugs while taking warfarin sodium (Coumadin).
- Advise patient to check with physician before taking any medication, including over-the-counter drugs.
- Advise patient to continue wearing antiembolism stockings as long as directed.
- Instruct patient to avoid laxatives, which affect vitamin K absorption (vitamin K promotes coagulation).
- Teach patient to avoid sitting with legs crossed or for prolonged periods.
- Recommend that patient change position regularly when traveling, walk occasionally, and do active exercises of legs and ankles.
- Advise patient to drink plenty of liquids.
- Teach patient to report dark, tarry stools immediately.
- Recommend that patient wear identification stating that he or she is taking anticoagulants.

P

For more information, see Chapter 23 in Smeltzer and Bare: *Brunner and Suddarth's Textbook of Medical-Surgical Nursing*, 11th edition. Philadelphia: Lippincott Williams & Wilkins, 2008.

Pulmonary Heart Disease (Cor Pulmonale)

Cor pulmonale is a condition in which the right ventricle enlarges (with or without right heart failure) as a result of diseases that affect the structure or function of the lung or its vasculature.

A mean pulmonary artery pressure of 45 mm Hg or more may occur. The most frequent cause is chronic obstructive pulmonary disease (COPD). Other causes are conditions that restrict or compromise ventilatory function (massive obesity, deformities of the thoracic cage) or that reduce the pulmonary vascular bed (pulmonary embolus), causing primary pulmonary hypertension. Certain disorders of the nervous system, respiratory muscles, chest wall, and pulmonary arterial tree may also be responsible for cor pulmonale. Prognosis depends on reversing the hypertensive process.

Clinical Manifestations

Symptoms are usually those of the underlying lung disease.

- Clinical features include COPD, shortness of breath, and cough.
- Right ventricular failure develops (edema of the feet and legs, distended neck veins, enlarged palpable liver, pleural effusion, ascites, and a heart murmur).
- Headache, confusion, and somnolence from carbon dioxide narcosis may occur.

Medical Management

Objectives of treatment are to improve ventilation and to treat both the underlying lung disease and the manifestations of heart disease.

- Oxygen is given to reduce pulmonary arterial pressure and pulmonary vascular resistance. Continuous (24-h/day) oxygen therapy is provided for severe hypoxia.
- Blood oxygen levels are assessed with pulse oximetry and arterial blood gas (ABG) analysis.
- Bronchial hygiene, bronchodilators, and chest physical therapy may be instituted.
- If respiratory failure occurs, intubation and mechanical ventilation may be necessary.

- If heart failure occurs, hypoxemia and hypercapnia must be relieved to improve cardiac output.
- Peripheral edema and circulatory load on the right side of the heart are reduced with bed rest, sodium restriction, and diuretics.
- If indicated (eg, in left ventricular failure), digitalis may be given.
- The electrocardiogram (ECG) is monitored.
- Pulmonary infection must be treated promptly (it will exacerbate hypoxemia and cor pulmonale).

Nursing Management

See Nursing Management of Heart Failure for additional information.

- If required, assist with intubation and mechanical ventilation. Support patient physically and emotionally.
- Assess respiratory and cardiac status.
- Instruct patient about the importance of close monitoring and adherence to the therapeutic regimen, especially oxygen.
- Explore and address factors that affect the patient's adherence to the treatment regimen.
- Advise patient and family that management is long-term and that most care and monitoring will be performed at home for this chronic disorder.
- Advise patient to avoid activities that irritate airway if COPD exists.
- Administer continuous oxygen and instruct how to use.
- Urge patient to stop smoking, if appropriate; refer patient to smoking cessation or community support group.
- Counsel patient about nutrition if a sodium-restricted diet or a diuretic medication is part of treatment.
- If patient's physical condition warrants close assessment or if patient cannot manage self-care, refer the patient for home care.

> **NURSING ALERT** If the patient has coincident left
> ventricular failure, supraventricular dysrhythmia, or right
> ventricular failure and is not responsive to other therapy,
> administer digitalis, if prescribed, with extreme caution
> because pulmonary heart disease appears to enhance
> susceptibility to digitalis toxicity.

For more information, see Chapter 23 in Smeltzer and Bare: *Brunner and Suddarth's Textbook of Medical-Surgical Nursing*, 11th edition. Philadelphia: Lippincott Williams & Wilkins, 2008.

Pulmonary Hypertension

Pulmonary hypertension is a condition that is not clinically evident until late in the disease. The systolic pulmonary arterial pressure exceeds 30 mm Hg, and the mean pulmonary artery pressure is higher than 25 mm Hg at rest or 30 mm Hg with activity. There are two forms: primary (idiopathic) and secondary. Primary pulmonary hypertension is uncommon; diagnosis is made by exclusion. The exact cause is unknown. The clinical presentation exists with no evidence of pulmonary and cardiac disease or pulmonary embolism. It occurs most often in women between ages 20 and 40 and is usually fatal within 5 years of diagnosis. Secondary pulmonary hypertension is more common and results from existing cardiac or pulmonary disease. The prognosis depends on the severity of the underlying disorder and the changes in the pulmonary vascular bed.

Pathophysiology

A common cause is pulmonary artery constriction due to hypoxia from chronic obstructive pulmonary disease (COPD). When the pulmonary vascular bed is destroyed or obstructed, its ability to handle the blood volume received is impaired. The increased blood flow increases the pulmonary artery pressure and pulmonary vascular resistance and pressure (hypertension).

Clinical Manifestations

- Dyspnea, the main symptom, is noticed first with exertion and then at rest.
- Substernal chest pain is common (25% to 50% of patients).
- Weakness, fatigability, syncope, and occasional hemoptysis may occur.
- Signs of right-sided heart failure (peripheral edema, ascites, distended neck veins, liver engorgement, crackles, heart murmur) are noted.
- Electrocardiogram (ECG) changes (right ventricular hypertrophy) are seen, with right axis deviation and tall, peaked P waves in inferior leads and tall anterior R waves and ST-segment depression or T-wave inversion anteriorly.
- PaO_2 is decreased (hypoxemia).

Assessment and Diagnostic Methods

- Chest x-ray films
- ECG
- Cardiac catheterization (elevated pulmonary arterial pressure)
- Ventilation-perfusion scan or pulmonary angiography (detects defects in pulmonary vasculature)
- Pulmonary function studies (normal or slight decreased vital capacity, lung compliance, and diffusing capacity)
- Lung biopsy (thoracotomy or thoracoscopy)
- Echocardiogram, open-lung biopsy (in some cases)

Medical Management

Objective of treatment is to manage the underlying cardiac or pulmonary condition. In all cases, management includes continuous oxygen therapy for progressive disease to decrease vasoconstriction and reduce pulmonary hypertension.

Treatment When Hypertension Results From Cor Pulmonale

- Fluid restriction
- Cardiac glycosides (digitalis)
- Calcium channel blockers for vasodilation
- Rest
- Diuretics to decrease fluid accumulation

Treatment When Hypertension Results From Primary Pulmonary Hypertension

- Vasodilators (calcium channel blockers, intravenous prostacyclin); also bosentan, an endothelin receptor antagonist.
- Anticoagulants (warfarin [Coumadin])
- Heart-lung transplantation when not responsive to other therapies

Nursing Management

- Identify patients at high risk for developing pulmonary hypertension (ie, those with COPD, pulmonary emboli, congenital heart disease, and mitral valve disease).
- Be alert for signs and symptoms.
- Administer prescribed oxygen therapy appropriately.
- Inform and instruct patient and family about home oxygen supplementation.

For more information, see Chapter 23 in Smeltzer and Bare: *Brunner and Suddarth's Textbook of Medical-Surgical Nursing*, 11th edition. Philadelphia: Lippincott Williams & Wilkins, 2008.

Pyelonephritis, Acute

Pyelonephritis, an upper urinary tract infection, is a bacterial infection of the renal pelvis, tubules, and interstitial tissue of one or both kidneys. Bacteria reach the bladder through the urethra and ascend to the kidney. It is frequently secondary to urine backup into the ureters (ureterovesical reflux), usually at the time of voiding. Urinary tract obstruction (eg, strictures, urinary stones, tumors, and prostatic hypertrophy) is another cause. Pyelonephritis may be acute or chronic.

Clinical Manifestations

- Chills and fever, flank pain, costovertebral angle tenderness, nausea, vomiting, headache, malaise
- Leukocytosis, bacteria and white blood cells in the urine, symptoms of lower urinary tract involvement (dysuria and frequency) are common.
- Enlarged kidneys

Assessment and Diagnostic Methods

- Ultrasound or computed tomography (CT) scan
- Urine culture and sensitivity tests
- Radionuclide imaging with gallium if other studies not conclusive

Medical Management

- Intensive antimicrobial therapy: 2 to 3 days of parenteral therapy if patient is dehydrated, has nausea or vomiting, shows signs of sepsis, or is pregnant; followed with oral agents once patient is afebrile and showing clinical improvement; 2-week course of antibiotics for outpatients
- Continuous antimicrobial treatment after initial regimen until there is no evidence of infection, all causative factors have been treated or controlled, and kidney function has stabilized
- Hydration (oral or parenteral) to flush urinary tract

Nursing Management

The plan of care is the same as that for upper urinary tract infections.

For more information, see Chapter 45 in Smeltzer and Bare: *Brunner and Suddarth's Textbook of Medical-Surgical Nursing*, 11th edition. Philadelphia: Lippincott Williams & Wilkins, 2008.

Pyelonephritis, Chronic

Repeated bouts of acute pyelonephritis may lead to chronic pyelonephritis (chronic interstitial nephritis). Complications of chronic pyelonephritis include end-stage renal disease from progressive loss of nephrons secondary to chronic inflammation and scarring, hypertension, and formation of kidney stones (from chronic infection with urea-splitting organisms, resulting in stone formation).

Clinical Manifestations

- Patient usually has no symptoms of infection unless an acute exacerbation occurs.
- Fatigue, headache, and poor appetite may occur.
- Polyuria, excessive thirst, and weight loss may result.
- Persistent and recurring infection may produce progressive scarring resulting in renal failure; however, evidence suggests chronic pyelonephritis is less frequently a cause of chronic renal failure.

Assessment and Diagnostic Methods

- Intravenous urography
- Measurement of blood urea nitrogen (BUN), creatinine levels, and creatinine clearance

Medical Management

Goal of treatment is to eradicate bacteria from the urine.

- Antimicrobial medication is based on pathogen identified by culture.
- Nitrofurantoin or a combination of trimethoprim and sulfamethoxazole (TMP-SMZ) to suppress bacterial growth

Nursing Management

The plan of care is the same as that for upper urinary tract infections.

- Recognize patients at risk for infection.
- If patient is hospitalized, encourage fluids (3 to 4 L/day) unless contraindicated.
- Monitor and record intake and output.
- Assess body temperature every 4 hours and treat elevations as prescribed.
- Teach preventive measures and early recognition of symptoms.
- Instruct patient to complete full prescription of antibiotics and have a follow-up urine culture 2 weeks after completion of antibiotic therapy (additional weeks of antibiotics will be needed if relapse occurs).
- Monitor with serum creatinine determinations and blood counts for duration of long-term therapy.
- Monitor for and teach patient signs of compromised renal function in excretion of antimicrobial agents, particularly with nephrotoxic antimicrobial agents.

P

For more information, see Chapter 45 in Smeltzer and Bare: *Brunner and Suddarth's Textbook of Medical-Surgical Nursing*, 11th edition. Philadelphia: Lippincott Williams & Wilkins, 2008.

R

Raynaud's Disease

Raynaud's disease is a form of intermittent arteriolar vasoconstriction that affects the fingers and toes. The cause is unknown, but episodes may be associated with immunologic disorders (scleroderma, systemic lupus erythematosus, rheumatoid arthritis, obstructive arterial disease). Episodes may be triggered by emotional factors or by unusual sensitivity to cold. Raynaud's disease is most common in women between the ages of 16 and 40 years and is seen much more frequently in cold climates and during the winter months. The term "Raynaud's phenomenon," as opposed to Raynaud's disease, is currently used to refer to localized, intermittent episodes of vasoconstriction of small arteries of the feet and hands, causing color and temperature changes. It is generally unilateral and affects only one or two digits. It is always associated with an underlying systemic disease. The prognosis for Raynaud's disease varies: some patients slowly improve, some grow slowly worse, and others show no change.

Clinical Manifestations

- Coldness, pain, and pallor brought on by sudden vasoconstriction followed by cyanosis followed by vasodilation and hyperemia (exaggerated reflow) with a resultant red color (rubor); the progression follows the characteristic color change white, blue, red.
- Numbness, tingling, and burning pain occur as color changes.
- Involvement tends to be bilateral and symmetric.

Medical Management

The prime objective in controlling Raynaud's disease is avoiding the stimuli (cold, tobacco) that provoke vasoconstriction.

Calcium-channel blockers may be effective in relieving symptoms. Sympathectomy (interruption of sympathetic nerves by removal of sympathetic ganglia or division of their branches) may be helpful.

Nursing Management

- Instruct patient to avoid situations that may be upsetting, stressful, or unsafe.
- Reassure patient that serious complications (gangrene and amputation) are not usual.
- Emphasize the importance of avoiding nicotine (smoking cessation without use of nicotine patches); assist in finding support group.
- Advise patient to minimize exposure to cold, remain indoors as much as possible, and wear protective clothing when outdoors during cold weather.
- Advise patient to handle sharp objects carefully to avoid injuring the fingers.
- Caution about postural hypotension (results from drugs and is increased by alcohol, exercise, and hot weather).

For more information, see Chapter 31 in Smeltzer and Bare: *Brunner and Suddarth's Textbook of Medical-Surgical Nursing*, 11th edition. Philadelphia: Lippincott Williams & Wilkins, 2008.

R

Regional Enteritis (Crohn's Disease)

Regional enteritis is a subacute and chronic inflammation that extends through all layers of the bowel wall. It commonly occurs in adolescents or young adults and is seen frequently in the older population (50 to 80 years), but it can occur at any time of life. Although the most common areas in which it is found are the distal ileum and colon, it can occur anywhere along the gastrointestinal tract. Fistulas, fissures, and abscesses form as the inflammation extends into the peritoneum. In advanced cases, the intestinal mucosa has a cobblestone-like appearance. As the disease advances, the bowel wall thickens and becomes fibrotic and the intestinal lumen narrows. The clinical course and symptoms vary. In some patients, periods of remission and exacerbation occur; in others, the disease follows a fulminating course.

Clinical Manifestations

- Onset of symptoms is usually insidious, with prominent abdominal pain and diarrhea unrelieved by defecation.
- Diarrhea is present in 90% of patients.
- Crampy pains occur after meals; the patient tends to limit intake, causing weight loss, malnutrition, and secondary anemia.
- Chronic diarrhea may occur, resulting in an uncomfortable person who is thin and emaciated from inadequate food intake and constant fluid loss. The inflamed intestine may perforate and form intra-abdominal and anal abscesses.
- Fever and leukocytosis occur.
- Abscesses, fistulas, and fissures are common.
- Symptoms extend beyond the gastrointestinal tract to include joint problems (arthritis), skin lesions (erythema nodosum), ocular disorders (conjunctivitis), and oral ulcers.

Assessment and Diagnostic Methods

- Barium study of the upper gastrointestinal tract is the most conclusive diagnostic aid; shows the classic "string sign" of the terminal ileum (constriction of a segment of intestine) as well as cobblestone appearance, fistulas, and fissures.
- Proctosigmoidoscopic examination, computed tomography (CT) scan
- Stool examination for occult blood and steatorrhea
- Complete blood count (decreased Hgb and Hct), sedimentation rate (elevated), albumin, and protein levels (usually decreased due to malnutrition)

Medical Management

See Medical Management under Ulcerative Colitis for additional information.

Nursing Management

See Nursing Process: The Patient With Inflammatory Bowel Disease under Ulcerative Colitis for additional information.

For more information, see Chapter 38 in Smeltzer and Bare: *Brunner and Suddarth's Textbook of Medical-Surgical Nursing*, 11th edition. Philadelphia: Lippincott Williams & Wilkins, 2008.

Renal Failure, Acute

Renal failure results when the kidneys are unable to remove metabolic waste and perform their regulatory functions. Acute renal failure (ARF) is a sudden and almost complete loss of kidney function (decreased glomerular filtration rate [GFR]). Three major categories of ARF are prerenal (hypoperfusion, as from volume depletion disorders, extreme vasodilation, or impaired cardiac performance); intrarenal (parenchymal damage to the glomeruli or kidney tubules, as from burns, crush injuries, infections, transfusion reaction, or nephrotoxicity, which may lead to acute tubular necrosis [ATN]); and postrenal (urinary tract obstruction, as from calculi, tumor, strictures, prostatic hyperplasia, or blood clots).

R

Clinical Stages

- Initiation period: initial insult and oliguria
- Oliguric period (urine volume less than 400 mL/d): uremic symptoms first appear and hyperkalemia may develop
- Diuresis period: gradual increase in urine output signaling beginning of glomerular filtration's recovery. Laboratory values stabilize and start to decrease.

- Recovery period: improving renal function (may take 3 to 12 months)

Clinical Manifestations

- Critical illness and lethargy with persistent nausea, vomiting, and diarrhea
- Skin and mucous membranes are dry; breath has odor of urine (uremic fetor).
- Central nervous system manifestations: drowsiness, headache, muscle twitching, seizures
- Urine output scanty to normal; urine may be bloody with low specific gravity
- Steady rise in BUN may occur depending on degree of catabolism; serum creatinine values increase with disease progression.
- Hyperkalemia may lead to dysrhythmias and cardiac arrest.
- Progressive acidosis, increase in serum phosphate concentrations, and low serum calcium levels may be noted.
- Anemia from blood loss due to uremic gastrointestinal lesions, reduced red blood cell life-span, and reduced erythropoietin production

Assessment and Diagnostic Methods

- BUN, creatinine, electrolyte analyses
- Urine output measurements
- Renal ultrasonography, CT and MRI scans

🌿 Gerontologic Considerations

- With normal aging, changes in kidney function increase susceptibility to kidney dysfunction and renal failure.
- Alterations in renal blood flow, GFR, and renal clearance increase the risk for drug-associated changes in renal function; administer all medications with caution.
- Because the older kidney is less able to respond to fluid and electrolyte changes, renal problems need to be recognized and treated quickly to avoid kidney damage.

- When elderly patients must undergo extensive diagnostic tests or when new medications (eg, diuretics) are added, take precautions to prevent dehydration leading to ARF.
- The mortality rate for ARF is slightly higher in elderly patients. Its etiology includes prerenal causes (eg, dehydration) and intrarenal causes (eg, nephrotoxic agents, such as nonsteroidal anti-inflammatory drugs and contrast agents).
- Diabetes mellitus increases the risk for contrast agent-induced renal failure because of preexisting renal insufficiency and imposed fluid restriction.

Medical Management

Treatment objectives are to restore normal chemical balance and prevent complications until renal tissues are repaired and renal function is restored. Possible causes of damage are identified and treated.

- Fluid balance is managed based on daily weight, serial measurements of central venous pressure, serum and urine concentrations, fluid losses, blood pressure, and clinical status. Fluid excesses are treated with mannitol, furosemide, or ethacrynic acid to initiate diuresis and prevent or minimize subsequent renal failure.
- Blood flow is restored to the kidneys with the use of intravenous fluids, albumin, or blood product transfusions.
- Dialysis (hemodialysis, hemofiltration, or peritoneal dialysis) is started to prevent complications of uremia, including hyperkalemia, pericarditis, and seizures.
- Ion exchange resins (orally or by retention enema)
- Intravenous glucose and insulin or calcium glutamate as an emergency and temporary measure to treat hyperkalemia
- Sodium bicarbonate to elevate plasma pH
- Parenteral erythropoietin (Epogen) to treat reduced erythropoietin production and prevent anemia
- Shock and infection are treated if present.
- Arterial blood gases are monitored when severe acidosis is present.

R

- If respiratory problems develop, ventilatory measures are started.
- Phosphate-binding agents such as aluminum hydroxide to control elevated serum phosphate concentrations
- Dietary protein is limited to about 1 g/kg during oliguric phase to minimize protein breakdown and to prevent accumulation of toxic end products.
- Caloric requirements are met with high-carbohydrate feedings; parenteral nutrition (PN)
- Foods and fluids containing potassium and phosphorus are restricted; potassium intake is limited to 40 to 60 mEq/d. Sodium intake is restricted to 2 g/d.
- Blood chemistries are evaluated to determine amount of replacement sodium, potassium, and water during oliguric phase.
- After the diuretic phase, high-protein, high-calorie diet is given with gradual resumption of activities.

NURSING PROCESS: The Patient with Acute Renal Failure

Assessment

- Take nursing history and perform physical assessment, particularly for patients at risk for ARF.
- Monitor intake and output for indications of failing renal function.
- Assess diagnostic test values and monitor patient's response to therapy regularly for signs of progress or deterioration.
- Direct attention to patient's primary disorder; monitor for complications.

Diagnosis

Nursing Diagnoses

- Fluid volume excess related to decreased urine output
- Activity intolerance related to fatigue, toxins, and fluid buildup

- Risk for impaired skin integrity related to edema, toxins, or impaired tissue perfusion
- Risk for infection related to intravenous lines or catheters or uremic toxins
- Deficient knowledge regarding condition and its treatment

Collaborative Problems/Potential Complications

- Pericarditis
- Anemia
- Bone disease
- Hyperkalemia, or risk for hyperkalemia

Planning and Goals

Major goals include ideal fluid balance, body weight, and electrolyte levels, increased knowledge about condition and treatment, participation in activities as tolerated, and absence of complications.

Nursing Interventions

- Stay focused on the primary disorder, and monitor for complications.
- Assist in emergency treatment of fluid and electrolyte imbalances.
- Assess progress and response to treatment; provide physical and emotional support.
- Keep family informed about condition and provide support.

Monitoring Fluid and Electrolyte Levels

- Screen parenteral fluids, all oral intake, and all medications for hidden sources of potassium.
- Monitor cardiac function and musculoskeletal status for signs of hyperkalemia. Monitor serum electrolyte levels and ECG for peaked T waves.
- Pay careful attention to parenteral and oral intake, urine output, gastric and stool output, wound drainage and perspiration, changes in body weight, edema, distention of

jugular veins, changes in heart and breath sounds, and increasing difficulty breathing.
- Auscultate lungs for moist crackles.
- Assess for generalized edema by examining presacral and pretibial areas regularly.
- Report indicators of deteriorating fluid and electrolyte status immediately. Prepare for emergency treatment of hyperkalemia. Prepare patient for dialysis as indicated to correct fluid and electrolyte imbalances.

Reducing Metabolic Rate

- Reduce exertion and metabolic rate during most acute stage with bed rest.
- Prevent or treat fever and infection promptly.

Promoting Pulmonary Function

Assist patient to turn, cough, and take deep breaths frequently. Encourage and assist patient to move and turn.

Avoiding Infection

- Practice asepsis when working with invasive lines and catheters.
- Avoid using an indwelling catheter if possible.

Providing Skin Care

- Perform meticulous skin care.
- Massage bony prominences, turn patient frequently, encourage bathing with tepid water for comfort, and prevent skin breakdown.

Providing Support During Dialysis

- Assist, explain, and support patient and family; do not overlook psychological needs and concerns.
- Explain rationale of treatment to patient and family. Repeat explanations and clarify answers as needed.
- Encourage family to touch and talk to patient during dialysis.

- Continually assess patient for complications (eg, pericarditis, bone disease, anemia) and their precipitating causes.

For more information, see Chapter 44 in Smeltzer and Bare: *Brunner and Suddarth's Textbook of Medical-Surgical Nursing*, 11th edition. Philadelphia: Lippincott Williams & Wilkins, 2008.

Renal Failure, Chronic (End-Stage Renal Disease)

Chronic renal failure, or end-stage renal disease (ESRD), is a progressive, irreversible deterioration in renal function in which the body's ability to maintain metabolic and fluid and electrolyte balance fails, resulting in uremia or azotemia. It may be caused by diabetes, hypertension, chronic glomerulonephritis, pyelonephritis, hereditary lesions (eg, polycystic disease), vascular disorders, obstruction of the urinary tract, infections, or toxic agents. Environmental and occupational agents that have been implicated in chronic renal failure include lead, cadmium, mercury, and chromium. Dialysis or kidney transplantation eventually becomes necessary for survival. The rate of decline and progression of ESRD is related to the underlying disorder, urinary excretion of protein, and the presence of hypertension.

Clinical Manifestations

- Cardiovascular: hypertension, pitting edema (feet, hands, sacrum), periorbital edema, pericardial friction rub, engorged neck veins, pericarditis, pericardial effusion, pericardial tamponade, hyperkalemia, hyperlipidemia
- Integumentary: gray-bronze skin color, dry flaky skin, severe pruritus, ecchymosis, purpura, thin brittle nails, coarse thinning hair
- Pulmonary: crackles; thick, tenacious sputum; depressed cough reflex; pleuritic pain; shortness of breath; tachypnea;

Kussmaul-type respirations; uremic pneumonitis ("uremic lung")

- Gastrointestinal: ammonia odor to breath (fetor uremicus), metallic taste, mouth ulcerations and bleeding, anorexia, nausea and vomiting, hiccups, constipation or diarrhea, bleeding from gastrointestinal tract
- Neurologic: weakness and fatigue, confusion, inability to concentrate, disorientation, tremors, seizures, asterixis, restlessness of legs, burning of soles of feet, behavior changes
- Musculoskeletal: muscle cramps, loss of muscle strength, renal osteodystrophy, bone pain, fractures, foot drop
- Reproductive: amenorrhea, testicular atrophy, infertility, decreased libido
- Hematologic: anemia, thrombocytopenia

🌿 Gerontologic Considerations

Diabetes mellitus and hypertension are the leading causes of chronic renal failure in elderly patients. The symptoms of other disorders (heart failure, dementia) can mask the symptoms of renal disease and delay or prevent diagnosis and treatment. The patient often complains of signs and symptoms of nephrotic syndrome, such as edema and proteinuria. The elderly patient may develop nonspecific signs of disturbed renal function and fluid and electrolyte imbalances. Hemodialysis and peritoneal dialysis have been used effectively in elderly patients. Concomitant disorders have made transplantation a less common treatment for the elderly. Conservative management, including nutritional therapy, fluid control, and medications (such as phosphate binders), may be used if dialysis or transplantation is not suitable.

Medical Management

Goals of management are to retain kidney function and maintain homeostasis for as long as possible. All factors that contribute to ESRD and those that are reversible (eg, obstruction) are identified and treated.

- Complications can be prevented or delayed by administering prescribed antihypertensives, cardiovascular agents, anticonvulsants, erythropoietin (Epogen), iron supplements, phosphate-binding agents (antacids), and calcium supplements.
- Dietary intervention is needed, with careful regulation of protein intake, fluid intake to balance fluid losses, and sodium intake, and with some restriction of potassium.
- Adequate intake of calories and vitamins is ensured. Calories are supplied with carbohydrates and fats to prevent wasting.
- Protein is restricted; protein must be of high biologic value (dairy products, eggs, meats).
- Vitamin supplementation
- Fluid allowance is 500 to 600 mL of fluid or more than the 24-hour urine output.

Pharmacologic Management

- Hyperphosphatemia and hypocalcemia are treated with aluminum-based antacids or calcium carbonate; both must be given with food.
- Hypertension is managed by intravascular volume control and antihypertensive medication.
- Heart failure and pulmonary edema are treated with fluid restriction, low-sodium diet, diuretics, inotropic agents (eg, digitalis or dobutamine), and dialysis.
- Metabolic acidosis is treated, if necessary, with sodium bicarbonate supplements or dialysis.
- Hyperkalemia is treated with dialysis; medications are monitored for potassium content; patient is placed on potassium-restricted diet; Kayexalate is administered as needed.
- Patient is observed for early evidence of neurologic abnormalities (eg, slight twitching, headache, delirium, or seizure activity).
- The onset of seizures, type, duration, and general effect on patient are recorded; physician is notified immediately and patient is protected from injury with padded side rails.

R

- Intravenous diazepam (Valium) or phenytoin (Dilantin) is administered to control seizures.
- Anemia is treated with recombinant human erythropoietin (Epogen); hematocrit is monitored frequently.
- Heparin is adjusted as necessary to prevent clotting of dialysis lines during treatments.
- Serum iron and transferrin levels are monitored to assess iron states (iron is necessary for adequate response to erythropoietin).
- Blood pressure and serum potassium levels are monitored.
- Patient is referred to a dialysis and transplantation center early in the course of progressive renal disease. Dialysis is initiated when patient cannot maintain a reasonable lifestyle with conservative treatment.

NURSING PROCESS: The Patient with Chronic Renal Failure

Assessment

- Assess fluid status and help patient limit fluid intake to prescribed limit.
- Assess nutritional status and address factors contributing to nutritional imbalance.
- Assess patient's understanding about the condition and it treatment, explain renal function, and assist patient to identify ways to incorporate lifestyle changes related to illness and treatment.
- Assess factors contributing to fatigue.
- Assess patient's and family's responses and reaction to illness and treatment. Encourage open discussion of concerns about changes produced by disease and treatment.
- Assess for and monitor collaborative problems (eg, hyperkalemia, pericarditis, pericardial effusion and pericardial tamponade, hypertension, anemia, bone disease, and metastatic calcifications).

Diagnosis

Nursing Diagnoses

- Excess fluid volume related to decreased urine output, dietary excesses, and retention of sodium and water
- Imbalanced nutrition: Less than body requirements related to anorexia, nausea and vomiting, dietary restrictions, and altered oral mucous membranes
- Deficient knowledge regarding condition and treatment regimen

Planning and Goals

Goals for the patient are fluid balance, optimal nutritional status, and knowledge about the disease and treatment regimen.

Nursing Interventions

Managing Excess Fluid Volume

- Assess fluid status and identify potential sources of imbalance.
- Monitor patient's progress and compliance with treatment regimen.

Promoting Balanced Nutrition

- Implement a dietary program to ensure proper nutritional intake within the limits of the treatment regimen.
- Provide a referral for a nutritional consultation.

Educating the Patient and Family

Teaching Patients Self-Care

- Provide ongoing explanations and information to patient and family concerning ESRD, treatment options, and potential complications.
- Refer patient for dietary counseling and assist with nutritional planning.
- Assist patient with an activity plan to conserve energy and maximize activity tolerance.

R

- Teach patient and family what problems to report: signs of worsening renal failure, hyperkalemia, access problems.
- Provide medication teaching and show patient undergoing hemodialysis how to assess vascular access for patency and precautions to take (no venipunctures or blood pressure on access arm).

Continuing Care

- Provide assistance and emotional support to patient and family in dealing with dialysis and its long-term implications.
- Stress the importance of follow-up examinations and treatment.
- Refer patient to home care nurse for continued monitoring and support.

Evaluation

Expected Patient Outcomes

- Demonstrates fluid balance
- Maintains adequate nutritional intake
- Tolerates activities of daily living
- Experiences absence of complications

For more information, see Chapter 44 in Smeltzer and Bare: *Brunner and Suddarth's Textbook of Medical-Surgical Nursing*, 11th edition. Philadelphia: Lippincott Williams & Wilkins, 2008.

R

Seborrheic Dermatoses

Seborrhea is an excessive production of sebum (secretion of sebaceous glands). Seborrheic dermatitis is a chronic inflammatory disease of the skin with a predilection for areas that are well supplied with sebaceous glands or that lie between folds of the skin, where the bacterial count is high. Seborrheic dermatitis has a genetic predisposition; hormones, nutritional status, infection, and emotional stress influence its course. There are remissions and exacerbations of this condition. Areas most often affected are the face, scalp, cheeks, ears, axillae, and various skin folds.

Clinical Manifestations

Two forms can occur: an oily form and a dry form. Either form may start in childhood with fine scaling of the scalp or other areas.

Oily Form

Moist or greasy patches of sallow, greasy-appearing skin, with or without scaling, and slight erythema (redness); small pustules or papulopustules on trunk resembling acne

Dry Form

Flaky desquamation of the scalp (dandruff); asymptomatic mild forms or scaling often accompanied by pruritus, leading to scratching and secondary complications (ie, infection and excoriation)

Medical Management

Because there is no known cure for seborrhea, the objectives of therapy are to control the disorder and allow the skin to repair itself. Treatment measures include:

- Administering topical corticosteroid cream to body and face (use with caution near eyes)
- Aerating skin and careful cleansing of creases or folds to prevent candidal yeast infection (evaluate patients with persistent candidiasis for diabetes)
- Shampooing hair daily or at least three times weekly with medicated shampoos. Two or three different types of shampoo are used in rotation to prevent the seborrhea from becoming resistant to a particular shampoo.

Nursing Management

- Advise patient to remove external irritants and to avoid excess heat and perspiration; rubbing and scratching prolong the disorder.
- Instruct patient to avoid secondary infections by airing the skin and keeping skin folds clean and dry.
- Caution patient that seborrheic dermatitis is a chronic problem that tends to recur. The goal is to keep it under control.
- Encourage patient to adhere to treatment program.
- Treat patients with sensitivity and an awareness of their need to express their feelings when they become discouraged by the disorder's effect on body image.

S

For more information, see Chapter 56 in Smeltzer and Bare: *Brunner and Suddarth's Textbook of Medical-Surgical Nursing*, 11th edition. Philadelphia: Lippincott Williams & Wilkins, 2008.

Shock, Cardiogenic

Cardiogenic shock occurs when the heart's ability to pump blood is impaired, leading to an inadequate supply of oxygen for the heart and tissues. The result is a marked reduction in cardiac output, with inadequate perfusion to the heart, brain, and kidneys. Causes of cardiogenic shock are either coronary or noncoronary. Coronary cardiogenic shock is more common and is seen most often in patients with myocardial infarction. Noncoronary causes include tension pneumothorax, severe metabolic problems, such as hypoxemia, acidosis, hypoglycemia, hypocalcemia, cardiac tamponade, cardiomyopathy, valvular damage, and dysrhythmias.

Clinical Manifestations

- Dysrhythmias are common and result from a decrease in oxygen to the myocardium.
- Angina pain may be experienced.
- Hemodynamic instability
- Classic signs include low blood pressure, rapid and weak pulse.
- Cerebral hypoxia manifested by confusion and agitation
- Decreased urinary output and cold, clammy skin

Medical Management

Goals of medical treatment include limiting further myocardial damage, preserving the healthy myocardium, and improving the heart's ability to pump effectively. The oxygen needs of the heart muscle are addressed. Hemodynamic monitoring is performed and pharmacologic therapy (eg, dopamine, nitroglycerine, dobutamine, and various antiarrhythmic medications) may be used.

- First-line treatment of cardiogenic shock includes supplying supplemental oxygen, controlling chest pain, administering vasoactive medications, controlling heart rate with medications or pacemakers, and providing selective fluid support.
- Mechanical cardiac support, such as intra-aortic balloon counterpulsation, ventricular assist systems, or extracorporeal cardiopulmonary bypass, may be necessary.
- Coronary cardiogenic shock is treated with thrombolytic therapy, angioplasty, or coronary artery bypass graft surgery.

- Noncoronary cardiogenic shock is treated with cardiac valve replacement or correction of dysrhythmia.

Nursing Management

Prevention

- Early on, identify patients at risk for cardiogenic shock.
- Promote adequate oxygenation of the heart muscle, and decrease cardiac workload (conserve energy, relieve pain, administer oxygen).

Hemodynamic Monitoring

- Monitor hemodynamic and cardiac status: maintain arterial lines and electrocardiogram (ECG) equipment.
- Anticipate need for medications, intravenous fluids, and other equipment.
- Document and promptly report changes in hemodynamic, cardiac, and pulmonary status.

Fluid Administration

- Provide for safe and accurate administration of intravenous fluids and medications.Neurologic assessment is essential after thrombolytic therapy. Monitor for possible infiltration with intravenous infusions.
- Monitor urine output, blood urea nitrogen, and serum creatinine level to detect possible decrease in renal function.

Intra-Aortic Balloon Counterpulsation

- Provide ongoing timing adjustments of the balloon pump for maximum effectiveness.
- Perform frequent checks of neurovascular status of lower extremities.

S

Safety and Comfort

Take an active role in ensuring patient's safety and comfort and in reducing anxiety.

For more information, see Chapter 15 in Smeltzer and Bare: *Brunner and Suddarth's Textbook of Medical-Surgical Nursing*, 11th edition. Philadelphia: Lippincott Williams & Wilkins, 2008.

Shock, Hypovolemic

In hypovolemic shock, the most common type of shock, a loss of effective circulating blood volume occurs. Hypovolemic shock is caused by external fluid losses from hemorrhage, internal fluid shifts (eg, severe dehydration, severe edema, or ascites), and fluid losses from prolonged vomiting or diarrhea. Decreased blood volume results in decreased venous return, decreased stroke volume and cardiac output, and decreased tissue perfusion.

Clinical Manifestations

- Fall in venous pressure, rise in peripheral resistance, tachycardia
- Cold, moist skin; pallor; thirst; diaphoresis
- Altered sensorium, oliguria, metabolic acidosis, tachypnea
- Most dependable criterion: level of arterial blood pressure

Medical Management

Goals of treatment are to restore intravascular volume, redistribute fluid volume, and correct the underlying cause. If the patient is hemorrhaging, bleeding is stopped by applying pressure or by surgery. Diarrhea and vomiting are treated with medications.

Fluid and Blood Replacement

- Dual IV lines are inserted to administer fluid, medications, and/or blood.
- Lactated Ringer's solution, colloids, and 0.9% sodium chloride solution (normal saline) are administered to restore intravascular volume.
- Blood products are used only if other alternatives are unavailable or blood loss is extensive and rapid; autotransfusion methods may be considered for closed cavity hemorrhage.

Redistribution of Fluids

Patient is positioned properly to assist in fluid redistribution (modified Trendelenburg). Military antishock trousers (MAST) are used in extreme emergency situations when bleeding cannot be controlled.

Pharmacologic Therapy

The same medications are used that are given in cardiogenic shock. The type of medication depends on the underlying cause.

Nursing Management

- Closely monitor patients at risk for fluid deficits (younger than 1 year or older than 65 years of age).
- Assist with fluid replacement before intravascular volume is depleted.
- Ensure safe administration of prescribed fluids and medications, and document effects.
- Monitor and report signs of complications and effects of treatment. Monitor patient closely for adverse effects.
- Monitor for cardiovascular overload and pulmonary edema: hemodynamic pressure, vital signs, arterial blood gases, and fluid intake and output.

- Reduce fear and anxiety about the need for oxygen mask by giving patient explanations and frequent reassurance.

For more information, see Chapter 15 in Smeltzer and Bare: *Brunner and Suddarth's Textbook of Medical-Surgical Nursing*, 11th edition. Philadelphia: Lippincott Williams & Wilkins, 2008.

Shock, Septic

Septic shock, the most common type of circulatory shock, is caused by widespread infection. Gram-negative bacteria are the most common pathogens. Other infectious agents, such as gram-positive bacteria (increasingly) and viruses and fungi, can also cause septic shock.

Risk Factors

Conditions placing patients at risk for septic shock are immunosuppression, extremes of age (younger than 1 year and older than 65 years of age), alcoholism, malnourishment, extensive trauma or burns, chronic illness, diabetes, malignancy, and invasive procedures.

Pathophysiology

Microorganism invasion causes an immune response. This immune response activates biochemical mediators associated with an inflammatory response and produces a variety of effects leading to shock. The resulting increased capillary permeability, with fluid loss from the capillaries and vasodilation, results in inadequate perfusion of oxygen and nutrients to the tissues and cells.

S

Clinical Manifestations

First Phase: Hyperdynamic or "Progressive" Phase

- High cardiac output with vasodilation
- Hyperthermia (febrile) with warm, flushed skin, bounding pulses
- Heart and respiratory rates elevated
- Blood pressure may remain within normal limits
- Subtle changes in mental status
- Urinary output decreased or normal
- Gastrointestinal status compromised (eg, decreased bowel sounds, nausea, vomiting, or diarrhea)

Later Phase: Hypodynamic or "Irreversible" Phase

- Low cardiac output with vasoconstriction
- Decreased blood pressure
- Skin cool and pale
- Temperature normal or below normal
- Heart and respiratory rates rapid
- Anuria and multiple organ dysfunction progressing to failure

Gerontologic Considerations

Septic shock may be manifested by atypical or confusing clinical signs. Suspect septic shock in any elderly person who develops an unexplained acute confused state, tachypnea, or hypotension.

Medical Management

- Urine, blood, sputum, and wound drainage specimens are collected to identify and eliminate the cause of infection.
- Broad-spectrum antibiotic therapy begins immediately, and potential routes of infection are eliminated (intravenous

lines rerouted if necessary). Abscesses are drained and necrotic areas débrided.

- Fluid replacement is instituted and aggressive nutritional supplementation (high protein) is provided. Enteral feedings are preferred.
- Treatment with recombinant human activated protein C (APC), an antithrombotic, anti-inflammatory, and profibrinolytic agent proved to reduce mortality.

Nursing Management

- Identify patients at risk for sepsis and septic shock.
- Carry out all invasive procedures with correct aseptic technique and follow with careful hand washing.
- Monitor for signs of infection at intravenous lines, arterial and venous puncture sites, surgical incisions, trauma wounds, urinary catheters, and pressure ulcers.
- Reduce patient's temperature when ordered for temperatures above 104.8°F (40.8°C) or if the patient is uncomfortable by administering salicylates, ice bags, and hypothermia blankets; monitor closely for shivering.
- Administer prescribed intravenous fluids and medications.
- Monitor and report blood levels (antibiotic, blood urea nitrogen, creatinine, white blood count).
- Monitor hemodynamic status, fluid intake and output, and nutritional status.
- Monitor daily weights and serum albumin levels to determine daily protein requirements.

S

For more information, see Chapter 15 in Smeltzer and Bare: *Brunner and Suddarth's Textbook of Medical-Surgical Nursing*, 11th edition. Philadelphia: Lippincott Williams & Wilkins, 2008.

Spinal Cord Injury

Spinal cord injuries are a major health problem. Most spinal cord injuries result from motor vehicle crashes. Other causes include falls, sporting and industrial accidents, and gunshot wounds. Over half of the victims are 16 to 30 years of age. Males are affected four times more often than females. Another risk factor is substance abuse (alcohol and drugs). There is a high frequency of associated injuries and medical complications. The vertebrae most frequently involved in spinal cord injuries are the 5th, 6th, and 7th cervical, the 12th thoracic, and the 1st lumbar. These vertebrae are the most susceptible because there is a greater range of mobility in the vertebral column in these areas. Damage to the spinal cord ranges from transient concussion (patient recovers fully), to contusion, laceration, and compression of the cord substance (either alone or in combination), to complete transection of the cord (paralysis below the level of injury). Injury can be categorized as primary (usually permanent) or secondary (nerve fibers swell and disintegrate as a result of ischemia, hypoxia, edema, and hemorrhagic lesions). Whereas a primary injury is permanent, a secondary injury may be reversible if treated within 4 to 6 hours of the initial injury. The type of injury refers to the extent of injury to the spinal cord itself.

Incomplete spinal cord lesions are classified according to the area of spinal cord damage: central, lateral, anterior, or peripheral. A complete spinal cord injury can result in paraplegia (paralysis of the lower body) or quadriplegia (paralysis of all four extremities).

Clinical Manifestations

The consequences of spinal cord injury depend on the type and level of injury of the cord.

Neurologic Level

The neurologic level refers to the lowest level at which sensory and motor functions are normal. Signs and symptoms include:

- Total sensory and motor paralysis below the neurologic level
- Loss of bladder and bowel control (usually with urinary retention and bladder distention)
- Loss of sweating and vasomotor tone below the neurologic level

- Marked reduction of blood pressure from loss of peripheral vascular resistance
- If conscious, patient reports acute pain in back or neck; patient may speak of fear that the neck or back is broken.

Respiratory Problems

- Related to compromised respiratory function; severity depends on level of injury
- Acute respiratory failure is the leading cause of death in high cervical cord injury.

Assessment and Diagnostic Methods

Detailed neurologic examination, x-ray examinations (lateral cervical spine x-rays, MRI, CT myelography), ECG (bradycardia and asystole are common in acute spinal injuries)

Complications

Spinal shock, a serious complication of spinal cord injury, is a sudden depression of reflex activity in the spinal cord (areflexia) below the level of injury. The muscles innervated by the part of the cord segment situated below the level of the lesion become completely paralyzed and flaccid, and the reflexes are absent. Blood pressure and heart rate fall as vital organs are affected. Parts of the body below the level of the cord lesion are paralyzed and without sensation.

S

Emergency Management

- Immediate patient management at the accident scene is crucial. Improper handling can cause further damage and loss of neurologic function.
- Consider any victim of a motor vehicle crash, a contact sports injury, a fall, or any direct trauma to the head and neck as having a spinal cord injury until ruled out.
- Initial care includes rapid assessment, immobilization, extrication, stabilization or control of life-threatening

injuries, and transportation to an appropriate medical facility.

- Maintain patient in an extended position (not sitting); no body part should be twisted or turned.
- The standard of care is referral to a regional spinal injury center or trauma center for treatment in first 24 hours.

Medical Management
Acute Phase

Goals of management are to prevent further spinal cord injury and to observe for symptoms of progressive neurologic deficits. The patient is resuscitated as necessary, and oxygenation and cardiovascular stability are maintained. High-dose corticosteroids (methylprednisolone) may be administered to counteract spinal cord edema. Regeneration therapy using fetal tissue is under investigation.

Oxygen is administered to maintain a high arterial PO_2. Extreme care is taken to avoid flexing or extending the neck if endotracheal intubation is necessary. Diaphragm pacing (electrical stimulation of the phrenic nerve) may be considered for patients with a high cervical lesion.

Spinal cord injury requires immobilization, reduction of dislocations, and stabilization of the vertebral column. The cervical fracture is reduced and the cervical spine aligned with a form of skeletal traction (using skeletal tongs or calipers or the halo-vest technique). Weights are hung freely so as not to interfere with the traction.

Early surgery reduces the need for traction. Laminectomy may be performed to reduce spinal fracture or dislocation or to decompress the spinal cord.

Management of Complications
Spinal and Neurogenic Shock

- Intestinal decompression is used to treat bowel distention and paralytic ileus caused by depression of reflexes. This loss of sympathetic innervation causes a variety of other clinical manifestations, including neurogenic shock signaled by decreased cardiac output, venous pooling in the extremities, and peripheral vasodilation.

- Patient who does not perspire on paralyzed portion of body requires close observation for early detection of an abrupt onset of fever.
- Body defenses are maintained and supported until the spinal shock abates and the system has recovered from the traumatic insult (up to 4 months).
- Special attention is paid to the respiratory system (may not be enough intrathoracic pressure to cough effectively). Special problem include decreased vital capacity, decreased oxygen levels, and pulmonary edema.
- Chest physiotherapy and suctioning are implemented to help clear pulmonary secretions. Patient is monitored for respiratory complications (respiratory failure, pneumonia).

Deep Vein Thrombosis and Other Complications

- Patient is observed for deep vein thrombosis (DVT), a complication of immobility (eg, pulmonary embolism). Symptoms include pleuritic chest pain, anxiety, shortness of breath, and abnormal blood gas values.
- Low-dose anticoagulation therapy is initiated to prevent DVT and pulmonary embolism. A permanent indwelling filter may be placed in the vena cava to prevent dislodged clots (emboli) from migrating to the lungs and causing pulmonary emboli. Thigh and calf measurements are assessed daily and thigh-high elastic stockings or pneumatic compression devices are applied to help prevent DVT.
- Patient is monitored for autonomic hyperreflexia (characterized by pounding headache, profuse sweating, nasal congestion, piloerection [gooseflesh], bradycardia, and hypertension).
- Constant surveillance is maintained for signs and symptoms of pressure ulcers and infection (urinary, respiratory, local infection at pin sites).

NURSING ALERT Perform a careful baseline neurologic examination and document findings. Monitor constantly for any changes in motor or sensory function and any symptoms of progressive neurologic damage. Immediately report any decrease in function.

NURSING PROCESS: The Patient with Acute Spinal Cord Injury

Assessment

- Observe breathing pattern; assess strength of cough; auscultate lungs.
- Test motor ability by asking patient to spread fingers, squeeze examiner's hand, and move toes or turn the feet.
- Evaluate sensation by pinching the skin or pricking it with a tongue blade, starting at shoulder and working down both sides. Ask patient where sensation is felt.
- Assess for spinal shock.
- Palpate bladder for signs of urine retention and overdistention.
- Assess for gastric dilation and ileus due to atonic bowel.
- Monitor temperature (hyperthermia may result due to autonomic disruption).

Diagnosis

Nursing Diagnoses

- Ineffective breathing patterns related to weakness or paralysis of abdominal and intercostal muscles and inability to clear secretions
- Ineffective airway clearance related to weakness of intercostal muscles
- Impaired bed and physical mobility related to motor and sensory impairment
- Disturbed sensory perception related to immobility and sensory loss

- Risk for impaired skin integrity related to immobility or sensory loss
- Impaired urinary elimination related to inability to void spontaneously
- Constipation related to presence of atonic bowel as a result of autonomic disruption
- Acute pain and discomfort related to treatment and prolonged immobility

Collaborative Problems/Potential Complications

- DVT
- Orthostatic hypotension
- Autonomic hyperreflexia

Planning and Goals

Major patient goals may include improved breathing pattern, improved mobility, maintenance of skin integrity, relief of urinary retention, improved bowel function, comfort, improved sensory and perceptual awareness, and absence of complications.

Nursing Interventions

Promoting Adequate Breathing

- Detect potential respiratory failure by observing patient, measuring vital capacity, and monitoring oxygen saturation through pulse oximetry and arterial blood gas values.
- Prevent retention of secretions and resultant atelectasis with early and vigorous attention to clearing bronchial and pharyngeal secretions.
- Suction with caution, because this procedure can stimulate the vagus nerve, producing bradycardia and cardiac arrest.
- Initiate chest physical therapy and assisted coughing to mobilize secretions.
- Supervise breathing exercises to increase strength and endurance of inspiratory muscles, particularly the diaphragm.
- Ensure proper humidification and hydration to maintain thin secretions.

- Assess for signs of respiratory infection: cough, fever, and dyspnea.
- Discourage smoking.
- Monitor respiratory status frequently.

Improving Mobility

- Maintain proper body alignment at all times. Place patient in dorsal or supine position.
- Turn patient every 2 hours; monitor for hypotension in patients with lesions above the midthoracic level. Assist patient out of bed as soon as spinal column is stabilized.
- Do not turn patient who is not on a turning frame unless physician indicates that it is safe to do so.
- Apply splints (various types) to prevent footdrop and trochanter rolls to prevent external rotation of the hip joints; reapply every 2 hours.
- Perform passive range-of-motion exercises within 48 to 72 hours after injury to avoid complications such as contractures and atrophy.
- Provide a full range of motion at least four or five times daily to toes, metatarsals, ankles, knees, and hips.

Promoting Adaptation to Disturbed Sensory Perception

- Stimulate the area above the level of the injury through touch, aromas, flavorful food, conversation, and music.
- Provide prism glasses to enable patient to see from supine position.
- Encourage use of hearing aids, if applicable.
- Provide emotional support; teach patient strategies to compensate for or cope with sensory deficits.

Maintaining Skin Integrity

- Change patient's position every 2 hours, and inspect the skin, particularly under cervical collar.
- Assess for redness or breaks in skin over pressure points; check perineum for soilage; observe catheter for adequate drainage; assess general body alignment and comfort.

- Wash skin every few hours with a mild soap, rinse well, and blot dry. Keep pressure-sensitive areas well lubricated and soft with bland cream or lotion; gently perform massage using a circular motion.
- Teach patient about pressure ulcers and encourage participation in preventive measures.

 NURSING ALERT Never massage calves or thighs because doing so may dislodge an undetected deep vein thrombus.

Promoting Urinary Elimination

- Perform intermittent catheterization to avoid overstretching the bladder and infection. If this is not feasible, insert an indwelling catheter.
- Show family members how to catheterize, and encourage them to participate in this facet of care.
- Teach patient to record fluid intake, voiding pattern, amounts of residual urine after catheterization, quality of urine, and any unusual feelings.

Improving Bowel Function

- Monitor reactions to gastric intubation.
- Provide a high-calorie, high-protein, and high-fiber diet. Food amount may be gradually increased after bowel sounds resume.
- Administer prescribed stool softener to counteract effects of immobility and pain medications, and institute a bowel program as early as possible.

Providing Comfort

- Reassure patient in halo traction that he or she will adapt to steel frame (ie, feeling caged in and hearing noises).
- Cleanse pin sites daily, and observe for redness, drainage, and pain; observe for loosening; keep a torque screwdriver readily available.
- Assess skull for signs of infection, including drainage around halo-vest tongs.

S

- Check back of head periodically for signs of pressure. Massage at intervals, taking care not to move the neck.
- Shave hair around tongs to facilitate inspection. Avoid probing under encrusted areas.
- Inspect skin under halo vest for excessive perspiration, redness, and skin blistering, especially on bony prominences.
- Open vest at the sides to allow torso to be washed. Do not allow vest to become wet; do not use powder inside vest.

Monitoring and Managing Potential Complications

Thrombophlebitis

Refer to Medical Management in text on thrombophlebitis.

Orthostatic Hypotension

Reduce frequency of hypotensive episodes by administering prescribed vasopressor medications. Provide compression stockings; allow time for slow position changes, and use tilt tables as appropriate. Close monitoring of vital signs before and during position changes is essential.

Autonomic Hyperreflexia

- Perform a rapid assessment to identify and alleviate the cause of autonomic hyperreflexia and remove the trigger.
- Place patient immediately in a sitting position to lower blood pressure.
- Catheterize the patient to empty bladder immediately.
- Examine rectum for fecal mass after symptoms subside. Apply topical anesthetic for 10 to 15 minutes before removing fecal mass.
- Examine skin for areas of pressure, irritation, or broken skin.
- As prescribed, administer a ganglionic blocking agent such as hydralazine (Apresoline) if the above measures do not relieve hypertension and excruciating headache.
- Label chart clearly and visibly, noting the risk for autonomic hyperreflexia.

- Instruct patient in prevention and management measures. Inform patient with lesion above T6 that hyperreflexic episode can occur years after initial injury. Document risk for autonomic hyperreflexia in the medical record.

Promoting Home and Community-Based Care

Teaching Patients Self-Care

- Shift emphasis from ensuring that patient is stable and free of complications to specific assessment and planning for independence and the skills necessary for activities of daily living.
- Coordinate management team, and serve as liaison with rehabilitation centers and home care agencies.
- Special teaching for women of childbearing age includes discussion of pregnancy and complications imposed by SCI as well as preconception counseling.

Continuing Care

- Support and assist patient and family in assuming responsibility for increasing care and provide assistance in dealing with psychological impact of spinal cord injury and its consequences.
- Refer for home care nursing support as indicated or desired.
- Refer patient to mental health care professional as indicated.

Evaluation

Expected Patient Outcomes

- Demonstrates improvement in gas exchange and clearance of secretions
- Moves within limits of dysfunction, and demonstrates completion of exercises within functional limitations
- Demonstrates adaptation to sensory and perceptual alterations
- Demonstrates optimal skin integrity
- Regains urinary bladder function
- Regains bowel function

- Reports absence of pain and discomfort
- Is free of complications

For more information, see Chapter 63 in Smeltzer and Bare: *Brunner and Suddarth's Textbook of Medical-Surgical Nursing*, 11th edition. Philadelphia: Lippincott Williams & Wilkins, 2008.

Syndrome of Inappropriate Antidiuretic Hormone Secretion

The syndrome of inappropriate antidiuretic hormone (SIADH) secretion refers to excessive antidiuretic hormone (ADH) secretion from the pituitary gland. Patients with this disorder cannot excrete a dilute urine. They retain fluids and develop a sodium deficiency (dilutional hyponatremia). SIADH is often of nonendocrine origin. The syndrome may occur in patients with bronchogenic carcinoma (malignant lung cells synthesize and release ADH). Other causes include severe pneumonia, pneumothorax, other disorders of the lungs, and malignant tumors that affect other organs. Disorders of the central nervous system (head injury, brain surgery or tumor, or infection) are thought to produce SIADH by direct stimulation of the pituitary gland. Some medications (vincristine, diuretics, phenothiazines, tricyclic antidepressants) have been implicated in SIADH.

Medical Management

SIADH is generally managed by eliminating the underlying cause if possible and restricting fluid intake. Diuretics are used with fluid restriction to treat severe hyponatremia.

Nursing Management

- Monitor fluid intake and output, daily weight, urine and blood chemistries, and neurologic status.

- Provide supportive measures and explanations of procedures and treatments to assist patient to deal with this disorder.

For more information, see Chapter 42 in Smeltzer and Bare: *Brunner and Suddarth's Textbook of Medical-Surgical Nursing*, 11th edition. Philadelphia: Lippincott Williams & Wilkins, 2008.

Systemic Lupus Erythematosus

Systemic lupus erythematosus (SLE) is a chronic, inflammatory autoimmune collagen disease resulting from disturbed immune regulation that causes an exaggerated production of autoantibodies.

Pathophysiology

This disturbance is brought about by some combination of genetic, hormonal (as evidenced by the usual onset during the childbearing years), and environmental factors (sunlight, thermal burns). Certain medications, such as hydralazine (Apresoline), procainamide (Pronestyl), isoniazid, chlorpromazine (Thorazine), and some anticonvulsants, have been implicated in chemical- or drug-induced SLE. In SLE, the increase in autoantibody production is thought to result from abnormal suppressor T-cell function, leading to immune complex deposition and tissue damage. Inflammation stimulates antigens, which in turn stimulate additional antibodies, and the cycle repeats (remissions and exacerbations).

Clinical Manifestations

Onset is insidious or acute. SLE can go undiagnosed for many years. The clinical course is one of exacerbations and remissions. Multisystem features include nephritis, cardiopulmonary disease, rashes, and more indirect evidence of systemic inflammation (fever, fatigue, and weight loss).

- Musculoskeletal system: arthralgias and arthritis (synovitis) are common presenting features. Joint swelling, tenderness, and pain on movement are common, accompanied by morning stiffness.
- Integumentary system: Several different types are seen (eg, subacute cutaneous lupus erythematosus [SCLE], discoid lupus erythematosus [DLE]). A butterfly rash across the bridge of the nose and cheeks occurs in fewer than half of patients and may be a precursor to systemic involvement. Lesions worsen during exacerbations ("flares") and may be provoked by sunlight or artificial ultraviolet light. Oral ulcers may involve buccal mucosa or hard palate.
- Cardiovascular system: Pericarditis is the most common clinical cardiac manifestation. Papular, erythematosus, and purpuric lesions may occur on fingertips, elbows, toes, and extensor surfaces of forearms or lateral sides of hands and may progress to necrosis.
- Other systemic manifestations: Pleuritis or pleural effusions may occur; lymphadenopathy occurs in half of all SLE patients; and renal involvement (glomeruli) may lead to systemic hypertension. SLE has varied and frequent neuropsychiatric presentations, generally demonstrated by subtle changes in behavior or cognitive ability. Depression and psychosis are common.

Assessment and Diagnostic Findings

Diagnosis is based on a complete history, physical examination, and analysis of blood work. No single laboratory test confirms SLE. Blood testing reveals moderate to severe anemia, thrombocytopenia, leukocytosis, or leukopenia and positive antinuclear antibodies. Other diagnostic immunologic tests support but do not confirm the diagnosis. Hematuria may be found on urinalysis.

Medical Management

Treatment includes management of acute and chronic disease. Goals of treatment include preventing progressive loss of organ function, reducing the likelihood of acute disease, minimizing disease-related disabilities, and preventing complications from therapy. Monitoring is performed to assess disease activity and therapeutic effectiveness.

Pharmacologic Therapy

*   Nonsteroidal anti-inflammatory drugs (NSAIDs) are used with corticosteroids to minimize corticosteroid requirements.
*   Corticosteroids are used topically for cutaneous manifestations.
*   Bolus intravenous administration of corticosteroids is an alternative to traditional high-dose oral use.
*   Cutaneous, musculoskeletal, and mild systemic features of SLE are managed with antimalarial drugs.
*   Immunosuppressive agents are generally reserved for the most serious forms of SLE.

Nursing Management

The nursing care of the patient with SLE is generally the same as that for the patient with rheumatic disease (see Nursing Management under Arthritis, Rheumatoid). The primary nursing diagnoses address fatigue, impaired skin integrity, disturbed body image, and deficient knowledge. Additional management measures follow:

*   Perform a thorough, systematic physical assessment, inspecting skin for erythematosus rashes and cutaneous erythematosus plaques with an adherent scale on scalp, face, or neck.
*   Note areas of hyperpigmentation or depigmentation, depending on the phase and type of the disease, and

question patient about skin changes, specifically about sensitivity to sunlight or artificial ultraviolet light.

- Inspect scalp for alopecia and examine mouth and throat for ulcerations; provide appropriate oral care.
- Check for pericardial friction rub and abnormal lung sounds (pleural effusion).
- Assess for vascular involvement: papular erythematosus and purpuric lesions.
- Observe for signs of musculoskeletal involvement: joint swelling, tenderness, warmth, pain on movement, and stiffness. Joint involvement is often symmetric.
- Observe for edema and hematuria, indicative of renal involvement.
- Direct neurologic assessment at identifying and describing central nervous system involvement.
- Question family members regarding behavioral changes, neuroses, or psychoses.
- Note signs of depression and reports of seizures, chorea, or other central nervous system manifestations.
- Assess knowledge of disease process and self-management.
- Assess patient's perception of and methods of coping with fatigue, body image changes, and other problems caused by disease. Assist patient to develop effective coping strategies.

For more information, see Chapter 54 in Smeltzer and Bare: *Brunner and Suddarth's Textbook of Medical-Surgical Nursing*, 11th edition. Philadelphia: Lippincott Williams & Wilkins, 2008.

S

Thrombocytopenia

Thrombocytopenia (low platelet level) is the most common cause of abnormal bleeding.

Pathophysiology

Thrombocytopenia can result from decreased production of platelets within the bone marrow or from increased destruction or consumption of platelets. Causes include failure of production as a result of certain anemias, septicemia, and cytotoxic medications; increased destruction as a result of idiopathic thrombocytopenia purpura, lupus erythematosus, malignant lymphoma, medications (digoxin, phenytoin, aspirin), and postviral infections; and increased utilization, such as results from disseminated intravascular coagulopathy (DIC). Another cause is sequestration; approximately one third of the circulating platelets are within the spleen, so a greatly enlarged spleen results in increased sequestration of platelets.

Clinical Manifestations

- With platelet count below 50,000/mm^3: bleeding and petechiae
- With platelet count below 20,000/mm^3: nosebleeds, gingival bleeding, excessive menstrual bleeding, and hemorrhage after surgery or dental extractions
- With platelet count below 5,000/mm^3: spontaneous fatal central nervous system hemorrhage or gastrointestinal hemorrhage

743

Assessment and Diagnostic Findings

- Bone marrow aspiration and biopsy, if platelet deficiency is secondary to decreased production
- Increased megakaryocytes (the cells from which platelets originate) and normal platelet production in bone marrow, when platelet destruction is the cause

Medical Management

The management of secondary thrombocytopenia is usually treatment of the underlying disease. Platelet transfusions are used to raise platelet count if platelet production is impaired; if excessive platelet destruction is the cause, the patient is treated as indicated for idiopathic thrombocytopenia purpura. For some patients a splenectomy can be therapeutic, although it may not be an option for other patients.

Nursing Management

Interventions focus on preventing injury (eg, use soft toothbrush and electric razors, minimize needlestick procedures), stopping or slowing bleeding (eg, pressure, cold), and administering medications and platelets as ordered, as well as patient teaching. See Nursing Management under Idiopathic Thrombocytopenia Purpura for additional information.

For more information, see Chapter 33 in Smeltzer and Bare: *Brunner and Suddarth's Textbook of Medical-Surgical Nursing*, 11th edition. Philadelphia: Lippincott Williams & Wilkins, 2008.

Thyroiditis, Acute

Thyroiditis (inflammation of the thyroid) can be acute, subacute, or chronic. Each type is characterized by inflammation, fibrosis, or lymphocytic infiltration of the thyroid gland. Acute thyroiditis is a rare disorder caused by infection of the thyroid gland. The causes are bacteria (*Staphylococcus aureus* most common), fungi, mycobacteria, or parasites. Subacute cases may be granulomatous thyroiditis (de Quervain's thyroiditis) or painless thyroiditis (silent thyroiditis or subacute lymphocytic thyroiditis). This form often occurs in the postpartum period and is thought to be an autoimmune reaction.

Clinical Manifestations
Acute Thyroiditis

- Anterior neck pain and swelling, fever, dysphagia, and dysphonia
- Pharyngitis or pharyngeal pain
- Warmth, erythema, and tenderness of the thyroid gland

Subacute Thyroiditis

- Thyroid enlarges symmetrically and occasionally is painful.
- Overlying skin is often reddened and warm.
- Swallowing may be difficult and uncomfortable.
- Irritability, nervousness, insomnia, and weight loss (manifestations of hyperthyroidism) are common.
- Chills and fever may occur.

Management
Acute Thyroiditis

- Antimicrobial agents and fluid replacement
- Surgical incision and drainage if abscess is present

Subacute Thyroiditis

- Control of inflammation; nonsteroidal anti-inflammatory drugs (NSAIDs) to relieve neck pain
- Beta-blocking agents to control symptoms of hyperthyroidism

T

- Oral corticosteroids to relieve pain and reduce swelling; do not usually affect the underlying cause
- Follow-up monitoring

For more information, see Chapter 42 in Smeltzer and Bare: *Brunner and Suddarth's Textbook of Medical-Surgical Nursing*, 11th edition. Philadelphia: Lippincott Williams & Wilkins, 2008.

Thyroiditis, Chronic (Hashimoto's Thyroiditis)

Chronic thyroiditis occurs most frequently in women 30 to 50 years of age and is termed Hashimoto's disease. Diagnosis is based on the histologic appearance of the inflamed gland. The chronic forms are usually not accompanied by pain, pressure symptoms, or fever, and thyroid activity is usually normal or low. Cell-mediated immunity plays a significant role in the pathogenesis of chronic thyroiditis. A genetic predisposition also appears to be significant in its etiology. If untreated, the disease slowly progresses to hypothyroidism.

Management

Objectives of treatment are to reduce the size of the thyroid gland and to prevent myxedema.

- Thyroid hormone therapy is prescribed to reduce thyroid activity and production of thyroglobulin.
- Thyroid hormone is given when hypothyroid symptoms are present.
- Surgery is performed when pressure symptoms persist.

For more information, see Chapter 42 in Smeltzer and Bare: *Brunner and Suddarth's Textbook of Medical-Surgical Nursing*, 11th edition. Philadelphia: Lippincott Williams & Wilkins, 2008.

Thyroid Storm (Thyrotoxic Crisis)

Thyroid storm (thyrotoxic crisis) is a form of severe hyperthyroidism, usually of abrupt onset and characterized by high fever (hyperpyrexia), extreme tachycardia, and altered mental state, which frequently appears as delirium. Thyroid storm is a life-threatening condition that is usually precipitated by stress, such as injury, infection, surgery, tooth extraction, insulin reaction, diabetic acidosis, pregnancy, digitalis intoxication, abrupt withdrawal of antithyroid drugs, or vigorous palpation of the thyroid. These factors precipitate thyroid storm in the partially controlled or completely untreated hyperthyroid patient. Untreated thyroid storm is almost always fatal, but with proper treatment the mortality rate can be reduced substantially.

Clinical Manifestations

- Extreme tachycardia (more than 130 beats/min)
- High fever (hyperpyrexia) above 38.5°C (101.3°F)
- Exaggerated symptoms of hyperthyroidism
- Disturbances of a major system, such as gastrointestinal (weight loss, diarrhea, abdominal pain), neurologic or mental state (psychoses, somnolence, coma), or cardiovascular (edema, chest pain, dyspnea, palpitations)

Medical Management

Immediate objectives are to reduce body temperature and heart rate and prevent vascular collapse. This is accomplished with a hypothermia mattress or blanket, ice packs, cool environment, hydrocortisone, and acetaminophen (Tylenol).

- Humidified oxygen is administered to improve tissue oxygenation and meet high metabolic demands, and respiratory status is monitored by arterial blood gas analysis or pulse oximetry.

- Intravenous fluids containing dextrose are administered to replace glycogen stores.
- Hydrocortisone is given to treat shock or adrenal insufficiency.
- Propylthiouracil (PTU) or methimazole is given to impede formation of thyroid hormone.
- Iodine is administered to decrease output of thyroxine (T4) from thyroid gland.
- Sympatholytic agents are given for cardiac problems. Propranolol, combined with digitalis, has been effective in reducing cardiac symptoms.

> **!** **NURSING ALERT** Salicylates are not used in the management of thyroid storm because they displace thyroid hormone from binding proteins and worsen the hypermetabolism.

Nursing Management

Observe patient carefully and provide aggressive and supportive nursing care during and after acute stage of illness. Care provided for the patient with hyperthyroidism is the basis for nursing management of patients with thyroid storm.

For more information, see Chapter 42 in Smeltzer and Bare: *Brunner and Suddarth's Textbook of Medical-Surgical Nursing*, 11th edition. Philadelphia: Lippincott Williams & Wilkins, 2008.

Toxic Epidermal Necrolysis and Stevens-Johnson Syndrome

Toxic epidermal necrolysis and Stevens-Johnson syndrome are potentially fatal skin disorders and the most severe forms of erythema multiforme. Both conditions are triggered by medications or are secondary to a viral infection. Antibiotics, anticonvulsants, butazones, and sulfonamides are the medications most commonly implicated. The complete body surface may be involved, with widespread areas of erythema and blisters. Sepsis and keratoconjunctivitis are possible complications.

Clinical Manifestations

- Initial signs are conjunctival burning or itching, cutaneous tenderness, fever, headache, cough, sore throat, extreme malaise, and myalgia (aches and pains).
- Rapid onset of erythema follows, involving the skin surface and mucous membranes; large, flaccid bullae in some areas; in other areas, large sheets of epidermis are shed, exposing underlying dermis; fingernails, toenails, eyebrows, and eyelashes may all be shed, along with surrounding epidermis.
- Excruciatingly tender skin and loss of skin lead to a weeping surface similar to that of a total-body second-degree burn; this condition may be referred to as scalded skin syndrome.
- In severe cases of mucosal involvement, there may be danger of damage to the larynx, bronchi, and esophagus from ulcerations.

Assessment and Diagnostic Methods

- Histologic studies of frozen skin cells
- Cytodiagnosis of cells from a freshly denuded area
- Immunofluorescent studies for atypical epidermal autoantibodies

Medical Management

Treatment goals include control of fluid and electrolyte balance, prevention of sepsis, and prevention of ophthalmic complications. The mainstay of treatment is supportive care.

- All nonessential medications are discontinued immediately.
- Patient is treated in a regional burn center.

- Surgical débridement or hydrotherapy is used initially to remove involved skin.
- Cultures are performed of nasopharynx, eyes, ears, blood, urine, skin, and unruptured blisters to identify pathogens.
- Intravenous fluids are prescribed to maintain fluid and electrolyte balance.
- Fluid replacement is accomplished by nasogastric tube and orally as soon as possible.
- Systemic corticosteroids are given early in the disease process (controversial).
- Skin is protected with topical agents.
- Topical antibacterial and anesthetic agents are used to prevent wound sepsis.
- Temporary biologic dressings (pigskin, amniotic membrane) or plastic semipermeable dressings (Vigilon) are applied.
- Meticulous oropharyngeal and eye care is essential when there is severe involvement of mucous membranes and eyes.

NURSING PROCESS: The Patient with Toxic Epidermal Necrolysis

Assessment

- Inspect appearance and extent of involvement of skin. Monitor blister drainage for amount, color, and odor.
- Inspect oral cavity for blistering and erosive lesions daily. Determine patient's ability to drink fluids and speak normally.
- Assess eyes daily for itching, burning, and dryness.
- Monitor vital signs, paying special attention to fever and respiratory status and secretions.
- Monitor urine volume, specific gravity, and color.
- Inspect intravenous insertion sites for local signs of infection.
- Record daily weight.
- Question patient about fatigue and pain levels.
- Assess level of anxiety and coping mechanisms; identify new effective coping skills.

Diagnosis

Nursing Diagnoses

- Impaired tissue integrity (oral, eye, and skin) related to epidermal shedding
- Deficient fluid volume and electrolyte losses related to loss of fluids from denuded skin
- Risk for imbalanced body temperature (hypothermia) related to heat loss, secondary to skin loss
- Acute pain related to denuded skin, oral lesions, and possible infection
- Anxiety related to the physical appearance and prognosis

Collaborative Problems/Potential Complications

- Sepsis
- Conjunctival retraction, scars, and corneal lesions

Planning and Goals

Major goals may include skin and oral tissue healing, fluid balance, prevention of heat loss, relief of pain, reduction of anxiety, and absence of complications.

Nursing Interventions

Maintaining Skin and Mucous Membrane Integrity

- Place patient on a circular turning frame bed to prevent skin from becoming denuded.
- Apply prescribed topical agents to reduce wound bacteria.
- Apply warm compresses gently, if prescribed, to denuded areas.
- Use topical antibacterial agent in conjunction with hydrotherapy; monitor treatment, and encourage patient to exercise extremities during hydrotherapy.
- Perform oral hygiene carefully. Use prescribed mouthwashes frequently to rid mouth of debris, soothe ulcerative areas, and control odor. Inspect oral cavity frequently, note changes, and report. Apply petrolatum to lips.

T

Attaining Fluid Balance

- Observe for signs of hypovolemia: vital signs, urine output, and sensorium.
- Evaluate laboratory tests, and report abnormal results.
- Weigh patient daily.
- Provide fluid replacement.
- Provide enteral nourishment or, if necessary, parenteral nutrition.
- Record intake and output and daily calorie count.

Preventing Hypothermia

- Maintain patient's comfort and body temperature with cotton blankets, ceiling-mounted heat lamps, or heat shields.
- Work rapidly and efficiently when large wounds are exposed for wound care to minimize shivering and heat loss.
- Monitor patient's temperature carefully and frequently.

Relieving Pain

- Assess for presence and character of pain, behavioral responses, and factors that influence pain.
- Administer prescribed analgesic agents, and observe for pain relief and side effects.
- Administer analgesic agents before painful treatments.
- Provide explanations and speak soothingly to patient during treatments to allay anxiety, which may intensify pain.
- Provide measures to promote rest and sleep; provide emotional support and reassurance to achieve pain control.
- Teach self-management techniques for pain relief, such as progressive muscle relaxation and imagery.

Reducing Anxiety

- Assess emotional state (anxiety, fear of dying, and depression); reassure patient that these reactions are normal.
- Give support, be honest, and offer hope that the situation will improve.
- Encourage patient to express feelings to someone he or she trusts.

- Listen to patient's concerns; provide skillful, compassionate care.
- Provide emotional support during the long recovery period with psychiatric nurse, chaplain, psychologist, or psychiatrist.

Monitoring and Managing Potential Complications

- Sepsis: Monitor vital signs and note changes to allow early detection of infection. Maintain strict asepsis. If a large portion of the body is involved, place patient in private room with protective isolation.
- Conjunctival retraction, scars, and corneal lesions: Inspect eyes for progression of disease to keratoconjunctivitis (itching, burning, and dryness). Administer eye lubricant. Use eye patches. Encourage patient to avoid rubbing eyes. Document and report progression of symptoms.

Evaluation

Expected Patient Outcomes

- Achieves increasing skin and oral tissue healing
- Attains fluid balance
- Attains thermoregulation
- Reports lessening of pain
- Appears less anxious
- Experiences no complication, such as sepsis and impaired vision

---

For more information, see Chapter 56 in Smeltzer and Bare: *Brunner and Suddarth's Textbook of Medical-Surgical Nursing*, 11th edition. Philadelphia: Lippincott Williams & Wilkins, 2008.

Transient Ischemic Attack

Transient ischemic attack (TIA) is a temporary episode of neurologic dysfunction commonly manifested by a sudden loss of motor, sensory, or visual function. It may last a few seconds or minutes but no longer than 24 hours. Complete recovery usually occurs between attacks. A TIA may serve as a warning of impending stroke; stroke often occurs within the first month after the first attack. The cause is a temporary impairment of blood flow to a specific region of the brain. Reasons may include atherosclerosis of the vessels supplying the brain, obstruction of cerebral microcirculation by a small embolus, a fall in cerebral perfusion pressure, and cardiac dysrhythmias. Risk factors include hypertension, insulin-dependent diabetes mellitus, cardiac disease, history of smoking, family history of stroke, and chronic alcoholism.

Clinical Manifestations

Signs and symptoms depend on the location of the affected vessel. Interrupted anterior circulation can result in amaurosis fugax (fleeting blindness) occurring without warning. Sudden, painless loss of vision of one eye, aphasia, or contralateral weakness may also occur. If ischemia occurs in the vertebral basilar system, vertigo, diplopia, numbness or paresthesia, dysphagia, or ataxia may occur.

Assessment and Diagnostic Methods

- Carotid phonoangiography allows auscultation, direct visualization, and photographic recording of carotid bruits.
- Oculoplethysmography measures pulsation in blood flow through the ophthalmic artery.
- Carotid angiography visualizes intracranial and cervical vessels.
- Digital subtraction angiography is used to define carotid artery obstruction.

Prevention

Treatment of hypertension and hyperglycemia; smoking cessation; sometimes carotid endarterectomy and/or anticoagulant therapy.

Medical Management

Pharmacologic Therapy

Anticoagulant therapy may prevent future attacks if patient is not a candidate for surgical intervention, and platelet-inhibiting drugs (aspirin) may decrease the risk for cerebral infarction. Some patients also are treated with cholesterol-lowering medication to decrease plaque formation in blood vessels.

Surgical Management

Common surgical procedures are endarterectomy and angioplasty.

Nursing Management

- Keep flowchart of neurologic status after procedures. Notify neurosurgeon immediately if deficits develop.
- Be aware of primary complications of carotid endarterectomy: stroke, cranial nerve injuries, infection or hematoma of the wound, and carotid artery disruption.
- Maintain adequate blood pressure in immediate postoperative period.
- Avoid hypotension to prevent cerebral ischemia and thrombosis.
- Prevent excessive hypertension, which may precipitate cerebral hemorrhage; use sodium nitroprusside.
- Assess for difficulty in swallowing, hoarseness, or other signs of cranial nerve dysfunction; have a tracheostomy set available.
- Monitor cardiac status closely because of high incidence of coronary artery disease.
- Be aware of long-term complications: recurrent stroke and myocardial infarction.
- Educate patient about preventing TIA in the future.

For more information, see Chapter 62 in Smeltzer and Bare: *Brunner and Suddarth's Textbook of Medical-Surgical Nursing*, 11th edition. Philadelphia: Lippincott Williams & Wilkins, 2008.

Trigeminal Neuralgia (Tic Douloureux)

Trigeminal neuralgia, a condition affecting the fifth cranial nerve, is characterized by unilateral paroxysms of shooting and stabbing pain in the area innervated by the second and third branches of the trigeminal nerve. Each pain episode can be described as abrupt, lasting from a few seconds to minutes, and producing contraction of some of the facial muscles (ie, sudden closing of the eye or a twitch of the mouth)-hence the name tic douloureux (painful twitch). Early attacks, appearing most often in the fifth decade of life, are usually mild and brief. Pain-free intervals may last minutes, hours, days, or longer. With advancing years, the painful episodes tend to become more frequent and agonizing. The patient lives in constant fear of attacks.

Pathophysiology

Although the cause is not certain, chronic compression or irritation of the trigeminal nerve or degenerative changes in the gasserian ganglion are suggested causes. The disorder occurs more commonly in patients with multiple sclerosis (women more than men) than in the general population.

Clinical Manifestations

- Pain is felt in the skin, not in the deeper structures, and is more severe at the peripheral areas of distribution of the affected nerve, notably over the lip, chin, and nostrils and in the teeth.
- Paroxysms are aroused by any stimulation of terminals of the affected nerve branches (eg, washing the face, shaving, brushing teeth, eating, and drinking). Patients may avoid these activities (behavior provides a cue to diagnosis).
- Drafts of cold air and direct pressure against the nerve trunk may cause pain.

- Trigger points are areas where the slightest touch immediately starts a paroxysm.

Assessment and Diagnostic Methods

Diagnosis is based on characteristic behavior: avoiding stimulating trigger point areas (eg, trying not to touch or wash the face, shave, chew, or do anything else that might cause an attack).

Medical Management
Pharmacologic Therapy

- Antiseizure agents—carbamazepine (Tegretol) and phenytoin (Dilantin)—reduce transmission of impulses at certain nerve terminals and relieve pain in most patients. Carbamazepine is given with meals, in doses gradually increased until relief is obtained. The patient is observed for side effects, including nausea, dizziness, drowsiness, and hepatic dysfunction, and carbamazepine levels are monitored to avoid toxicity. Gabapentin and baclofen are also used to treat pain.

Surgical Management

Percutaneous radiofrequency trigeminal gangliolysis (interruption of the gasserian ganglion) is the surgical procedure of choice and can provide permanent pain relief in most patients. Small unmyelinated and thinly myelinated fibers that conduct pain are thermally destroyed (touch and proprioceptive function intact). Stereotactic MRI is used to guide gamma knife radiosurgery in some treatment centers.

In microvascular decompression of the trigeminal nerve, an intracranial approach (craniotomy) to decompress the trigeminal nerve is used. This procedure relieves facial pain while preserving normal sensation. In the patient who has trigeminal neuralgia and multiple sclerosis and who is refractory to medical pain management, the surgical treatment of choice is trigeminal rhizotomy

Percutaneous balloon neurocompression may be used to compress the trigeminal nerve and provide immediate pain relief, but muscle weakness and facial weakness may follow.

Nursing Interventions

- Monitor patient for bone marrow depression during long-term carbamazepine therapy (aplastic anemia).
- Monitor patient for phenytoin side effects, including nausea, dizziness, nystagmus, somnolence, ataxia, gum hyperplasia, and skin rashes or eruptions.
- Assist patient to recognize the factors that trigger excruciating facial pain (eg, hot or cold food or water, jarring motions). Teach patient how to lessen these discomforts by using cotton pads and room-temperature water to wash face.
- Instruct patient to rinse mouth after eating when tooth brushing causes pain.
- Advise patient to take food and fluids at room temperature, to chew on unaffected side, and to ingest soft foods.
- Recognize that anxiety, depression, and insomnia often accompany chronic painful conditions, and use appropriate interventions and referrals.
- Provide postoperative care by performing neurologic checks to assess facial motor and sensory deficits. Instruct patient not to rub the eye if the surgery results in sensory deficits to the affected side of the face, because pain will not be felt in the event there is injury. Assess the eye for irritation or redness. Insert artificial tears, if prescribed, to prevent dryness to affected eye. Caution patient not to chew on the affected side until numbness diminishes. Observe patient carefully for any difficulty in eating and swallowing foods of different consistencies.

For more information, see Chapter 64 in Smeltzer and Bare: *Brunner and Suddarth's Textbook of Medical-Surgical Nursing*, 11th edition. Philadelphia: Lippincott Williams & Wilkins, 2008.

Tuberculosis, Pulmonary

Tuberculosis (TB), an infectious disease primarily affecting the lung parenchyma, is most often caused by *Mycobacterium tuberculosis*. It may spread to almost any part of the body, including the meninges, kidney, bones, and lymph nodes. The initial infection usually occurs 2 to 10 weeks after exposure. The patient may then develop active disease because of a compromised or inadequate immune system response. The active process may be prolonged and characterized by long remissions when the disease is arrested, only to be followed by periods of renewed activity. TB is a worldwide public health problem and the leading cause of death among HIV-positive patients. Mortality and morbidity rates continue to rise.

TB is transmitted when a person with active pulmonary disease expels the organisms. A susceptible person inhales the droplets and becomes infected. Bacteria are transmitted to the alveoli and multiply. An inflammatory reaction results in exudate in the alveoli and bronchopneumonia, granulomas, and fibrous tissue. Onset is usually insidious.

Risk Factors

- Close contact with someone who has active TB
- Injection drug use and alcoholism
- Residence in overcrowded, substandard housing or institutions (eg, long-term care patients, psychiatric patients, prison inmates)
- Immunocompromise (eg, elderly, cancer, corticosteroid therapy, and HIV)
- Patients with preexisting medical conditions, including diabetes, chronic renal failure, silicosis, and malnourishment
- Immigrants from countries with a high incidence of TB (eg, Haiti, southeast Asia)
- People lacking adequate health care (eg, homeless or impoverished, minorities, children, and young adults)

- Occupation (eg, health care workers, particularly those performing high-risk activities)

Clinical Manifestations

- Low-grade fever, fatigue, anorexia, weight loss, night sweats, chest pain, and cough
- Nonproductive cough, which may progress to mucopurulent sputum with hemoptysis

Assessment and Diagnostic Methods

- TB skin test (Mantoux test)
- Sputum culture
- Chest x-ray

🌿 Gerontologic Considerations

Elderly patients may have atypical manifestations, such as unusual behavior or disturbed mental status, fever, anorexia, and weight loss. TB is increasingly encountered in the nursing home population. In many elderly people the TB skin test produces no reaction.

Medical Management

Prevention is the ideal form of management. People at high risk for TB are identified; if indicated, isoniazid (INH) is given prophylactically in a single daily dose for 6 to 12 months. The goals of management for the patient with active TB are to relieve pulmonary and systemic symptoms; to return the patient to health, work, and family life as quickly as possible; and to prevent transmission of the infection.

Pharmacologic Therapy

- First-line medications: INH, rifampin, ethambutol, and pyrazinamide daily for 8 weeks and continuing for up to 6 to 7 months

- Second-line medications: capreomycin, ethionamide, para-aminosalicylate sodium, and cycloserine
- Vitamin B6 (pyridoxine) usually administered with INH

NURSING PROCESS: The Patient with Tuberculosis

Assessment

- Perform complete history and physical examination.
- Perform respiratory assessment: fever, anorexia, weight loss, night sweats, fatigue, cough, and sputum production.
- Assess changes in temperature, respiratory rate, amount and color of secretions, frequency and severity of cough, and chest pain.
- Evaluate breath sounds for consolidation (diminished, bronchial, or bronchovesicular sounds, crackles), fremitus, egophony, and percussion (dullness).
- Assess for enlarged, painful lymph nodes.
- Assess patient's living arrangements.
- Assess patient's emotional readiness to learn and perceptions and understanding of TB and treatment.
- Review results of physical and laboratory evaluations.

Diagnosis

Nursing Diagnoses

- Ineffective airway clearance related to copious tracheobronchial secretions
- Activity intolerance
- Imbalanced nutrition: Less than body requirements
- Noncompliance with treatment regimens
- Deficient knowledge of preventive health measures and treatment regimen

Collaborative Problems/Potential Complications

- Malnutrition
- Side effects of medication therapy: hepatitis, neurologic changes (deafness or neuritis), rash, gastrointestinal upset

- Multidrug resistance
- Spread of TB infection (miliary TB)

Planning and Goals

Patient goals include patent airway, knowledge about the disease and treatment regimen, compliance with treatment regimen, increased activity tolerance, and absence of complications.

Nursing Interventions

Promoting Airway Clearance

- Instruct about best position to facilitate drainage.
- Encourage increased fluid intake.

Promoting Activity and Adequate Nutrition

- Plan a progressive activity schedule with the patient to increase activity tolerance and muscle strength.
- Devise a complementary plan to encourage adequate nutrition. A nutritional regimen of small, frequent meals and nutritional supplements may be helpful in meeting daily caloric requirements.

Advocating Compliance and Prevention

- Explain that TB is a communicable disease and that taking medications is the most effective way of preventing transmission.
- Instruct about hygiene measures, including mouth care, covering mouth and nose when coughing and sneezing, proper disposal of tissues, and hand washing.
- Instruct about medications, schedule, and side effects.

Monitoring and Managing Potential Complications

- Strategize with health care team to ensure adequate nutritional intake and availability of nutritious foods and high-calorie nutritional supplements.

T

- Assess for side effects of medication therapy and signs of multidrug resistance.
- Encourage patient to obtain liver and kidney function follow-up studies.
- Monitor sputum culture results to evaluate effectiveness of therapy.
- Teach patient to take medications on empty stomach or 1 hour before meals, because food interferes with drug absorption.
- Teach patients taking INH to avoid foods containing tyramine and histamine (tuna fish, aged cheese, yeast extract).
- Inform patient that rifampin may discolor tears and contact lenses. Eyeglasses may be substituted for contact lenses.
- Instruct patient about risk of drug resistance if regimen is not followed continuously; failure to comply results in multidrug resistance.
- Caution about the spread of TB infection from lungs to other body sites, a consequence of late reactivation of dormant infection.

Promoting Home and Community-Based Care
Teaching Patients Self-Care

- Assess patient's ability to continue therapy at home.
- Instruct patient and family about infection control procedures: cover mouth when coughing; use disposable tissues, place in paper bag, and discard.
- Teach and use universal precautions for body fluids, including sputum.
- Demonstrate and stress good hand hygiene.

Continuing Care

- Evaluate patient's environment to identify other potentially infected people, and arrange follow-up screening for them.
- Emphasize importance of keeping scheduled appointments with health care providers.

Evaluation

Expected Patient Outcomes

- Maintains patent airway by managing secretions
- Increases activity and nutritional status
- Demonstrates adequate level of knowledge
- Adheres to treatment regimen by taking medications as prescribed
- Takes steps to minimize side effects
- Participates in preventive measures
- Exhibits no complications

For more information, see Chapter 23 in Smeltzer and Bare: *Brunner and Suddarth's Textbook of Medical-Surgical Nursing*, 11th edition. Philadelphia: Lippincott Williams & Wilkins, 2008.

T

Ulcerative Colitis

Ulcerative colitis is a recurrent ulcerative and inflammatory disease of the mucosal and submucosal layer of the colon and rectum. It is a serious disease, accompanied by systemic complications and a high mortality rate; eventually, 10% to 15% of the patients develop carcinoma of the colon. It is characterized by multiple ulcerations, diffuse inflammations, and desquamation of the colonic epithelium, with alternating periods of exacerbation and remission. Bleeding occurs from the ulceration and the mucosa becomes edematous and inflamed, with continuous lesions and abscesses. Ulcerative colitis most commonly affects Caucasian people, including people of Jewish heritage, and peaks in the third to fifth decade of life.

Clinical Manifestations

- Predominant symptoms: diarrhea, abdominal pain, intermittent tenesmus, ineffective straining at stool, and rectal bleeding
- Pallor, if bleeding is severe
- Anorexia, weight loss, fever, vomiting, dehydration, cramping, and feeling an urgent need to defecate (may report passing 10 to 20 liquid stools daily)
- Hypocalcemia and anemia
- Rebound tenderness in right lower quadrant
- Skin lesions, eye lesions (uveitis), joint abnormalities, and liver disease

Assessment and Diagnostic Methods

- Assess for tachypnea, tachycardia, hypotension, fever, and pallor.

- Stool examination to rule out dysentery, occult blood test
- Abdominal x-rays, CT, MRI
- Sigmoidoscopy and barium enema
- Blood studies (low hematocrit and hemoglobin, high white blood cell count, decreased albumin level, electrolyte imbalance)

 NURSING ALERT Do not use cathartics in preparing patient for procedures: cathartic preparations may exacerbate the condition.

Medical Management

Medical treatment for both regional enteritis and ulcerative colitis is aimed at reducing inflammation, suppressing inappropriate immune responses, and providing rest for the diseased bowel so that healing may take place.

Nutritional Therapy

Initial therapy consists of diet and fluid management with oral fluids; low-residue, high-protein, high-calorie diets; supplemental vitamin therapy; and iron replacement. Fluid and electrolyte balance may be corrected by intravenous therapy. Additional treatment measures include smoking cessation and avoiding foods that exacerbate symptoms, such as milk and cold foods. Parenteral nutrition (PN) may be provided as indicated.

Pharmacologic Therapy

- Sedative, antidiarrheal, and antiperistaltic medications
- Sulfonamides: sulfasalazine (Azulfidine) or sulfisoxazole (Gantrisin), which are effective for mild or moderate inflammation
- Antibiotics for secondary infections
- Adrenocorticotropic hormone (ACTH) and corticosteroids
- Aminosalicylates (topical and oral), including newer sulfa-free (mesalamine [Asacol, Pentasa])
- Immunomodulator agents (eg, Imuran)

Psychotherapy

Psychotherapy is aimed at determining the factors that distress the patient, coping with these factors, and attempting to resolve conflicts.

Surgical Management

When nonsurgical measures fail to relieve the severe symptoms of inflammatory bowel disease, surgery may be recommended (segmental, subtotal, or total colectomy). A fecal diversion may be needed, such as ileostomy, continent ileal reservoir (Kock pouch), or ileoanal anastomosis. Strictureplasty or fecal diversions may be needed (eg, ileal reservoir, ileoanal anastomosis). Proctocolectomy with ileostomy (excision of colon, rectum, and anus) may be performed if rectum is severely involved. A recently developed option may be intestinal transplantation, especially for children and young adults who have lost intestinal function because of the disease.

NURSING PROCESS: The Patient with Inflammatory Bowel Disease

Both regional enteritis (Crohn's disease) and ulcerative colitis are categorized as inflammatory bowel diseases. Box U-1 lists assessment findings that help distinguish one from the other.

Assessment (Subjective)

- Determine the onset and duration of abdominal pain; presence of diarrhea, tenesmus, nausea, anorexia, and weight loss.
- Explore dietary pattern, including amounts of alcohol, caffeine, and nicotine used daily or weekly.
- Ask about family history of inflammatory bowel disease.
- Inquire about allergies, especially to milk or lactose.
- Determine bowel elimination patterns, including character, frequency, and presence of blood, pus, fat, or mucus.
- Ask about sleep pattern disturbances if diarrhea or pain occurs at night.

BOX U–1   Nursing Assessment Findings in Ulcerative Colitis and Regional Enteritis

Ulcerative Colitis

- Dominant sign is rectal bleeding.
- Distended abdomen with rebound tenderness may be present.

Regional Enteritis

- Most prominent symptom is intermittent pain associated with diarrhea that does not decrease with defecation.
- Pain usually localized in the right lower quadrant
- Abdominal tenderness noted on palpation
- Periumbilical regional pain suggesting involvement of terminal ileum

Assessment (Objective)

- Auscultate for bowel sounds and their characteristics. Listen for hyperactive bowel sounds.
- Palpate for distention, tenderness, or pain.
- Inspect skin for evidence of fistula tracts or symptoms of dehydration; inspect stool for blood.

Diagnosis

Nursing Diagnoses

- Diarrhea related to inflammatory process
- Acute pain related to increased peristalsis and gastrointestinal inflammation
- Deficient fluid volume and Imbalanced nutrition related to anorexia, nausea, and diarrhea
- Activity intolerance related to fluid losses and insufficient nutrition
- Anxiety related to impending surgery
- Ineffective individual coping related to repeated episodes of diarrhea

U

- Risk for impaired skin integrity related to malnutrition and diarrhea
- Risk for ineffective management of therapeutic regimen related to insufficient knowledge concerning process and management of disease

Collaborative Problems/Potential Complications

- Cardiac dysrhythmias related to electrolyte depletion
- Gastrointestinal bleeding with fluid volume loss
- Perforation of bowel
- Electrolyte imbalance

Planning and Goals

Major goals may include normal bowel elimination, relief of abdominal pain and cramping, prevention of fluid volume deficit, optimal nutrition and weight, avoidance of fatigue, reduction of anxiety, effective coping, prevention of skin breakdown, knowledge and understanding of the disease process and therapeutic regimen, and absence of complications.

Nursing Interventions

Maintaining Normal Elimination Patterns

- Determine if there is a relationship between diarrhea and certain foods, activities, or emotional stress.
- Identify any precipitating factors as well as stool frequency, consistency, and amount.
- Provide ready access to bathroom or bedpan; keep environment clean and odor-free.
- Administer antidiarrheal agents as prescribed, and record frequency and consistency of stools after therapy has started.
- Encourage bed rest to decrease peristalsis.

Relieving Pain

- Describe character of pain (dull, burning, or cramplike) and its onset, pattern, and medication relief.

- Administer anticholinergic medications 30 minutes before a meal to decrease intestinal motility.
- Give analgesic agents as prescribed; reduce pain by position changes, local application of heat (as prescribed), diversional activities, and prevention of fatigue.

Maintaining Fluid Balance

- Record intake and output, including wound or fistula drainage.
- Monitor weight daily.
- Assess for signs of fluid volume deficit: dry skin and mucous membranes, decreased skin turgor, oliguria, exhaustion, decreased temperature, increased hematocrit.
- Evaluate urine specific gravity, and note hypotension.
- Encourage oral intake; monitor intravenous flow rate.
- Initiate measures to decrease diarrhea: dietary restrictions, stress reduction, and antidiarrheal agents.

Promoting Nutritional Measures

- Use PN when symptoms are severe.
- Record fluid intake and output and daily weights during PN therapy; test for glucose daily.
- Give feedings high in protein and low in fat and residue after PN therapy; note intolerance (eg, vomiting, diarrhea, distention).
- Provide small, frequent, low-residue feedings if oral foods are tolerated.
- Restrict activities to conserve energy, reduce peristalsis, and reduce calorie requirements.

Promoting Rest and Activity Tolerance

- Recommend intermittent rest periods during the day; schedule or restrict activities to conserve energy and reduce metabolic rate.
- Encourage activity within limits; advise bed rest with active or passive exercises for a patient who is febrile, has frequent stools, or is bleeding.

Reducing Anxiety

- Establish rapport by being attentive and displaying a calm, confident manner.
- Provide time for patient to ask questions and express feelings.
- Note nonverbal indicators of anxiety (restlessness, tense facial expressions).
- Tailor information about impending surgery to patient's level of understanding and desire for detail.

Promoting Coping Skills

- Provide understanding and emotional support to patient who feels isolated, helpless, and out of control.
- Recognize that behavior may be affected by a number of factors unrelated to inherent emotional characteristics.
- Support patient's attempts to deal with stresses.
- Communicate that patient's feelings are understood; encourage patient to discuss any disturbing matters.
- Use stress-reduction measures: relaxation techniques, breathing exercises, and biofeedback.
- Refer for professional counseling as needed.

Preventing Skin Breakdown

- Examine skin, especially perianal skin.
- Provide perianal care after each bowel movement.
- Give immediate care to reddened or irritated areas over bony prominences.
- Use pressure-relieving devices to avoid skin breakdown.
- Consult with a wound care specialist or enterostomal therapist as indicated.

U

Monitoring and Managing Potential Complications

- Monitor serum electrolyte levels; administer replacements.
- Report dysrhythmias or change in level of consciousness.
- Monitor rectal bleeding, and give blood and volume expanders.
- Monitor blood pressure; obtain laboratory blood studies.

- Monitor for indications of perforation: acute increase in abdominal pain, rigid abdomen, vomiting, or hypotension.
- Monitor for signs of obstruction and toxic megacolon: abdominal distention, decreased or absent bowel sounds, changes in mental status, fever, tachycardia, hypotension, dehydration, and electrolyte imbalance.

Promoting Home and Community-Based Care
Teaching Patients Self-Care

- Assess need for additional information about medical management (medications, diet) and surgical interventions.
- Provide information about nutritional management (bland, low-residue, high-protein, high-calorie, and high-vitamin diet).
- Give rationale for using steroids and anti-inflammatory, antibacterial, antidiarrheal, and antispasmodic agents.
- Emphasize importance of taking medications as prescribed and not abruptly discontinuing regimen (especially steroids, because serious medical problems may result).
- Explain procedure and preoperative and postoperative care if surgery is required. Review ileostomy care as necessary. Obtain information from the National Foundation for Ileitis and Colitis.

Continuing Care

- Refer for home care nurse if nutritional status is compromised and patient is receiving PN.
- Explain that disease can be controlled and patient can lead a healthy life between exacerbations.
- Encourage patient to rest as needed and modify activities according to energy levels during a flare-up. Advise patient to limit tasks that impose strain on the lower abdominal muscles and to sleep close to bathroom because of frequent diarrhea. Suggest room deodorizers for odor control.
- Instruct about medications and the need to take them on schedule while at home. Recommend use of medication reminders (containers that separate pills according to day and time).

- Recommend low-residue, high-protein, high-calorie diet during an acute phase. Encourage patient to keep a record of foods that irritate bowel and to eliminate them from diet. Recommend intake of eight glasses of water per day.
- Provide support for prolonged nature of disease because it is a strain on family life and financial resources. Arrange for individual and family counseling as indicated.
- Provide time for patient to express fears and frustrations.

Evaluation

Expected Patient Outcomes

- Reports decrease in frequency of diarrheal stools
- Experiences less pain
- Maintains fluid volume balance
- Attains optimal nutrition
- Maintains skin integrity
- Prevents fatigue
- Experiences less anxiety
- Copes successfully with diagnosis
- Acquires an understanding of the disease process
- Recovers without complications

For more information, see Chapter 38 in Smeltzer and Bare: *Brunner and Suddarth's Textbook of Medical-Surgical Nursing*, 11th edition. Philadelphia: Lippincott Williams & Wilkins, 2008.

Unconscious Patient

Unconsciousness is an altered level of consciousness (LOC) in which the patient is unresponsive to and unaware of environmental stimuli, usually for a short duration. Coma is a clinical state—an unarousable unresponsive condition—in which the patient is unaware of self or the environment for prolonged periods (days to months, or even years). Akinetic mutism is a state of unresponsiveness to the environment in which the patient makes no movement or sound but sometimes has his or her eyes open. A persistent vegetative state is one in which the patient is described as wakeful, without cognitive or affective mental function. The causes of unconsciousness may be neurologic (head injury, stroke), toxicologic (drug overdose, alcohol intoxication), or metabolic (hepatic or renal failure, diabetic ketoacidosis). Locked-in syndrome consists of tetraplegia, inablity to speak, and minimal eye movement.

Assessment and Diagnostic Methods

- Neurologic examination (CT, MRI, PET, EEG) to identify cause of loss of consciousness
- Laboratory tests: major chemical profile, serum ammonia, blood urea nitrogen, osmolality, prothrombin time, serum ketones, alcohol and drug screen, arterial blood gases

Medical Management

The first priority is a patent and secure airway (intubation or tracheostomy). Then circulatory status (carotid pulse, heart rate and impulse, blood pressure) is assessed and adequate oxygenation maintained. An intravenous line is established to maintain fluid balance status, and nutritional support is provided (feeding tube or gastrostomy). Neurologic care is based on specific pathology. Other measures include drug therapy and measures to prevent complications.

NURSING PROCESS: The Unconscious Patient

U

Assessment

- Assess level of responsiveness (consciousness) using the Glasgow Coma Scale. Assess also the patient's ability to respond verbally. Evaluate pupil size, equality, and reaction to light; note movement of eyes.
- Assess facial symmetry and swallowing reflexes, and elicit deep tendon reflexes.

- Assess for spontaneous, purposeful, or nonpurposeful responses: decorticate posturing (arms flexed, adducted, and internally rotated, and legs in extension) or decerebrate posturing (extremities extended and reflexes exaggerated).
- Rule out paralysis or stroke as cause of flaccidity.
- Examine respiratory status, eye signs, reflexes, and body functions (circulation, respiration, elimination, fluid and electrolyte balance) in a systematic manner.
- Suspect a toxic or metabolic disorder if patient is comatose and pupillary light reflex is preserved.
- Assume that neurologic disease is present if patient is comatose and localized signs are severe.

Diagnosis

Nursing Diagnoses

- Ineffective airway clearance related to inability to clear respiratory secretions
- Risk for fluid volume deficit related to inability to ingest fluids
- Impaired oral mucous membranes related to mouth breathing, absence of pharyngeal reflex, and inability to ingest fluids
- Risk for impaired skin integrity related to immobility or restlessness
- Impaired tissue integrity of cornea related to diminished or absent corneal reflex
- Ineffective thermoregulation related to damage to hypothalamic center
- Impaired bowel elimination (diarrhea or constipation) or urinary elimination (incontinence or retention) related to unconscious state
- Dysfunctional family processes related to health crisis of unconsciousness

Collaborative Problems/Potential Complications

- Respiratory distress or failure
- Pneumonia
- Pressure ulcer

U

- Aspiration
- Deep vein thrombosis
- Contractures

Planning and Goals

Goals of care during the unconscious period may include patient protection by ensuring a clear airway, fluid volume balance, intact oral mucous membranes, normal skin integrity, absence of corneal irritation, thermoregulation, absence of urinary retention and infection, absence of diarrhea or fecal impaction, intact family or support system, freedom from injury, and absence of complications.

Nursing Interventions

Maintaining the Airway

- Establish an adequate airway, and ensure ventilation.
- Position patient in a lateral or semiprone position; do not allow patient to remain on back.
- Remove secretions to reduce danger of aspiration; elevate head of bed to a 30-degree angle to prevent aspiration; provide frequent suctioning and oral hygiene.
- Auscultate chest every 8 hours for crackles, wheezes, or absence of breath sounds.
- Maintain patency of endotracheal tube or tracheostomy; monitor arterial blood gases; maintain ventilator settings.
- Promote pulmonary hygiene with chest physiotherapy and postural drainage.

Providing Safety and Protection

U

- Provide padded side rails for protection; maintain head of bed in raised position.
- Use every measure available and appropriate for calming a disturbed patient; avoid physical restraints if possible to prevent rise in intracranial pressure.
- Protect the patient's dignity and privacy; act as the patient's advocate.

Attaining Fluid and Nutritional Balance

- Assess for hydration status: examine mucous membranes; assess skin for tissue turgor.
- Meet fluid needs by giving required intravenous fluids and then nasogastric or gastrostomy feedings.
- Give intravenous fluids and blood transfusions slowly if patient has an intracranial condition.
- Never give oral fluids to a patient who cannot swallow; insert feeding tube for administration of enteral feedings.

Maintaining Healthy Oral Mucous Membranes

- Inspect mouth for dryness, inflammation, and crusting; cleanse and rinse carefully to remove secretions and crusts and keep membranes moist; apply petrolatum to lips.
- Assess sides of mouth and lips for ulceration if patient has an endotracheal tube. Move tube to opposite side of mouth daily.

Maintaining Skin Integrity

- Follow a regular schedule of turning and repositioning to prevent ischemic necrosis over pressure areas, and to provide kinesthetic, proprioceptive, and vestibular stimulation.
- Give passive exercise of extremities to prevent contractures; use a splint or foam boots to prevent footdrop and eliminate pressure on toes.
- Keep hip joints and legs in proper alignment with supporting trochanter rolls.
- Position arms in abduction, fingers lightly flexed, and hands in slight supination.

U

Maintaining Corneal Integrity

- Cleanse eyes with cotton balls moistened with sterile normal saline to remove debris and discharge.
- Instill artificial tears every 2 hours, as prescribed.
- Use cold compresses as prescribed for periocular edema after cranial surgery. Avoid contact with cornea.

- Use eye patches cautiously because of potential for further corneal abrasions.

Attaining Thermoregulation

- Adjust environment to promote normal body temperature.
- Use prescribed measures to treat hyperthermia: remove bedding, except light sheet; give antipyretic agents; avoid shivering, which may be due to chlorpromazine (Thorazine).

 NURSING ALERT Take rectal or tympanic (unless contraindicated) body temperature.

Preventing Urinary Retention

- Palpate or scan bladder at intervals to detect urinary retention.
- Insert indwelling catheter if there are signs of urinary retention; observe for fever and cloudy urine; inspect urethral orifice for drainage.
- Use external penile catheter (condom catheter) for male patients and absorbent pads for female patients if they can urinate spontaneously.
- Initiate bladder training program as soon as conscious.
- Monitor frequently for skin irritation and breakdown; implement appropriate skin care.

Promoting Bowel Function

- Evaluate abdominal distention by listening for bowel sounds and measuring abdominal girth.
- Monitor number and consistency of bowel movements; perform rectal examination for signs of fecal impaction; patient may require enema every other day to empty lower colon.
- Enemas may be contraindicated if Valsalva maneuver increases intracranial pressure.
- Administer stool softeners and glycerin suppositories as indicated.

Supporting the Family

- Reinforce and clarify information about patient's condition to permit family members to mobilize their own adaptive capacities.
- Encourage ventilation of feelings and concerns.
- Support family in decision-making process concerning posthospital management and placement.

Promoting Sensory Stimulation

- Provide continuing sensory stimulation to help patient overcome profound sensory deprivation. Explain to family that periods of agitation may be a sign of increasing patient awareness of the environment.
- Make efforts to maintain usual day and night patterns of activity and sleep; orient patient to time and place every 8 hours.
- Touch and talk to patient; encourage family and friends to do the same; avoid making any negative comments about patient's status in patient's presence. Avoid overstimulating patient.
- Introduce sounds from patient's home and workplace if possible by means of audio and video tapes.
- Read favorite books and provide familiar radio and television programs to enrich environment.

Attaining Self-Care and Meeting Family Needs

Begin to teach activities of daily living as soon as consciousness returns. Support, encourage, and supervise family and patient's efforts.

Monitoring and Managing Potential Complications

U

- Monitor vital signs and respiratory function for signs of respiratory failure or distress.
- Assess for adequate red blood cells to carry oxygen: total blood count and arterial blood gases.
- If pneumonia develops, obtain culture specimens to identify organism for selection of appropriate antibiotic.

- Monitor for evidence of impaired skin integrity, and implement strategies to prevent skin breakdown and pressure ulcers.
- Address factors that contribute to impaired skin integrity, and undertake strategies to promote healing if pressure ulcers do develop.
- Monitor for signs and symptoms of deep vein thrombosis (redness and swelling).

Evaluation

Expected Patient Outcomes

- Maintains clear airway and demonstrates appropriate breath sounds
- Experiences no injuries
- Attains or maintains healthy oral mucous membranes
- Attains or maintains adequate fluid status
- Demonstrates normal range of serum electrolytes
- Maintains normal skin integrity
- Has no corneal irritation
- Attains or maintains thermoregulation
- Has no urinary retention
- Avoids other complications

For more information, see Chapter 61 in Smeltzer and Bare: *Brunner and Suddarth's Textbook of Medical-Surgical Nursing*, 11th edition. Philadelphia: Lippincott Williams & Wilkins, 2008.

Urolithiasis

U

Urolithiasis refers to stones (calculi) in the urinary tract. Stones are formed in the urinary tract when the urinary concentration of substances such as calcium oxalate, calcium phosphate, and uric acid increases. Calculi vary in size from minute granular deposits to the size of an orange. Factors that favor formation of stones include infection, urinary stasis, immobility, and altered calcium metabolism (hypercalcemia and hypercalciuria). The problem occurs predominantly in the third to fifth decades and affects men more often than women.

Clinical Manifestations

Manifestations depend on the presence of obstruction, infection, and edema. Symptoms range from mild to excruciating pain and discomfort.

Stones in Renal Pelvis

- Intense, deep ache in costovertebral region
- Hematuria and pyuria
- Pain that radiates anteriorly and downward toward bladder in female and toward testes in male
- Acute pain, nausea, vomiting, costovertebral area tenderness (renal colic)
- Abdominal discomfort, diarrhea

Ureteral Colic (Stones Lodged in Ureter)

- Acute, excruciating, colicky, wavelike pain, radiating down the thigh to the genitalia
- Frequent desire to void, but little urine passed; usually contains blood because of the abrasive action of the stone (known as ureteral colic)

Stones Lodged in Bladder

- Symptoms of irritation associated with urinary tract infection and hematuria
- Urinary retention, if stone obstructs bladder neck
- Possible sepsis if infection is present with stone

Assessment and Diagnostic Methods

- Most stones are radiopaque and can be detected by radiography.

U

- Diagnosis is confirmed by kidney, ureter, and bladder (KUB) studies, intravenous urography, or retrograde pyelography.
- Chemical analysis is performed to determine stone composition.

Medical Management

Basic goals are to eradicate the stone, determine the stone type, prevent nephron destruction, control infection, and relieve any obstruction that may be present.

Stone Removal Procedures

- Cystoscopic examination and passage of small ureteral catheter
- Chemical analysis of stones to determine composition
- Extracorporeal shock wave lithotripsy (ESWL)
- Percutaneous nephrostomy; endourologic methods
- Electrohydraulic lithotripsy
- Ureteroscopy: stones fragmented with use of laser, electrohydraulic lithotripsy, or ultrasound and then removed
- Chemolysis (stone dissolution): alternative for those who are poor risks for other therapies, refuse other methods, or have easily dissolved stones (struvite)
- Surgical removal is performed in only 1% to 2% of patients.

Pharmacologic and Nutritional Therapy

- Analgesic agents (morphine or meperidine to prevent shock and syncope) and nonsteroidal anti-inflammatory drugs (NSAIDs)
- Increased fluid intake to assist in stone passage, unless patient is vomiting
- Increased round-the-clock fluid intake to dilute urine and ensure high urinary output
- For calcium stones: reduced dietary protein and sodium intake; liberal fluid intake; medications to acidify urine, such as ammonium chloride, sodium cellulose phosphate

(Calcibind), and thiazide diuretics if parathormone production is increased

- For phosphate stones: diet low in phosphorus; aluminum hydroxide gel
- For uric stones: low-purine and limited protein diet; allopurinol (Zyloprim); alkalinization of urine
- For cystine stones: low-protein diet; alkalinization of urine; penicillamine
- For oxalate stones: dilute urine; limit oxalate intake (green, leafy vegetables such as spinach; strawberries; rhubarb; wheat bran; chocolate; tea; and peanuts)

NURSING PROCESS: The Patient with Urolithiasis (Kidney Stones)

Assessment

- Assess for pain and discomfort, including severity, location, and radiation of pain.
- Assess for associated symptoms, including nausea, vomiting, diarrhea, and abdominal distention.
- Observe for signs of urinary tract infection (chills, fever, dysuria, frequency, and hesitancy) and obstruction (frequent urination of small amounts, oliguria, or anuria).
- Observe urine for blood; strain for stones or gravel.
- Focus history on factors that predispose patient to urinary tract stones or that may have precipitated current episode of renal or ureteral colic.
- Assess patient's knowledge about renal stones and measures to prevent recurrence.

Diagnosis

Nursing Diagnoses

- Acute pain related to inflammation, obstruction, and abrasion of the urinary tract
- Deficient knowledge regarding prevention of recurrence of renal stones

Collaborative Problems/Potential Complications

- Infection and sepsis (from urinary tract infection and pyelonephritis)
- Obstruction of the urinary tract by a stone or edema, with subsequent acute renal failure

Planning and Goals

Major goals may include relief of pain and discomfort, prevention of recurrence of renal stones, and prevention of complications.

Nursing Interventions

Relieving Pain

- Administer narcotic analgesics as prescribed. Suggest hot baths or application of moist heat to flank areas.
- Encourage and assist patient to assume a position of comfort.
- Assist patient to ambulate to obtain some pain relief.
- Monitor pain closely and report promptly increases in severity.
- Prepare patient for treatment (eg, lithotripsy, ureteroscopy, surgery) if pain is unrelieved.

Monitoring and Managing Complications

- Instruct patient to report decreased urine volume and bloody or cloudy urine.
- Monitor total urine output and patterns of voiding.
- Encourage increased fluid intake and ambulation.
- Begin intravenous fluids if patient cannot take adequate oral fluids.
- Observe patient constantly to detect spontaneous passage of a stone.
- Strain urine through gauze.
- Crush any blood clots passed in urine, and inspect sides of urinal and bedpan for clinging stones.
- Instruct patient to report any increase in pain; administer analgesic agents.
- Monitor vital signs for early indications of infection.

Promoting Home and Community-Based Care

Teaching Patients Self-Care

- Explain causes of kidney stones and ways to prevent recurrence.
- Show patient how to monitor and interpret urine pH.
- Encourage patient to drink enough to excrete 3,000 to 4,000 mL of urine every 24 hours.
- Instruct patient to avoid sudden increases in environmental temperatures and activities that produce excessive sweating and dehydration.
- Give detailed verbal and written information about specific foods to avoid.
- Explain actions and importance of medications prescribed to prevent stone formation.
- Teach signs and symptoms of stone formation, obstruction, and infection; advise patient to report these to physician promptly.

Providing Home and Follow-Up Care After ESWL

- Instruct patient to increase fluid intake to assist passage of stone fragments (may take 6 weeks to several months after procedure).
- Instruct patient about signs and symptoms of complications: fever, decreasing urinary output, and pain.
- Inform patient that hematuria is anticipated but should subside in 24 hours.
- Give appropriate dietary instructions based on composition of stones.
- Encourage regimen to avoid further stone formation; advise patient to adhere to prescribed diet.
- Teach patient to take sufficient fluids in the evening to prevent urine from becoming too concentrated at night.
- Recommend that patient have urine cultures every 1 to 2 months the first year and periodically thereafter.
- Recommend that recurrent urinary infection be treated vigorously.
- Encourage increased mobility whenever possible, and discourage ingestion of vitamin (especially vitamin D) and mineral supplements.

U

- Instruct patient about signs and symptoms of postoperative complications that warrant physician notification.
- Emphasize to family and patient the importance of follow-up to assess kidney function and to ensure removal of all kidney stones.

Evaluation

Expected Patient Outcomes

- Reports relief of pain
- Experiences no complications
- States increased knowledge of health-seeking behaviors to prevent recurrence

---

For more information, see Chapter 45 in Smeltzer and Bare: *Brunner and Suddarth's Textbook of Medical-Surgical Nursing,* 11th edition. Philadelphia: Lippincott Williams & Wilkins, 2008.

U

V

Vein Disorders

Venous Thrombosis, Thrombophlebitis, Phlebothrombosis, and Deep Vein Thrombosis

Although the vein disorders described here do not necessarily present an identical pathology, for clinical purposes these terms are often used interchangeably. The exact cause of venous thrombosis remains unclear, although three factors (Virchow's triad) are believed to play a significant role in its development: stasis of blood, injury to the vessel wall, and altered blood coagulation.

Thrombophlebitis is an inflammation of the walls of the veins, often accompanied by the formation of a clot. When a clot develops initially in the veins as a result of stasis or hypercoagulability, but without inflammation, the process is referred to as phlebothrombosis.

Venous thrombosis can occur in any vein but is most frequent in the veins of the lower extremities. Both superficial and deep veins of the legs may be affected. Damage to the lining of blood vessels creates a site for clot formation, and increased blood coagulability occurs in patients who abruptly stop taking anticoagulant medications and also occurs with oral contraceptive use and several blood dyscrasias. The danger associated with venous thrombosis is that parts of a clot can become detached and produce an embolic occlusion of the pulmonary blood vessels. Venous thrombosis is less common in the upper extremity than in the lower extremity.

V

Risk Factors

- Obesity
- Advanced age
- Oral contraceptive use

Clinical Manifestations

- Half of all patients have no symptoms; signs and symptoms are nonspecific.
- Edema and swelling of the extremity resulting from obstruction of the deep veins of the leg
- Skin over the affected leg may become warmer; superficial veins may become more prominent (cordlike venous segment).
- Bilateral swelling may be difficult to detect (lack of size difference).
- Tenderness occurs later and is detected by gently palpating the leg.
- Homans' sign (pain in the calf after sharp dorsiflexion of the foot) is not specific for deep vein thrombosis (DVT) because it can be elicited in any painful condition of the calf.
- In some cases, signs of a pulmonary embolus are the first indication of DVT.
- Thrombus of superficial veins produces pain or tenderness, redness, and warmth in the involved area.
- In massive iliofemoral venous thrombosis (phlegmasia cerulea dolens), the entire extremity becomes massively swollen, tense, painful, and cool to touch.

Assessment and Diagnostic Methods

- History revealing risk factors such as varicose veins or neoplastic disease
- Doppler ultrasonography, impedance plethysmography, duplex imaging
- ^{125}I-labeled fibrinogen scanning, contrast phlebography (venography)

Prevention

Prevention is dependent on identifying risk factors for thrombus and on educating the patient about appropriate interventions.

Medical Management

Objectives of management are to prevent the thrombus from growing and fragmenting, resolve the current thrombus, and prevent recurrence.

Pharmacologic Therapy

- Heparin is administered for 5 to 7 days by intermittent or continuous intravenous infusion. Dosage is regulated by partial thromboplastin time (PTT), international normalized ratio (INR), and platelet counts. Low-molecular-weight heparin is given in one or two injections daily; it is more expensive than unfractionated heparin but safer.
- Oral anticoagulants (eg, warfarin [Coumadin]) are given with heparin therapy.
- Thrombolytic (fibrinolytic) therapy is given within the first 3 days after acute thrombosis. Drugs such as streptokinase, urokinase, and tissue plasminogen activator are used.
- Throughout therapy, PTT, prothrombin time, hemoglobin, hematocrit, platelet count, and fibrinogen level are monitored frequently. Drug therapy is discontinued if bleeding occurs and cannot be stopped.
- Fondaparinux given subcutaneously for prophylaxis during major orthopedic surgery (hip replacement, etc.)

Surgical Management

Thrombectomy is the treatment of choice when anticoagulant or thrombolytic therapy is contraindicated, the danger of pulmonary embolism is extreme, and permanent damage to the extremity will probably result. A vena cava filter may be placed to trap emboli and prevent pulmonary complications.

V

Nursing Management

Assessment

- Assess for early signs of venous disorders in lower extremities.
- Take history of varicose veins, hypercoagulation, neoplastic disease, cardiovascular disease, or recent major surgery or injury. Obese people, elderly people, and women taking oral contraceptives are at risk.
- Question patient about leg pain, heaviness, and any functional impairment or edema.
- Inspect legs from groin to feet, noting asymmetry and measuring and recording calf circumference (one early indication of edema is engorgement of the space behind the ankle).
- Note any increase in temperature in the affected leg.
- Identify areas of tenderness and any thromboses.
- Advise patient to remove elastic stockings for a brief interval at least twice daily and at night; to inspect skin for signs of irritation; to examine calves for possible tenderness; and to report any skin changes or signs of tenderness.

Nursing Interventions

Providing Comfort

- Intermittent pneumatic compression devices can be used with elastic stockings for prevention of DVT. Ensure that prescribed pressures are not exceeded, and assess for comfort.
- Recommend bed rest. Advise patient to elevate affected extremity. Provide elastic stockings, and administer analgesic agents for pain. For DVT advise bed rest for 5 to 7 days after diagnosis.
- Use elastic stocking when patient begins to ambulate; apply and monitor carefully to prevent it from rolling down to form a tourniquet (which restricts circulation).
- Encourage walking (better than standing or sitting for long periods).

- Recommend bed exercises, such as dorsiflexion of the foot against a footboard.
- Apply warm, moist packs to affected extremity to reduce discomfort.
- Provide additional pain relief with mild analgesic agents as prescribed.

> **NURSING ALERT** Elderly patients may be unable to apply elastic stockings properly. Teach the family member who is to assist the patient to apply the stockings so that they do not cause undue pressure on any part of the feet or legs.

Positioning the Body and Encouraging Exercise

- Elevate feet and lower legs periodically above heart level when on bed rest.
- Perform active and passive leg exercises, particularly those involving calf muscles, to increase venous flow preoperatively and postoperatively.
- Provide early ambulation to help prevent venous stasis.
- Encourage deep-breathing exercises because they produce increased negative pressure in the thorax, which assists in emptying the large veins.

Monitoring and Managing Potential Complications

- Monitor urinalysis for hematuria (first sign of anticoagulant toxicity).
- Monitor anticoagulant therapy closely and regularly. Prepare to reverse anticoagulant effects by administering protamine sulfate for heparin or vitamin K and fresh-frozen plasma for warfarin.
- Monitor for heparin-induced thrombocytopenia. Note platelet counts regularly and report counts less than 100,000/mL or a greater than 25% decrease in platelet count. Report the need for increasing doses of heparin to maintain therapeutic levels. Note thromboembolic or

hemorrhagic complications. Report a patient history of heparin sensitivity.

- Closely monitor the medication schedule, because oral anticoagulants interact with many other medications and herbal and nutritional supplements.
- Teach patient which medications potentiate oral anticoagulants: salicylates, anabolic steroids, chloral hydrate, glucagon, chloramphenicol, neomycin, quinidine, vitamin E, and phenylbutazone (Butazolidin). Medications that decrease the anticoagulant effect include phenytoin, barbiturates, diuretics, and estrogen. Identify medication interactions for patients taking specific oral anticoagulants.

Teaching Patients Self-Care

- Teach patient how to apply elastic stockings.
- Instruct patient on the purpose and importance of medication (correct dosage at specific times) and need for scheduled blood tests to regulate medications.

For more information, see Chapter 31 in Smeltzer and Bare: *Brunner and Suddarth's Textbook of Medical-Surgical Nursing*, 11th edition. Philadelphia: Lippincott Williams & Wilkins, 2008.

V

Appendix A

Selected Lab Values

BLOOD CHEMISTRY

TEST	CONVENTIONAL UNITS	SI UNITS
Alanine aminotransferase (ALT, formerly SGPT)	Males: 10-40 U/mL	Males: 0.17-0.68 μkat/L
	Females: 8-35 U/mL	Females: 0.14-0.60 μkat/L
Alkaline phosphatase	50-120 U/L	50-120 U/L
Ammonia (plasma)	15-45 μg/dL (varies with method)	11-32 μmol/L
Amylase	60-160 Somogyi U/dL	111-296 U/L
Aspartase amino transferase (AST, formerly SGOT)	Males: 10-40 U/L	Males: 0.34-0.68 μkat/L
	Females: 15-30 U/L	Females: 0.25-0.51 μkat/L
Bicarbonate	24-31 mEq/L	24-31 mmol/L
Bilirubin (total)	0.3-1.0 mg/dL	5-17 μmol/L
Direct	0.1-0.4 mg/dL	1.7-3.7 μmol/L
Indirect	0.1-0.4 mg/dL	3.4-11.2 μmol/L
Blood urea nitrogen (BUN)	8-20 mg/dL	2.9-7.1 mmol/L
Calcium	8.6-10.2 mg/dL	2.5-2.55 mmol/L
Carbon dioxide, arterial (whole blood) partial pressure ($PaCO_2$)	35-45 mm Hg	4.66-5.99 kPa
Chloride	97-107 mEq/L	97-107 mmol/L
Creatine kinase (CK) isoenzymes	32-267 U/L[†]	0.53-4.45 μkat/L[†]
Creatine kinase (MB)	<16 IU/L[†] or 4% of total CK	<0.27 μkat/L[†]
Creatinine (serum)	0.7-1.4 mg/dL[†]	64-124 μmol/L[‡]
Gamma-glutamyl-transpeptidase (GGT)	Males: 20-30 U/L	0.03-0.5 μkat/L
	Females: 1-24 U/L	0.02-0.4 μkat/L
Glucose (blood)	Fasting: 60-110 mg/dL	3.3-6.05 mmol/L
	Postprandial (2 h): 65-140 mg/dL	3.58-7.7 mmol/L

Test		
Glycosylated hemoglobin (HbA$_{1c}$)	3.9–6.9%	
Lactate dehydrogenase (LDH)	90–176 mU/mL	90–176 U/L
Lipids		
Cholesterol	<200 mg/dL (desirable)	<5.2 mmol/L
Triglycerides	<165 mg/dL	<1.65 g/L
Lipase	0–160 U/L†	0.266 µkat/L†
Magnesium	1.3–2.3 mg/dL	0.62–0.95 mmol/L
Osmolality	275–300 mOsm/kg	275–300 mmol/L
Phosphorus (inorganic)	2.5–4.5 mg/dL	0.8–1.45 mmol/L
Potassium	3.5–5.0 mEq/L	3.5–5.0 mmol/L
Prostate specific antigen (PSA)	0–4 ng/mL	0–4 µg/L
Protein total	6.0–8.0 g/dL	60–80 g/L
Albumin	3.5–5.5 g/dL	40–55 g/L
Globulin	1.7–3.3 g/dL	17–33 g/L
A/G ratio	1.0–2.2	1.0–2.2
Thyroid Tests		
Thyroxine (T$_4$) total	5.0–11.0 µg/dL	65–138 nmol/L
Thyroxine, free (FT$_4$)	0.8–2.7 ng/dL	10.3–35 pmol/L
Triiodothyronine (T$_3$) total	70–204 ng/dL	1.08–3.14 nmol/L
Thyroid stimulating hormone (TSH)	0.4–6.0 µU/mL	0.4–4.2 mIU/L
Thyroglobin	3–42 ng/mL	3–42 µg/L
Sodium	135–145 mEq/L	135–145 mmol/L
Uric acid	2.5–8 mg/dL	0.15–0.0 mmol/L

U, units
†Laboratory and/or method specific
‡Varies with age and muscle mass

795

HEMATOLOGY

TEST	CONVENTIONAL UNITS	SI UNITS
Erythrocyte count (RBC count)	M. 4.2-5.4 × 10⁶/µL	M. 4.2-5.4 × 10¹²/L
	F. 3.6-5.0 × 10⁶/µL	F. 3.6-5.0 × 10¹²/L
Hematocrit (Hct)	M. 40-50%	M. 0.40-0.50
	F. 37-47%	F. 0.37-0.47
Hemoglobin (Hb)	M. 14.0-16.5 g/dL	M. 140-165 g/L
	F. 12.0-15.0 g/dL	F. 120-150 g/L
Mean corpuscular hemoglobin (MHC)	27-34 pg/cell	0.40-0.53 fmol/cell
Mean corpuscular hemoglobin concentration (MCHC)	31-35 g/dL	310-350 g/L
Mean corpuscular volume (MCV)	80-100 fl	
Reticulocyte count	1.0-1.5% total RBC	
Leukocyte count (WBC count)	4.4-11.3 × 10³/µL	4.4-11.3 × 10⁹/L
Basophils	0-2%	
Eosinophils	0-3%	
Lymphocytes	24-40%	
Monocytes	4-9%	
Neutrophils (segmented [Segs])	47-63%	
Neutrophils (bands)	0-4%	

Appendix B

NANDA-Approved Nursing Diagnoses 2005–2006

Activity Intolerance
Activity Intolerance, Risk for
Adjustment, Impaired
Airway Clearance, Ineffective
Allergy Response, Latex
Allergy Response, Risk for Latex
Anxiety
Anxiety, Death
Aspiration, Risk for
Attachment, Risk for Impaired Parent/Infant/Child
Autonomic Dysreflexia
Autonomic Dysreflexia, Risk for
Body Image, Disturbed
Body Temperature, Risk for Imbalanced
Bowel Incontinence
Breastfeeding, Effective
Breastfeeding, Ineffective
Breastfeeding, Interrupted
Breathing Pattern, Ineffective
Cardiac Output, Decreased
Caregiver Role Strain
Caregiver Role Strain, Risk for
Communication, Impaired Verbal
Communication, Readiness for Enhanced
Conflict, Decisional (Specify)
Conflict, Parental Role
Confusion, Acute
Confusion, Chronic
Constipation

Constipation, Perceived
Constipation, Risk for
Coping, Ineffective
Coping, Defensive
Coping, Readiness for Enhanced
Coping, Ineffective Community
Coping, Readiness for Enhanced Community
Coping, Compromised Family
Coping, Disabled Family
Coping, Readiness for Enhanced Family
Death Syndrome, Risk for Sudden Infant
Denial, Ineffective
Dentition, Impaired
Development, Risk for Delayed
Diarrhea
Disuse Syndrome, Risk for
Diversional Activity, Deficient
Energy Field, Disturbed
Environmental Interpretation Syndrome, Impaired
Failure to Thrive, Adult
Falls, Risk for
Family Processes, Dysfunctional: Alcoholism
Family Processes, Interrupted
Family Processes, Readiness for Enhanced
Fatigue
Fear
Fluid Balance, Readiness for Enhanced
Fluid Volume, Deficient
Fluid Volume, Excess
Fluid Volume, Risk for Deficient
Fluid Volume, Risk for Imbalanced
Gas Exchange, Impaired
Grieving, Anticipatory
Grieving, Dysfunctional
Grieving, Risk for Dysfunctional
Growth and Development, Delayed
Growth, Risk for Disproportionate
Health Maintenance, Ineffective

Health-Seeking Behaviors (Specify)
Home Maintenance, Impaired
Hopelessness
Hyperthermia
Hypothermia
Identity, Disturbed Personal
Incontinence, Functional Urinary
Incontinence, Reflex Urinary
Incontinence, Stress Urinary
Incontinence, Total Urinary
Incontinence, Urge Urinary
Incontinence, Risk for Urge Urinary
Infant Behavior, Disorganized
Infant Behavior, Risk for Disorganized
Infant Behavior, Readiness for Enhanced Organized
Infant Feeding Pattern, Ineffective
Infection, Risk for
Injury, Risk for
Injury, Risk for Perioperative-Positioning
Intracranial Adaptive Capacity, Decreased
Knowledge, Deficient (Specify)
Knowledge, Readiness for Enhanced (Specify)
Lifestyle, Sedentary
Loneliness, Risk for
Memory, Impaired
Mobility, Impaired Bed
Mobility, Impaired Physical
Mobility, Impaired Wheelchair
Nausea
Neglect, Unilateral
Noncompliance
Nutrition, Imbalanced: Less Than Body Requirements
Nutrition, Imbalanced: More Than Body Requirements
Nutrition, Readiness for Enhanced
Nutrition, Risk for Imbalanced: More Than Body Requirements
Oral Mucous Membrane, Impaired
Pain, Acute
Pain, Chronic

Parenting, Readiness for Enhanced
Parenting, Impaired
Parenting, Risk for Impaired
Peripheral Neurovascular Dysfunction, Risk for
Poisoning, Risk for
Post-Trauma Syndrome
Post-Trauma Syndrome, Risk for
Powerlessness
Powerlessness, Risk for
Protection, Ineffective
Rape-Trauma Syndrome
Rape-Trauma Syndrome: Compound Reaction
Rape-Tauma Syndrome: Silent Reaction
Religiosity, Impaired
Religiosity, Readiness for Enhanced
Religiosity, Risk for Impaired
Relocation Stress Syndrome
Relocation Stress Syndrome, Risk for
Role Performance, Ineffective
Self-Care Deficit, Bathing/Hygiene
Self-Care Deficit, Dressing/Grooming
Self-Care Deficit, Feeding
Self-Care Deficit, Toileting
Self-Concept, Readiness for Enhanced
Self-Esteem, Chronic Low
Self-Esteem, Situational Low
Self-Esteem, Risk for Situational Low
Self-Mutilation
Self-Mutilation, Risk for
Sensory Perception, Disturbed (Specify: Visual, Auditory,
   Kinesthetic, Gustatory, Tactile, Olfactory)
Sexual Dysfunction
Sexuality Pattern, Ineffective
Skin Integrity, Impaired
Skin Integrity, Risk for Impaired
Sleep Deprivation
Sleep Pattern, Disturbed
Sleep, Readiness for Enhanced

Social Interaction, Impaired
Social Isolation
Sorrow, Chronic
Spiritual Distress
Spiritual Distress, Risk for
Spiritual Well-Being, Readiness for Enhanced
Suffocation, Risk for
Suicide, Risk for
Surgical Recovery, Delayed
Swallowing, Impaired
Therapeutic Regimen Management, Effective
Therapeutic Regimen Management, Ineffective
Therapeutic Regimen Management, Readiness for Enhanced
Therapeutic Regimen Management, Ineffective Community
Therapeutic Regimen Management, Ineffective Family
Thermoregulation, Ineffective
Thought Processes, Disturbed
Tissue Integrity, Impaired
Tissue Perfusion, Ineffective (Specify Type: Renal, Cerebral,
    Cardiopulmonary, Gastrointestinal, Peripheral)
Transfer Ability, Impaired
Trauma, Risk for
Urinary Elimination, Impaired
Urinary Elimination, Readiness for Enhanced
Urinary Retention
Ventilation, Impaired Spontaneous
Ventilatory Weaning Response, Dysfunctional
Violence, Risk for Other-Directed
Violence, Risk for Self-Directed
Walking, Impaired
Wandering

NANDA International (2005). *Nursing Diagnoses: Definitions & Classification 2005–2006*. Philadelphia.

Appendix C

Key Health Care Abbreviations and Acronyms

Note: These are examples and may differ slightly from facility to facility.

A

AAFP	American Academy of Family Physicians
AALPN	American Association of Licensed Practical Nurses
AAMI	age-associated memory impairment
AAP	American Academy of Pediatricians
AARP	American Association of Retired Persons
AB	abortion
Ab	antibody
ABCDE	airway and cervical spine, breathing, circulation, disability, exposure
ABG	arterial blood gas
ABP	acute bacterial prostatitis
AC	Adriamycin and Cytoxan
ACE	all-cotton elastic
ACE	angiotensin-converting enzyme
ACIP	Advisory Committee on Immunization Practices
ACLS	Advanced Cardiac Life Support
ACS	American Cancer Society; Ambulatory Care Sensitive
ACTH	adrenocorticotropic hormone
AD	advance directive
ADA	American Diabetes Association
ADAMHA	Alcohol, Drug Abuse, and Mental Health Administration
ADC	AIDS dementia complex

ADDH	attention deficit disorder with hyperactivity
ADH	antidiuretic hormone
ADHD	attention deficit hyperactivity disorder
ADL	activities of daily living
AEA	above-the-elbow amputation
AEB	as evidenced by
AED	automated external defibrillator
AFP	alpha-fetoprotein
Ag	antigen
AGA	appropriate for gestational age
AHA	American Hospital Association
AHCPR	Agency for Health Care Policy and Research
AI	adequate intake
AICD	automatic implantable cardioverter-defibrillator
AIDS	acquired immunodeficiency syndrome
AJN	*American Journal of Nursing*
AKA	above-the-knee amputation; also known as
ALL	acute lymphocytic leukemia
ALS	amyotrophic lateral sclerosis
ALT	aspartate aminotransferase (formerly SGOT)
AMA	American Medical Association; against medical advice
AML	acute myelogenous leukemia
ANA	American Nurses Association
ANCC	American Nurses Credentialing Center
ANP	atrial natriuretic peptide
ANS	autonomic nervous system
AP	apical pulse; anteroposterior; anterior-posterior (repair); assault precautions (attack)
APGAR	A = appearance (color); P = pulse (heart rate); G = grimace or reflexes (irritability); A = activity (muscle tone); R = respiratory effort
APHA	American Public Health Association
APIE	assessment, plan, intervention, evaluation
APTT	activated partial thromboplastin time
A-R	apical–radial (pulse)
ARC	American Red Cross
ARDD	alcohol-related developmental disability
ARDS	adult respiratory distress syndrome

ARND	alcohol-related neurodevelopmental disorder
AROM	active range of motion; artificial rupture of the membranes
ARRP	anatomic retropubic radical prostatectomy
ART	Accredited Record Technician
AS	sickle cell trait
ASA	acetylsalicylic acid (aspirin)
ASD	atrial septal defect; autism spectrum disorders
ASO	antistreptolysin O titer
AST	aspartate aminotransferase
ASU	Ambulatory Surgery Unit
ATF	Alcohol, Tobacco, and Firearms
ATLS	Advanced Trauma Life Support
ATN	acute tubular necrosis
ATP	adenosine triphosphate
AV	atrioventricular
AVPU	Alert, Verbal, Pain response, Unresponsive
AWOL	absent without leave
Ax	axillary

B

BAL in Oil	dimercaprol
BBB	blood–brain barrier
BBP	blood-borne pathogens
BCG	bacille Calmette-Guérin
BCLS	Basic Cardiac Life Support
BCP	birth control pill
BE	barium enema x-ray
BEA	below-the-elbow amputation
BIDS	bedtime insulin and daytime sulfonylureas
BKA	below-the-knee amputation
BLL	blood lead level
BLS	Basic Life Support
BM	bowel movement
BMI	Body Mass Index
BMT	bone marrow transplantation
BOA	born out of asepsis
BOH	Board of Health
BP	blood pressure

BPAD	bipolar affective disorder
BPD	bipolar disorder
BPH	benign prostatic hyperplasia
BPM	beats per minute
BPRS	Brief Psychiatric Rating Scale
BRAT	bananas, rice, applesauce, toast
BRM	biologic response modifiers
BRP	bathroom privileges
BS	bowel sounds
BSC	bedside commode
BSE	breast self-examination
BUN	blood urea nitrogen
C	
C	Celsius; centigrade
C & S	(blood) culture and sensitivity
C2, C3, etc.	cervical section of the spinal cord
Ca^{++}	calcium
$Ca_3[PO_4]_2$	calcium phosphate
CABG	coronary artery bypass grafting
$CaCl_2$	calcium chloride
$CaCO_3$	calcium carbonate
CAD	coronary artery disease
CAF	Cytoxan, Adriamycin, fluorouracil
CAPD	continuous ambulatory peritoneal dialysis
CAT	computerized adaptive testing
CBC	complete blood count
CBE	charting by exception
CBP	chronic bacterial prostatitis
cc	cubic centimeter
CC	chief complaint
CCP	clinical care pathway
CCU	coronary care unit
CCU/CICU	coronary care unit/coronary intensive care unit
CD	chemical dependency
CD4	helper T lymphocytes
CDC	Centers for Disease Control and Prevention
CDU	chemical dependency unit, clinical decision unit

CEA	carcinoembryonic antigen; cultured epithelial autografts
CEH	continuing education hour
CEU	continuing education unit
CF	cystic fibrosis
CHAP	Community Health Accreditation Program
CHC	community health center
CHD	coronary heart disease
CHF	congestive heart failure
CHHA	Certified Home Health Aide
CHO	carbohydrates
CIC	crisis intervention center
CICU	coronary intensive care unit
CK	creatine kinase
Cl	chloride
CLL	chronic lymphocytic leukemia
CLTC	Citizens for Long-Term Care
CM	case/care manager
CMF	Cytoxan, methotrexate, fluorouracil
CMG	cystometrogram
CML	chronic myelogenous leukemia
CMMS	Medicare and Medicaid Services
CMS	color, motion, sensitivity (circulation, mobility, sensation)
CMV	cytomegalovirus
CNM	Certified Nurse Midwife
CNO	Community Nursing Organization
CNS	central nervous system
CO	cardiac output
CO_2	carbon dioxide
COA	children of alcoholics; coarctation of the aorta
COAs	children of alcoholics
COLD	chronic obstructive lung disease
COPD	chronic obstructive pulmonary disease
COPs	Conditions of Participation (Medicare requirements)
COTA	Certified Occupational Therapy Assistant
CP	cardiopulmonary; cerebral palsy
CPAP	continuous positive airway pressure
CPD	cephalopelvic disproportion

CPK	creatine phosphokinase
CPM	continuous passive motion
CPR	cardiopulmonary resuscitation
CPT	chest physiotherapy
CQI	contiguous (or continuous) quality improvement
CRH	corticotropin-releasing hormone
CRNA	Certified Registered Nurse Anesthetist
CRNH	Certified Registered Nurse—Hospice
CRP	C-reactive protein
CRU	Coronary Rehabilitation Unit
Cryo	cryoprecipitate
CS	complete stroke; cardiac sphincter
CSF	cerebral spinal fluid; colony-stimulating factors
CSR, CSS	Central Supply Room, Central Service Supply
CT	computed tomography
CUC	chronic ulcerative colitis
CVA	cerebrovascular accident
CVP	central venous pressure
CVS	chorionic villus sampling
CXR	chest x-ray
D	
D & C	dilatation and curettage
D/2NS5%	dextrose in half-normal saline (0.45% NS)
D/C	discontinue
D5NS5%	dextrose in normal saline (0.9% NS)
D5W5%	dextrose in sterile water
DAPE	data, assessment, plan, evaluation
DARE	data, action, response, education
DAT	diet as tolerated
Db	decibel
DBP; dBP	diastolic blood pressure
DCH	District Court hold
DCT	distal convoluted tubule
DDST	Denver Developmental Screening Test
DEA	Drug Enforcement Agency
DEP	Department of Environmental Protection
DERM	dermatology

DES	diethylstilbestrol
DIC	disseminated intravascular coagulation
DISCUS	Dyskinesia Identification System-Condensed User Scale
DJD	degenerative joint disease
DKA	diabetic ketoacidosis
dL	deciliter
DMAT	Disaster Medical Assistance Team
DMD	Duchenne muscular dystrophy
DME	Durable Medical Equipment
DMSA	2, 3-dimercaptosuccinic acid
DNA	deoxyribonucleic acid
DNH	do not hospitalize
DNI	do not intubate
DNR	do not resuscitate
DOA	Department of Agriculture
DOH	Department of Health
DOL	Department of Labor
DRF	drip rate factor
DRG	diagnosis-related group
DRI	dietary reference intake
DSM-IV	*Diagnostic and Statistical Manual of Mental Disorders, Revision IV*
DT	diphtheria and tetanus toxoids
DTAD	drain tube attachment device
DtaP	diphtheria, tetanus, acellular pertussis
DTP	diphtheria and tetanus toxoids and pertussis vaccine
DVR	Division of Vocational Rehabilitation
DVT	deep vein thrombosis
E	
EAR	estimated average requirement
EC	emergency contraception
ECF	extended care facility; extracellular fluid
ECG (EKG)	electrocardiogram
ECT	electroconvulsive therapy
ED	emergency department; erectile dysfunction
EDC	estimated date of confinement

EDD	estimated date of delivery
EDTA	edetate calcium disodium
EEG	electroencephalogram
EGD	esophagogastroduodenoscopy
EHS	Employee Health Service
e-IPV	enhanced potency inactivated poliovirus vaccine
ELISA	enzyme-linked immunosorbent assay
EMB	ethambutol
EMG	electromyogram
EMS	Emergency Medical Services
EMT	Emergency Medical Technician
ENG	electronystagmography
EP	escape (elopement) precautions
EPA	Environmental Protection Agency
EPO	erythropoietin
EPS	electrophysiology study
EPSE	extrapyramidal side effects
ERCP	endoscopic retrograde cholangiopancreatography
ERG	electroretinogram
ERT	estrogen replacement therapy
ERV	expiratory reserve volume
ESR	erythrocyte sedimentation rate
ESRD	end-stage renal disease
ESWL	extracorporeal shock wave lithotripsy
ET	enterostomal therapist
ETOH	ethanol (alcohol)
ETOH W/D	alcohol withdrawal
F	
F	Fahrenheit
FADL	functional activities of daily living
FAM	fertility awareness method
FAS	fetal alcohol syndrome
FBP	fetal biophysical profile
FBS	fasting blood sugar (fasting blood glucose)
FDA	Food and Drug Administration
Fe^{++}	iron
FES	functional electrical stimulation
FFP	fresh-frozen plasma

FHC	family health center
FHR	fetal heart rate
FHT	fetal heart tones
FPG	fasting plasma glucose
FQHC	Federally Qualified Healthcare
FRC	functional residual capacity
FRV	functional residue volume
FSH	follicle-stimulating hormone
FTT	failure to thrive
5-FU	5-fluorouracil
FVD	fluid volume deficit
FVE	fluid volume excess
G	
G	gauge
GABHS	group A beta-hemolytic streptococcus
GCS	Glasgow Coma Scale
GDM	gestational diabetes mellitus
GERD	gastroesophageal reflux disease
GERI	geriatrics
GFR	glomerular filtration rate
GH	growth hormone
GHIH	growth hormone–inhibiting hormone
GI	gastrointestinal
GI tract	gastrointestinal tract
GnRH	gonadotropin-releasing hormone
G_6PD	glucose 6-phosphodehydrogenase
GRH, GHRH	growth hormone–releasing hormone
GTT	glucose tolerance test
G-Tube	gastrostomy (tube)
GU	genitourinary
GYN	gynecology
H	
H^+	hydrogen ion
H flu	*Haemophilus influenzae*
H_2CO_3	carbonic acid
H_2O, HOH	water

HAS	Health Services Administration
HAV	hepatitis A virus
HAZMAT	hazardous materials
Hb A$_{1c}$	glycosylated hemoglobin
HBD	hydroxybutyric dehydrogenase
HBO	hyperbaric oxygenation
HBV	hepatitis B virus
HCA	Health Care Assistant
HCFA	Health Care Financing Association (payor source)
HCG	human chorionic gonadotropin
HCl	hydrochloric acid
HCO$_3$$^-$	bicarbonate
Hct	hematocrit
HCTZ	hydrochlorothiazide
HCV	hepatitis C virus
HD	Hodgkin's disease; Huntington's disease
HDL	high-density lipoprotein
HDV	hepatitis D virus
HEV	hepatitis E virus
HFCS	high-fructose corn syrup
Hgb; Hb	hemoglobin
HGF	hematopoietic factor
HGV	hepatitis G virus
HHA	Home Health Aide
HHRG	Home Health Resource Group
HHS	Department of Health and Human Services
HI	homicidal ideation
Hib	*Haemophilus influenzae* type B conjugate vaccine
HICPAC	Hospital Infection Control Practices Advisory Committee
HIS	Indian Health Service
HIV	human immunodeficiency virus
HIV-RNA	viral load of HIV
HMO	health maintenance organization
HNP	herniated nucleus pulposus
HOSA	Health Occupations Students of America
hPL	human placental lactogen
HPO$_4$$^-$, H$_2PO_4$$^-$	phosphate

HPV	human papillomavirus
HR	heart rate
HRT	hormone replacement therapy
HS	hour of sleep
HSV-1	herpes simplex virus type 1
HSV-2	herpes simplex virus type 2
HTN	hypertension
HUS	hemolytic uremic syndrome
I	
IADL	instrumental activities of daily living
IBD	inflammatory bowel disease
IBS	irritable bowel syndrome
IBW	ideal body weight
IC	interstitial cystitis; inspiratory capacity
ICD	implantable cardioverter-defibrillator
ICF	intermediate care facility
ICN	International Council of Nurses
ICP	intracranial pressure
↑ICP	increased intracranial pressure
ICSH	interstitial cell-stimulating hormone
ICU	intensive care unit
ID	identification
IDDM	insulin-dependent diabetes mellitus
IDG	interdisciplinary group
IDT	interdisciplinary team
IFG	impaired fasting glucose
IFN	interferon
IG	immune globulins
Ig	immunoglobulin
IgE	immunoglobulin E
IgG	gamma immunoglobulin (gamma globulin)
IGH	impaired glucose homeostasis
IGT	impaired glucose tolerance
II	intellectual impairment
IICP	increased intracranial pressure
IL	interleukin
InFeD	iron dextran
INH	isoniazid

I & O	intake and output
IOL	intraocular lens
IOL implant	intraocular lens implant
IOP	intraocular pressure
IPPB	intermittent positive-pressure breathing
IQ	intelligence quotient
IR	infrared (rays)
IRV	inspiratory reserve volume
ITP	idiopathic thrombocytopenic purpura
IUD	intrauterine device
IV	intravenous
IVC	inferior vena cava
IVD	intervertebral disk disease
IVF	in vitro fertilization
IVIG	intravenous immune globulin
IVP	intravenous pyelogram
IVPB	intravenous piggyback

J	
J tube	jejunostomy tube
JCAHO	Joint Commission on Accreditation of Healthcare Organizations
JGA, JG apparatus	juxtaglomerular apparatus
JP	Jackson Pratt (drains)
JRA	juvenile rheumatoid arthritis

K	
K^+	potassium
Kcal; C	kilocalorie
KCl	potassium chloride
KOH	potassium hydroxide
KUB	kidney-ureters-bladder x-ray

L	
L1, L2, etc.	level of lumbar area of the spinal cord
LAD	left anterior descending
LASIK	laser-assisted in situ keratomileusis

LATCH	L = latch; A = audible swallowing; T = type of nipple; C = comfort (breast/nipple); H = hold (positioning)
LBW	low birthweight
LCA	left coronary artery
LCX	left circumflex
LDH	lactic dehydrogenase
LDL	low-density lipoprotein
LDRP	labor/delivery/recovery/postpartum room
LEEP	loop electrosurgical excision procedure
LEP	laparoscopic extraperitoneal approach
LES	lower esophageal sphincter
LFT	liver function tests
LGA	large for gestational age
LH	luteinizing hormone
LLQ	left lower quadrant
LMCA	left main coronary artery
LMP	last menstrual period
LNMP	last normal menstrual period
LOC	level of consciousness
LP	lumbar puncture
LPM, L/min	liters per minute
LPN/LVN	Licensed Practical Nurse/Licensed Vocational Nurse
LQR/LSR	locked quiet room, locked seclusion room
LS ratio	lecithin-sphingomyelin ratio
LSD	lysergic acid diethylamide
LT	leukotriene
LTB	laryngotracheobronchitis
LTC	long-term care
LUQ	left upper quadrant

M

MABP	mean arterial blood pressure
MAC	*Mycobacterium avium* complex
MAP	mean arterial pressure
MAR	Medication Administration Record
MAST	military antishock trousers

MCHB	Maternal Child Health Bureau
MD	muscular dystrophy
MDD	major depressive disorder
MDI	metered-dose inhaler
MDS	Minimum Data Set
mEq	milliequivalents
mEq/L	milliequivalents per liter
Mg; Mg^{++}	magnesium
MG	myasthenia gravis
mg/dL	milligrams per deciliter
MgSO$_4$	magnesium sulfate
MH, MHU	Mental Health Unit
MI & D	mentally ill and dangerous
MI	mental illness; myocardial infarction
MI-CD	mentally ill and chemically dependent
MICU	medical intensive care unit
MIF	melanocyte-inhibiting factor
MIS	Management Information Services/Systems
mL	milliliters
MMI	methimazole
MMPI	Minnesota Multiphasic Personality Inventory
MMR	measles, mumps, and rubella
MOM	milk of magnesia
MPD	multiple personality disorder
MRI	magnetic resonance imaging
MRSA	methicillin-resistant *Staphylococcus aureus*
MS	morphine sulfate; multiple sclerosis
MSAFP;	
** MS-AFP**	maternal serum alpha-fetoprotein test
MSDS	Material Safety Data Sheet
MSH	melanocyte-stimulating hormone
MSW	Medical Social Worker
MUA	medically underserved area
MVA	motor vehicle accident
N	
Na$^+$	sodium
NACHC	National Association of Community Health Centers

NaCl	sodium chloride
NAHC	National Association for Home Care
NAHCC	National Association of Health Care Centers
NANDA	North American Nursing Diagnosis Association
NaOH	sodium hydroxide
NAPNES	National Association of Practical Nurse Education and Services
Na_2SO_4	sodium sulfate
NCHS	National Center for Health Statistics
NCI	National Cancer Institute
NCLEX	National Council Licensure Examination
NCLEX-PN	National Council Licensure Examination for Practical Nurses
NCLEX-RN	National Council Licensure Examination for Registered Nurses
NCP	nursing care plan
NCSBN	National Council of State Boards of Nursing
NEC	necrotizing enterocolitis
NEURO	neurology
NF	National Formulary
NFLPN	National Federation of Licensed Practical Nurses
NG	nasogastric
NG tube	nasogastric tube
NHIC	National Health Information Center
NHL	non-Hodgkin's lymphoma
NHO	National Hospice Organization
NHP	nursing home placement
NHPCO	National Hospice and Palliative Care Organization
NICU	neonatal intensive care unit
NIDDM	non-insulin-dependent diabetes mellitus
NIH	National Institute of Health
NINR	National Institute of Nursing Research
NIOSH	National Institute of Occupational Safety and Health
NLN	National League for Nursing
NMR	nuclear magnetic resonance
NMS	neuroleptic malignant syndrome
NOS	not otherwise specified

NP	nurse practitioner
NPO	nothing by mouth
NPT	nocturnal penile tumescence
NRM	non-rebreathing mask
NS	normal saline or 0.9% sodium chloride
NSAID	nonsteroidal anti-inflammatory drug
NSC	National Safety Council
NST	nonstress test
NTG	nitroglycerine
O	
O_2	oxygen
OA	osteoarthritis
OASIS	Outcome and Assessment Information Set
OB	obstetrics
OB/GYN	obstetrician/gynecologist
OBRA	Omnibus Budget Reconciliation Act
OBS/OBD	organic brain syndrome/organic brain disorder
OBT	over-bed table
OCD	obsessive-compulsive disorder
OCT	oxytocin challenge test
OD	overdose; right eye (oculus dexter)
OFC	occipital-frontal circumference
OH^-	hydroxyl ion
OMH	Office for Migrant Health
ONS	Oncology Nursing Society
OOB	out of bed
OP	occiput posterior
O & P	ova (eggs) and parasites
OPD	outpatient department
OPHS	Office of Public Health and Science
OPV	(live) oral poliovirus vaccine
OR	operating room
ORIF	open reduction and internal fixation
ORS	oral rehydration solution
ORTHO	orthopedics
OS	left eye (oculus sinister)
O_2Sat	percent oxygen saturation

OSHA	Occupational Safety and Health Administration
OT	occupational therapy
OTC	over the counter
OTR	Occupational Therapist, Registered
OU	both eyes (oculi unitas)
P	
P	phosphorus
PA	Physician Assistant
PACE	Pre-Admission and Classification Examination
$PaCO_2$; pCO_2	carbon dioxide content of arterial blood
PACU	postanesthesia care unit
PaO_2; pO_2	oxygen content of arterial blood
Pap test	Papanicolaou test (smear)
PAR	postanesthesia recovery (room)
PBI	protein-bound iodine
PBSC	peripheral blood stem cell
PCA	patient-controlled analgesia; personal care attendant
PCM	protein-calorie malnutrition
PCN	penicillin
PCP	*Pneumocystis carinii* pneumonia; primary care provider
PCT	proximal convoluted tubule
PDA	patent ductus arteriosus; posterior descending artery
PDR	Physician's Desk Reference
PE	polyethylene (tube)
PEDS	pediatrics
PEG	percutaneous endoscopic gastrostomy
PEP	postexposure prophylaxis
PERRLA + C	pupils equal, round, react to light, accommodation OK and coordinated
PET	position emission tomography scan
PFT	pulmonary function test
pH	potential of hydrogen; power of hydrogen (hydrogen ion concentration)

PIA	prolonged infantile apnea
PIC	peripheral indwelling catheter
PICC	peripherally inserted central catheter
PICU	pediatric intensive care unit
PID	pelvic inflammatory disease
PIE	plan, intervention, evaluation
PIH	pregnancy-induced hypertension; prolactin-inhibiting hormone
PKU	phenylketonuria
PM&R	physical medicine and rehabilitation
PMI	point of maximal impulse
PMP	previous menstrual period
PMS	premenstrual syndrome
PNS	peripheral nervous system
PO	by mouth (per os)
POC	plan of care
POS	point of service
PPD	purified protein derivative
PPE	personal protective equipment
PPF	plasma protein fraction
PPG	postprandial glucose
PPIP	Put Prevention Into Practice
2hPP	2-hour postprandial
PPN	peripheral parenteral nutrition
PPO	preferred provider organization
PPROM	prolonged premature rupture of membranes
PPS	prospective payment system
PRH	prolactin-releasing hormone
PRK	photorefractive keratotomy
PRL	prolactin
PRM	partial-rebreathing mask
PRN	as needed
PROM	passive range of motion; premature rupture of membranes
PR/R	per rectum/rectal
PSA	prostate-specific antigen
PSDA	Patient Self-Determination Act
psi	per square inch
PSV	pressure support ventilation

PSYCH	psychiatry
PT	prothrombin time; physical therapy
PTA	Physical Therapist Assistant
PTCA	percutaneous transluminal coronary angioplasty
PTH	parathyroid hormone, parathormone
PTL	preterm labor
PTSD	posttraumatic stress disorder
PTT	partial thromboplastin time
PTU	propylthiouracil
PUBS	percutaneous umbilical blood sampling
PUS	prostate ultrasound
PVC	premature ventricular contraction
PZA	pyrazinamide

Q	
QA	quality assurance
QI	quality improvement

R	
RA	rheumatoid arthritis
RAA system	renin-angiotensin-aldosterone system
RACE	rescue, alarm, confine, extinguish
RAI	radioactive iodine
RAIU	radioactive iodine uptake
RAP	resident assessment protocol
RBC	red blood cell
RCA	right coronary artery
RDA	recommended dietary allowance
RDS	respiratory distress syndrome
REE	resting energy expenditure
REHAB	rehabilitation unit
REM	rapid eye movement
RF	rheumatoid factor
RGP	rigid gas-permeable plastic
Rh^+	Rh positive
Rh^-	Rh negative
RhoGAM	Rh immune globulin

RICE	rest, ice, compression, elevation
RIE	recorded in error
RIND	reversible ischemic neurologic deficit
RK	radial keratotomy
RLQ	right lower quadrant
RMP	rifampin
RN	registered nurse
RNA	ribonucleic acid
ROI	release of information
ROM	range of motion
ROP	retinopathy of prematurity; right occiput posterior
RP	retinitis pigmentosa
RPh	registered pharmacist
RPT	registered physical therapist
RR	recovery room
RRA	registered record administrator
RSV	respiratory syncytial virus
RT	respiratory therapy
R/T	related to
RUG	resource utilization group
RUQ	right upper quadrant
RV	residual volume
S	
S1	first heart sound
S2	second heart sound
S/A	suicide attempt
SA node	sinoatrial node; sinus node
SBE	subacute bacterial endocarditis
SBFT	small bowel follow-through x-ray
SBP; sBP	systolic blood pressure
SDSU	Same-Day Surgery Unit
S/G	suicide gesture
SGA	small for gestational age
SGOT	serum glutamic oxaloacetic transaminase
SI	suicidal ideation
SI units	International system of units (or Systeme International d'Unites)

SIADH	syndrome of inappropriate antidiuretic hormone
SIB	self-injurious behavior
SICU	surgical intensive care unit
SIDS	sudden infant death syndrome
SIE	stroke in evolution
SIMV	synchronized intermittent mandatory ventilation
SIRES	stabilize, identify toxin, reverse effect, eliminate toxin, support
SL	sublingual
SLD	specific learning disabilities
SLE	systemic lupus erythematosus
S/M	sadomasochism
SMBG	self-monitoring of blood glucose
SNF	skilled nursing facility
SNS	sympathetic nervous system
SO	significant other
SO$_4^-$	sulfate
SOAP	subjective, objective, assessment, plan
SOAPIER	subjective, objective, assessment, plan, intervention, evaluation, response
SOB	short of breath
SOBOE	short of breath on exertion
SP	suprapubic (catheter)
SP/GP	suicide precautions/general precautions
SPF	sun protective factor
SRO	single room occupancy
SROM	spontaneous rupture of the membranes
SSA	Social Security Administration
SSDI	Social Security Disability Insurance
SSE	soap suds enema
START	Simple Triage and Rapid Treatment
STAT	at once, immediately
STD	sexually transmitted disease
STH	somatotropic hormone (somatotropin)
STI	sexually transmitted infection
SV	stroke volume
SVC	superior vena cava
SVE	sterile vaginal examination
SVR	systemic vascular resistance

SX P	sexual precautions
SZ P	seizure precautions

T

T1, T2, etc.	level of injury in the thoracic area of the spinal cord
T3	triiodothyronine
T4	thyroxine
T&A	tonsillectomy and adenoidectomy
TAC	time, amount, character
TB	tuberculosis
TBI	traumatic brain injury
TBW	total body water
TCDB	turning, coughing, deep breathing
TCN	tetracycline
TD	tardive dyskinesia
TED	thromboembolic disease
TEE	transesophageal echocardiography
TENS	transcutaneous electrical nerve stimulation
TFT	thyroid function test
TGV	transposition of the great vessels
THA	total hip arthroplasty
THC	cannabis (marijuana and related drugs)
T-hold	transportation hold (police)
TIA	transient ischemic attack
TICU	trauma intensive care unit
Title XVIII	Medicare section of the Social Security Act
Title XIX	Medicaid section of the Social Security Act
Title XXII	source of COPs
TKA	total knee arthroplasty
TLC	total lung capacity
TLSO	thoracolumbar sacroorthosis
Tm	transport maximum
TMJ	temporal mandibular joint
TMR	transmyocardial revascularization
TO	telephone order
TOF	tetralogy of Fallot
TORCH	toxoplasmosis, other, rubella, cytomegalovirus, herpes simplex

t-PA	tissue plasminogen activator
TPA	total parenteral alimentation
TPN	total parenteral nutrition
TPR	temperature, pulse, and respiration
TR	therapeutic recreation
TS	Tourette syndrome
TSE	testicular self-examination
TSH	thyroid-stimulating hormone
TSLO	thoracic-lumbar-sacral orthosis
TSS	toxic shock syndrome
TURBT	transurethral resection of bladder tumor
TURP	transurethral resection of prostate
TV	tidal volume
TWE	tap water enema
T&X	type and crossmatch

U	
U-100	100 units per milliliter
UA	urinalysis
UAP	unlicensed assistive personnel
UL	tolerance upper intake level
UN	United Nations
UNICEF	United Nations Children's Fund
UNOS	United Network of Organ Sharing
UPP	urethral pressure profile
UPT	urine pregnancy test
URI	upper respiratory infection
UROL	urology
US	ultrasound
USD	U.S. Dispensatory
USDA	U.S. Department of Agriculture
USDHHS	U.S. Department of Health and Human Services
USP	U.S. Pharmacopoeia
USPHS	U.S. Public Health Service
UTI	urinary tract infection
UTox	urine toxicity screen (for drugs)
UV	ultraviolet (rays)

V	
VC	vital capacity
VCUG	voiding cystourethrogram
VLBW	very low birthweight
VMA	vanillylmandelic acid
VNA	Visiting Nurse Association
VO	verbal order
Vol	voluntarily admitted
VRE	vancomycin-resistant enterococci
V & S; vol. and spec.	volume and specific gravity (urine)
VSD	ventricular septal defect
W	
WA	while awake
WBC	white blood cell
W/C	wheelchair
WHO	World Health Organization
WIC	Women, Infants and Children
WISC-R	Weschler Intelligence Scale for Children—Revised
WNL	within normal limits

Index

Abdominal pain
  in hepatitis B, 440
  in Hodgkin's disease, 448
  in pheochromocytoma, 657
ABG analysis. *See* Arterial blood
    gas (ABG) analysis
Absolute neutrophil count
    (ANC), 498
Acetone breath, in diabetic
    ketoacidosis, 313
Acoustic neuroma, 110
Acquired immunodeficiency
    syndrome (AIDS), 1–18
  activity tolerance, 14–15
  alternative therapies, 7–8, 10
  assessment, 8–10
  assessment/diagnostic
    methods, 5
  clinical manifestations
    cancers, 4–5
    gastrointestinal, 2–3
    hematologic/lymphatic, 4
    integumentary, 4
    neurologic, 3
    reproductive (female), 4
    respiratory, 2
  cognitive management, 15
  diagnosis, 10–11
  and diarrhea, 316
  expected outcomes, 17–18
  fluid/electrolyte management, 9
  grief management, 15
  home/community-based care,
    16–17
  infection prevention, 13
  and Kaposi's sarcoma, 4, 494
  medical management, 5–8
  and meningitis, 525
  neurologic status, 9
  nursing interventions, 11–18
  nutrition management, 8, 14
  pain prevention, 14

  patient education, 10
  pharmacologic therapy, 6–7
  planning/goals, 11
  respiratory management, 9
  risk factors, 1–2
  self-care, 16–17
  skin/mucous membranes in, 9
  social management, 15
  supportive care, 7–8
  treatment decision factors, 5
Acral-lentiginous melanomas,
    220–221
Acromegaly, 660, 661
ACTH. *See* Adrenocorticotropic
    hormone (ACTH)
Activity tolerance
  in Addison's disease, 24
  in AIDS, 14–15
  in Alzheimer's disease, 29–30
  in burn injuries, 133
  in cardiomyopathies, 243
  in cerebral vascular accidents,
    255
  in COPD, 271
  for Cushing's syndrome, 290
  in heart failure, 425
  in hepatic cirrhosis, 276
  in hypothyroidism, 478, 479
  in myxedema, 479
  in pneumonia, 669
  in pulmonary tuberculosis,
    762
  in ulcerative colitis, 770
Acupuncture, for morbid obesity,
    565
Acute bacterial prostatitis, 676
Acute chest syndrome, 49–50, 52
Acute gastritis, 377–378
Acute lymphocytic leukemia
    (ALL), 504–505
Acute myeloid leukemia (AML),
    507–509

Acute respiratory distress
    syndrome (ARDS), 18–20
  assessment, 18–19
  clinical manifestations, 18
  diagnosis, 18–19
  in DIC, 323
  and diffuse, axonal injuries,
    416
  fluid balance management, 19
  medical management, 19
  nutrition management, 19
ADC. *See* AIDS dementia
    complex
Addison's disease, 21–25
  activity tolerance, 24
  Addisonian crisis, 21–22, 24
  assessment, 22, 23
  clinical manifestations, 21–22
  complications management, 24
  continuing care, 25
  diagnosis, 22, 23
  fluid balance management,
    23–24
  home/community-based care,
    25
  medical management, 22
  monitoring/management, 24
  planning/goals, 23
  self-care, 25
Adenocarcinoma
  kidneys, 185
  lungs, 200
  papillary, 233
  serous, of ovaries, 208–209
Adrenal insufficiency, 21
Adrenocorticotropic hormone
    (ACTH), 21
  and Cushing's disease, 286
African Americans, and
    glaucoma, 382
AIDS dementia complex (ADC), 3
Airway management
  in asthma, 86
  in cerebral vascular accidents,
    251
  in clinical unit, postoperative,
    635

  in COPD, 267, 270–271
  in diffuse, axonal injuries, 414,
    416, 418
  in epilepsy, 345
  in Guillain-Barré syndrome,
    397
  in hypothyroidism/myxedema,
    479
  in increased intracranial
    pressure, 489, 490
  in larynx cancer, 191–192
  in lung cancer, 202
  by nurse, in PACU, 632
  in peritonitis, 652
  in pneumonia, 668, 669
  in pulmonary tuberculosis,
    762
  in unconsciousness, 776
Alcohol dependence
  and chronic pancreatitis, 592
  and chronic pharyngitis, 655
  and epilepsy, 343
  and hepatic cirrhosis, 275
  and low back pain, 90
  and peptic ulcers, 610
Alcoholics Anonymous, 278
Alcohol-induced anemia, 47
Alkalosis, in bleeding esophageal
    varices, 354
ALL. *See* Acute lymphocytic
    leukemia (ALL)
Allergies, and asthma, 84
Alopecia, in cancer, 143
ALS. *See* Amyotrophic lateral
    sclerosis (ALS)
Alternative therapies
  for AIDS, 7–8, 10
  for morbid obesity, 565
  for sickle cell anemia, 52
Alzheimer's disease, 26–30
  activity/rest balancing, 29
  anxiety/agitation reduction, 29
  assessment, 27–28
    blood/CSF lab tests, 27
    EEG/MRI/CT scan, 27
    Mini-Mental Status
      Examination, 27

clinical manifestations, 26–27
cognitive function support, 28
diagnosis, 27, 28
home/community-based care, 30
medical management, 27
nutrition management, 29
outcomes expectations, 30
physical safety promotion, 28–29
planning/goals, 28
self-care promotion, 30
socialization needs promotion, 30
Amenorrhea
and hyperthyroidism, 462
and hypopituitarism, 474
and hypothyroidism, 476
and pituitary tumors, 660
American Cancer Society, 143
AML. *See* Acute myeloid leukemia (AML)
Amyotrophic lateral sclerosis (ALS), 31–33
assessment, 32
clinical manifestations, 31–32
diagnosis, 32
mechanical ventilation, 32
supportive/rehabilitative measures, 32
Anaphylaxis, 33–35
assessment, 34
clinical manifestations
mild, 33–34
moderate, 34
severe, 34
diagnosis, 34
medical management, 34–35
pharmacologic therapy, 35
prevention, 34
Type I hypersensitivity, 33
ANC. *See* Absolute neutrophil count (ANC)
Anemia, 35–40
and acute lymphocytic leukemia, 505

alcohol-induced, 47
assessment, 36–38
clinical manifestations, 36
collaborative problems, 38
community-based care, 40
complications, 38
diagnosis, 36–38
fatigue management, 39
gerontologic considerations, 37
and hepatic cirrhosis, 274
and Hodgkin's disease, 448
home/community-based care, 40
medical management, 37
normochromic/normocytic, in multiple myeloma, 533
nutrition management, 38, 39
outcome expectations, 40
perfusion management, 39
planning/goals, 38
Anemia, aplastic, 40–42
assessment/diagnosis, 41
causative factors, 40
clinical manifestations, 41
home/community-based care, 42
medical management, 41
nursing management, 41–42
prevention, 41
supportive therapy, 41
Anemia, iron-deficiency, 42–45
assessment, 43
clinical manifestations, 43
diagnosis, 43
medical management, 43–44
nursing management, 44–45
Anemia, megaloblastic, 45–48
assessment/diagnosis, 46
clinical manifestations, 46
medical management, 46
nursing management, 47–48
nutrition management
folic acid, 47
Vitamin B12, 46
pathophysiology, 45
Schilling test, 47

Anemia, sickle cell, 48–54
  assessment, 49, 50–51
  causation, 48
  clinical manifestations, 48–49
  collaborative problems, 51
  complications, 51
  diagnosis, 49, 51
  fluid balance management, 50
  home/community-based care,
    53
  infection management, 51, 52
  medical management, 49–50
  nursing interventions, 51–52
  outcome expectations, 54
  pain management, 50, 53
  pathophysiology, 48
  physical therapy, 50, 52
  planning/goals, 51
Aneurysms
  aortic, 54–57
  dissecting, in
    pheochromocytoma, 657
  mycotic, and infectious
    endocarditis, 337
  rebleeding, 60, 62
  rupture of, and ischemic
    strokes, 248
Anger management, and peptic
    ulcers, 611
Angina pectoris, 63–68
  and anemia, 38
  and arteriosclerosis, 76
  assessment, 64, 65
  and atherosclerosis, 76
  clinical manifestations, 63–64
  collaborative problems/
    complications, 66
  and coronary
    atherosclerosis/artery
    disease, 284
  diagnosis, 64, 66
  factors affecting, 63
  gerontologic considerations, 64
  medical management, 64–65
  nursing interventions, 66–67
  outcome expectations, 68
  pain management, 66–67

    pharmacologic therapy, 65
    planning/goals, 66
    self-care, 67
    surgical management, 65
    triggers of, 67
Angiograms
  for angina pectoris, 64
  for aortic aneurysm, 56
  for bleeding esophageal
    varices, 352
  cerebral
    for brain injury, 409
    for increased intracranial
      pressure, 487
    for migraine headaches, 403
  for pancreatic cancer, 211
  for renal tumors, 186
Angiomas, 110
Angle closure glaucoma, 382, 384
Angular cheilosis, in anemia, 36
Anorexia
  in Addison's disease, 21
  in AIDS, 3
  in diabetic ketoacidosis, 313
  in diarrhea, 316, 317
  in empyema, 334
  in fulminant hepatic failure,
    437
  in hepatitis A, 438
  and hyperthyroidism, 463
  in migraine headaches, 402
  in myocarditis, 561
  in pelvic infection, 601
  in pneumonia, 666
  in pulmonary emphysema, 333
  and radiation therapy, 449
Anticoagulation therapy, 691,
    693–694, 754
Antimicrobial therapy
  for bronchiectasis, 115
  for chronic bronchitis, 116
Antiretroviral therapy (ART), for
    AIDS, 6
Anxiety
  in brain injuries, 408
  in cardiac tamponade, 616
  in heart failure, 422, 424

in hypoparathyroidism, 472
in leukemia, 502
in mastoiditis, 518
in Ménière's disease, 523
in mitral valve prolapse, 532
in pheochromocytoma, 657
and pneumothorax, 671
Anxiety management
in acute respiratory distress
syndrome, 20
in Alzheimer's disease, 29
in angina pectoris, 67
in appendicitis, 72
in asthma, 86
in bone tumors, 102–103
in burn injuries, 121, 130
in cancer
of cervix, 170
of larynx, 191
of prostate, 217
of stomach, 228
of vulva, 237
in cardiomyopathies, 244
in constipation, 281
in diabetes mellitus, 306
in diarrhea, 319, 320
in DIC, 324
in gastritis, 379, 380
in heart failure, 427
in Huntington's disease, 452
in intracranial aneurysm, 61
in Ménière's disease, 524
in myocardial infarction, 558,
559
in pemphigus, 606
in peptic ulcer, 612, 613
perioperative nursing, 623
in pulmonary edema, 694
in skin cancer, 224
in toxic epidermal necrolysis,
752–753
in ulcerative colitis, 771
Aortic aneurysm, 54–57
and arteriosclerosis, 76
assessment, 56
and atherosclerosis, 76
clinical manifestations

abdominal aortic aneurysm,
55
dissecting aneurysm, 55–56
thoracic aortic aneurysm, 55
diagnosis, 56
nursing management, 57
surgical management, 56
Aortic insufficiency
(regurgitation), 68–69
assessment/diagnosis, 69
clinical manifestations, 68
medical management, 69
nursing management, 69
Aortic stenosis, 69–70
assessment/diagnosis, 70
clinical manifestations, 70
medical management, 70
Aphasia, and diffuse, axonal
injuries, 414
Aplastic anemia. See Anemia,
aplastic
Appendicitis, 71–73
assessment, 71–72
clinical manifestations, 71
complications, 72
diagnosis, 71–72
gerontologic considerations, 72
home/community-based care,
73
McBurney's point/Rovsing's
sign, 71
medical management, 72
nursing management, 72–73
and peritonitis, 651
self-care, 73
ARDS. See Acute respiratory
distress syndrome (ARDS)
ART. See Antiretroviral therapy
(ART)
Arterial blood gas (ABG) analysis
for asthma, 85
for chronic obstructive
pulmonary disease, 270,
272
for hepatic cirrhosis, 275
for hyperthyroidism, 467
for hypothyroidism, 477

Arterial embolism, 73–75
assessment/diagnosis, 74
clinical manifestations, 74
medical management, 74–75
nursing management, 75
Arterial hypoxemia, 18
Arterial thrombosis, 73–75
assessment/diagnosis, 74
clinical manifestations, 74
medical management, 74–75
nursing management, 75
Arteriography
for arterial embolism/
thrombosis, 74
for arteriosclerosis/
atherosclerosis, 77
for bone tumors, 100
for liver cancer, 196
renal, for hypertension, 457
Arteriosclerosis, 75–77, 285
clinical manifestations, 76
management, 76–77
risk factors, 76
Arteriovenous malformations
(AVMs), 248
Arthritis. *See* Rheumatoid
arthritis (RA)
Arthrocentesis, for rheumatoid
arthritis, 78
Asthma, 84–87
airway clearance management,
86
anxiety management, 86
assessment, 85, 86
and chronic obstructive
pulmonary disorder, 267
clinical manifestations, 84–85
continuing care, 87
diagnosis, 85, 86
home/community-based care,
87
medical management, 85
nursing interventions, 86–87
outcome expectations, 89
pharmacologic therapy, 85
planning/goals, 86
self-care, 87

Asthma: status asthmaticus
airway clearance management,
89
assessment/diagnosis, 88
clinical manifestations, 88
fluid balance management, 89
home/community-based care,
89
medical management, 88–89
nursing interventions, 88–89
self-care in, 89
Ataxia, and anemia, 39
Atelectasis
in chronic obstructive
pulmonary disorder, 267
in morbid obesity, 565
in pneumonia, 668, 669
Atherectomy
for angina pectoris, 65
for arteriosclerosis, 77
for atherosclerosis, 77
Atherosclerosis, 75–77
clinical manifestations, 76
management, 76–77
risk factors, 76
Atrial fibrillation, and mitral
stenosis, 531
Aura
in epilepsy, 344
in migraine headaches, 402
Auscultation, of chest
for emphysema, 335
for hiatal hernia, 445
AVMs. *See* Arteriovenous
malformations (AVMs)
Axial (sliding) hiatal hernia.
See Hiatal hernia
Azotemia, in acute
glomerulonephritis, 386

Back pain, in multiple myeloma,
533
Bacteremia, and pharyngitis, 653
Bacterial meningitis, 525, 526
Bacteriuria
and cystitis, 292
and epididymitis, 331

Balance difficulties
  in mastoiditis, 517
  in multiple sclerosis, 535
Barium swallow
  for bleeding esophageal
      varices, 352
  for hiatal hernia, 444
Battle's sign, 408
B-cell lymphomas, 4, 5
Bell's palsy, 94–96
  complications, 95
  medical management, 94–95
  nursing management, 95–96
  self-care, 95
Benign bone tumors, 98–99
Benign prostatic hyperplasia
      (BPH), 96–98
  clinical manifestations, 96–97
  medical management, 97–98
  nursing management, 98
  surgical management, 97–98
Biliary drainage, in cholecystitis,
      265–266
Biologic response modifier (BRM)
      therapy
  for cancer, 139
  nursing management of,
      155–156
Biologic therapy, 186
Biopsy
  bone, for osteomalacia, 570
  bone marrow, in multiple
      myeloma, 533
  for brain tumors, 112
  for cancer, 137
    of bladder, 157
    of cervix, 168
    of endometrium, 179
    of liver, 196
  endomyocardial
    for cardiomyopathies, 241
    for myocarditis, 561
  kidney
    for glomerulonephritis, 387
    for nephrotic syndrome, 562
  lymph node, for Hodgkin's
      disease, 449

  muscles, in muscular
      dystrophies, 542
  for pemphigus, 604
  for peptic ulcers, 609
  pleural
    for pleural effusion, 662
    for pleurisy, 664
  TNM classification, for larynx
      cancer, 188
  of tumor/mucosa, in bladder
      cancer, 157
Bladder control management
  in cerebral vascular accidents,
      257
  in multiple sclerosis, 537–538,
      540
Bladder disorders
  from cancer, 156–159
  from ischemic stroke, 250
Bleeding
  in cancer, 139–140, 148
  of cervix, 168
  in cerebral vascular accidents,
      252
  in cholecystitis, 265
  in DIC, 321
  in diverticular disorders, 329
  of esophageal varices, 351–355
  gastrointestinal
    in anemia, 36
    in colorectal cancer, 175
    in hepatic cirrhosis, 275
  in hemophilia, 430, 432
  in hepatic cirrhosis, 276
  in idiopathic
      thrombocytopenia
      purpura, 483.484
  in leukemia, 498, 499–500,
      507
  in morbid obesity, 565
  in musculoskeletal trauma,
      545, 546
  in peptic ulcers, 609
  in polycythemia, 674
  in thrombocytopenia, 743
  uterine, and endometriosis,
      341

Blindness, and glaucoma, 382
Blood glucose, in diabetes
  mellitus, 309
Blood pressure. *See also*
  Hypertension;
  Hypotension
  elevated, in
    pheochromocytoma, 657
  falling, in cardiac tamponade,
    616
Blood tests
  for Alzheimer's disease, 27
  for anaphylaxis, 34
  for glomerulonephritis, 390
  for HHNS, 453
  for Hodgkin's disease, 449
  for migraine headaches, 403
  for osteomyelitis, 573
  for regional enteritis, 706
Blood transfusions
  for bleeding esophageal
    varices, 353, 354
  for sickle cell anemia, 49
Blue-toe syndrome, 55
BMI. *See* Body mass index (BMI)
Body image management
  in cancer, 141, 145–146
    of cervix, 170
    colorectal, 177–178
  in Cushing's syndrome, 290
  in leukemia, 502
Body mass index (BMI), 564
Body temperature management
  in burn injury, 124
  in clinical unit, postoperative,
    636–637
  in diffuse axonal injuries, 417
  in exfoliative dermatitis, 356
  in hyperthyroidism, 462, 466
  in hypothyroidism, 476
  in hypothyroidism/myxedema,
    478, 479
Bone cysts, 98
Bone marrow transplantation
  for acute myeloid leukemia,
    509
  for anemia, aplastic, 41

  for anemia, sickle cell, 49
  nursing management, 154–155
  for ovarian cancer, 210
Bone scans
  for bone tumors, 100
  for osteomyelitis, 573
Bone tumors, 98–104. *See also*
  Osteomyelitis
  assessment, 100, 101
  benign, 99
  clinical manifestations, 99–100
  collaborative
    problems/complications,
    101
  community-based care, 104
  diagnosis, 100, 101
  home care, 104
  malignant, 98–99
    chondrosarcoma, 98
    osteogenic sarcoma, 98
  medical management,
    100–104
  nursing interventions,
    102–104
  nutrition management, 101,
    103
  pain management, 102
  patient education, 102
  planning/goals, 101–102
  problem prevention, 103
Borborygmus
  in constipation, 279
  in diarrhea, 316
Bowel management
  in AIDS, 13
  in appendicitis, 72
  in cerebral vascular accidents,
    257
  in diarrhea, 317
  in hyperthyroidism, 462
  in hypothyroidism, 480
  in leukemia, 500
  in multiple sclerosis, 537–538,
    540
  in osteoporosis, 580
  in Parkinson's disease, 598
  in spinal cord injury, 735

in ulcerative colitis, 769
in unconsciousness, 778
Bowel obstruction
    large, 104–106
    small, 106–107
Bowel perforation, in colorectal
        cancer, 175
BPH. *See* Benign prostatic
        hyperplasia (BPH)
Bradycardia
    and brain injuries, 409, 490
    and cardiac arrest, 239
    and glaucoma, 383
    and myocarditis, 561
Bradykinesia, in Parkinson's
        disease, 594
Brain abscess, 108–109
    in acute otitis media, 582
Brain damage
    and cardiac arrest, 240
    and intracranial pressure, 407
Brain infarctions, and Alzheimer's
        disease, 26
Brain injuries, 407–410. *See also*
        Diffuse axonal injuries
    assessment/diagnosis, 409
    clinical manifestations,
        408–409
    concussion, 409
    contusion, 410
    medical management, 409
    nursing management, 409–410
    stem herniation, in ICP, 489
Brain tumors, 109–113. *See also*
        Chromophobic tumors;
        Eosinophilic tumors
    assessment, 112
    clinical manifestations
        generalized symptoms, 111
        localized symptoms,
            111–112
    diagnosis, 112
    medical management,
        112–113
    nursing management, 112–113
    surgical management,
        112–113

types
    acoustic neuroma, 110
    angiomas, 110
    gliomas, 110
    meningiomas, 110
    metastatic, 109–110
    pituitary adenomas, 110
    primary, 109
Breast cancer
    assessment, 160, 162
        postoperative, 162
        preoperative, 162
    clinical manifestations,
        160–161
    collaborative
        problems/complications,
        163
    diagnosis, 160, 162–163
    home/community-based care,
        166–167
    infection, 163
    and lymphedema, 163
    medical management,
        161–162
    nursing interventions,
        164–166
    nursing management,
        162–163
    outcome expectations, 167
    pain management, 165
    patient education, 164
    planning/goals, 163
    prevention strategies, 160
    protective factors, 159
    risk factors, 159
    skin integrity maintenance,
        164–165
    staging of, 160–161
Breath, shortness of
    and coronary
        atherosclerosis/artery
        disease, 284
    and hypertension, 458
    and mitral regurgitation, 529
    and mitral valve prolapse,
        532
    and pleural effusion, 662

BRM therapy. *See* Biologic
    response modifier (BRM)
    therapy
Bronchiectasis, 114–115
Bronchitis, chronic, 115–117
Bronchogenic carcinoma.
    See Lung cancer
Bronchopulmonary infections, in
    COPD, 271
Bronchoscopy, in lung abscess,
    512
Bronchospasm, and
    hypoparathyroidism, 472
Brudzinski's sign, in bacterial
    meningitis, 526
Buerger's disease (thromboangiitis
    obliterans), 117–119
Buffalo hump, in Cushing's
    syndrome, 286
Bulbar muscle impairment, 32
Bullous impetigo, 485
Burn injuries, 119–135
    acute/intermediate phase
        anxiety management, 129,
            130
        assessment, 126
        collaborative problems/
            complications, 127,
            130–131
        diagnosis, 126–127
        fluid/electrolyte
            management, 127–128
        home/community-based
            care, 131
        infection prevention, 128
        medical management,
            126–132
        mobility promotion,
            129–130
        nursing interventions,
            127–132
        nutrition management, 128
        outcome expectations, 131
        pain management, 129
        planning/goals, 127
    emergent/resuscitative phase
        anxiety management, 121

        assessment, 121–122
        collaborative problems/
            complications, 125
        diagnosis, 122–123
        fluid/electrolyte
            management, 124
        medical management,
            121–125
        nursing interventions,
            123–125
        pain management, 124
        planning/goals, 123
    gerontologic considerations,
        120–121
    rehabilitation/long-term phase
        activity tolerance
            promotion, 133
        assessment, 132
        collaborative problems/
            complications, 133
        diagnosis, 133
        home/community-based
            care, 134–135
        nursing interventions,
            133–135
        planning/goals, 133
        self-care, 134–135
        self-image promotion,
            133
Bypass, coronary artery, 556

Cachexia. *See* Wasting syndrome
Calcitriol (Vitamin D), in
    osteomalacia, 569, 570
Cancer
    and AIDS, 4–5
    and alopecia, 143
    assessment, 137, 139
    bleeding management,
        139–140, 148
    body image management, 141,
        145–146
    chemotherapy, 138
    clinical manifestations,
        136–137
    collaborative problems/
        complications, 141, 147

fatigue management, 140–141, 145

fluid balance management, 143

grief management, 146–147

Hodgkin's disease, 447

home/community-based care, 148–149

and infection, 139

Kaposi's sarcoma (KS), 494–496

medical management, 138–150

nursing interventions, 142–150

nursing management

biological response modifiers, 155–156

bone marrow transplantation, 154–155

cancer surgery, 150

chemotherapy, 152–153

hyperthermia, 155

photodynamic therapy, 156

radiation therapy, 151–152

nutrition management, 140, 144

pain management, 140–141, 144–145

pathophysiology, 136

planning/goals, 142

and pruritus, 678

radiation therapy, 138

self-care, 148–149

self-esteem management, 145–146

sepsis shock management, 147–148

skin breakdown, 140

stomatitis management, 142

supportive programs, 143

tissue integrity maintenance, 142

TMN classification system, 137–138

tumors, primary/metastatic, 98

types

bladder, 156–159

breast, 137, 159–167

cervical, 168–172

colon, 156

colorectal, 137

endometrial, 179–180

esophageal, 180–185

Hodgkin's disease, 447–450

kidney, 185–187

larynx, 188–195

liver, 195–199, 442

lung, 200–202

oral cavity, 203–208

oropharyngeal, 137

ovarian, 208–210

pancreatic, 210–213

prostate, 156

rectal, in men, 156

skin, 220–226

stomach, 226–230

testicular, 137, 231–232

thyroid, 233–234

vaginal, 234–235

Candidiasis, in AIDS, 2, 7

CAP. *See* Community-acquired pneumonia (CAP)

Carcinomas

adenocarcinomas

kidneys, 185

lungs, 200

cholangiocellular (CCC), 195–196

choriocarcinomas, 231

embryonal, 231

hepatocellular (HCC), 195–196

small cell (oat cell), 200

teratocarcinomas, 231

yolk sac, 231

Cardiac arrest, 239–240, 557

Cardiac failure

in angina pectoris, 66

in sickle cell anemia, 50, 52

Cardiac rehabilitation, 559

Cardiac tamponade.
 See also Pericarditis
 in angina pectoris, 66
 clinical manifestations, 616
 in heart failure, 424
 surgical management, 617
Cardiogenic shock
 in angina pectoris, 66
 clinical manifestations, 721
 fluid balance management, 722
 in heart failure, 424
 hemodynamic monitoring, 722
 intra-aortic balloon
  counterpulsation, 722
 medical management,
  721–722
 nursing management,
  722–723
 preventive measures, 722
Cardiomegaly
 and glomerulonephritis, 386,
  389
 and sickle cell anemia, 49, 50
Cardiomyopathies, 240–245
 anxiety management, 244
 assessment, 241, 242
 classifications, 240–241
  arrhythmogenic, 241
  dilated/congested, 240–241
  hypertrophic, 241
  restrictive, 241
  unclassified, 241
 clinical manifestations, 241
 collaborative problems/
  complications, 243
 diagnosis, 241, 242–243
 home/community-based care,
  244–245
 medical management,
  241–245
 in muscular dystrophies, 542
 nursing interventions,
  243–245
 outcome expectations, 245
 pathophysiology, 241
Cardiopulmonary resuscitation
 (CPR)

for anaphylaxis, 34
for cardiac arrest, 240
Cardiovascular disorders
 and epistaxis, 350
 and morbid obesity, 564
Cast care, in musculoskeletal
 trauma, 547
Cataracts, 245–247
Catheterization
 for arterial embolism/
  thrombosis, 74
 avoidance of, in leukemia, 500
 for benign prostatic
  hyperplasia, 97
 cardiac
  for angina pectoris, 64
  for aortic insufficiency, 69
  for cardiomyopathies, 241
  for heart failure, 422
  for mitral stenosis, 531
 left heart, for aortic stenosis,
  70
 percutaneous, in lung abscess,
  512
CCC. *See* Cholangiocellular
 carcinoma (CCC)
Cecostomy, for large bowel
 obstruction, 105
Central nervous system,
 infarctions of, 321
Central venous pressure (CVP)
 elevated, in cardiac
  tamponade, 616
Centrilobular pulmonary
 emphysema, 333
Cephalgia. *See* Headaches
Cerebral embolism, 243
Cerebral hypoxia
 and CVA, 250, 251
 and heart failure, 427
Cerebral vascular accident (CVA),
 248–260
 assessment, 250, 251
 bladder control management,
  257
 bowel function management,
  257

clinical manifestations
bladder dysfunction, 250
cognitive/psychological
effects, 250
communication loss, 249
motor loss, 249
perceptual
disturbances/sensory loss,
249
cognitive management,
257–258
communication goals, 258
complications management,
251, 254
coping improvement,
258–259
deformity prevention,
254–255
depression management,
260
diagnosis, 250, 253–254
dysphagia management, 257
exercise management, 255
home/community-based care,
259–260
medical management, 251
mobility management,
254–255
nursing interventions,
254–260
outcome expectations, 260
pain management, 256
planning/goals, 254
prevention of, 250
risk factors, 248–249
self-care, 256
sensory-perceptual difficulties
management, 256–257
sexual function/dysfunction,
258
skin integrity management,
258
t-PA therapy, 251
acute phase assessment,
252–253
postacute phase assessment,
252–253

Cerebrospinal fluid (CSF)
and diffuse, axonal injuries,
416
drainage of, and brain injury,
408
electrophoresis study, in
multiple sclerosis, 536
and increased intracranial
pressure, 486
tests
for Alzheimer's disease, 27
for brain tumors, 112
for multiple sclerosis, 536
Cervical adenitis, and
pharyngitis, 653
Cervical cancer, 168–172
anxiety management, 170
assessment, 168–169
bleeding, 168
body image management,
170
clinical manifestations, 168
collaborative problems/
complications, 170, 171
diagnosis, 168–169
home/community-based care,
171–172
outcome expectations, 172
pain management, 171
self-care, 171–172
Cervical lymphadenopathy, 233
Cervical motion tenderness, in
pelvic infection, 601
CHD. *See* Coronary heart disease
(CHD)
Chemotherapy
for brain tumors, 112
for cancer, 138
of bladder, 158
of breast, 161
of esophagus, 181
of liver, 197
nursing management,
152–153
of ovaries, 210, 212
of prostate, 215
for Hodgkin's disease, 449

Chemotherapy (*Contd.*)
  for leukemia
    acute lymphocytic, 505
    acute myeloid, 508
    chronic lymphocytic,
      506
  photochemotherapy, for
    psoriasis, 684
  and pruritus, 678
  for renal tumors, 186
  for stomach cancer, 227
Chest pain
  in AIDS, 2
  in coronary
    atherosclerosis/artery
    disease, 284
  in mitral valve prolapse, 532
  in thyroid storm, 747
Chest radiograph, for
    cardiomyopathies, 241
Childhood leukemia. *See* Acute
    lymphocytic leukemia
Chills
  and exfoliative dermatitis,
    355
  and pleural effusion, 662
  and pneumonia, 666
Chlamydia trachomatis, in
    epididymitis, 331
Cholangiocellular carcinoma
    (CCC), 196
Cholecystectomy
  complications management,
    266
  home/community-based care,
    266–277
  nursing management
    assessment, 264
    collaborative problems/
      complications, 265
    diagnosis, 264–265
    planning/goals, 265
  nutrition management, 265
  outcome expectation, 267
  pain management, 265
Cholecystitis. *See* Cholelithiasis/
    cholecystitis

Cholelithiasis/cholecystitis
  assessment, 262
  clinical manifestations,
    261–262
  diagnosis, 262
  gerontologic considerations,
    262
  medical management,
    262–263
  nutrition management, 263
  pharmacologic therapy, 263
  surgical management,
    263–264
Cholesteatoma, 516, 583
Chondrosarcoma, 98
Choreiform (dance-like)
    movements
  and Huntington's disease,
    450–451
Choriocarcinomas, 231
Chromophobic tumors, 660
Chronic bacterial prostatitis, 677
Chronic gastritis, 378
Chronic lymphocytic leukemia
    (CLL), 506–507
Chronic myelogenous leukemia
    (CML), 509–511
Chronic obstructive pulmonary
    disease (COPD), 267–274
  activity tolerance in, 271
  assessment, 269
  clinical manifestations, 268
  collaborative problems/
    complications, 270, 273
  complications, 267
  diagnosis, 269
  gas exchange improvement,
    270
  gerontologic considerations,
    268
  home/community-based care,
    271
  and hypertension, 700
  medical management,
    268–274
  nursing interventions,
    270–274

outcome expectations, 273–274
oxygen administration, 268
patient education, 272
planning/goals in, 270
and pneumonia, 666
risk factors, 268
self-care, 271–272
Chronic prostatitis, 676
Cigarette smoking
aversion to, in hepatitis A, 438
and chronic pharyngitis, 655
and gastritis, 380
and osteoporosis, 579
and peptic ulcers, 610
and perioperative nursing management, 624
and pulmonary emphysema, 332
and Raynaud's disease, 704
and transient ischemic attack, 754
Circulatory shock, in Addison's disease, 21
Cirrhosis, hepatic, 274–278
activity tolerance in, 276
assessment, 275, 276
clinical manifestations, 274–275
collaborative problems/ complications, 276, 277–278
diagnosis, 276
and esophageal varices, bleeding, 351
and hepatitis C, 442
home/community-based care, 278
medical management, 275–278
nursing interventions, 276–278
nutrition management, 275, 277
outcome expectations, 278
planning/goals, 276

Claudication
in peripheral arterial occlusive disease, 648
in polycythemia, 674
Clavicle fractures, 365
CLL. *See* Chronic lymphocytic leukemia (CLL)
Closed fractures, 364
Cluster headaches, 401, 406
CMF/CAF regimen, for breast cancer, 161
CML. *See* Chronic myeloid leukemia (CML)
CMV retinitis, in AIDS, 7
Cochlear disease, 521
Cognitive management
for Alzheimer's disease, 28
for anemia, 38, 39
for cerebral vascular accidents, 257–258
for Cushing's syndrome, 290
for diffuse, axonal injuries, 417–418
for hip fractures, 374
for hypothyroidism/ myxedema, 480
for ischemic strokes, 250
for multiple sclerosis, 538, 540
Colonoscopy
for diverticular disorders, 326
for large bowel obstruction, 105
Colorectal cancer, 137, 172–179
assessment, 173, 175
body image management, 177–178
clinical manifestations, 173
collaborative problems/ complications, 175, 178
diagnosis, 173, 175
fluid balance management, 177
gerontologic considerations, 173–174
home/community-based care, 178
medical management, 174–179

Colorectal cancer (*Contd.*)
  nursing interventions,
      176–179
  nutrition management,
      176–177
  outcome expectations, 179
  and polyps, 172
  surgical management, 174
Coma, hepatic, 434–436
Communication management
  in cerebral vascular accidents,
      258
  in Guillain-Barré syndrome,
      399
  in mastoiditis, 518
  in myasthenia gravis, 552
  in oral cavity cancer, 207
  in Parkinson's disease, 599
Community-acquired pneumonia
      (CAP), 665
Community-based care
  for acute pancreatitis, 591
  for Addison's disease, 35
  for AIDS, 16–17
  for Alzheimer's disease, 30
  for anemia, 40
  for anemia, aplastic, 42
  for anemia, sickle cell, 53
  for appendicitis, 73
  for asthma, 87
  for bone tumors, 104
  burn injuries, 133, 134–135
  for burn injuries, 131
  for cancer, 148–149
      of breasts, 166–167
      of cervix, 171–172
      colorectal, 178
      of esophagus, 184
      of larynx, 194
      of oral cavity, 207–208
      of prostate, 219–220
      of stomach, 230
      of vulva, 239
  for cardiomyopathies,
      244–245
  for cerebral vascular accidents,
      259–260
  for cholecystectomy, 266–267
  for chronic obstructive
      pulmonary disease, 271
  for cystitis, 296
  for diffuse, axonal injuries,
      419
  for epilepsy, 349
  for Guillain-Barré syndrome,
      399–400
  for heart failure, 428–429
  for hepatic cirrhosis, 278
  for hiatal hernia, 446–447
  for hip fractures, 375–376
  for hypertension, 466
  for hyperthyroidism,
      467–468
  for hypothyroidism/
      myxedema, 481
  for leukemia, 503
  for mastoiditis, 519
  for Ménière's disease, 525
  for migraine headaches,
      405–406
  in morbid obesity, 565
  for multiple sclerosis, 541
  for myasthenia gravis,
      553–554
  for myocardial infarction, 559
  in osteomyelitis, 575–576
  for Parkinson's disease,
      599–600
  for pemphigus, 607
  for peptic ulcers, 614
  for peripheral arterial occlusive
      disease, 650–651
  for pneumonia, 670
  postoperative, 645–646
  for psoriasis, 686
  for pulmonary edema,
      694–695
  for pulmonary tuberculosis,
      763
  for rheumatoid arthritis, 83
  for spinal cord injury, 737
  for status asthmaticus, 89
  for ulcerative colitis, 772–773
  for urolithiasis, 785–786

Complications
  of acute pancreatitis, 588
  of anemia, 38, 39
  of anemia, sickle cell, 51
  of angina pectoris, 66
  of appendicitis, 72
  of Bell's palsy, 95
  of bleeding esophageal varices,
      354
  bone tumors, 101
  of brain abscesses, 109
  of burn injuries, 123, 125,
      127, 130–131
  of cancer, 141–142, 147
    of breast, 163, 166
    of cervix, 170, 171
    colorectal, 178
    of larynx, 190, 193–194
    of prostate, 217
    of skin, 224
    of vulva, 237
  of cardiomyopathies, 243
  of cerebral vascular accidents,
      251, 254
  of cholecystectomy, 265
  of chronic obstructive
      pulmonary disorder, 270,
      273
  in clinical unit, monitoring/
      prevention, 642
  of Cushing's syndrome,
      290–291
  of cystitis, 295
  of diabetes mellitus, 301–302,
      305
  of diarrhea, 317, 319
  of DIC, 323
  of diffuse axonal injuries, 414,
      415, 418
  of diverticular disorders, 329
  of epilepsy, 347
  of fractures, 359–360,
      362–363
  of gastritis, 379
  of Guillain-Barré syndrome,
      397
  of heart failure, 424, 428
  of hemophilia, 432
  of hepatic cirrhosis, 276,
      277–278
  of hip fractures, 372, 374–375
  of hypertension, 458
  of hyperthyroidism, 465, 467
  of hypothyroidism, 477
  of hypothyroidism/myxedema,
      480
  of increased intracranial
      pressure, 489–490, 492
  of infective endocarditis, 337
  of intracranial aneurysm, 61
  of Ménière's disease, 524
  of multiple sclerosis, 536
  of muscular dystrophies, 543
  of myasthenia gravis
    cholinergic crisis, 549, 551,
        552–553
    myasthenic crisis, 549, 551,
        552–553
  of myocardial infarction, 557,
      559
  of pemphigus, 605, 606
  of peptic ulcer, 612, 613
  of pericarditis, 618, 619
  of peripheral arterial occlusive
      disease, 650
  of pharyngitis, 653
  of pneumonia, 668, 669–670
  of psoriasis, 684
  of pulmonary emphysema,
      333
  of pulmonary tuberculosis,
      761–762, 762–763
  of renal failure, acute, 711
  of rheumatoid arthritis, 80,
      82
  of spinal cord injury, 729,
      733
  of toxic epidermal necrolysis,
      751, 753
  of ulcerative colitis, 769,
      771–772
  of unconsciousness, 775–776,
      779–780
  of urolithiasis, 784

Computed tomography (CT) scan
  for Alzheimer's disease, 27
  for aortic aneurysm, 56
  for bleeding esophageal
      varices, 352
  for bone tumors, 100
  for brain abscess, 108
  for brain injuries, 409
  for brain tumors, 112
  for bronchiectasis, 114
  for cancer, 137
      of bladder, 157
      of larynx, 188
      of liver, 196
      of lungs, 201
      or cervix, 168
      of ovaries, 209
      of pancreas, 211
      of prostate, 214
      of skin, 222
      of thyroid, 233–234
  for Cushing's syndrome, 287
  for diverticular disorders, 326
  for empyema, 335
  for epilepsy, 345
  for hepatic cirrhosis, 275
  for Hodgkin's disease, 449
  for Huntington's disease, 450,
      451
  for increased intracranial
      pressure, 487
  for ischemic stroke, 250
  for low back pain, 91
  for lung abscess, 512
  for migraine headaches, 403
  for pericarditis, 616
  for peritonitis, 652
  for pituitary tumors, 661
  for pulmonary emphysema,
      333
  for renal tumors, 186
  for stomach cancer, 227
Concussion, 409
Confusion
  in cardiac tamponade, 616
  in hepatic encephalopathy,
      434
  and hypoglycemia, 469
  in Parkinson's disease, 595
  in pneumonia, 668
Congestive heart failure.
      See Heart failure
Constipation
  anxiety management, 281
  causative factors, 279
  and fecal impaction, 280
  and hepatic cirrhosis, 274
  in hypothyroidism, 478
  in large bowel obstruction,
      105
  in multiple sclerosis, 536
  in osteoporosis, 579
  in Parkinson's disease, 595
  in peptic ulcers, 609
Contact dermatitis, 281–283
Contusions, 410, 545
Convulsions, and
      hypoparathyroidism,
      473
COPD. See Chronic obstructive
      pulmonary disease
      (COPD)
Coping management
  in cerebral vascular accidents,
      258–259
  in epilepsies, 348
  in hip fractures, 374
  in hyperthyroidism, 466
  in multiple sclerosis, 540
  in Parkinson's disease, 599
  in ulcerative colitis, 771
Cor pulmonale. See Heart failure;
      Pulmonary heart disease
Corneal integrity, in
      unconsciousness, 777
Coronary atherosclerosis/
      coronary artery disease,
      283–286, 299
Coronary heart disease (CHD),
      283
Corticosteroids
  and cataracts, 245, 247
  and Cushing's syndrome,
      288

Cough
  in AIDS, 2
  in aortic aneurysm, 55
  and bronchiectasis, 114
  in cerebral vascular accidents, 257
  in cholecystitis, 264
  in chronic bronchitis, 116
  in chronic obstructive pulmonary disorder, 268
  in empyema, 334
  in Guillain-Barré syndrome, 397
  in lung abscess, 511, 512
  in mitral regurgitation, 529
  in mitral stenosis, 530
  in pleural effusion, 662
  in pneumonia, 666
  in pulmonary emphysema, 333
CPR. *See* Cardiopulmonary resuscitation (CPR)
Cramps, abdominal, and diarrhea, 316
Cranial arteritis, 406–407
Cretinism, 475
Crohn's disease. *See* Regional enteritis
Cryosurgery
  for liver cancer, 197
  for prostate cancer, 215
Cryotherapy, for cervical cancer, 169
Cryptococcal infections, in AIDS, 7
Cryptococcus neoformans, 3
CSF. *See* Cerebrospinal fluid (CSF)
CT scan. *See* Computed tomography (CT) scan
Cushing's syndrome, 286–292
  and ACTH, 286
  assessment, 287, 288
  and basophilic tumors, 660
  body image management, 290
  and brain tumors, 111

clinical manifestations, 286–287
  collaborative problems/ complications, 289, 290–291
  diagnosis, 287, 288–289
  and increased intracranial pressure, 487
  infections in, 288
  medical management, 287
  outcome expectations, 291
  rest/activity management, 290
  self-care, 289, 291
  skin care management, 289–290
CVA. *See* Cerebral vascular accident (CVA)
Cyanosis
  in Addison's disease, 21
  in aortic aneurysm, 55
  in pneumothorax, 672
Cystectomy, for bladder cancer, 158
Cystitis (lower urinary tract infection), 292–296
  assessment, 292–293, 294
  clinical manifestations, 292
  collaborative problems/ complications, 295
  diagnosis, 292–293, 294–295
  fluid balance management, 295
  gerontologic considerations, 293
  home/community-based care, 296
  nutrition management, 295
  outcome expectations, 296
  pharmacologic therapy, 293
  planning/goals, 295
  recurrent, management of, 293–294

Death anxiety
  in myocardial infarction, 557
  in pheochromocytoma, 657

Deep vein thrombosis (DVT),
787–792
clinical manifestations, 788
in clinical unit, monitoring/
prevention, 642
diagnosis, 790
and Guillain-Barré syndrome,
396, 398
medical management, 789
nursing management, 790–792
pharmacologic therapy, 789
prevention, 789
risk factors, 788
in spinal cord injury, 731
surgical management, 789
Deformity prevention, in cerebral
vascular accidents, 254
Degenerative joint disease.
See Osteoarthritis
Dehydration
and diabetic ketoacidosis,
313–314
and diarrhea, 319
and hepatic encephalopathy,
434
and HHNS, 453
and sickle cell anemia, 52
Dementias
and Huntington's disease,
450
neurologic
Alzheimer's disease, 26–30
in Parkinson's disease, 595
Dental/oral hygiene management
in hemophilia, 431
in Hodgkin's disease, 449
in idiopathic
thrombocytopenia
purpura, 484
in leukemia, 500, 501
in lung abscess, 512
in muscular dystrophies, 543
Dependent pedal edema, 536
Depression
in Addison's disease, 21
in AIDS, 5, 7
in cardiomyopathies, 244

in cerebral vascular accidents,
260
in endometriosis, 341
in Huntington's disease, 451
in hypoparathyroidism, 472
in hypothyroidism, 476
in ischemic strokes, 250
in larynx cancer, 191
in low back pain, 90
in migraine headaches, 402
in morbid obesity, 564
in muscular dystrophies, 543
in Parkinson's disease, 595
Dermatitis
contact, 281–283
exfoliative, 355–357
DEXA. *See* Dual-energy x-ray
absorptiometry (DEXA)
Dexamethasone suppression test,
287
Diabetes insipidus, 297–299
fluid balance management, 298
and increased intracranial
pressure, 489
and macrovascular/
microvascular disease,
302
and vasopressin replacement,
298
Diabetes mellitus
and angina pectoris, 63
anxiety management, 306
assessment, 304
caloric requirements, 303
and cataracts, 245
collaborative problems/
complications, 305,
306–307
complications, 301–302
and coronary artery disease,
283, 299
and coronary atherosclerosis,
283
in Cushing's syndrome, 287
diagnosis, 304–305
electrolyte/fluid balance
management, 305

and exercise, 308–309
gestational, 300
and glycosylated hemoglobin, 309
and HHNS, 454
and hypoglycemia, 471
insulin
administration, 310
problems with, 310–311
ketone measurement, 309
medical management, 302–303
and myocardial infarction, 555
nursing interventions, 305–312
nutrition management, 303, 307–308
and obesity, 301
oral hypoglycemic agents, 311
and osteomyelitis, 572
and pancreatic cancer, 210
patient education, 307
planning/goals, 305
and pruritus, 678
self blood glucose monitoring, 309
self-care, 307
types of
Type 1, 299–300
Type 2, 300
Diabetic ketoacidosis (DKA)
acid-base balance management, 315
assessment, 313
causes, 213
and diabetes mellitus, 299, 301, 305
diagnosis, 313
electrolyte management, 312, 314
fluid management, 313–315
and hyperglycemia, 312
medical management, 313–314
nursing management, 314–316

Dialysis
for acute renal failure, 712–713
for glomerulonephritis, 387
Diaphoresis
in asthma, 84
in hypovolemic shock, 723
Diarrhea
in AIDS, 2, 3, 7, 10
anxiety management, 319, 320
assessment, 317, 318
in cancer, 140
clinical manifestations, 316–317
complications, 317, 319
control of, 319
diagnosis, 317, 318
and endometriosis, 341
fluid/electrolyte management, 319–320
and hepatic cirrhosis, 274
in leukemia, 498
medical management, 317–320
in migraine headaches, 402
in morbid obesity, 565
in peptic ulcers, 609
and radiation therapy, 449
in regional enteritis, 706
in thyroid storm, 747
types of, 316
DIC. *See* Disseminated intravascular coagulopathy (DIC)
Diffuse axonal injuries, 410–420
airway management, 416
assessment
eye signs, 413–414
Glasgow Coma Scale, 413
motor functions, 413–414
vital signs, 413
cognitive management, 417–418
complications, 414, 415, 418
diagnosis, 414–415
expected outcomes, 420
fluid balance management, 416

Diffuse axonal injuries (*Contd.*)
  home/community-based care,
    419
  medical management, 411,
    412
  nursing management, 413–420
  nutrition management, 415,
    416
  planning/goals, 415
  self-care, 419
  skin integrity maintenance,
    417
  sleep management, 418
  temperature management, 417
  types
    epidural hematoma, 411
    intracerebral hemorrhage,
      412
    intracranial hemorrhage,
      410–411
    subdural hematoma,
      411–412
Digestive disturbances
  in constipation, 279
  in glomerulonephritis, 389
Digital rectal examination (DRE)
  for benign prostatic
    hyperplasia, 97
  for prostate cancer, 214
Dilation and curettage (D & C),
    168
Diplopia
  in myasthenia gravis, 552
  in pituitary tumors, 660
Dislocations, in musculoskeletal
    trauma, 546
Dissecting aneurysm, 55–56
Disseminated intravascular
    coagulopathy (DIC),
    321–325
  in acute pancreatitis, 585
  assessment, 322
  clinical manifestations,
    321–322
  collaborative problems/
    complications, 323
  diagnosis, 322–323

  fluid balance management,
    324
  hemodynamic status
    maintenance, 323
  medical management,
    322–325
  nursing interventions,
    323–325
  outcome expectations, 325
  pathophysiology, 321
  planning/goals, 323
  and skin integrity, 324
  and thrombocytopenia, 321,
    743
Diverticular disorders, 325–330,
    651
Diverticulitis, 325
  assessment, 328
  clinical manifestations, 326
  diagnosis, 328
Diverticulosis, 325
  clinical manifestations, 326
  management, 327–328
  surgical management, 328
Dizziness
  in brain injuries, 408
  in glomerulonephritis, 389
  in hypertension, 458
  in Ménière's disease, 523
  in migraine headaches, 402
  in mitral valve prolapse, 532
  in polycythemia, 674
DKA. *See* Diabetic ketoacidosis
    (DKA)
Double vision. *See* Monocular
    diplopia
DRE. *See* Digital rectal
    examination (DRE)
Drowsiness
  and diarrhea, 317
  in migraine headaches, 402
Dry mouth. *See* Xerostomia
Dual-energy x-ray absorptiometry
    (DEXA), 577–578
Duodenal ulcer. *See* Peptic ulcer
Duodenography, for pancreatic
    cancer, 211

DVT. *See* Deep vein thrombosis
(DVT)
Dysarthria, in myasthenia gravis,
552
Dyscrasias, of blood, and
epistaxis, 350
Dyspepsia
chronic, and hepatic cirrhosis,
274
and hepatitis B, 440, 441
Dysphagia
in acute thyroiditis, 745
in cerebral vascular accidents,
257
in esophageal cancer, 181
in hiatal hernia, 444
in hypoparathyroidism, 472
in myasthenia gravis, 552
Dysphonia, in Parkinson's
disease, 595
Dyspnea
in acute respiratory distress
syndrome, 18
in AIDS, 2
in anemia, 36
in anemia, aplastic, 41
in aortic aneurysm, 55
in asthma, 84
in cardiac tamponade, 616
in chronic obstructive
pulmonary disorder, 268,
270
in empyema, 334
exertional, and aortic
insufficiency, 68
in glomerulonephritis, 386
in mitral regurgitation, 529
in mitral stenosis, 530
paroxysmal nocturnal, and
aortic insufficiency, 68
in pericarditis, 616
in pleural effusion, 662
in pneumothorax, 671
in polycythemia, 674
in pulmonary emphysema,
333
in thyroid storm, 747

Dysrhythmias
in angina pectoris, 66
in aortic insufficiency, 69
in cardiomyopathies, 242,
243
in cerebral vascular accidents,
251
in epilepsy, 343
in heart failure, 424
in hyperthyroidism, 462
in hypoparathyroidism, 472
in ischemic stroke, 248
and mitral regurgitation, 529
in myocardial infarction, 557
in myocarditis, 561
in pheochromocytoma, 657
in rheumatic endocarditis, 339
in sickle cell anemia, 49

Ear disorders
cholesteatoma, 516
endolymphatic hydrops, 520
Ménière's disease, 520–525
cochlear disease, 521
vestibular disease, 521
otitis media, 516
acute, 581–582
chronic, 583–584
otorrhea, 516
postauricular pain, in
mastoiditis, 516
Eastern European ancestry, and
KS, 494
ECCE. *See* Extracapsular cataract
extraction (ECCE)
Ecchymosis
in acute pancreatitis, 585
in brain injury, 408
ECG. *See* Electrocardiogram
(ECG)
Echocardiography
for angina pectoris, 64
for arterial embolism/
thrombosis, 74
for cardiomyopathies, 241
for heart failure, 422
for ischemic stroke, 250

Echocardiography (*Contd.*)
  for mitral regurgitation,
    529–530
  for mitral stenosis, 531
  for pericarditis, 616
  transesophageal
    in aortic aneurysm, 56
    in arterial embolism/
      thrombosis, 74
    for mitral regurgitation,
      530
Eczema, and asthma, 84
Edema
  in asthma, 84
  cerebral
    in diabetes mellitus, 305
    in fulminant hepatic failure,
      437
  in chronic otitis media, 583
  dependent pedal, in multiple
    sclerosis, 536
  facial, in glomerulonephritis,
    386
  in hepatic cirrhosis, 274
  lower extremities, and heart
    failure, 422
  in mastoiditis, 517
  in nephrotic syndrome, 562
  pulmonary, 66, 386, 421, 557,
    687–689
  in thyroid storm, 747
  of trachea, and larynx cancer,
    190
EEG. *See* Electroencephalography
    (EEG)
EGD. *See* Esophagogastroduo-
    denoscopy
    (EGD)
Elbow fractures, 366–367
Elderly. *See* Gerontologic
    considerations
Electrocardiogram (ECG)
  for angina pectoris, 64
  for aortic stenosis, 70
  for arterial embolism/
    thrombosis, 74
  for cardiomyopathies, 241

for glomerulonephritis, 390
for Guillain-Barré syndrome,
    396
for hypertension, 457
for hyperthyroidism, 467
for ischemic stroke, 250
for mitral stenosis, 531
for pericarditis, 616
Electroencephalography (EEG)
  for Alzheimer's disease, 27
  for aortic insufficiency, 69
  for brain tumors, 112
  for epilepsy, 345
  for hepatic coma/hematic
    encephalopathy, 434
  for myocardial infarction, 555
Electrolyte management
  in acute pancreatitis, 590
  in Addison's disease, 25
  in AIDS, 9
  in bleeding esophageal varices,
    354
  burn injuries
    emergent/resuscitative
      phase, 124
  in colorectal cancer, 177
  in diabetes mellitus, 304
  in diabetic ketoacidosis, 312,
    313, 315
  in diarrhea, 319–320
  in exfoliative dermatitis, 356
  for large bowel obstruction,
    105
  in leukemia, 501–502
  in pemphigus, 607
  in renal failure, acute,
    711–712
  in small bowel obstruction,
    106
Electromyographic (EMG)
    studies
  for amyotrophic lateral
    sclerosis, 32
  for low back pain, 91
  for migraine headaches, 403
Electronystagmogram, for
    Ménière's disease, 521

Electrophoresis
of CSF, for multiple sclerosis,
536
in nephrotic syndrome, 562
Elephantiasis, and lymphedema,
513–515
Embolism
arterial, 73–75
cerebral, in cardiomyopathies,
243
in heart failure, 424
pulmonary, 689–695
in DIC, 323
in Guillain-Barré syndrome,
396
Embryonal carcinomas, 231
EMG studies.
See Electromyographic
(EMG) studies
Emotional disturbances
in Huntington's disease, 450,
451
in hypertension, 456
in hyperthyroidism,
461–462
Emphysema, pulmonary,
332–334
age onset, 332
assessment, 333
causes of, 332
classifications
centrilobular, 333
panlobular, 333
clinical manifestations, 333
complications, 333
diagnosis, 333
medical management, 334
and pneumothorax, 671
Empyema, 334–336
Encephalitis, in AIDS, 7
Encephalopathy
hepatic, 276, 277, 434–436
portal, 434
recurrent, 436
Endarterectomy, percutaneous
coronary
for angina pectoris, 65

Endocarditis, infective, 336–339
assessment/diagnosis, 337
clinical manifestations, 337
complications, 337
hospital acquisition of, 336
medical management, 338
nursing management, 338–339
risk factors, 336
Endocarditis, rheumatic,
339–341
Endolymphatic hydrops
Endolymphatic hydrops, in
Ménière's disease, 520
Endometrial cancer, 179–180
Endometriosis, 341–343
Endoscopic retrograde cholan-
giopancreatography
(ERCP)
for cholecystitis, 262
for chronic pancreatitis, 592
for pancreatic cancer, 211
Endoscopy
for bleeding esophageal
varices, 352
for cancer, 137, 201
fiberoptic, in peptic ulcers, 608
End-state renal disease. *See* Renal
failure, chronic
Enterovirus family, 437
Eosinophilic tumors, 660
Epidermoid cell carcinoma, 200
Epididymitis, 331–332
Epidural hematoma, 411
Epidural hemorrhages, 248
Epigastric distress, in
cholecystitis, 261
Epilepsies, 343–350. *See also*
Status epilepticus
airway management, 345
assessment, 345, 346
causes, 343
clinical manifestations
complex partial seizures,
344
grand mal seizures, 344
postictal state, 345
simple partial seizures, 344

Epilepsies (*Contd.*)
  collaborative problems/
      complications, 347
  coping management, 348
  diagnosis, 345, 346–347
  and diffuse, axonal injuries,
      414
  home/community-based care,
      349
  medical management,
      345–350
  nursing interventions,
      347–349
  outcome expectations, 349
  pharmacologic therapy,
      345–346
  planning/goals, 347
  seizure fear control, 348
  and status epilepticus, 347
  surgical management, 346
Epistaxis (nosebleed), 350–351
  in glomerulonephritis, 389
Epstein-Barr virus
  and acute glomerulonephritis,
      386
  and Hodgkin's disease, 447
ERCP. *See* Endoscopic retrograde
      cholangiopancreatography
      (ERCP)
Erythema
  in acute thyroiditis, 745
  in chronic otitis media, 583
  in mastoiditis, 517
Erythromyalgia, in polycythemia,
      675
Escherichia coli
  and bone infections, 572
  and epididymitis, 331
  and peritonitis, 651
  and prostatitis, 676
Esophageal cancer, 180–185
  assessment, 181, 182
  and chemotherapy, 181
  clinical manifestations, 181
  diagnosis, 181, 182
  home/community-based care,
      184

medical management, 181
nursing interventions,
    182–184
nutrition management,
    183–184
outcome expectations,
    184–185
planning/goals, 182
risk factors, 180–181
surgical preparation, 183
wound healing promotion,
    183
Esophageal ulcer. *See* Peptic ulcer
Esophageal varices, bleeding,
    351–355
Esophagectomy, for esophageal
    cancer, 181
Esophagitis, from radiation
    therapy, 449
Esophagogastroduodenoscopy
    (EGD)
  for esophageal cancer, 181
Estrogen, and osteoporosis, 577
Excretory urography, in bladder
    cancer, 157
Exercise management
  in cerebral vascular accidents,
      255
  in diabetes mellitus, 302,
      308–309
  in Guillain-Barré syndrome,
      396
  in multiple sclerosis, 539
  in muscular dystrophies, 543
  in myocarditis, 561
  in osteoporosis, 578
Exfoliative dermatitis, 355–357
Exophthalmos, and
    hyperthyroidism, 462
Extracapsular cataract extraction
    (ECCE), 246
Extremities
  peripheral arterial occlusive
      disease, 648
  swelling, in osteomyelitis, 573
Eyelid ptosis, in myasthenia
    gravis, 552

Fatigue
   in Addison's disease, 21
   in anemia, 39
   in anemia, aplastic, 42
   and aortic insufficiency, 68
   in cancer, 145
      of lungs, 202
   in constipation, 279
   in coronary
      atherosclerosis/artery
      disease, 284
   in diabetes mellitus, 300
   in heart failure, 424, 425
   in hypothyroidism/myxedema,
      475
   in leukemia, 502
   in low back pain, 90
   in mitral regurgitation, 529
   in mitral stenosis, 530
   in mitral valve prolapse, 532
   in multiple sclerosis, 535
   in nephrotic syndrome, 562
   in peripheral arterial occlusive
      disease, 648
   in pulmonary emphysema, 333
   in rheumatoid arthritis, 78, 81
Fecal impaction, 279, 280, 543
Femur fractures, 370
Fetor hepaticus, in hepatic coma,
      434
Fever
   in acute pancreatitis, 585
   in acute thyroiditis, 745
   in Addison's disease, 21
   in AIDS, 2
   in chronic lymphocytic
      leukemia, 506
   in empyema, 334
   in exfoliative dermatitis, 355
   in leukemia, 498
   in lung abscess, 511
   in meningococcal meningitis,
      527
   in myocarditis, 560
   in pelvic infection, 601
   in pericarditis, 616
   in pharyngitis, 654

   in pleural effusion, 662
   in pneumonia, 666
   in regional enteritis, 706
   in sickle cell anemia, 49
   in thyroid storm, 747
   in ulcerative colitis, 765
Fibromas, 98
Fibula fractures, 370–371
Finger fractures, 368
Fissures, anal, and constipation,
      279
Flank pain, facial, 386
Fluid balance management
   in acute pancreatitis, 590
   in acute respiratory distress
      syndrome, 19
   in Addison's disease, 22, 23–24
   in AIDS, 9
   in appendicitis, 72
   burn injuries
      acute/intermediate phase,
         127–128
      emergent/resuscitative
         phase, 124
   in cancer, 143
      colorectal, 177
      of oral cavity, 206
   in cardiogenic shock, 722
   in chronic renal failure, 717
   in clinical unit, postoperative,
      640
   in cute respiratory distress
      syndrome, 19
   in cystitis, 295
   in diabetes insipidus, 298
   in diabetes mellitus, 304
   in diabetic ketoacidosis, 313,
      314–315
   in diarrhea, 319–320
   in DIC, 324
   in diffuse axonal injuries, 416
   in diverticular disorders, 329
   in exfoliative dermatitis, 356
   in gastritis, 379, 381
   in Guillain-Barré syndrome,
      398
   in hepatic cirrhosis, 276

Fluid balance management
(*Contd.*)
in HHNS, 453, 454
in hypothyroidism, 477
in hypovolemic shock, 724
in increased intracranial
pressure, 491
in large bowel obstruction, 105
in larynx cancer, 192–193
in leukemia, 498, 501–502
in Ménière's disease, 524
in meningitis, 528
in pemphigus, 607
perioperative nursing,
623–624
in pneumonia, 669
in renal failure, acute, 711–712
in sickle cell anemia, 50
in small bowel obstruction,
106
in status asthmaticus, 89
in toxic epidermal necrolysis,
752
in ulcerative colitis, 770
in unconsciousness, 777
Fluoroscopy
for cancer, 137
for hiatal hernia, 444
Flushing, in pheochromocytoma,
657
Focal nerve palsies, 414
Focal nerve palsy, 414
Folic acid, for anemia,
megaloblastic, 47
Fowler's position
in acute pancreatitis, 589
in angina pectoris, 66
in appendicitis, 73
in cholecystitis, 265
in hiatal hernia, 446
in larynx cancer, 191
in pelvic infection, 602
in pneumonia, 669
in vulvar cancer, 237
Fractures, 358–376
assessment, 361
clinical manifestations, 359

closed, management of, 364
complications, 359–360,
362–363
diagnosis, 361
emergency management,
361–362
gerontologic considerations,
361
healing of, 363–364
of hip (*See* Hip fractures)
medical management,
361–363
in multiple myeloma, 533
nursing management, 363–376
open, management of,
364–365
reduction of, 362
site specific
clavicle, 365
elbow, 366–367
femur, 370
hand/fingers, 368
hip (*See* Hip fractures)
humerus, 365–366
pelvis, 368–369
rib, 368
tibia/fibula, 370–371
wrist, 367–368
of skull, 408
types, 358–359
closed, 364
open, 364–365
Friction rub, in pericarditis, 616
Fulminant hepatic failure,
436–437

Gallbladder, and cholecystitis,
261
Gallop rhythm, in myocarditis,
561
Gallstones. *See* Cholelithiasis/
cholecystitis
Ganglionectomy, for Buerger's
disease, 118
Gangrene
in Buerger's disease, 118
in DIC, 323

Gastric cancer. *See* Stomach
    cancer
Gastric ulcer. *See* Peptic ulcer
Gastrinoma. *See* Zollinger-Ellison
    syndrome
Gastritis, 377–381
    anxiety management in, 379,
        380
    assessment, 379
    clinical manifestations
        acute, 377–3378
        chronic, 378
    collaborative problems/
        complications, 379
    diagnosis, 379
    fluid balance management,
        379, 381
    intravenous therapy, 380
    nursing interventions,
        380–381
    nutrition management, 380
    pain management, 380, 381
    planning/goals, 380
    self-care, 381
Gastroesophageal reflux, in hiatal
    hernia, 444
Gastrointestinal disorders
    in Addison's disease, 21
    in AIDS, 2–3
    in anemia, megaloblastic, 48
    bleeding
        in anemia, 36
        in colorectal cancer, 175
    bleeding, in hemophilia, 430
    in exfoliative dermatitis, 355,
        356
    in muscular dystrophies, 543
Gastrointestinal series, upper,
    209
Gene therapy, 210
Genetic counseling, in muscular
    dystrophies, 543
Gene-transfer therapy, 113
Gerontologic considerations
    for acute pancreatitis, 586
    for anemia, 37
    for angina pectoris, 64

for appendicitis, 72
for arteriosclerosis, 76
for atherosclerosis, 76
for Buerger's disease, 118
for burn injuries, 120–121
for cholelithiasis/cholecystitis,
    262
for chronic obstructive
    pulmonary disorder, 268
for colorectal cancer, 173–174
for coronary atherosclerosis/
    artery disease, 285
for cystitis, 293
for diabetes mellitus, 302
for diverticular disorders, 327
for fractures, 361
for glaucoma, 383
for glomerulonephritis, 386
for hepatitis B, 440
for hypertension, 459–460
for hyperthyroidism, 462–463
for hypoglycemia, 469
for hypothyroidism, 476
for leukemia, 497–498
for multiple myeloma, 533
for myocardial infarction, 555
for osteomalacia, 570
for osteoporosis, 577–578
perioperative nursing
    management, 622
and perioperative nursing
    management, 629
for pneumonia, 666–667
postoperative nursing
    management, 646–647
for pulmonary tuberculosis,
    760
for renal failure
    acute, 708–709
    chronic, 714
for septic shock, 726
Gestational diabetes mellitus, 300
Gigantism, 660
Glasgow Coma Scale
    for diffuse axonal injuries, 413
    for increased intracranial
        pressure, 488

Glaucoma, 382–386
  assessment/diagnosis, 383
  clinical manifestations,
      382–383
  gerontologic considerations,
      383
  and intraocular pressure, 382,
      383, 384, 385
  medical management,
      383–384
  nursing management, 385–386
  pharmacologic therapy, 384
  surgical management,
      384–385
    iridotomy, 384
    ophthalmic laser
        trabeculoplasty, 384
  types
    angle closure, 382, 384
    open angle, 382
Gliomas, 110
Glomerulonephritis
  acute, 386–388
  chronic, 388–391
Glucose intolerance, in Cushing's
    syndrome, 286
Glucose tolerance test
  for chronic pancreatitis, 592
  for pancreatic cancer, 211
Glycosylated hemoglobin, 309
Gonioscopy, for glaucoma, 383
Gonorrhea, and epididymitis,
    331
Gout, 391–394
  assessment, 393
  clinical manifestations
    acute gouty arthritis, 392
    hyperuricemia, 392
    tophi, 392–393
    urolithiasis, risk for, 393
  diagnosis, 393
  medical management, 393
  nursing management, 393–394
  pathophysiology, 391
Grand mal seizures, 344
Graves' disease.
    See Hyperthyroidism

Grief management
  in AIDS, 15
  in cancer, 146–147
  in leukemia, 502
Griess nitrate reduction test, in
    cystitis, 292
Guillain-Barré syndrome,
    394–400
  assessment, 395–396
  clinical manifestations,
      394–395
  collaborative problems/
      complications, 397
  communication management
      in, 399
  diagnosis, 395–397
  exercise management, 396
  fluid balance management,
      398–399
  home/community-based care,
      399–400
  medical management,
      396–400
  mobility management, 398
  nursing interventions,
      397–400
  nutrition management,
      398–399
  outcome expectations,
      395–396
  pathophysiology, 394
  patient education, 399
  pharmacologic therapy, 396
  planning/goals, 397
  and respiratory failure,
      397–398
Gynecomastia (breast
    enlargement), 356

HAART. *See* Highly active
    antiretroviral therapy
    (HAART)
Haemophilus influenzae, and acute
    otitis media, 581
Hair loss
  and hypopituitarism, 474
  and hypothyroidism, 476

Hallucinations, in Huntington's disease, 451

Hand/finger fractures, 368

HAP. *See* Hospital-acquired pneumonia (HAP)

Hashimoto's thyroiditis, 475, 746

HCC. *See* Hepatocellular carcinoma (HCC)

HDL. *See* High-density lipoproteins (HDL)

Head injury (brain injury), 407–410

Headaches (cephalgia), 401–407
  in acute glomerulonephritis, 386
  in acute lymphocytic leukemia, 505
  in bacterial meningitis, 526
  in brain abscess, 108
  in brain injuries, 408
  in brain tumors, 111
  classifications
    primary, 401
    secondary, 401
  cluster, 406
  in constipation, 279
  in diabetic ketoacidosis, 313
  in glomerulonephritis, 389
  in hypertension, 458
  in increased intracranial pressure, 488
  migraines (*See* Migraine headaches)
  in myocarditis, 561
  in nephrotic syndrome, 562
  in pelvic infection, 601
  in pheochromocytoma, 657
  in pituitary tumors, 660
  in pneumonia, 666
  in polycythemia, 674
  in pulmonary emphysema, 333
  tension, 407

Heart failure (cor pulmonale), 420–429. *See also* Pulmonary heart disease

  and anemia, 38
  in angina pectoris, 66
  anxiety management, 427
  assessment, 423–424
  clinical manifestations, 421–422
    left-sided, 421–422
    right-sided, 422
  complications, 424, 428
  diagnosis, 424
  fatigue management, 425–426
  fluid management, 426
  and HHNS, 454
  home/community-based care, 428–429
  in Huntington's disease, 451
  and hypertension, 457
  and hyperthyroidism, 462
  and infective endocarditis, 337
  medical management, 422–423
  in myocardial infarction, 557
  in myocarditis, 561
  nursing interventions, 425–429
  outcome expectations, 429
  pharmacologic therapy, 423
  planning/goals, 425
  in rheumatic endocarditis, 339
  surgical management, 423

Heartburn
  in gastritis, 379
  in hiatal hernia, 444

Helicobacter pylori
  and gastritis, 377
  and idiopathic thrombocytopenia purpura, 482–483
  and peptic ulcer, 608, 609

Hemangioblastomas, and ischemic strokes, 248

Hematemesis, in bleeding esophageal varices, 352

Hematologic disorders, in AIDS, 4

Hematoma
  in brain injury
    epidural, 411
    subdural, 411–412
  in breast cancer, 163
  in hemophilia, 430
  in musculoskeletal trauma,
    545
Hematuria
  and bladder cancer, 157
  and cystitis, 292
  and glomerulonephritis, 387
  microscopic, in nephrotic
    syndrome, 562
  and prostate cancer, 216
  and renal tumors, 185
  spontaneous, and hemophilia,
    430
Hemolysis, chronic, and sickle
    cell anemia, 51
Hemolytic anemia, 36
Hemophilia, 429–434
  assessment/diagnosis, 430,
    431
  complications, 432
  dental hygiene management in,
    431
  home/community-based care,
    433
  and intracerebral hemorrhage/
    hematomas, 412
  medical management, 431
  nursing interventions,
    432–434
  outcome expectations,
    433–434
  pain management, 432
  planning/goals, 432
  type A, 430
  type B, 430
Hemoptysis, in mitral stenosis,
    530
Hemorrhages
  in cancer, 141, 148
  in DIC, 322
  epidural, 248
  in esophageal cancer, 181

from esophageal varices,
    351–355
  in gastritis, 379
  in hemophilia, 430
  in hepatic cirrhosis, 276
  intracerebral, 248
  intracranial, 410–411
  in larynx cancer, 190
  monitoring/prevention, in
    clinical unit, 643–644
  in myocardial infarction, 554
  of retina, in
    glomerulonephritis, 389
  subarachnoid, 248
  upper gastric, in peptic ulcers,
    612, 613
Hemorrhagic stroke, 248
Hemorrhoids, and constipation,
    279
Hemothorax, and pneumothorax,
    670–673
Hepatic coma, 434–436
Hepatic encephalopathy, 276,
    277, 434–436
  in bleeding esophageal varices,
    354
Hepatic failure, fulminant,
    436–437
Hepatitis A, 437–439
Hepatitis B virus (HBV), 196,
    439–442
  and acute glomerulonephritis,
    386
Hepatitis C, 442
Hepatitis D, 442–443
Hepatitis E, 443
Hepatitis G, 443
Hepatocellular carcinoma (HCC),
    195–196
Hepatomegaly, and heart failure,
    422
Hepatoportography, for bleeding
    esophageal varices, 352
Herpes simplex, in AIDS, 4
Herpes zoster
  in AIDS, 4
  in Hodgkin's disease, 448

HHNS. *See* Hyperglycemic
hyperosmolar nonketotic
syndrome (HHNS)
Hiatal hernia, 443–447
assessment/diagnosis, 444, 445
clinical manifestations, 444
home/community-based care,
446–447
medical management,
444–445
nutrition management,
445–446
pain management, 446
types
axial (sliding), 443
paraesophageal, 443, 444
High-density lipoproteins (HDL),
and exercise, 308
Highly active antiretroviral
therapy (HAART), 5–6
Hip fractures, 371–376
assessment, 371
cognitive management, 374
collaborative problems/
complications, 372
complications, 372, 374–375
coping management, 374
diagnosis, 371–372
function/stability management,
373
and hip replacement, 372
home/community-based care,
375–376
nursing interventions,
372–376
outcome expectations, 376
pain management, 372–373
planning/goals, 372
urinary elimination
management, 374
wound healing in, 373
Hip replacement, 372
HIV encephalopathy. *See* AIDS
dementia complex
Hoarseness
and hypothyroidism, 476
and pharyngitis, 654

Hodgkin's disease, 447–450
assessment/diagnosis, 448–449
clinical manifestations, 448
medical management, 449
nursing management, 449–450
Home care
for acute pancreatitis, 591
for Addison's disease, 35
for AIDS, 16–17
for Alzheimer's disease, 30
for anemia, 40, 42, 53
for appendicitis, 73
for asthma, 87
for burn injuries, 131,
134–135
for cancer, 148–149
of breast, 166–167
of cervix, 171–172
colorectal, 178
of esophagus, 184
of larynx, 194
of oral cavity, 207–208
of prostate, 219–220
of stomach, 230
of vulva, 239
for cardiomyopathies,
244–245
for cerebral vascular accidents,
259–260
for cholecystectomy, 266–267
for chronic obstructive
pulmonary disease, 271
for cystitis, 296
for diffuse axonal injuries, 419
for epilepsy, 349
for Guillain-Barré syndrome,
399–400
for heart failure, 428–429
for hemophilia, 433
for hepatic cirrhosis, 278
for hiatal hernia, 446–447
for hip fractures, 375–376
for hypertension, 466
for hyperthyroidism, 467–468
for hypothyroidism/
myxedema, 481
for leukemia, 503

Home care (*Contd.*)
for mastoiditis, 519
for Ménière's disease, 525
for migraine headaches, 405–406
for morbid obesity, 565
for multiple sclerosis, 541
in muscular dystrophies, 543
for myasthenia gravis, 553–554
for myocardial infarction, 559
for osteomyelitis, 575–576
for Parkinson's disease, 599–600
for pemphigus, 607
for peptic ulcers, 614
for peripheral arterial occlusive disease, 650–651
for pneumonia, 670
postoperative, 645–646
and postoperative nursing management, 633
for psoriasis, 686
for pulmonary edema, 694–695
for pulmonary tuberculosis, 763
for rheumatoid arthritis, 83
for spinal cord injury, 737
for status asthmaticus, 89
for ulcerative colitis, 772–773
for urolithiasis, 785–786
Hormonal therapy
for cancer
of breasts, 161
of endometrium, 179
of prostate, 215
for endometriosis, 342
for Hashimoto's thyroiditis, 746
for hypothyroidism, 477–478
for leukemia, 500
for osteoporosis, 579
for renal tumors, 186
Hospital-acquired pneumonia (HAP), 665

Human immunodeficiency virus (HIV), 1–18
and acute glomerulonephritis, 386
and hemophilia, 433
and Kaposi's sarcoma, 494
and tuberculosis, 759
Humerus fractures, 365–366
Humoral immunodeficiency, 114
Hunger, and hypoglycemia, 469
Huntington's disease, 450–452
choreiform movements, 450–451
Hydrocephalus, and intracranial aneurysm, 60, 61
Hydrostatic therapy, for bladder cancer, 158
Hyperadrenalism, 659
Hypercalcemia
in acute pancreatitis, 585
in bone tumors, 100, 101
monitoring/management, 103
in cancer, 141
in liver cancer, 196
in multiple myeloma, 533
in osteomyelitis, 572
in pancreatic cancer, 211
Hypercapnia, and pulmonary emphysema, 333
Hypercholesterolemia, 196
Hyperglycemia
and diabetes mellitus, 299, 305
and diabetic ketoacidosis, 312
and pheochromocytoma, 657
and transient ischemic attack, 754
Hyperglycemic hyperosmolar nonketotic syndrome (HHNS), 299, 301, 453–454
Hyperhidrosis, in pheochromocytoma, 657
Hyperkalemia
and Addison's disease, 22
and diabetic ketoacidosis, 315

Hyperlipidemia
  in acute pancreatitis, 585
  and coronary atherosclerosis/
      artery disease, 283
Hyperphosphatemia, 715
Hyperplasia, in myasthenia
      gravis, 550
Hyperproliferative anemia.
      See Anemia, aplastic
Hypertension, 455–461
  in arteriosclerosis, 76
  assessment/diagnosis, 457, 458
  in atherosclerosis, 76
  and brain injuries, 408
  and cerebral vascular
      accidents, 251
  and chronic renal failure, 715
  clinical manifestations,
      456–457
  collaborative problems/
      complications, 458
  and constipation, 279
  from cor pulmonale, 698–700
  in Cushing's syndrome, 287
  emergency hypertensive crisis,
      456
  genetic factor, 456
  gerontologic considerations,
      459–460
  and glomerulonephritis, 386
  home/community-based care,
      466
  and intracerebral hemorrhage/
      hematomas, 412
  and ischemic strokes, 248
  medical management,
      457–458
  nursing interventions,
      459–461
  nutrition management, 460
  outcome expectations, 461
  patient education, 459
  and pituitary tumors, 660
  planning/goals, 458
  portal, and esophageal varices,
      bleeding, 251
  pulmonary, 698–700
    risk factors, 455
    self-care, 460
    in transient ischemic attack,
        754
    types
      cor pulmonale, 700
      essential (primary),
          455–456, 700
      isolated systolic, 459
      secondary, 456
Hypertension, pulmonary, 49,
      52
Hyperthermia
  and brain injuries, 408
  and leukemia, 499
  and liver cancer, 197
Hyperthyroidism (Graves'
      disease), 461–468
  adjunctive therapy, 464
  assessment/diagnosis, 462, 465
  body temperature
      management, 466
  collaborative problems/
      complications, 465, 467
  coping management, 466
  gerontologic considerations,
      462–463
  home/community-based care,
      467–468
  and LATS, 461
  medical management, 463
  nursing interventions,
      466–468
  nutrition management, 466
  outcome expectations, 468
  pharmacologic therapy, 464
  planning/goals, 465
  self-esteem management, 466
  surgical intervention, 464
  in thyroid storm, 747
Hyperuricemia
  in exfoliative dermatitis, 356
  and gout, 392
Hyperventilation, and diabetic
      ketoacidosis, 313
Hypnosis, for morbid obesity,
      565

Hypocalcemia
   and chronic renal failure, 715
   and hypoparathyroidism, 473
Hypoglycemia (insulin reaction),
      468–472
   and Addison's disease, 22
   assessment/diagnosis, 469
   causes, 469
   and diabetes mellitus, 301,
      305
   in fulminant hepatic failure,
      437
   gerontologic considerations,
      469
   and hypopituitarism, 474
   in liver cancer, 196
   medical management,
      470–471
   nursing management, 471–472
   nutrition management, 470,
      471
   symptom types
      adrenergic, 469
      central nervous system, 469
   types
      mild, 469
      moderate, 469–470
      severe, 470
   unconsciousness in, 471
Hypokalemia, and diabetes
      mellitus, 305
Hypokinesia, in Parkinson's
      disease, 595
Hypometabolism, and
      hypopituitarism, 474
Hyponatremia
   and Addison's disease, 22
   and intracranial aneurysm, 60
Hypoparathyroidism, 472–474
   assessment/diagnosis, 473
   and cataracts, 245
   causes, 472
   clinical manifestations, 472
   medical management, 473
   nursing management, 473–474
   nutrition management, 473,
      474

Hypopituitarism, 474–475, 660
Hypoproteinemia, and exfoliative
      dermatitis, 355
Hypotension
   in Addison's disease, 21
   in cerebral vascular accidents,
      251
   in diabetic ketoacidosis, 313
   and diarrhea, 317
   and Guillain-Barré syndrome,
      398
   and hemophilia, 432
   in HHNS, 453
   monitoring/prevention, in
      clinical unit, 642
   orthostatic
      in Parkinson's disease, 595
      in spinal cord injury, 736
   in peptic ulcers, 613
   in pneumonia, 668
   in pneumothorax, 672
   postural
      in pheochromocytoma, 657
      in Raynaud's disease, 705
   and ulcerative colitis, 765
Hypothermia
   in brain injuries, 408
   in toxic epidermal necrolysis,
      752
Hypothyroidism/myxedema,
      475–476, 475–481
   assessment/diagnosis, 478
   body temperature
      management, 478, 479
   bowel function management,
      480
   clinical manifestations,
      475–476
   cognitive management, 480
   complications, 477, 480
   emotional support
      management, 480
   fluid balance management, 477
   gerontologic considerations,
      476
   home/community-based care,
      481

hormonal therapy, 477–478
and hyperthyroidism, 465
medical management, 477–478
nursing interventions, 479–481
outcome expectations, 481
pharmacologic therapy, 477
planning/goals, 479
Hypovolemia
in hemophilia, 431
and peritonitis, 651
Hypovolemic shock
clinical manifestations, 723
fluid balance management, 724
medical management, 723–724
nursing management, 724–725
pharmacologic therapy, 724
Hypoxemia
and diffuse, axonal injuries, 418
and pneumothorax, 672
and pulmonary emphysema, 333
Hypoxia
in acute pancreatitis, 585
cerebral
and CVA, 250, 251
and heart failure, 427
and hemophilia, 432
and larynx cancer, 190
and sickle cell anemia, 52
Hysterectomy
in cervical cancer, 169–170
in ovarian cancer, 209

ICCE. *See* Intracapsular cataract extraction (ICCE)
ICP. *See* Increased intracranial pressure (ICP)
Idiopathic thrombocytopenia purpura (ITP), 482–484
Ileus, paralytic, and diarrhea, 316

Imaging studies. *See* Angiograms; Computed tomography (CT) scan; Magnetic resonance imaging (MRI); Positron-emission tomography; Ultrasonography; X-ray studies
Immunoelectrophoresis, in nephrotic syndrome, 562
Immunomodulators, for AIDS, 7
Immunosuppressive therapy
for anemia, aplastic, 41
for infective endocarditis, 336
for Kaposi's sarcoma, 494
for myasthenia gravis, 550
for nephrotic syndrome, 563
for pemphigus, 604
Immunotherapy, for renal tumors, 186
Impetigo, 484–486
Impotence
and hypopituitarism, 474
and sickle cell anemia, 53
Incontinence, and cystitis, 292
Increased intracranial pressure (ICP), 407, 486–492
airway management, 489, 490
assessment, 487, 488–489
clinical manifestations, 486–487
collaborative problems/complications, 489–490, 492
diagnosis, 487, 489
fluid balance management, 491
infection prevention, 491
in intracerebral hemorrhage/hematoma, 412
medical management, 487–488
in meningitis, 525
pharmacologic therapy, 488
and SIADH, 489
and unconsciousness, 488–492

Indigestion, in hepatitis A, 438
Infarctions
 of brain, and Alzheimer's
  disease, 26
 of central nervous system, and
  DIC, 321
 pulmonary, and pleurisy, 663
Infections
 in AIDS, 6, 13
 in anemia, aplastic, 41
 in anemia, sickle cell, 51, 52
 in bone tumors, 101, 103–104
 bronchopulmonary, in COPD,
  271
 in burn injuries, 128
 in cancer, 139, 141
  of breast, 163
  of larynx, 190
  of oral cavity, 207
 in chronic lymphocytic
  leukemia, 506
 in Cushing's syndrome, 288,
  289
 dental, and brain abscess,
  108
 in epididymitis, 331
 in epistaxis, 350
 in fulminant hepatic failure,
  437
 hematogenous, in
  osteomyelitis, 573
 in Huntington's disease,
  451
 in increased intracranial
  pressure, 491
 in leukemia, 498, 500
 in mastoiditis, 517, 518
 in meningitis, 528
 in morbid obesity, 565
 in myocarditis, 560
 in pemphigus, 605
 in pharyngitis, 653
 in pruritus, 678
 in psoriasis, 684
 pulmonary, and bronchiectasis,
  114
 in renal failure, acute, 712

 respiratory tract, and
  bronchitis, 115
 in mitral stenosis, 530
 of urinary tract, 157
 in multiple sclerosis, 536
Infective endocarditis, 336–339
Influenza, 492–493
Injury reduction
 in Cushing's syndrome, 289
 in epilepsy, 347
 in hepatic cirrhosis, 277
 in multiple sclerosis, 539
 in osteoporosis, 580
Insulin
 administering, 310
 problems with, 310–311
 for Type 1 diabetes, 302
Integumentary disorders, in
  AIDS, 4, 9, 10, 12
Interferon, for renal tumors, 186
Intermittent positive-pressure
  breathing (IPPB)
 in chronic obstructive
  pulmonary disorder, 270
Intracapsular cataract extraction
  (ICCE), 246
Intracerebral hemorrhages, 248,
  412
Intracranial aneurysm, 58–63
 anxiety management, 61
 assessment, 58, 59–60
 clinical manifestations, 58
 complications, 61
 diagnosis, 58, 60
 medical management, 58–59
 nursing interventions, 60–62
 outcome expectations, 62–63
 planning/goals, 60
 self-care, 62
Intracranial hemorrhage,
  410–411
Intralesional therapy, for
  psoriasis, 683
Intraocular lens (IOL) implants,
  246
Intraocular pressure (IOP), 382,
  383, 384, 385

Intravenous pyelogram (IVP)
  for hypertension, 457
  for ovarian cancer, 209
Intravenous therapy
  for gastritis, 380
  for lung abscess, 513
  for small bowel obstruction, 107
Intravenous urography (IVU), in cervical cancer, 169
IOL implants. *See* Intraocular lens (IOL) implants
IOP. *See* Intraocular pressure (IOP)
IPPB. *See* Intermittent positive-pressure breathing (IPPB)
Iron-deficiency anemia, 36
Irritability
  and brain injuries, 408
  and hyperthyroidism, 461–462
  and hypoparathyroidism, 472
  and migraine headaches, 402
  and nephrotic syndrome, 562
Ischemia, and sickle cell anemia, 52
Ischemic strokes, 248–260
Itching. *See* Pruritus
ITP. *See* Idiopathic thrombocytopenia purpura (ITP)
IVP. *See* Intravenous pyelogram (IVP)
IVU. *See* Intravenous urography (IVU)

Jaundice
  in acute pancreatitis, 585
  in anemia, 36
  in anemia, sickle cell, 49
  in cholecystitis, 262, 265–266
  in fulminant hepatic failure, 437
  in hepatic cirrhosis, 274
  in hepatitis A, 438
  in hepatitis B, 440
  in Hodgkin's disease, 448

  in liver cancer, 196
  in ovarian cancer, 212
Joints. *See also* Osteoarthritis
  destruction of, and gout, 393
  dislocations, 545
  immobilization, in musculoskeletal trauma, 547
  pain in, and hemophilia, 430, 431
  in rheumatoid arthritis, 77–78
  subluxations of, 545

Kaposi's sarcoma (KS), 4, 494–496
  assessment/diagnosis, 495
  categories, 494
  and Eastern European ancestry, 494
  and HIV, 494
  medical management, 495
  nursing management, 495–496
  pharmacologic therapy, 495
Kernig's sign, in bacterial meningitis, 526
Kidney disorders
  cancer/tumors, 185–187
  and hypertension, 457
  and perioperative nursing management, 624
  urolithiasis (kidney stones), 780–786
Klebsiella
  and lung abscess, 511
  and peritonitis, 651
  and pneumonia, 665
KS. *See* Kaposi's sarcoma (KS)
Kussmaul respirations, and diabetic ketoacidosis, 313
Kyphosis, in osteomalacia, 570

Laparoscopy
  for pancreatic cancer, 211
  for prostate cancer, 216
Laryngoscopy, for larynx cancer, 188

Larynx cancer, 188–195
  airway management,
    191–192
  anxiety/depression
    management, 191
  assessment, 188, 190
  clinical manifestations, 188
  collaborative problems/
    complications, 190,
    193–194
  diagnosis, 188, 190
  fluid management, 192–193
  home/community-based care,
    194
  medical management,
    189–195
  nursing interventions,
    191–195
  nutrition management, 192
  outcome expectations, 195
  patient education, 191
  planning/goals, 191
  self-care, 194
  speech rehabilitation, 192
Laser therapy
  for cervical cancer, 169
  for esophageal cancer, 181
Latent tetany, and
  hypoparathyroidism,
  472
LATS. *See* Long-acting thyroid
  stimulator (LATS)
Left ventricular dilation/
  hypertrophy, 68
Left-sided heart failure
  backward failure, 421–422
  forward failure, 422
Leg ulcers, in sickle cell anemia,
  53
Lentigo-maligna melanomas,
  220, 222
Lesions
  necrotic, of lung parenchyma,
    511
  oral, in pemphigus, 604
  of skin
    in cancer, 143–144

    in impetigo, 485
    in psoriasis, 681
  subcutaneous, and KS, 494
Lethargy
  and brain injuries, 408
  and increased intracranial
    pressure, 487
Leukemia, 497–504
  acute myeloid (AML),
    507–509
  anxiety management, 502
  assessment, 497, 498
  bleeding management,
    499–500
  body image management, 502
  chronic lymphocytic (CLL),
    506–507
  chronic myelogenous (CML),
    509–511
  clinical manifestations, 497
  diagnosis, 497, 498–499
  electrolyte management,
    501–502
  fatigue management, 502
  fluid balance management,
    498, 501–502
  gerontologic considerations,
    497–498
  home/community-based care,
    503
  infection prevention, 500
  and intracerebral hemorrhage/
    hematomas, 412
  mucositis management, 500
  nursing interventions,
    499–504
  nutrition management, 498,
    501
  oral hygiene management,
    500, 501
  outcome expectations, 504
  pain management, 501
  planning/goals, 499
  spirituality management, 503
  terminal care, 503–504
Leukocyte esterase test, in
  cystitis, 292

Leukocytosis
  and Addison's disease, 22
  in liver cancer, 196
  in regional enteritis, 706
Leukopenia
  and acute lymphocytic
      leukemia, 505
  in multiple myeloma, 533
Libido, loss of, in Cushing's
      syndrome, 287
Lightheadedness
  and hypoglycemia, 469
  in mitral valve prolapse,
      532
Liver cancer, 195–199, 197
  assessment/diagnosis, 196
  chemotherapy for, 197
  clinical manifestations, 196
  medical management,
      197–199
  nonsurgical modalities, 197
  nursing management,
      198–199
  percutaneous biliary drainage,
      197
  radiation therapy, 197
  surgical management, 198
  transplantation in, 198
Liver disorders
  cancer, 195–199
  cirrhosis, 195–196
      hepatic, 274–278
  enlargement, in hepatitis B,
      440
  hepatitis B/C, 196
  and perioperative nursing
      management, 624
Liver function tests
  for bleeding esophageal
      varices, 352
  for hepatic cirrhosis, 275
Living wills, 32
Long-acting thyroid stimulator
      (LATS), 461
Loop electrosurgical excision
      procedure (LEEP), for
      cervical cancer, 169

Low back pain, 90–94
  assessment, 90–91
  body mechanics promotion,
      93–94
  clinical manifestations, 90
  diagnosis, 90–91, 92
  medical management, 91–94
  nursing interventions, 92–94
  nutrition management, 92, 93
  outcome expectations, 94
  pain management, 92
  pharmacologic therapy, 91
  planning/goals, 92
  socialization management, 93
Lumpectomy, for breast cancer,
      161
Lung abscess, 511–513
Lung cancer, 200–202
  assessment/diagnosis, 201
  causation, 200
  clinical manifestations,
      200–201
  fatigue management, 202
  medical management, 201
  nursing management, 202
  types of, 200
Lung crackles, and
      glomerulonephritis, 389
Lyme disease, and meningitis,
      525
Lymphadenopathy, cervical, 233
Lymphadenopathy, in chronic
      lymphocytic leukemia,
      506
Lymphangiography, for prostate
      cancer, 214
Lymphatic disorders
  in AIDS, 4
  in anemia, aplastic, 41
  in breast cancer, 163
  Hodgkin's disease, 447–450
Lymphedema
  and elephantiasis, 513–515
  and Kaposi's sarcoma, 494
Lymphocytosis, in chronic
      lymphocytic leukemia,
      506

Lymphokine-activated killer (LAK) cells, for renal tumors, 186
Lymphomas
  B-cell, 4, 5
  and exfoliative dermatitis, 355
  non-Hodgkin's, in AIDS, 4

MAC. See Mycobacterium avium complex (MAC)
Macrovascular disease, and diabetes mellitus, 302
Magnetic resonance imaging (MRI)
  for Alzheimer's disease, 27
  for amyotrophic lateral sclerosis, 32
  in aortic aneurysm, 56
  for aortic insufficiency, 69
  for bone tumors, 100
  for brain abscess, 108
  for brain injuries, 409
  for brain tumors, 112
  for cancer, 137
    of cervix, 168–169
    of larynx, 188
    of liver, 196
    of lungs, 201
    of thyroid, 233–234
  for Cushing's syndrome, 287
  for epilepsy, 345
  for hepatic cirrhosis, 275
  for Huntington's disease, 450, 451
  for increased intracranial pressure, 487
  for ischemic stroke, 250
  for low back pain, 91
  for migraine headaches, 403
  for multiple sclerosis, 536
  for osteomyelitis, 573
  for pancreatic cancer, 211
  for pericarditis, 616
  for pituitary tumors, 661
MAI. See Mycobacterium avium intracellulare (MAI)

Malabsorption, in chronic pancreatitis, 592
Malaise
  in acute glomerulonephritis, 386
  in hepatitis B, 440
  in myocarditis, 561
  in nephrotic syndrome, 562
  in pelvic infection, 601
  in pharyngitis, 654
Malignant melanoma. See Skin cancer
Malnutrition
  and Alzheimer's disease, 26
  and impetigo, 484
Mastoiditis, 516–520
  in acute otitis media, 582
  anxiety management, 518
  assessment/diagnosis, 517
  and brain abscess, 108
  clinical manifestations, 516
  hearing/communication management, 518
  home/community-based care, 519
  infection management, 517, 518
  medical management, 516
  outcome expectations, 520
  pain management, 518
  patient education, 519
  and pharyngitis, 653
  planning/goals, 517–518
  sensory perception management, 519
  surgical management, 516
McBurney's point, and appendicitis, 71
Medications. See Pharmacologic therapy
Megaloblastic anemia. See Anemia, megaloblastic
Melanomas
  acral-lentiginous, 220–221
  lentigo-maligna, 220
  nodular, 220
  superficial spreading, 220, 221

Melena, in bleeding esophageal varices, 352
Memory defects
and diffuse, axonal injuries, 414
and hypoglycemia, 469
Ménière's disease, 520–525
anxiety management, 524
assessment, 521, 522–523
clinical manifestations
cochlear disease, 521
vestibular disease, 521
complications, 524
diagnosis, 521, 523
disability adjustment, 524
fluid balance management, 524
home/community-based care, 525
medical management, 521–522
nursing interventions, 523–525
nutrition management, 522
pharmacologic therapy, 522
planning/goals, 523
surgical management, 522
Meningiomas, 110
Meningitis, 525–529
in acute otitis media, 582
assessment/diagnosis, 527
clinical manifestations, 526–527
fluid balance management, 528
and increased intracranial pressure, 525
infection control, 528
medical management, 527–528
nursing management, 528–529
pathophysiology, 525–526
pharmacologic therapy, 527–528
and pharyngitis, 653
prevention, 527
types
bacterial, 525, 526
meningococcal, 526–527

Meningococcal meningitis, 526–527
Menorrhagia, and hypothyroidism, 476
Metabolic disorders
and chronic renal failure, 715
and headaches, 401
hypermetabolism, in pheochromocytoma, 657
in hypovolemic shock, 723
in morbid obesity, 565
MG. See Myasthenia gravis (MG)
MI. See Myocardial infarction (MI)
Microvascular disease, and diabetes mellitus, 302
MIDCAB. See Minimally invasive direct coronary artery bypass (MIDCAB)
Migraine headaches
assessment, 403, 404–405
clinical manifestations, 402–403
diagnosis, 403, 405
and ischemic strokes, 248
medical management, 403–407
acute attack, 403–404
nursing interventions, 405–406
outcome expectations, 406
pain management in, 405
pharmacologic therapy, 404
phases
aura phase, 402
headache phase, 402–403
prodrome phase, 402
recovery phase, 403–404
planning/goals, 405
Minimally invasive direct coronary artery bypass (MIDCAB)
for angina pectoris, 65
for myocardial infarction, 556
Mini-Mental Status Examination, for Alzheimer's disease, 27

Mitral valve disorders
  mitral regurgitation
    (insufficiency), 529–530
  mitral stenosis, 530–531
  mitral valve prolapse, 531–533
  and rheumatic endocarditis,
    339
Mobility management
  in burn injuries, 129–130
  in cerebral vascular accidents,
    254–255
  in clinical unit, postoperative,
    639–640
  in Guillain-Barré syndrome,
    398
  in low back pain, 93
  in multiple sclerosis, 539
  in myasthenia gravis, 551–552
  in osteomyelitis, 575
  in Parkinson's disease, 598
  and perioperative nursing
    management, 625
  in rheumatoid arthritis, 81
  in spinal cord injury, 734
Monocular diplopia (double
  vision), 245
Moraxella catarrhalis, and acute
  otitis media, 581
Morbid obesity, 564–566
Mortality
  and acute pancreatitis, 586
  and cholecystitis, 262
MRI. *See* Magnetic resonance
  imaging (MRI)
Mucositis management
  in cancer, of oral cavity, 206
  in leukemia, 498, 499, 500
Mucous membranes
  in AIDS, 9
  oral, in unconsciousness,
    777
Multiple myeloma, 533–534
Multiple organ dysfunction
  syndrome, 591
Multiple sclerosis, 534–542
  assessment/diagnosis, 536,
    538

  bowel/bladder function
    management, 537–538,
    540
  clinical manifestations,
    535–536
  cognitive management, 538,
    540
  complications, 536
  coping management, 540
  disease course, 535
  home/community-based care,
    541
  injury prevention, 539
  medical management,
    537–538
  mobility management, 539
  nursing interventions,
    539–542
  outcome expectations, 541
  pathophysiology, 535
  pharmacologic therapy, 537
  planning/goals, 538–539
  relapses, 536
  self-care, 540–541
  sensory perception
    management, 540
  sexual function/dysfunction,
    538, 541
  speech management, 541
  swallowing management,
    541
Muscular dystrophies, 542–544
Musculoskeletal system
  primary neoplasms
    bone cysts, 98
    fibromas, 98
    osteochondroma, 98
    osteoid osteoma, 98
    rhabdomyoma, 98
  trauma, 544–548
    assessment/diagnosis, 546
    cast care, 547
    clinical manifestations, 546
    medical management,
      546–547
    nursing management,
      547–548

pain management, 547
stages, 547
types, 545
Myalgia, in pneumonia, 666
Myasthenia gravis
aspiration prevention, 552
communication management,
552
eye care in, 552
home/community-based care,
553–554
mobility management,
551–552
outcome expectation, 555
respiratory management, 551
self-care, 553–554
Myasthenia gravis (MG),
548–554
assessment, 549, 550
clinical manifestations, 548
complications
cholinergic crisis, 549
myasthenic crisis, 549
diagnosis, 549, 550–551
medical management,
549–550
anticholinesterase
medications, 550
immunosuppressive therapy,
550
Mycobacterium avium complex
(MAC), 2
*Mycobacterium avium
intracellulare* (MAI), 2
Mycotic aneurysms, 337
Myelography, for bone tumors,
100
Myocardial infarction (MI),
554–560
and angina pectoris, 66
anxiety management, 558, 559
and arteriosclerosis, 76
assessment, 555, 556–557
and atherosclerosis, 76
cardiac rehabilitation for, 559
clinical manifestations,
554–555

complications, 557
diagnosis, 555, 557
gerontologic considerations,
555
home/community-based care,
559
medical management,
555–556
nursing interventions,
558–559
outcome expectations,
559–560
oxygen administration, 555,
558
pain management, 558
pharmacologic therapy, 556
planning/goals, 557–558
Myocardial ischemia, 284
Myocardial rupture
in angina pectoris, 66
in myocardial infarction,
557
Myocarditis, 560–561
Myringotomy (tympanotomy), in
acute otitis media, 582
Myxedema, and hypothyroidism,
475–481

N. meningitidis (meningococcal
meningitis), 525–526
Nausea
in acute pancreatitis, 585
in diabetes mellitus, 301
in diabetic ketoacidosis, 313
in endometriosis, 341
in gastritis, 379
in glaucoma, 383
monitoring of, in PACU,
632
in myocarditis, 561
in pelvic infection, 601
in peritonitis, 652
in pheochromocytoma, 657
and radiation therapy, 449
Necrosis
of pancreas, 590
of pituitary, 474

Neoplasms
  malignant, in cancer, 136, 220
  primary
    bone cysts, 98
    fibromas, 98
    osteochondroma, 98
    osteoid osteoma, 98
    rhabdomyoma, 98
Nephrectomy, radical, for renal
      tumors, 186
Nephritis, and pharyngitis, 653
Nephrotic syndrome, 562–563
Nephrotomograms, for renal
      tumors, 186
Nervousness, and hypoglycemia,
      469
Neurologic disorders
  in AIDS, 3, 9
  in anemia, megaloblastic,
      47
Neurologic examination, for
      brain injuries, 409
Neuromas, acoustic, 110
Neuropathies
  in cerebral vascular accidents,
      254
  in diabetes mellitus, 299
  peripheral, and
      glomerulonephritis, 389
Night sweats, in empyema, 334
Nocturia
  and cystitis, 292
  and glomerulonephritis, 389
  and heart failure, 422
  and hypertension, 458
Nodular melanomas, 220, 222
Noncardiogenic pulmonary
      edema. See Acute
      respiratory distress
      syndrome
Non-Hodgkin's lymphoma, 4
Nosebleed (epistaxis), 350–351
  and hypertension, 458
NSAID drops, for cataracts, 247
Nuchal rigidity (neck stiffness),
      in bacterial meningitis,
      526

Numbness
  in diabetes mellitus, 300
  in extremities, in peripheral
      arterial occlusive disease,
      648
  in migraine headaches, 402
  in multiple sclerosis, 535
  in Raynaud's disease, 704
Nurses, postoperative anesthesia
      care unit, 631–632
Nursing management. See
      Perioperative nursing
      management;
      Postoperative nursing
      management
Nutrition management
  in acute pancreatitis, 589
  in acute respiratory distress
      syndrome, 19
  in AIDS, 8, 14
  in Alzheimer's disease, 29
  in anemia, 38, 39
    iron-deficiency, 44
    megaloblastic, 47
  in bone tumors, 101, 103
  in burn injuries, 128
  in cancer, 140, 144
    colorectal, 176–177
    of larynx, 192–193
    of oral cavity, 206
    of stomach, 228–229
  in cholelithiasis/cholecystitis,
      263, 265
  in chronic renal failure, 717
  in clinical unit, postoperative,
      637–638
  in cystitis, 295
  in diabetes mellitus, 303,
      307–308
  in diffuse axonal injuries, 415,
      416
  in esophageal cancer, 183–184
  in gastritis, 380
  in glomerulonephritis, 387
  in gout, 393
  in Guillain-Barré syndrome,
      398–399

in hepatic cirrhosis, 275, 277
in hepatic coma/hepatic encephalopathy, 436
in hepatitis A, 439
in hepatitis B, 441
in hiatal hernia, 445–446
in hypertension, 460
in hyperthyroidism, 466
in hypoglycemia, 471
in hypoparathyroidism, 473, 474
in leukemia, 498, 501
in low back pain, 02, 93
in Ménière's disease, 522
in nephrotic syndrome, 563
in peptic ulcer, 610, 612–613
perioperative nursing, 623
in pneumonia, 669
in pulmonary tuberculosis, 762
for skin integrity promotion, 128–129
in ulcerative colitis, 766, 770
in unconsciousness, 777
in urolithiasis, 782–783

OA. *See* Osteoarthritis (OA)
Obesity
and coronary atherosclerosis/ artery disease, 283
and Cushing's syndrome, 286
and diabetes mellitus, 301
and low back pain, 90
morbid, 564–566
and osteoarthritis, 567
and pituitary tumors, 660
Occupational therapy, for anemia, megaloblastic, 47
Oliguria
in heart failure, 422
in hypovolemic shock, 723
Open angle glaucoma, 382
Open fractures, 364–365
Open pneumothorax, 673
Ophthalmoscopy
for cataracts, 246
for glaucoma, 383

Oral cavity cancer, 203–208
assessment, 203, 204
clinical manifestations, 203
communication management, 207
diagnosis, 203, 204
fluid management, 206
home/community-based care, 207–208
infection management, 207
medical management, 203–208
mouth care management, 205–206
nutrition management, 206
outcome expectations, 208
planning/goals, 204
risk factors, 203
Oropharyngeal cancer, 137
Orthopnea, and aortic insufficiency, 68
Orthostatic hypotension, in Parkinson's disease, 595
Osmotic diuresis, in HHNS, 453
Osteoarthritis (OA), 567–569
assessment/diagnosis, 567
categories
primary (idiopathic), 567
secondary, 567
clinical manifestations, 567
medical management, 568
nursing management, 569
pharmacologic therapy, 568
Osteochondroma, 98
Osteogenic sarcoma, 98
Osteoid osteoma, 98
Osteomalacia, 569–572
assessment, 570, 571
clinical manifestations, 570
diagnosis, 570, 571
gerontologic considerations, 570
nursing interventions, 571–572
pain management, 571
risk factors, 569
and Vitamin D, 569, 570

Osteomyelitis, 572–576
  assessment, 573, 574
  diagnosis, 573
  and diffuse axonal injuries, 414
  and hematogenous infection, 573
  home/community-based care, 575–576
  infection management, 575
  medical management, 573–574
  mobility management, 575
  nursing interventions, 574–576
  outcome expectations, 576
  pain management, 574–575
  planning/goals, 574
Osteoporosis, 576–581
  assessment, 577, 578
  bowel management, 580
  diagnosis, 577, 579
  exercise management, 578
  gerontologic considerations, 577–578
  and hyperthyroidism, 462
  and idiopathic thrombocytopenia purpura, 484
  injury reduction, 580
  medical management, 578
  nursing interventions, 579–580
  outcome expectations, 581
  pain management, 580
  patient education, 579
  and pituitary tumors, 660
  planning/goals, 579
  risk factors, 577, 578
  vertebral fractures, 578
  Vitamin D in, 577, 580
Otitis media. *See also* Myringotomy
  acute, 581–582
  and brain abscess, 108
  chronic, 583–584
  and mastoiditis, 516
  and pharyngitis, 653

Otorrhea (middle ear discharge)
Otorrhea (middle ear discharge), in mastoiditis, 516, 517
Ovarian cancer, 208–210
Oxygen administration
  in anaphylaxis, 34–35
  in bleeding esophageal varices, 353
  in cardiomyopathies, 243
  in cerebral vascular accidents, 251, 254
  in chronic obstructive pulmonary disorder, 268, 272
  in epilepsy, 345
  in migraine headaches, 404
  in myocardial infarction, 555, 558
  in peritonitis, 652
  in pneumonia, 667
  in pulmonary edema, 688, 694
  in thyroid storm, 747

PACU. *See* Postanesthesia care unit (PACU)
Pain management
  in acute pancreatitis, 589
  in AIDS, 14
  in angina pectoris, 66–67
  in bone tumors, 102
  in Buerger's disease, 117–118
  in burn injuries
    acute/intermediate phase, 129
    emergent/resuscitative phase, 124
  in cancer
    of breast, 165
    of cervix, 171
    of kidneys, 187
    of oral cavity, 206
    of ovaries, 212
    of prostate, 217
    of skin, 224
    of stomach, 229
  in cerebral vascular accidents, 256

in cholecystectomy, 265
in clinical unit, postoperative, 636
in diverticular disorders, 329
in gastritis, 380, 381
in hemophilia, 432
in hiatal hernia, 446
in hip fractures, 372–373
in leukemia, 501
in low back pain, 92
in mastoiditis, 518
in migraine headaches, 405
in multiple sclerosis, 535
in musculoskeletal trauma, 547
in myocardial infarction, 558
oral, in pemphigus, 605–606
in osteomalacia, 577
in osteomyelitis, 574–575
in osteoporosis, 580
in peptic ulcers, 609, 612–613
in pericarditis, 618–619
in pulmonary edema, 694
in renal tumors, 185
in rheumatoid arthritis, 80–81
in sickle cell anemia, 50, 53
in toxic epidermal necrolysis, 752
in ulcerative colitis, 769–770
in urolithiasis, 784
Palpitations
in hypoglycemia, 469
in mitral regurgitation, 529
in mitral valve prolapse, 532
in thyroid storm, 747
Palsies, focal nerve, 414
Pancreatic cancer, 210–213
Pancreatitis, acute, 585–591
assessment/diagnosis, 586, 588
clinical manifestations, 585–586
collaborative problems/ complications, 588
pancreatic cancer, 210–211
pancreatic necrosis, 590

shock/multiple organ dysfunction syndrome, 591
fluid/electrolyte management, 590
gerontologic considerations, 586
home/community-based care, 591
medical management
acute phase, 587
postacute phase, 587
nursing interventions, 589–591
nutrition management, 589
outcome expectations, 591
pain management, 589
and pancreatic cancer, 210–211
planning/goals, 588
Pancreatitis, chronic, 592–593
Panhypopituitarism (Simmond's disease), 474
Panlobular pulmonary emphysema, 333
Pap smear, in cervical cancer, 168
Papillary adenocarcinoma, 233
Papilledema, and brain tumors, 111
Paraesophageal hiatal hernia. See Hiatal hernia
Paresthesias
and anemia, 38, 39
and diarrhea, 317
and polycythemia, 674
Parkinson's disease, 594–600
assessment, 595, 596–597
assistive devices management, 598
bowel management, 598
clinical manifestations, 594–595
communication management, 599
diagnosis, 595, 597
home/community-based care, 599–600

Parkinson's disease (*Contd.*)
  medical management, 595
  mobility management, 598
  nursing interventions,
    598–600
  outcome expectations, 600
  pathophysiology, 594
  pharmacologic therapy, 596
  planning/goals, 597–598
  swallowing management, 599
Paroxysmal hemicrania, 401
Paroxysmal nocturna dyspnea, 68
Partial thromboplastin time
    (PTT), in DIC, 321
Patient education
  in AIDS, 10
  in bone tumors, 102
  in breast cancer, 164
  in COPD, 272
  in diabetes mellitus, 307
  in Guillain-Barré syndrome,
    399
  in hypertension, 459
  in large bowel obstruction,
    105
  in larynx cancer, 191
  in mastoiditis, 519
  in mitral valve prolapse, 532
  in multiple myeloma, 534
  in myasthenia gravis, 551
  in osteoporosis, 579
  and perioperative nursing
    management, 626
  in rheumatoid arthritis, 82, 83
  in sickle cell anemia, 52
  in skin cancer, 225
PCI. *See* Percutaneous coronary
    intervention (PCI)
PEEP. *See* Positive end-expiratory
    pressure (PEEP)
Pelvic infection (pelvic
    inflammatory disease),
    600–603
Pelvis fractures, 368–369
Pemphigus, 603–607
  anxiety management, 606
  assessment/diagnosis, 604, 605

clinical manifestations, 604
collaborative problems/
    complications, 605
fluid/electrolyte management,
    607
home/community-based care,
    607
medical management,
    604–607
nursing interventions,
    605–606
oral discomfort management,
    605–606
outcome expectations, 607
pathophysiology, 603–604
planning/goals, 605
skin integrity management,
    606
Peptic ulcer, 607–615
  anxiety management, 612, 613
  assessment, 609, 611–612
  clinical manifestations, 609
  collaborative problems/
    complications, 612, 613
  diagnosis, 609, 612
  home/community-based care,
    614
  nursing interventions,
    612–615
  nutrition management,
    612–613
  outcome expectations, 615
  pain management, 609,
    612–613
  perforation management, 613
  planning/goals, 612
  predisposition factors, 608
  surgical management, 611
Percutaneous biliary drainage
  for cancer
    of liver, 197
    of pancreas, 211
Percutaneous coronary
    intervention (PCI), 556
Percutaneous transhepatic
    cholangiography (PTC),
    262

Percutaneous transluminal
coronary angioplasty
(PTCA)
for angina pectoris, 65
for arteriosclerosis/
atherosclerosis, 77
Perforation, in peptic ulcers,
613
Perfusion management
in anemia, 39
in angina pectoris, 66
in DIC, 324
in diffuse axonal injuries,
414
in heart failure, 421
in increased intracranial
pressure, 490–491
in intracranial aneurysm,
60–61
in myocardial infarction, 558
Pericardial effusion
in angina pectoris, 66
in cancer, 141
in heart failure, 424
in myocardial infarction, 557
in pericarditis, 618, 619
Pericarditis, 615–619
assessment/diagnosis, 618
clinical manifestations, 616
collaborative problems/
complications, 618, 619
medical management,
616–617
in myocardial infarction, 557
and myocarditis, 560
nursing interventions,
618–619
outcome expectations, 619
pain management, 618–619
pharmacologic therapy, 617
planning/goals, 618
Perimetry, for glaucoma, 383
Perioperative nursing
management, 619–630
of ambulatory surgical
patients, 626
anxiety management, 623

assessment
ambulatory surgery, 622
inpatient surgery, 621–622
diagnoses, 622
elderly patients, special needs,
629
fluid balance management,
623–624
gerontologic consideration,
622
hepatic/renal function support,
624–625
and mobility management, 625
nursing interventions,
623–630
nursing management, 620
nutrition management,
623–624
operating room transport, 628
outcome expectations, 630
patient education, 626
bowel surgery preparation,
627–628
deep breathing/coughing
exercises, 627
pain management, 627
surgery preparation, 628
planning/goals, 622
preoperative concerns,
619–620
and spirituality management,
625–626
Peripheral arterial occlusive
disease, 647–651
assessment/diagnosis, 649
circulation promotion/
maintenance, 649–650
clinical manifestations, 648
complications management,
650
home/community-based care,
650–651
medical management, 649
nursing management, 649–651
Peripheral neuropathy
AIDS-related, 3
and glomerulonephritis, 389

Peritonitis, 651–653
  in appendicitis, 72
  in cholecystitis, 262
  in colorectal cancer, 175
  in diverticular disorders, 329
  in morbid obesity, 565
  peritoneal aspiration, 652
  in sepsis, 651
Peritonsillar abscess, and
      pharyngitis, 653
PET. *See* Positron-emission
      tomography (PET)
Pharmacologic therapy
  for AIDS, 6–7
  for anaphylaxis, 35
  for angina pectoris, 65
  for asthma, 85
  in bleeding esophageal varices,
      353
  for cholelithiasis/cholecystitis,
      263
  for chronic myelogenous
      leukemia, 510
  for cystitis, 293
  for endometriosis, 342
  for epilepsy, 345–346
  for glaucoma, 384
  for glomerulonephritis, 387
  for Guillain-Barré syndrome,
      396
  for heart failure, 423
  for hyperthyroidism, 464
  for hypothyroidism/
      myxedema, 477
  for hypovolemic shock, 724
  for idiopathic
      thrombocytopenia
      purpura, 483
  for impetigo, 485
  for increased intracranial
      pressure, 488
  for Kaposi's sarcoma, 495
  for low back pain, 91
  for lung abscess, 512–513
  for lymphedema/elephantiasis,
      514
  for Ménière's disease, 522
  for meningitis, 527–528
  for migraine headaches, 404
  for morbid obesity, 564
  for multiple sclerosis, 537
  for myocardial infarction, 556
  for nephrotic syndrome, 563
  for osteoarthritis, 568
  for Parkinson's disease, 596
  for peptic ulcers, 610–611
  for pericarditis, 617
  for pulmonary edema, 688
  for pulmonary tuberculosis,
      760–761
  for renal failure, chronic,
      715–716
  for systemic lupus
      erythematosus, 741
  for transient ischemic attack,
      755
  for trigeminal neuralgia, 757
  for ulcerative colitis, 766
  for urolithiasis, 782–783
  for vein disorders, 789
Pharyngitis
  acute, 653–655
  chronic, 655–656
Pheochromocytoma, 656–659
  assessment/diagnosis,
      657–658
  clinical manifestations, 657
  five H's of, 657
  medical management, 658
  nursing management, 658–659
  paroxysmal form, 657
Phlebothrombosis, 787–792
  clinical manifestations, 788
  diagnosis, 790
  medical management, 789
  nursing management, 790–792
  pharmacologic therapy, 789
  prevention, 789
  risk factors, 788
  surgical management, 789
Phlebotomy, for polycythemia,
      675
Photochemotherapy, for
      psoriasis, 683–684

Photodynamic therapy
  for brain tumors, 113
  for cancer, 156
    of breast, 161
Photophobia
  in bacterial meningitis, 526
  and hypoparathyroidism, 472
Physical therapy
  for anemia, megaloblastic, 47
  for anemia, sickle cell, 50, 52
  for chronic obstructive
      pulmonary disease, 270
  for Guillain-Barré syndrome,
      398
  for myasthenia gravis, 551
Pituitary adenomas, and brain
      tumors, 111
Pituitary disorders
  hypopituitarism, 474–475,
      660
  panhypopituitarism, 474
  pituitary adenomas, 111
  pituitary tumors, 659–661
  postpartum pituitary necrosis,
      474
Plasmapheresis
  for glomerulonephritis, 387
  for myasthenia gravis, 550
  for pemphigus, 604
Pleural effusion, 661–663, 668
Pleural pain, in empyema, 334
Pleurisy, 663–665
PML. *See* Progressive multifocal
      leukoencephalopathy
      (PML)
Pneumonia, 665–670
  activity tolerance, 669
  airway management, 668, 669
  and Alzheimer's disease, 26
  assessment, 666, 667–668
  in chronic obstructive
      pulmonary disorder,
      267
  clinical manifestations, 666
  collaborative problems/
      complications, 668,
      669–670

community-acquired (CAP),
    665
  diagnosis, 666, 668
  and diffuse axonal injuries,
      416, 418
  fluid balance management,
      669
  gerontologic considerations,
      666–667
  home care, 670
  home/community-based care,
      670
  hospital-acquired (HAP), 665
  in Huntington's disease, 451
  medical management, 667
  in morbid obesity, 565
  in multiple sclerosis, 536
  nursing interventions,
      669–670
  nutrition management, 669
  pathophysiology, 665
  and pharyngitis, 653
  planning/goals, 668
  and pleural effusion, 662
  and pleurisy, 663
  Pneumocystis carinii
      pneumonia, 6
  in rheumatic endocarditis,
      339
Pneumothorax
  in COPD, 267
  and hemothorax, 670–673
  open, 673
  tension, 672
Polycythemia, 674–675
  and pituitary tumors, 660
  primary, 674
  secondary, 674
Polydipsia
  and diabetes insipidus, 297
  and diabetes mellitus, 300
  and diabetic ketoacidosis, 313
Polyphagia, and diabetes
      mellitus, 300
Polyradiculoneuritis
      (Guillain-Barré
      syndrome), 394–400

Polyuria
  and diabetes insipidus, 297
  and diabetes mellitus, 300
  and diabetic ketoacidosis, 313
  and pheochromocytoma, 657
  and pituitary tumors, 660
Portal encephalopathy, 434
Positive end-expiratory pressure
    (PEEP)
  for acute respiratory distress
      syndrome, 19
  for pulmonary edema, 688
Positron-emission tomography
    (PET)
  for brain tumors, 112
  for cancer, 137
  for Hodgkin's disease, 449
  for increased intracranial
      pressure, 487
  for larynx cancer, 188
  for liver cancer, 196
  for Parkinson's disease, 595
Postanesthesia care unit (PACU),
    630–631
Postoperative nursing
    management, 630–647
  airway management, 635
  body temperature
      management, 636–637
  cardiovascular stability
      maintenance, 635–636
  in clinical unit, 634–646
  complications, monitoring/
      prevention, 642–645
    of DVT, 642
    of hemorrhages, 643–644
    of hypotension/shock,
        642–643
    wound management,
        644–645
  emotional support promotion,
      641
  environmental safety
      maintenance, 641
  fluid management, 640
  gastrointestinal assessment,
      637–638

  gerontologic considerations,
      646–647
  and home care, 633
  home/community-based care,
      645–646
  mental status assessment, 637
  mobility management,
      639–640
  nurses role, 631–632
  nutrition management,
      637–638
  pain management, 636
  in postanesthesia care unit
      (PACU), 630–631
  for pulmonary edema, 694
  in same day surgery, 632–633
  self-care promotion, 640–641
  voluntary voiding assessment/
      management, 638–639
Postpartum pituitary necrosis
    (Sheehan's syndrome),
    474
Pregnancy, ectopic, and pelvic
    infection, 603
Prevention
  of cardiogenic shock, 722
  of diabetes mellitus, 301
  of hepatitis B, 440
  of pulmonary edema, 690, 693
Priapism, in sickle cell anemia, 53
Primary polycythemia, 674
Proctosigmoidoscopy
  for ovarian cancer, 209
  for regional enteritis, 706
Progressive multifocal
    leukoencephalopathy
    (PML), 3
Prolonged prothrombin time
    (PT), in DIC, 321
Prostate cancer, 213–220
  assessment, 214, 216
  clinical manifestations,
      213–214
  collaborative problems/
      complications, 217,
      218–219
  diagnosis, 214, 216

digital rectal examination in, 214
home/community-based care, 219–220
hormone therapy, 215
medical management, 214–220
outcome expectations, 220
pain management in, 217
PSA levels in, 214
radiation therapy, 215
radical prostatectomy, 214–215
nursing process, 216–220
patient preparation, 218
transurethral resection in, 215–216
Prostate disorders
benign prostatic hyperplasia, 96–98
cancer, 156, 213–220
and epididymitis, 331
Prostate-specific antigen (PSA) levels, 214
Prostatitis, 676–678
Prostration, and exfoliative dermatitis, 355
Proteinuria, and glomerulonephritis, 387
Proteus, and bone infections, 572
Pruritus (itching), 678–680
in Hodgkin's disease, 448
in hyperthyroidism, 462
in polycythemia, 675
Pseudomonas
and bone infections, 572
and peritonitis, 651
and pneumonia, 665
Psoriasis, 680–686
assessment, 681, 684
clinical manifestations, 681
collaborative problems/ complications, 684
diagnosis, 681, 684
and exfoliative dermatitis, 355
home/community-based care, 686

medical management, 682–684
intralesional therapy, 683
photochemotherapy, 683–684
systemic therapy: oral/injectable, 683
topical therapy, 682
nursing interventions, 684–686
outcome expectations, 686
pathophysiology, 680–681
planning/goals, 684
psychological considerations, 681
and rheumatoid arthritis, 680
skin integrity management, 685
Psychological support
in lung cancer, 202
in psoriasis, 681
in stomach cancer, 229
Psychosis, in Parkinson's disease, 595
PT. *See* Prolonged prothrombin time (PT)
PTC. *See* Percutaneous transhepatic cholangiography (PTC)
PTCA. *See* Percutaneous transluminal coronary angioplasty (PTCA)
PTT. *See* Partial thromboplastin time (PTT)
Pulmonary edema, 687–689
acute, in angina pectoris, 66
anxiety management, 694
assessment/diagnosis, 687–688
clinical manifestations, 687
and glomerulonephritis, 386
and heart failure, 421
home/community-based care, 694–695
medical management, 688
nursing management, 689
pain management, 694

Pulmonary edema (*Contd.*)
pharmacologic therapy, 688
postoperative nursing care,
694
Pulmonary embolism, 689–695
assessment, 690, 692
clinical manifestations, 690
diagnosis, 690, 692–693
in DIC, 323
medical management
anticoagulation therapy,
691, 693–694
thrombolytic therapy,
691–692, 693–694
nursing interventions,
693–695
planning/goals, 693
preventive measures, 690,
693
surgical management, 692
Pulmonary heart disease,
695–698
clinical manifestations, 696
medical management,
696–697
nursing management,
697–698
Pulmonary hypertension,
698–700
Pulmonary resection
(lobectomy), in lung
abscess, 512
Pulse, irregular
and mitral regurgitation,
529
and mitral stenosis, 531
Pulse oximetry
for hyperthyroidism, 467
by nurse, in PACU, 632
for pulmonary emphysema,
333
Pulsus alternans, in myocarditis,
560
Purpura, in aplastic anemia, 41
Pyelonephritis
acute, 701–702
chronic, 702–703

Pyloric obstruction, in gastritis,
379
Pyrosis (heartburn), in peptic
ulcers, 609
Pyuria
and cystitis, 292
and epididymitis, 331

RA. *See* Rheumatoid arthritis (RA)
Radiation exposure, and
cataracts, 245
Radiation therapy
for brain tumors, 113
for cancer, 138
of bladder, 158
of head/neck, 475
of kidneys, 186
of larynx, 189
of liver, 197
of lungs, 201
nursing management,
151–152
or esophagus, 197
of ovaries, 210, 212
of prostate, 215
for esophagitis, 449
external beam, for breast
cancer, 161
for Hodgkin's disease, 449
for hypopituitarism, 474
for pruritus, 678
Radical mastectomy, for breast
cancer, 161
Radioactive iodine studies,
233
Radiography
abdominal, for cholecystitis,
262
for empyema, 335
for heart failure, 422
for hiatal hernia, 444
for lung abscess, 512
for Ménière's disease, 521
for osteomalacia, 570
for rheumatoid arthritis, 78
for sickle cell anemia, 50
for stomach cancer, 227

Radioimmunoconjugate, for
cancer, 137
Radioisotope scans, for hepatic
cirrhosis, 275
Radionuclide imaging
for aortic insufficiency, 69
for cancer, of skin, 222
Rash (*N. meningitidis*), in bacterial
meningitis, 526
Raynaud's disease, 78,
704–705
Rectal cancer, in men, 156
Recurrent encephalopathy,
436
Reed-Sternberg cell, and
Hodgkin's disease, 447,
449
Regional enteritis (Crohn's
disease), 705–707
Regurgitation, in hiatal hernia,
444
Renal disorders
adenocarcinoma, 185
cancer, 185–187
in DIC, 321, 323
glomerulonephritis
acute, 386–388
chronic, 388–391
and gout, 393
and leukemia, 498, 499
and sickle cell anemia, 52
Renal failure
in acute pancreatitis, 585
in fulminant hepatic failure,
437
in glomerulonephritis, 386,
389
in osteomalacia, 569
in pheochromocytoma, 657
Renal failure, acute, 707–713
assessment, 708, 710
clinical manifestations, 708
clinical stages, 707–708
collaborative
problems/complications,
711
diagnosis, 708, 710–711

dialysis support, 712–713
fluid/electrolyte management,
711–712
gerontologic considerations,
708–709
infection management, 712
medical management,
709–710
metabolic reduction, 712
nursing interventions,
711–713
pulmonary function
promotion, 712
Renal failure, chronic, 713–718
assessment, 716
clinical manifestations,
713–714
diagnosis, 717
fluid/nutrition management,
717
gerontologic considerations,
714
medical management,
714–715
nursing interventions,
717–718
outcome expectations, 718
pharmacologic therapy,
715–716
planning/goals, 717
Renal function tests, 214
Renal insufficiency, in
glomerulonephritis, 389
Reproductive disorders (female),
in AIDS, 4
Respiratory disorders
in AIDS, 2, 9, 10, 11–12
in muscular dystrophies,
543
in myasthenia gravis, 550
in pneumonia, 666
in spinal cord injury, 729
Respiratory distress, and larynx
cancer, 192
Respiratory failure, in
Guillain-Barré syndrome,
397–398

Respiratory management
  in acute pancreatitis, 589–590
  in myasthenia gravis, 551
  in myocardial infarction, 558
  in perioperative nursing, 624
  in spinal cord injury, 733–734
Rest
  for Cushing's syndrome, 290
  for hepatic cirrhosis, 276–278
  for hepatitis A, 439
  for musculoskeletal trauma,
    546
  for myocarditis, 561
  for nephrotic syndrome, 562
  for pelvic infection, 602
Rest, ice, compression, elevation
    (RICE), 546
Restlessness, in cardiac
    tamponade, 616
Retinal disturbance, in
    hypertension, 456
Retinal hemorrhages, in aplastic
    anemia, 41
Retroperitoneal adenopathy, in
    Hodgkin's disease, 448
Retroviruses, 1
Rhabdomyoma, 98
Rheumatic endocarditis, 339–341
Rheumatic fever, and pharyngitis,
    653
Rheumatoid arthritis (RA), 77–84
  assessment, 78, 79
  clinical manifestations, 77–78
  complications, 80, 82
  continuing care in, 83
  diagnosis, 78, 80
  fatigue management, 81
  home/community-based care,
    83
  joint involvement, 77–78
  medical management, 78–79
  mobility management, 81
  nursing interventions, 80–84
  outcome expectations, 84
  pain management in, 80–81
  patient education, 82, 83
  planning/goals, 80

planning/goals in, 80
  and psoriasis, 680
  self-care in, 82, 83
  sleep management, 81, 82
Rib fractures, 368
RICE. See Rest, ice, compression,
    elevation (RICE)
Right-sided heart failure, 422
Risk factors
  for AIDS, 1–2
  for arteriosclerosis, 76
  for cancer
    of breast, 159
    of breasts, 159
    of endometrium, 179
    of esophagus, 180–181
    of lungs, 200
    of oral cavity, 203
    of pancreas, 210
    of skin, 221
  for cerebral vascular accidents,
    248–249
  for chronic obstructive
    pulmonary disorder, 268
  for coronary atherosclerosis/
    artery disease, 283–284
  for hypertension, 455
  for infective endocarditis, 336
  for osteomalacia, 569
  for osteoporosis, 577, 578
  for pulmonary tuberculosis,
    759–760
  for septic shock, 725
  for vein disorders, 788
Rovsing's sign, and appendicitis,
    71

Sarcomas
  chondrosarcoma, 98
  Kaposi's sarcoma, 4
  osteogenic sarcoma, 98
Scalp injuries, 408
Schilling test, for megaloblastic
    anemia, 47
Schistosomiasis, chronic, 156
Seborrheic dermatoses, 719–720
Secondary polycythemia, 674

Seizures
  and chronic renal failure, 715
  epilepsies
    complex partial, 344
    grand mal, 344
    postictal, 345
    simple partial, 344
  and hypoglycemia, 469
  and hypoparathyroidism, 472
  and intracranial aneurysm, 60, 61
Self-care
  in acute pancreatitis, 591
  in Addison's disease, 25
  in AIDS, 16–17
  in Alzheimer's disease, 30
  in anaphylaxis, 35
  in anemia, iron-deficiency, 44
  in anemia, sickle cell, 52–53
  in angina pectoris, 67
  in asthma, 87
  in Bell's palsy, 95
  in burn injuries, 134–135
  in cancer, 148–149
    of breast, 166–167
    of cervix, 171–172
    of larynx, 194
    of oral cavity, 206
  in cardiomyopathies, 244
  in cerebral vascular accidents, 256
  in chronic obstructive pulmonary disease, 271–272
  in chronic renal failure, 717–718
  in clinical unit, postoperative, 640–641
  in constipation, 281
  in Cushing's syndrome, 289, 291
  in diabetes mellitus, 307
  in diabetic ketoacidosis, 315–316
  in diffuse axonal injuries, 419
  in fractures, 375–376
  in gastritis, 381
  in Guillain-Barré syndrome, 399–400
  in heart failure, 428–429
  in hypertension, 466
  in intracranial aneurysm, 60–62
  in leukemia, 502
  in mastoiditis, 519
  in migraine headaches, 405–406
  in morbid obesity, 565
  in multiple sclerosis, 540–541
  in musculoskeletal trauma, 547
  in myasthenia gravis, 553–554
  in myocardial infarction, 559
  in osteomalacia, 572
  in Parkinson's disease, 598, 599–600
  in pelvic infection, 602
  in peptic ulcers, 614
  in pulmonary tuberculosis, 763–764
  in rheumatoid arthritis, 82, 83
  in status asthmaticus, 89
  in unconsciousness, 779
  in urolithiasis, 785–786
Self-esteem management
  in burn injuries, 134
  in cancer, 145–146
    of larynx, 193
  in hyperthyroidism, 466
  in morbid obesity, 564
Sensory perception management
  in cerebral vascular accident, 256–257
  in mastoiditis, 519
  in multiple sclerosis, 540
  in spinal cord injury, 734
  in unconsciousness, 779
Sepsis
  in cancer, 141, 147–148
  in colorectal cancer, 175
  in DIC, 322
  in osteomyelitis, 573
  in pemphigus, 605
  in peritonitis, 651

Septic shock, 725–727
  clinical manifestations
    hyperdynamic (progressive)
      phase, 726
    hypodynamic (irreversible)
      phase, 726
  gerontologic considerations,
    726
  medical management,
    726–727
  nursing management, 727
  pathophysiology, 725
  risk factors, 725
Serous adenocarcinoma,
  208–209
Serum markers, in nephrotic
  syndrome, 562
Sexual function/dysfunction
  in cancer
    of breast, 165–166
    of prostate, 219
    of vulva, 238
  in cerebral vascular accidents,
    254, 258
  in Cushing's syndrome, 289
  in hypothyroidism, 476
  in multiple sclerosis, 538,
    541
Sexually transmitted diseases
  (STDs), 293
Sheehan's syndrome. *See*
    Postpartum pituitary
    necrosis
Shock
  cardiogenic, 720–723
  hypovolemic, 613, 723–725
  monitoring/prevention, in
    clinical unit, 642
  septic, 725–727
Shoulder pain, in cerebral
  vascular accidents,
  256
SIADH. *see* Syndrome of
    inappropriate antidiuretic
    hormone (SIADH)
Sickle cell anemia. *See* Anemia,
    sickle cell

Simmond's disease
    (panhypopituitarism),
    474
Sinusitis
  and brain abscess, 108
  and pharyngitis, 653
Skeletal disorders, in pituitary
    tumors, 660
Skin cancer, 137, 220–226
  anxiety management in, 224
  assessment, 222, 223–224
  clinical manifestations
    acral-lentiginous melanoma,
      222
    lentigo-maligna melanoma,
      222
    nodular melanoma, 222
    superficial spreading
      melanoma, 221
  collaborative problems/
    complications, 224, 225
  diagnosis, 222, 224
  medical management,
    223–226
  nursing management,
    223–226
  outcome expectations,
    225–226
  pain management in, 224
  patient education in, 225
  planning/goals in, 224
  risk factors, 221
Skin disorders
  contact dermatitis, 281–283
  exfoliative dermatitis, 355–357
  impetigo, 484–486
  pemphigus, 603–607
  pigmentation, in
    glomerulonephritis, 389
  seborrheic dermatoses,
    719–720
  in ulcerative colitis, 771
Skin integrity
  in acute renal failure, 712
  in burn injuries, 128–129
  in cancer, 140, 143–144
    of breast, 164–165

colorectal, 175
  of vulva, 238
in cerebral vascular accidents,
    258
in cholecystitis, 264, 265–266
in contact dermatitis, 281
in Cushing's syndrome,
    289–290
in diarrhea, 320
in DIC, 322, 324
in diffuse axonal injuries, 417
in hepatic cirrhosis, 277
in hip fractures, 373
in mastoiditis, 517–518
in musculoskeletal trauma,
    547
in pemphigus, 606
in psoriasis, 685
in spinal cord injury, 734–735
in toxic epidermal necrolysis,
    751
in unconsciousness, 777
Skull injuries, 408
Sleep apnea, in morbid obesity,
    564
Sleep disorders, in Parkinson's
    disease, 595
Sleep management, in diffuse,
    axonal injuries, 418
Small cell (oat cell) carcinoma,
    200
Smoking cessation
  for Buerger's disease, 117, 118
  for chronic bronchitis, 116
Snellen visual acuity test, for
    cataracts, 246
Socialization management
  in Alzheimer's disease, 30
  in low back pain, 92, 93
Sodium retention, in Cushing's
    syndrome, 287
Speech management, in multiple
    sclerosis, 541
Speech rehabilitation
  in cerebral vascular accidents,
    258
  in larynx cancer, 192

Spinal cord injury, 727–738
  assessment, 729, 732
  bowel management, 735
  clinical manifestations
    neurologic level, 728–729
    respiratory problems, 729
  complications, 729, 733
    autonomic hyperreflexia,
      736
    deep vein thrombosis, 731
    orthostatic hypotension, 736
    spinal/neurogenic shock,
      730–731
    thrombophlebitis, 736
  compression, in cancer, 141
  diagnosis, 729, 732–733
  emergency management,
      729–730
  home/community-based care,
      737
  medical management, 730
  mobility management, 734
  nursing interventions,
      733–738
  outcome expectations,
      737–738
  planning/goals, 733
  respiratory management,
      733–734
  sensory perception
      management, 734
  skin integrity management,
      734–735
  urinary elimination
      management, 735
Spinal fusion, in muscular
    dystrophies, 543
Spirituality management
  in leukemia, 503
  and perioperative nursing
      management, 625–626
Spirometry, incentive
  in Guillain-Barré syndrome,
      397, 398
  in sickle cell anemia, 50
Spleen disorders, in anemia,
    aplastic, 41

Splenomegaly
  in chronic lymphocytic
    leukemia, 506
  and hepatic cirrhosis, 274
  and Hodgkin's disease, 448
Splenoportography, for bleeding
    esophageal varices, 352
Spontaneous hematuria, 430
Sprains, 545
Squamous cell carcinoma
  and lung cancer, 200
  and vulvar cancer, 235
Staphylococcus aureus
  and bone infections, 572
  and bullous impetigo, 485
  and lung abscess, 511
  and pneumonia, 665
Staphylococcus pneumoniae, 665
  and pneumonia, 665
Status epilepticus, 347
Stents, intracoronary
  for angina pectoris, 65
  for arteriosclerosis/
    atherosclerosis, 77
Steroid therapy, for chronic
    bronchitis, 116
Stevens-Johnson syndrome.
    See Toxic epidermal
    necrolysis
Stomach cancer, 226–230
  anxiety management in, 228
  assessment, 227–228
  clinical manifestations, 226
  diagnosis, 227, 228
  home/community-based care
    in, 230
  medical management,
    227–230
  nursing interventions,
    228–230
  nutrition management,
    228–229
  planning/goals, 228
Stomal obstruction, in morbid
    obesity, 565
Stomatitis management, in
    cancer, 142, 206

Stool
  analysis
    in hepatitis A, 438
    in peptic ulcers, 609
  clay colored, in cholecystitis,
    262
Strains, 545
Streptococcal infections
  and acute glomerulonephritis,
    386
  and impetigo, 484
Streptococcus pneumoniae
  and acute otitis media, 581
  and pharyngitis, 653
Stress management
  in breast cancer, 164
  and low back pain, 90
Stress testing, for angina pectoris,
    64
Stroke
  in DIC, 323
  hemorrhagic, 248
  and hypertension, 457
  ischemic, 248–260
  and sickle cell anemia, 52
Subacute thyroiditis, 745
Subarachnoid hemorrhages,
    248
Subdural hematoma, 411–412
Subluxations, of joints, 545, 546
Superficial spreading melanoma,
    220, 221
Supplementation
  for anemia, iron-deficiency,
    44
  for anemia, megaloblastic
    folic acid, 47
    Vitamin B12, 46
  for bleeding esophageal
    varices, 354
  for cancer, 144
    of stomach, 229
  for hepatic cirrhosis, 277
  Saw palmetto, for BPH, 97
Supportive care
  for AIDS, 7–8
  for leukemia, 509

Surgical management
 in angina pectoris, 65
 in aortic aneurysm, 56
 in appendicitis, 72
 in benign prostatic
  hyperplasia, 97–98
 in bleeding esophageal varices,
  353
 in brain tumors, 112–113
 for cardiac tamponade, 617
 in cholelithiasis/cholecystitis,
  263–264
 in colorectal cancer, 174
 in diverticulosis, 328
 in endometriosis, 342
 in glaucoma, 384–385
 in heart failure, 423
 in liver cancer, 198–199
 in lymphedema/elephantiasis,
  514–515
 in Ménière's disease, 522
 in morbid obesity, 565
 in osteoarthritis, 568–569
 in Parkinson's disease, 596
 in peptic ulcers, 611
 in pulmonary edema, 692
 in transient ischemic attack,
  755
 in trigeminal neuralgia,
  757–758
 in ulcerative colitis, 767
 in vein disorders, 789
Swallowing difficulties
 in cancer, 140
 in cerebral vascular accidents,
  257
 in chronic pharyngitis, 655
 in Guillain-Barré syndrome,
  397–398
 in multiple sclerosis, 541
 in Parkinson's disease, 599
Sweating
 in chronic lymphocytic
  leukemia, 506
 in glaucoma, 383
 in hypoglycemia, 469
 in Parkinson's disease, 595

Syncope, in mitral valve prolapse,
  532
Syndrome of inappropriate
  antidiuretic hormone
  (SIADH), 489, 528,
  738–739
Systemic lupus erythematosus,
  739–742
 assessment/diagnosis, 740
 clinical manifestations,
  739–740
 medical management, 741
 nursing management, 741–742
 pathophysiology, 739
 pharmacologic therapy, 741
Systolic murmur, in myocarditis,
  561

Tachycardia
 in acute pancreatitis, 585
 in anemia, 36
 in asthma, 84
 in cardiac arrest, 239
 in dissecting aneurysm, 55
 in heart failure, 422
 in hemophilia, 432
 in HHNS, 453
 in hyperthyroidism, 462
 in hypoglycemia, 469
 in hypovolemic shock, 723
 in larynx cancer, 192
 in myocardial infarction, 554,
  555
 in myocarditis, 560
 in peptic ulcers, 613
 in pheochromocytoma, 657
 in pneumonia, 666
 in pneumothorax, 672
 in sickle cell anemia, 49
 in thyroid storm, 747
 in ulcerative colitis, 765
Tachypnea
 in acute pancreatitis, 585
 in acute respiratory distress
  syndrome, 18
 in cardiac tamponade, 616
 in hypovolemic shock, 723

Tachypnea (*Contd.*)
  in larynx cancer, 192
  in myocardial infarction, 555
  in pneumonia, 666
  in pneumothorax, 671
  in pulmonary emphysema, 333
  in ulcerative colitis, 765
TB. *See* Tuberculosis, pulmonary (TB)
TBI. *See* Traumatic brain injury (TBI)
Telangiectases, spider, and hepatic cirrhosis, 274
Tension headaches, 401, 407
Tension pneumothorax, 672
Teratocarcinomas, 231
Terminal care, in leukemia, 503–504
Testicular cancer, 137, 231–232
Testicular tumor, 331
Tetany, latent, and hypoparathyroidism, 472
Thoracentesis
  in empyema, 335
  in pleural effusion, 662
  in pleurisy, 664
  in pneumonia, 670
Thoracic aortic aneurysm, 55
Throat cultures, for pharyngitis, 654
Thromboangiitis obliterans. *See* Buerger's disease
Thrombocytopenia, 743–744
  in DIC, 321, 743
  and intracerebral hemorrhage/hematomas, 412
  in leukemia
    acute lymphocytic, 505
    chronic lymphocytic, 506
  in multiple myeloma, 533
  pathophysiology, 743
Thromboembolism
  in heart failure, 424
  in morbid obesity, 565
  in myocardial infarction, 557

Thrombolytic therapy, 691–692, 693–694
Thrombophlebitis, 787–792
  clinical manifestations, 788
  diagnosis, 790
  medical management, 789
  nursing management, 790–792
  pharmacologic therapy, 789
  prevention, 789
  risk factors, 788
  in spinal cord injury, 736
  superficial
    in Buerger's disease, 117
    in polycythemia, 674
  surgical management, 789
Thrombosis
  arterial, 73–75
  and Guillain-Barré syndrome, 396
  and sickle cell anemia, 51
Thymectomy, for myasthenia gravis, 550
Thyroid cancer, 233–234
Thyroid panel, for migraine headaches, 403
Thyroid storm (thyrotoxic crisis), 747–748
Thyroiditis
  acute, 744–746
  chronic (*See* Hashimoto's thyroiditis)
  subacute, 745
Thyrotoxicosis
  and hyperthyroidism, 465
  in myocardial infarction, 554
TIA. *See* Transient ischemic shock (TIA)
Tibia/fibula fractures, 370–371
Tic douloureux. *See* Trigeminal neuralgia
Tinnitus
  in Ménière's disease, 520
  in polycythemia, 674
Tissue integrity maintenance, in cancer, 142

Tissue plasminogen activator
(t-PA) therapy
for cerebral vascular accidents,
251
acute phase assessment,
252–253
postacute phase assessment,
253
TMN classification system
laboratory values, 138
staging, 137–138
Tophi, and gout, 392–393
Topical therapy, for psoriasis, 682
Toxic epidermal necrolysis,
748–753
anxiety management, 752–753
assessment, 749, 750
clinical manifestations, 749
collaborative problems/
complications, 751, 753
diagnosis, 749, 751
fluid balance management, 752
hypothermia prevention, 752
medical management,
749–750
nursing interventions,
751–753
outcome expectations, 753
pain management, 752
planning/goals, 751
skin integrity management,
751
Toxoplasma gondii, 3
t-PA therapy. *See* Tissue
plasminogen activator
(t-PA) therapy
Transient ischemic shock (TIA),
753–755
Transplantation
bone marrow
for anemia, aplastic, 41
for anemia, sickle cell, 49
nursing management,
154–155
for ovarian cancer, 210
and Kaposi's sarcoma, 495
of liver, 198, 437

Transurethral resection of
prostate (TUR/TURP),
157, 215–216
Trauma
and epistaxis, 350
and head injuries, 407
and ischemic strokes, 248
Traumatic brain injury (TBI),
407
Tremors
in hypoglycemia, 469
in Parkinson's disease, 594
in pheochromocytoma, 657
Trigeminal neuralgia (tic
douloureux), 756–758
clinical manifestations,
756–757
medical management,
757–758
nursing interventions, 758
pathophysiology, 756
Tuberculosis, pulmonary (TB),
759–764
activity promotion, 762
AIDS-related, 2, 3, 759
airway management, 762
assessment/diagnosis, 760,
761
clinical manifestations, 760
collaborative problems/
complications, 761–762,
762–763
gerontologic considerations,
760
home/community-based care,
763
medical management,
760–761
nursing interventions,
762–764
nutrition management, 762
outcome expectations, 764
planning/goals, 762
and pleurisy, 663
risk factors, 759–760
Tumor lysis syndrome, and
leukemia, 499

Tumors
of brain, 109–113
chromophobic, 660
eosinophilic, 660
in gastric triangle, 608
of kidneys, 185–187
nasal, and epistaxis, 350
pheochromocytoma, 656–659
pituitary, 659–661
primary/metastatic, 98
stages of, 138
testicular, and epididymitis,
331
TMN classification system
laboratory values, 138
staging, 137–138
TUR/TURP. *See* Transurethral
resection of prostate
Tympanoplasty, for mastoiditis,
518
Tympanotomy. *See* Myringotomy
Type 1 diabetes, 299–300
and insulin, 302
Type 2 diabetes, 300
and weight loss, 302, 303

Ulcerative colitis, 765–773
anxiety management, 771
assessment, 765–766,
767–768
bowel management, 769
clinical manifestations, 765
collaborative
problems/complications,
769, 771–772
coping management, 771
diagnosis, 765–766, 768–769
fluid balance management,
770
home/community-based care,
772–773
medical management, 766
nursing interventions,
769–773
nutrition management, 766,
770
outcome expectations, 773

pain management, 769–770
planning/goals, 769
Ulcers
peptic, 607–615
perforated, and peritonitis, 651
pressure, and Guillain-Barré
syndrome, 398
pressure, in multiple sclerosis,
536
stress, 608
Ultrasonography
for aortic aneurysm, 56
for arterial embolism/
thrombosis, 74
A-scan, for cataracts, 246
for bleeding esophageal
varices, 352
for cancer, 137
of bladder, 157
of endometrium, 179
of liver, 196
of ovaries, 209
of thyroid, 233–234
for Cushing's syndrome, 287
for hepatic cirrhosis, 275
for increased intracranial
pressure, 487
for ischemic stroke, 250
for pleural effusion, 662
for prostate cancer, 214
quantitative (QUS), for
osteoporosis, 577
for renal tumors, 186
Unconsciousness, 773–780
airway management, 776
assessment/diagnosis, 774–775
bowel management, 778
collaborative problems/
complications, 775–776,
779–780
corneal integrity maintenance,
777–778
family support, 779
fluid balance management, 777
in hypoglycemia, 471
in increased intracranial
pressure, 488–492

medical management, 774
nursing interventions,
776–780
nutrition management, 777
outcome expectations, 780
planning/goals, 776
sensory perception
management, 779
urinary management, 778
Urinalysis
for benign prostatic
hyperplasia, 97
for bladder cancer, 157
for cystitis, 292, 296
for glomerulonephritis, 390
for hypertension, 457
for ketones, in diabetes
mellitus, 309
Urinary elimination management
in hip fractures, 374
in spinal cord injury, 735
in unconsciousness, 778
Urinary tract infections (UTI)
in bladder cancer, 157
in epididymitis, 331
lower (cystitis), 292–296
in prostatitis, 676
Urography
intravenous
for ovarian cancer, 209
for renal tumors, 186
for prostate cancer, 214
Urolithiasis (kidney stones),
780–786
assessment/diagnosis,
781–782, 783
clinical manifestations
bladder stones, 781
renal pelvis stones, 781
ureter stones, 781
collaborative problems/
complications, 784
home/community-based care,
785–786
medical management, 782
nursing interventions,
784–786

nutrition management,
782–783
outcome expectations, 786
pain management, 784
pharmacologic therapy,
782–783
planning/goals, 784
risk for, and gout, 393
stone removal procedures,
782
Urticaria, and asthma, 84
Uterine bleeding, and
endometriosis, 341
UTI. *See* Urinary tract infections
(UTI)

Vaccination
for chronic bronchitis, 116
for influenza, 493
for meningitis, 527
for pneumonia, 667
Vaginal cancer, 234–235
Vaginal discharge, in pelvic
infection, 601
Valvuloplasty commissurotomy
in aortic insufficiency, 69
in mitral stenosis, 531
Varicella zoster, and acute
glomerulonephritis, 386
Vascular damage, in
hypertension, 456
Vascular myelopathy, in AIDS, 3
Vasospasm
and intracranial aneurysm, 60,
61
and ischemic strokes, 248
and myocardial infarction, 554
Venous stasis, and KS, 494
Venous thrombosis, 787–792
assessment, 788, 790
clinical manifestations, 788
diagnosis, 790
medical management, 789
nursing management, 790–792
pharmacologic therapy, 789
risk factors, 788
surgical management, 789

Ventilation, mechanical, for amyotrophic lateral sclerosis, 32

Ventricular fibrillation, and cardiac arrest, 239

Vertigo, 521
in mastoiditis, 517
in Ménière's disease, 520, 523
in pheochromocytoma, 657

Vestibular disease, 521

Viral diseases
and Bell's palsy, 94
Enterovirus family in Hepatitis A, 437
Epstein-Barr virus, 386
Hepatitis B, 439–442
herpes simplex, 4
herpes zoster, 4
and idiopathic thrombocytopenia purpura, 482
influenza, 492–493
retroviruses, 1

Virilization, in females, in Cushing's syndrome, 287

Visual changes
in diabetes mellitus, 300
in diabetic ketoacidosis, 313
in glaucoma, 382
in hypertension, 458
in migraine headaches, 402
in multiple sclerosis, 535, 538
in pituitary tumors, 660

Vitamins
for anemia, megaloblastic, 47
for bleeding esophageal varices, 354
D (calcitriol)
in osteomalacia, 569, 570
in osteoporosis, 577, 580
for hepatic cirrhosis, 277
for hypoparathyroidism, 474

Vocal disorders, in aortic aneurysm, 55

Vomiting
in acute lymphocytic leukemia, 505
in acute pancreatitis, 585
in brain tumors, 111
in cancer, 140
in cholecystitis, 266
in diabetes mellitus, 301
in diabetic ketoacidosis, 313
in gastritis, 379
in glaucoma, 383
monitoring of, in PACU, 632
in morbid obesity, 565
in myocarditis, 561
in pelvic infection, 601
in peptic ulcers, 609, 611
in peritonitis, 652
in pheochromocytoma, 657
in radiation therapy, 449

Vulvar cancer, 235–239
anxiety management, 237
assessment, 236
clinical manifestations, 236
collaborative problems/complications, 237, 238
diagnosis, 236, 237
home/community-based care, 239
pain management, 237
planning/goals, 237
vulvectomy for, 236–239

Wasting syndrome (cachexia), in AIDS, 3, 16

Weakness
in extremities, in migraine headaches, 402
in mitral regurgitation, 529
in multiple sclerosis, 535
in peripheral arterial occlusive disease, 648
in pituitary tumors, 660

Weber's test, for Ménière's disease, 521

Weight gain, in Cushing's syndrome, 286

Weight loss
  in chronic lymphocytic
      leukemia, 506
  in chronic obstructive
      pulmonary disorder, 268
  in chronic pancreatitis, 592
  in empyema, 334
  in glomerulonephritis, 389
  in Hodgkin's disease, 448
  in hyperthyroidism, 462, 463
  in hypopituitarism, 474
  in pulmonary emphysema, 333
  in thyroid storm, 747
  in Type 2 diabetes, 302, 303
Weight management
  for diabetes mellitus, 301
  for gout, 394
  for hepatic cirrhosis, 275
  for low back pain, 93
Wound care
  in acute pancreatitis, 590
  in clinical unit, postoperative,
      644–645
  in esophageal cancer, 183
Wrist fractures, 367–368

Xerostomia (dry mouth), in oral
      cavity cancer, 205–206
X-ray studies
  abdominal, for diverticular
      disorders, 326
  abdominal, for peritonitis,
      652
  for bone tumors, 100
  for brain abscess, 108
  chest, and pulmonary
      emphysema, 333
  chest, for glomerulonephritis,
      390
  chest, for Hodgkin's disease,
      449
  chest, for pleurisy, 664

Yolk sac carcinomas, 231

Zollinger-Ellison syndrome
      (gastrinoma)
  and diarrhea, 316
  in peptic ulcer, 608, 610
  surgery for, 611